Ophthalmic Epidemiology

Ophthalmic Epidemiology
Current Concepts to Digital Strategies

Edited by

Ching-Yu Cheng, MD, MPH, PhD
Professor, Duke-NUS Medical School, Singapore
Principal Clinician Scientist, Singapore Eye Research Institute
Senior Clinician Scientist, Singapore National Eye Centre

Tien Yin Wong, MD, PhD
Arthur Lim Professor of Ophthalmology
Medical Director, Singapore National Eye Centre
Chairman, Singapore Eye Research Institute
Vice Dean, Duke-NUS Medical School, Singapore

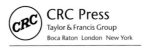

CRC Press
Taylor & Francis Group
Boca Raton London New York

CRC Press is an imprint of the
Taylor & Francis Group, an **informa** business

First edition published 2022
by CRC Press
6000 Broken Sound Parkway NW, Suite 300, Boca Raton, FL 33487-2742

and by CRC Press
4 Park Square, Milton Park, Abingdon, Oxon, OX14 4RN

CRC Press is an imprint of Taylor & Francis Group, LLC

© 2022 Taylor & Francis Group, LLC

ISBN: 9781138505889 (hbk)
ISBN: 9781032247595 (pbk)
ISBN: 9781315146737 (ebk)

DOI: 10.1201/9781315146737

Typeset in Palatino
by Newgen Publishing UK

Contents

Preface

In the past decades, epidemiological research in ophthalmology has provided us with much important information on the prevalence, incidence, risk factors, and impact of eye diseases. Ophthalmologic epidemiology will continue to play a major role in the practice of public health and clinical ophthalmology in the coming decade. However, the recent advances in new technologies are transforming the ways of data generation, collection, and analysis, as well as the practice of epidemiology.

For instance, the generation of *'big data'* derived from electronic medical records, digital technologies, omics platforms, and clinical imaging is deepening our understanding of the complex social, environmental, and biological determinants of eye diseases. Moreover, the adoption of novel approaches in data analysis, such as machine and deep learning analytics, is enabling better automation and quantitation to extract critical features from complex datasets. These advances have a great potential to lead to improved prevention, detection, and management of eye diseases in populations. On the other hand, the reach of epidemiology is extending beyond disease prevalence estimates and etiologic research to translational research, including but not limited to community intervention and outcomes research.

In this book, we invited authors around the world with expertise in ophthalmic epidemiology, digital health, telemedicine, statistical and big-data analysis, and health outcome evaluation, to embrace the above-mentioned trends, harness technological advances, discuss the latest epidemiological approaches, and provide updates on major eye diseases, in order to lead and shape the future direction of ophthalmic epidemiology.

We would like to thank all the authors who have contributed chapters to this book, in particular during the COVID-19 pandemic.

About the Editors

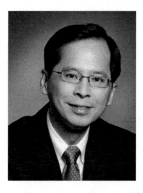

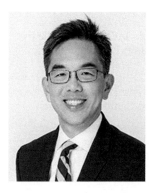

Ching-Yu Cheng's academic career has been dedicated to understanding and characterizing the epidemiology and genetics of major blinding eye diseases, such as glaucoma and age-related macular degeneration. He directs the Singapore Epidemiology of Eye Diseases (SEED) program, a large multi-disciplinary research program focusing on epidemiology, imaging, and genetics in eye diseases in Singapore. The SEED program includes one of the largest epidemiological databases for eye diseases in the world. Its achievements have become visible via both a number of high-impact publications in prestigious journals and the surging amount of new knowledge in prevention of blindness. The data collected from the SEED program have been widely used by leading international agencies.

Professor Cheng has received a number of prestigious awards, including the Clinician Scientist Award from the National Medical Research Council, Singapore; the Asia-Pacific Academy of Ophthalmology Outstanding Service in Prevention of Blindness Award; and the American Academy of Ophthalmology Achievement Award.

Tien Yin Wong is a retinal specialist and physician-scientist, balancing clinical practice with a research and innovation portfolio on retinal diseases and ocular imaging, including artificial intelligence (AI). He has published more than 1,400 peer-reviewed papers (h-index of 148, 2018, 2020 Highly Cited Researcher). He has given more than 500 invited named, plenary, and symposium lectures globally, and received >US$100 million in grant funding. He is a two-times recipient of the Singapore Translational Researcher (STaR) Award. For his contributions, Professor Wong has been recognized with the Commonwealth Health Minister's Award, the Arnall Patz Medal from the Macula Society, the Alcon Research Institute Award, the Jose Rizal Medal from the Asia Pacific Academy of Ophthalmology, and others. He has received the National Outstanding Clinician Scientist Award, the President's Science Award, and the President's Science and Technology Award, the highest awards for healthcare and scientific contribution in Singapore. He is an elected international member of the US National Academy of Medicine.

Contributors

Alléxya Affonso
Department of Ophthalmic Oncology, Cole Eye Institute, Cleveland Clinic, United States

Marcus Ang
Department of Cornea and Refractive Service, Singapore National Eye Center, Singapore

Ophthalmology & Visual Sciences Academic Clinical Program (Eye ACP), Duke-NUS Medical School, Singapore

Abdus Samad Ansari
Department of Academic Ophthalmology, King's College London, United Kingdom

Catey Bunce
School of Population Health and Environmental Sciences, Faculty of Life Sciences and Medicine, King's College London, United Kingdom

Ving Fai Chan
Centre for Public Health, School of Medicine, Dentistry and Biomedical Sciences, Queen's University Belfast, United Kingdom

College of Health Sciences, University of KwaZulu Natal, South Africa

Shruti Chandra
National Institute of Health Research Moorfields Biomedical Research Centre, Moorfields Eye Hospital NHS Foundation Trust and UCL Institute of Ophthalmology, United Kingdom

Ching-Yu Cheng
Ocular Epidemiology Research Group, Singapore Eye Research Institute, Singapore National Eye Centre, Singapore

Ophthalmology & Visual Sciences Academic Clinical Program (Eye ACP), Duke-NUS Medical School, Singapore

Grace May Chuang
Singapore Eye Research Institute, Singapore National Eye Centre, Singapore
Duke-NUS Medical School, Singapore

Nathan Congdon
School of Medicine, Dentistry and Biomedical Sciences, Institute of Clinical Sciences, Queen's University Belfast, United Kingdom

Zhongshan Ophthalmic Center, Sun Yat-Sen University, China

Gabriela Czanner
Applied Statistics, Faculty of Engineering and Technology, Liverpool John Moores University, United Kingdom

Shuan Dai
Queensland Children's Hospital School of Clinical Medicine, University of Queensland, Brisbane, Australia

Faculty of Medicine, The University of Queensland, Brisbane, Queensland, Australia

Department of Ophthalmology, Queensland Children's Hospital, Brisbane, Queensland, Australia

Rashmi Deshmukh
Department of Ophthalmology, Queen's Medical Centre, Nottingham, United Kingdom

Jennifer Evans
Centre for Public Health, School of Medicine, Dentistry and Biomedical Sciences, Queen's University Belfast, United Kingdom

International Centre for Eye Health, London School of Hygiene and Tropical Medicine, United Kingdom

Centre for Public Health, Queen's University Belfast, United Kingdom

Eva K. Fenwick
Population Health Research Group, Singapore Eye Research Institute, Singapore National Eye Centre, Singapore

Ophthalmology & Visual Sciences Academic Clinical Program (Eye ACP), Duke-NUS Medical School, Singapore

Jakob Grauslund
Department of Ophthalmology, Odense University Hospital, Odense, Denmark

Department of Clinical Research, University of Southern Denmark, Odense, Denmark

Steno Diabetes Center Odense, Odense University Hospital, Odense, Denmark

Department of Ophthalmology, Vestfold Hospital Trust, Tønsberg, Norway

Preeti Gupta
Population Health Research Group, Singapore Eye Research Institute, Singapore National Eye Centre, Singapore

Ophthalmology & Visual Sciences Academic Clinical Program (Eye ACP), Duke-NUS Medical School, Singapore

Mingguang He
Centre for Eye Research Australia, University of Melbourne, Royal Victorian Eye and Ear Hospital, Australia

State Key Laboratory of Ophthalmology, Zhongshan Ophthalmic Center, Sun Yat-Sen University, China

De-Kuang Hwang
Department of Ophthalmology, Taipei Veterans General Hospital, Taiwan

School of Medicine, National Yang Ming Chiao Tung University, Taiwan

Yih-Shiou Hwang
Department of Ophthalmology, Chang Gung Memorial Hospital, Linkou Medical Center, Taiwan

College of Medicine, Chang Gung University, Taiwan

Department of Ophthalmology, Chang Gung Memorial Hospital, Xiamen, China

Pirro G. Hysi
Department of Twin Research and Genetic Epidemiology, King's College London, United Kingdom

Jost B. Jonas
Department of Ophthalmology, Medical Faculty Mannheim, Heidelberg University, Germany

Institute of Molecular and Clinical Ophthalmology Basel, Switzerland

Ka Wai Kam
Department of Ophthalmology & Visual Sciences, The Chinese University of Hong Kong, Hong Kong

Department of Ophthalmology & Visual Sciences, Prince of Wales Hospital, Hong Kong

Emmanuel Kemel
GREGHEC Department of Economics and Decision Sciences, CNRS and HEC, Paris, France

Victor Koh
Department of Ophthalmology, National University Hospital, Singapore

Department of Ophthalmology, Yong Loo Lin School of Medicine, National University of Singapore, Singapore

Tianjing Li
Department of Ophthalmology, School of Medicine, University of Colorado Anschutz Medical Campus, United States

Ryan E. K. Man
Population Health Research Group, Singapore Eye Research Institute, Singapore National Eye Centre, Singapore

Ophthalmology & Visual Sciences Academic Clinical Program (Eye ACP), Duke-NUS Medical School, Singapore

Revathy Mani
School of Optometry and Vision Science, UNSW Sydney, Australia

Alexander Melendez
Department of Ophthalmic Oncology, Cole Eye Institute, Cleveland Clinic, United States

Rubens Belfort Neto
Department of Ophthalmic Oncology, Cole Eye Institute, Cleveland Clinic, United States

Department of Ophthalmology and Visual Sciences, Paulista School of Medicine, Federal University of São Paulo, Brazil

Luke Nicholson
National Institute of Health Research Moorfields Biomedical Research Centre,

Moorfields Eye Hospital NHS Foundation Trust and UCL Institute of Ophthalmology, United Kingdom

Simon Nusinovici
Ocular Epidemiology Research Group, Singapore Eye Research Institute, Singapore National Eye Centre, Singapore

Ophthalmology & Visual Sciences Academic Clinical Program (Eye ACP), Duke-NUS Medical School, Singapore

Olusola Olawoye
School of Medicine, Dentistry and Biomedical Sciences, Institute of Clinical Sciences, Queen's University Belfast, United Kingdom

Department of Ophthalmology, College of Medicine, University of Ibadan, Nigeria

Shinji Ono
Department of Ophthalmology, Asahikawa Medical University, Asahikawa, Japan

Songhomitra Panda-Jonas
Privatpraxis Prof Jonas und Dr Panda-Jonas, Heidelberg, Germany

Chi Pui Pang
Department of Ophthalmology & Visual Sciences, The Chinese University of Hong Kong, Hong Kong

Prabhath Piyasena
School of Medicine, Dentistry and Biomedical Sciences, Institute of Clinical Sciences, Queen's University, United Kingdom

Pradeep Ramulu
Johns Hopkins University, School of Medicine, Baltimore, United States

Malin Lundberg Rasmussen
Department of Ophthalmology, Odense University Hospital, Odense, Denmark

Department of Clinical Research, University of Southern Denmark, Odense, Denmark

Vishal Raval
The Operation Eyesight Universal Institute for Eye Cancer, L V Prasad Eye Institute, India

Department of Ophthalmic Oncology, Cole Eye Institute, Cleveland Clinic, United States

Priya Adhisesha Reddy
School of Medicine, Dentistry and Biomedical Sciences, Institute of Clinical Sciences, Queen's University Belfast, United Kingdom

Seva Foundation, United States

Charumathi Sabanayagam
Ocular Epidemiology Research Group, Singapore Eye Research Institute, Singapore National Eye Centre, Singapore

Ophthalmology & Visual Sciences Academic Clinical Program (Eye ACP), Duke-NUS Medical School, Singapore

Jane Scheetz
Centre for Eye Research Australia, University of Melbourne, Royal Victorian Eye and Ear Hospital, Australia

Samantha Simkin
Department of Ophthalmology, New Zealand National Eye Centre, Faculty of Medical and Health Sciences, The University of Auckland, New Zealand

Arun D. Singh
Department of Ophthalmic Oncology, Cole Eye Institute, Cleveland Clinic, United States

Sobha Sivaprasad
National Institute of Health Research Moorfields Biomedical Research Centre, Moorfields Eye Hospital NHS Foundation Trust and UCL Institute of Ophthalmology, United Kingdom

Zhi Da Soh
Ocular Epidemiology Research Group, Singapore Eye Research Institute, Singapore National Eye Centre, Singapore

Department of Ophthalmology, Yong Loo Lin School of Medicine, National University of Singapore, Singapore

Hansell Soto
Department of Ophthalmic Oncology, Cole Eye Institute, Cleveland Clinic, United States

Fiona Stapleton
School of Optometry and Vision Science, UNSW Sydney, Australia

Zachary Tan
Centre for Eye Research Australia, University of Melbourne, Royal Victorian Eye and Ear Hospital, Australia

Faculty of Medicine, The University of Queensland, Brisbane, Queensland, Australia

Yih-Chung Tham
Ocular Epidemiology Research Group, Singapore Eye Research Institute, Singapore National Eye Centre, Singapore

Ophthalmology & Visual Sciences Academic Clinical Program (Eye ACP), Duke-NUS Medical School, Singapore

Alexandre Thiery
Department of Statistics and Applied Probability, National University of Singapore, Singapore

Daniel S. W. Ting
Department of Surgical Retina, Singapore National Eye Center, Singapore

Ophthalmology & Visual Sciences Academic Clinical Program (Eye ACP), Duke-NUS Medical School, Singapore

Darren S. J. Ting
Academic Ophthalmology, Division of Clinical
Neuroscience, School of Medicine, University of
Nottingham, United Kingdom

Department of Ophthalmology, Queen's
Medical Centre, Nottingham, United Kingdom

Rachel Marjorie Wei Wen Tseng
Ocular Epidemiology Research Group,
Singapore Eye Research Institute, Singapore
National Eye Centre, Singapore

Ashwin Venkatesh
University of Cambridge, United Kingdom

Gianni Virgili
Eye Clinic, Department of Neuroscience,
Psychology, Pharmacology and Child Health
(NEUROFARBA), University of Florence, Italy

Centre for Public Health, School of Medicine,
Dentistry and Biomedical Sciences, Queen's
University Belfast, United Kingdom

Tien Yin Wong
Singapore National Eye Centre, Singapore

Ophthalmology & Visual Sciences Academic
Clinical Program (Eye ACP), Duke-NUS
Medical School, Singapore

Jason C. S. Yam
Department of Ophthalmology & Visual
Sciences, The Chinese University of Hong
Kong, Hong Kong

Department of Ophthalmology & Visual
Sciences, Prince of Wales Hospital, Hong Kong

Yasuo Yanagi
Ophthalmology & Visual Sciences Academic
Clinical Program (Eye ACP), Duke-NUS
Medical School, Singapore

Department of Ophthalmology and Micro-
Technology, Yokohama City University, Japan

PART I

CURRENT AND FUTURE EPIDEMIOLOGICAL APPROACHES TO OPHTHALMOLOGY

1 Use of Electronic Health Records, Disease Registries, and Health Insurance Databases in Ophthalmology

Rachel Marjorie Wei Wen Tseng, Grace May Chuang, Zhi Da Soh, and Yih-Chung Tham

1.1 BACKGROUND

With the advancement of artificial intelligence (AI) and the Internet of Things (IOT) in the era of the fourth industrial revolution (the Digital Revolution), Big Data has gained further recognition in propelling this revolution. In healthcare, Big Data commonly comes in the forms of electronic health records (EHRs), disease registries, and health insurance databases (1).

In ophthalmology, the role and use of Big Data have expanded exponentially in recent years. Given the advancements and enhancements in volume, variety, and velocity in Big Data (2), there is a lot of potential in Big Data to be further harnessed for research. These may include evaluation of diseases trends, patient compliance on visits or medications, and even the discovery of potential new biomarkers (3). More importantly, the use of these data presents new research approaches and opportunities in ophthalmology and may help to alleviate the cumbersome challenges in traditional data collection approaches.

EHRs and health insurance databases are the two major sources of Big Data in healthcare. Digital advancements in network connectivity, IOT, and improved computing power in recent years have further enabled the linkage of different EHRs to form subsections of data registries (2). Similarly, with improved digitalization, health insurance databases have also been created through mass de-identification, and classification of claims from both physicians and/or patients. Altogether, these Big Data sources present new opportunities which enable 'real-world' clinical findings to be more readily translated into clinical applications, potentially improving the quality and efficiency of eyecare services.

In this chapter, we describe the characteristics of EHRs, disease registries, and health insurance databases, and their current applications in ophthalmology research. Following that, we discuss the future outlook and challenges of these data types.

1.2 ELECTRONIC HEALTH RECORDS AND DISEASE REGISTRIES

1.2.1 What Are Electronic Health Records?

EHRs are databases which consist of patients' medical history, diagnosis, clinical test results, and other additional health data such as imaging and scan results (2). Since the transition from traditional to electronic medical records, there has been a substantial improvement in the accessibility of medical record data. Furthermore, EHRs are updated in real time, further enabling efficient sharing of medical information among authorized users and across different healthcare systems in some instances (4). Consequently, the smooth integration and streamlining of workflow ultimately allow for a more holistic and efficient delivery of care for patients (4).

EHR data from different facilities in the healthcare network are accumulated into a data repository, also known as an EHR data warehouse. In order to centralize the data for each patient, identification numbers are created in the EHR to allow for the merging of medical records from different patient registries (5).

1.2.2 What Are Disease Registries?

The approach of converging EHR data to disease registries has gained traction in recent years (6). In this approach, EHR data from multiple clinical settings are typically combined to form disease registries. This enables the capturing of longitudinal data and sorting of clinical data according to the need and purpose of respective disease registries (5). The establishment of data registries serves several purposes. Firstly, to predict trends of ocular diseases such as prevalence, incidence, and progression. Secondly, to act as a management guide for future screening and treatment (2). Thirdly, to further process the unstructured data present in EHRs for the convenience of clinical trials (5). Some data registries are established for general ocular diseases, while others are curated for specific ocular diseases.

Countries such as the USA, Germany, and the UK are actively contributing their EHRs to different data registries. Table 1.1 summarizes the ophthalmic data registries currently available. First, the Intelligent Research In Sight (IRIS) registry is known to be the first established ophthalmic clinical registry in the USA (7). The purpose of IRIS is to aid clinical performance from screening to follow-up and care interventions using participants' EHR data, including patient demographics, past medical history, diagnoses, and medications (7). Secondly, the Smart Eye database (SMEYEDAT) registry was established in Germany as a real-time ophthalmology data warehouse that combines patients' health records

DOI: 10.1201/9781315146737-2

Table 1.1 Summary of the ophthalmic data registries

Data registry	Country	Description	Data source	Target disease
IRIS (29)	USA	A national cloud-based registry that aims to streamline patient information on eye diseases and conditions to improve public health (29)	Multiple EHRs	General ocular diseases
SMEYEDAT (8)	Germany	A real-time ophthalmology data warehouse that integrates EMRs and imaging data from a hospital for data visualization and academic research (8)	EHRs from the University Eye Hospital Munich	General ocular diseases
SOURCE (2)	USA	An ophthalmology data repository that includes patient demographics, billing codes, free text data, diagnoses, and information from diagnostic tests for better classification of ocular diseases (2)	EPIC EHR system (EPIC Systems Corporation)	General ocular diseases
Save Sight Registries (42)	Multiple countries, including Switzerland, The Netherlands, Belgium, France, New Zealand, Spain, Singapore, and the UK	A mix of observational data registries that serve as management guides for various eye diseases (42)	EHRs from participating countries	Fight Retinal Blindness Registry: nAMD, CNV, diabetic retinopathy, retinal vein occlusion Fight Tumor Blindness Registry: Ocular melanoma Fight Glaucoma Blindness Registry: Glaucoma Fight Corneal Blindness Registry: Keratoconus and corneal transplantation failure

Abbreviations: EHRs, electronic health records; EMRs, electronic medical records; IRIS, Intelligent Research In Sight; SMEYEDAT, Smart Eye Database; SOURCE, Sight Outcomes Research Collaborative; nAMD, neovascular age-related macular degeneration; CNV, choroidal neovascularization.

and imaging data for all types of ocular diseases and conditions (8). Thirdly, the Sight Outcomes Research Collaborative (SOURCE) registry is a US-based registry which is built upon an EHR consortium of several academic medical centers in the USA (i.e., University of Michigan Kellogg Eye Center, Stanford University Byers Eye Institute, Moran Eye Center, etc.) (9). Data such as patient demographics, billing codes, imaging data, and diagnostic tests were included in this registry (9). On the other hand, the Save Sight Registry is a culmination of different registries (of different countries), including the Fight

Retinal Blindness Registry and Fight Tumour Blindness Registry. The Fight Retinal Blindness Registry in particular focuses on ocular diseases that affect the retina, such as diabetic retinopathy (DR) and retinal vein occlusion.

1.2.3 Applications of EHRs and Disease Registries in Ophthalmology

The integration of different sources of EHRs (either across different health systems or countries) has heralded the creation of disease registries, allowing researchers and physicians to further derive evidence-based findings. The amalgamation of large data from diverse sources in these registries provides unprecedented statistical power for studying rare but clinically significant diseases, health system efficiency, and in observing the effectiveness of various treatments over time. This section details examples on how the various disease registries have been applied to ophthalmic research.

The first disease registry that will be discussed is the IRIS registry which combines data from multiple EHRs in the USA for the purpose of streamlining information on ocular diseases. The studies that utilized the IRIS registry highlight the continuum of care approach that the data registry seeks to provide. These studies also show how Big Data, when properly curated, can support research by providing a collaborative platform for analysis of rare ocular diseases or clinical scenarios in ophthalmology. The first two examples described below show how the IRIS data registry has allowed researchers to evaluate the prevalence and risk factors of rare but clinically significant post-cataract surgery complications. The availability of large longitudinal data allows observation of disease trend, and the breadth of data allows for complex and in-depth analyses of real-world data.

Firstly, Pershing et al. evaluated the incidence and visual outcomes of endophthalmitis after cataract surgery (10). By evaluating over 8.5 million eyes with previous history of cataract surgery in the IRIS database, the authors found that acute endophthalmitis occurred in 0.04% of post-cataract surgery cases, with higher rates observed in younger patients, combined surgery, and anterior vitrectomy. The use of IRIS further allowed vision status to be tracked over time; the study showed that 44% of affected patients had visual acuity of 6/12 or better 3 months after the episode.

Another study by Mahr et al. evaluated the frequency of reoperation to remove retained lens fragments in the anterior chamber after cataract surgery. The authors reported that 0.18% (approximately 1 in 561 patients) underwent reoperation within a year, and higher risk of reoperation was observed among men, smokers, and patients who resided in the west of the USA (11). Without IRIS, information on these rare complications would have to rely on small cohorts, case series, or administrative claims systems, and it would take considerably more time and effort to gain insights on the prevalence, risk factors, and change in clinical features over time. In contrast, findings from IRIS in both studies are not only crucial in informing clinical practice and disease patterns; they are also relevant in benchmarking the quality of care in real-world clinical practice.

In addition, the IRIS data registry has been used to study treatment patterns for a variety of ocular conditions, including diabetic macular edema and amblyopia (12, 13). For example, Cantrell et al. observed the pattern and efficiency of administering anti-vascular endothelial growth factor (anti-VEGF) treatment in diabetic macular edema, and reported that only 15.6% of patients received anti-VEGF treatment following their diagnosis, of which the majority were treated with bevacizumab (12). In addition, Repka conducted a study on the prevalence and treatment outcomes of patients diagnosed with amblyopia, and observed that treatment for amblyopia was effective till 12 years of age and that treatment success rate varies with race (13). Specifically, African Americans and Hispanic or Latino children had lower success rates compared to white children (13).

The second disease registry that will be discussed is SOURCE, which combines data from medical centers that utilize the EPIC EHR system in the USA. Data from SOURCE have been applied in various ways, and notably for triaging patients. For instance, Bommakanti et al. conducted a cross-sectional study using SOURCE data to determine if Big Data could assist with the triaging of patients (i.e., whether appointments could be postponed as well as rescheduling and prioritization of appointments) during COVID-19 through the development of a risk stratification tool for patients with glaucoma (9). A scoring algorithm was created using the SOURCE data to rank patients according to those who should be prioritized and those whose appointments could be postponed or rescheduled (9). This was possible because of the wealth of information available from the SOURCE data, allowing for researchers to analyze morbidity and mortality, as well as risk for progression among the patients (9). Other algorithms were also created, including one by Stein et al. that could facilitate the accurate identification of patients with exfoliation syndrome by taking into account both structured and unstructured EHR data (14). The study resulted in a positive predictive value (correctly identifying patients with exfoliation syndrome) of 95%, and negative predictive value (correctly identifying patients without exfoliation syndrome) of 100%, and was deemed more accurate in its prediction than when relying on billing codes per se (14). Furthermore, 60% of exfoliation cases would have been missed had the algorithm relied solely on billing codes.

Lastly, the Save Sight Registry, which was developed as an extension to the Fight Retinal Blindness project, is a large-scale population-based treatment outcomes registry. This registry was developed to improve the quality of clinical management and to benchmark the standard of care for ocular conditions affecting the corneal, retinal, and optic nerves. For example, the usage of this registry allowed for long-term monitoring of neovascular age-related macular degeneration (nAMD), and real-world observation of changes in its disease pattern with intravitreal anti-VEGF treatment (15, 16). For example, Cornish et al. reported the 5-year differences in clinical presentation and response to treatment between the first and second eye to be affected by nAMD (15). Notable findings included the observation that progression from unilateral to bilateral manifestation occurred in approximately 50% of patients over 5 years, the observed 481 days of time-lapse before the second eye was affected, the poorer prognosis in the first treated eye despite more aggressive treatment, and the earlier disease recurrence in the second eye. These findings are crucial in understanding clinical practice and disease patterns in the real world, and mitigate against the shortcomings typically present in clinical trials such as small sample size, short follow-up duration, and lack of generalizability.

Another study by Teo et al. using the Fight Retinal Blindness Registry evaluated the impact of delayed anti-VGEF treatment in nAMD patients. The study concluded that both the quantity and timing of treatment were important for prognosis of nAMD (16). As shown in these studies, utilization of registry data helps to enhance clinical care by further providing evidence-based information on management strategies.

From studying the trends of ocular diseases to management strategies and identifying risk factors, these are the few ways in which disease registries have been useful in informing ophthalmologists, researchers, and the public on the current quality of care in ophthalmology. These large registry data, when properly curated, allow ophthalmologists to make better-informed decisions in clinical practice.

1.2.4 Applications of EHR-Linked Biobanks in Genomics

The completion of the Human Genome Project in 2003 has led to a massive increase in genetic studies and advances in the field of genomics. The growing demand for larger data sets to study variability in human traits calls for less costly, more time-efficient alternatives to obtaining study populations than through traditional prospective purpose-built cohorts of adequate sample size. With the increase in adoption of EHR and reduction in genome-sequencing costs, the integration of clinical profiles from EHR with genomics research has been making headway in many areas of medicine (17–19). This can be accomplished by linking patients' de-identified EHRs to biobanks that store clinical patient biospecimens for genomic analysis.

Since some disease phenotypes are inherently longitudinal, including many of the ocular diseases, integration of EHRs with genetic information from biobanks (Table 1.2) enables studies in phenotype variability and disease trajectory (20). In addition, it allows studies of large sample sizes, information on diverse populations including minority populations, and repetition and reinterpretation as new knowledge is presented. Herein, we describe how EHRs have been leveraged in genomic research and some of their applications in ophthalmology.

1.2.5 Overall Applications of EHR-Linked Genomics Research in Medicine

The rise of EHR-driven genomic research has allowed replication and confirmation of known genetic associations from previous studies, discovery of new associations, and construction of hypothesis-free and hypothesis-generating studies in many medical fields. One of the first genome-wide association studies (GWAS) to confirm previous findings using EHR-derived cohort was performed by Denny et al. in 2010; it investigated single-nucleotide polymorphisms (SNPs) associated with atrioventricular conduction. The researchers implemented a phenotype algorithm that utilized natural language processing, laboratory and billing code queries, and medication records from de-identified EHRs to define cases and controls for the study cohort. This led to the confirmation of four SNPs on a sodium-channel gene that was previously not implicated in cardiac pathophysiology (21). Since then, EHR-derived cohort genomic studies have been gaining traction in other medical fields, including ophthalmology, to uncover disease-associated loci.

Aside from replicating genetic findings, the integration of EHR and genomics also led to the development of a technique known as phenome-wide association study (PheWAS). Compared to GWAS, which consists solely of identifying the association between genetic variants and a phenotype, PheWAS simultaneously searches for associations between clinical phenotypes and a given genetic variant and can identify pleiotropy (22, 23). In addition, inputs other than SNPs are being explored. These include a set of SNPs, disease exposure, drug exposure, transcription factor-based motifs, or other functional annotation data, thereby expanding the functions of PheWAS in EHR-based research (24, 25). PheWAS is often used as an approach complementary to GWAS, and the integration

Table 1.2 Examples of well-known electronic health record-linked biobanks

Biobank	Starting year of recruitment	Country	Participant characteristics	Samples collected
UK Biobank	2006	UK	500,000 individuals aged 40–69 years (52)	Blood, urine, saliva
All of Us	2018	USA	Individuals living in the USA who are over 18 years old (53)	Blood, urine, saliva
BioVU Biobank (part of the eMERGE Network)	2007	USA	Patients at Vanderbilt University Medical Center (54, 55)	Blood
MyCode Community Health and DiscovEHR	2007	USA	Patients at Geisinger clinic (56)	Blood
Kaiser Permanente Research Bank	2007	USA	Kaiser Permanente members who are 18 years or older (57)	Blood
Million Veteran Program	2011	USA	US veterans receiving care through the Veterans Affairs Healthcare system (58)	Blood
deCODE	1996	Iceland	Icelandic population, UK Biobank sequencing (59)	Blood
Estonia Genome Center Biobank	2000	Estonia	Individuals 18 years or older of the Estonian population (60)	Blood
Danish National Biobank	2012	Denmark	Residents in Denmark (61)	Blood mostly
FinnGen	2017	Finland	Patients in Finnish healthcare (62)	Blood
Biobank Japan	2003	Japan	Patients identified with any of the 47 target diseases (63, 64)	Blood, tissues
China Kadoorie Biobank	2004	China	>510,000 adults to study chronic diseases (65)	Blood
Korea Biobank Project	2008	Korea	General population in Korea (66)	Blood

of these two tools has been explored in EHR-related research to validate findings, replicate known associations, identify pleiotropy, and predict disease development (26).

Overall, these applications highlight the potential of utilizing EHRs for hypothesis-free studies in a bid to unravel new associations between variants with disease risks and disease-related traits. Other methods to utilize biobank-linked EHR data include creating polygenic risk scores and phenotype risk scores (PheRSs) to predict disease risk and uncover underlying causative genetic variants (27, 28). In the following section, we describe some examples of EHR-linked biobanks applied in ophthalmology genomic research.

1.2.6 Examples of EHR-Linked Genomics Research in Ophthalmology

An earlier example involving the application of a phenotyping algorithm to select for a study cohort from EHRs was demonstrated by Ritchie et al. In this study, the team used a cataract algorithm, which utilized EHR procedure and diagnostic codes with cataracts as the phenotype, to extract study samples from across several study sites within the Electronic Medical Records and Genomics (eMERGE) network, including Marshfield Clinic, Group Health Research Institute, Vanderbilt University, and Mayo Clinic. Patient samples within the network had undergone genome-wide genotyping. Using phenotypic and genotypic data extracted from the eMERGE network, Ritchie and his team performed a GWAS to explore single-locus tests of associations from selected age-related cataract cases and controls. Results included the detection of several potential cataract susceptibility loci, such as SNPs within or in close proximity to genes implicated in encoding for proteins in neurofilament structure, transcription factors, and fructose intolerance. This study highlights the utility of repurposing EHR-linked biobank data to perform genotype–phenotype association studies in the field of ophthalmology, considering that patient data can be extracted across a network of study sites and reused to perform more genotype–phenotype association studies (29). While this was the first GWAS regarding age-related cataract, it called for further validation and replication of results by studies with larger sample sizes, in addition to refinement of electronic phenotyping methods.

In another study, Choquet et al. demonstrated the capability of EHR data and its linkage to genetic data to enhance genomics research. The team conducted a GWAS using longitudinal intraocular pressure (IOP) measurements derived from EHRs of 69,756 study individuals of the Genetic Epidemiology Research in Adult Health and Aging (GERA) cohort, to identify IOP-associated loci (30). This was part of the Kaiser Permanente Research Program on Genes, Environment, and Health (RPGEH) in northern California, and participants of the GERA cohort had previously provided saliva samples for genotyping and consented to linkage to their clinical data from EHRs. With access to their health records, researchers could obtain IOP measurements from GERA subjects' clinical visits, averaging 5.8 visits per person, which set it apart from previous studies that usually utilized only a single IOP measurement for each eye of the subject. The researchers found that incorporating IOP measurements from multiple visits, as derived from EHRs of the subjects, reduced risk of measurement error and improved power to identify new genetic loci associated with the disease. The diversity of data from the EHR–biobank-linked cohort also allowed representation of four ethnicity groups – non-Hispanic whites, Hispanic/Latinos, East Asians, and African Americans – in contrast to earlier genetics studies that focused mainly on individuals of European descent. The GWAS results identified 47 loci that were associated with IOP. Forty of the loci had not been identified previously, of which 14 were later replicated in an independent GWAS. Since elevated IOP is not only an important causative risk factor for glaucoma but is also modifiable, this finding can lead to potential development of treatments targeting the genetic aspect of disease.

In a recent study, Unlu et al. utilized biobanks, EHRs, and zebrafish models to study the genetics underlying eye diseases (31). By applying computational genetic analyses to the EHR-linked biobank BioVU, the researchers identified associations between expression of GRIK5 gene and eye diseases. GRIK5 had previously been studied mostly in the context of central nervous system signaling and is known to encode for the glutamate ionotropic receptor kainite-type subunit 5. Thus, its implication in 18 eye diseases, including retinal detachment, various forms of retinal defects, cataracts, and glaucoma, sheds light on a novel role of the gene. Unlu and colleagues applied gene editing to lower or deplete expression of GRIK5 in zebrafish and found smaller eyes and decreased vascular integrity, shown by increased vessel leakage and decreased blood vessels. With these results in mind, the researchers reviewed Vanderbilt's EHRs and insurance claims for confirmation of comorbidity of eye and vascular diseases.

From the study, it was found that decreased levels of GRIK5 expression were associated with eye diseases, including retinal detachment, other retinal disorders, cataracts, glaucoma, and also systematic vascular traits such as peripheral vascular disease and cerebrovascular disease. The results suggest that reduced GRIK5 expression plays a role in lowering the integrity of vasculature in the eye, which the authors infer can result in increased risks of late-onset ocular diseases such as cataracts, glaucoma, and retinal diseases. Taken together, by incorporating findings from biobank-based studies into animal studies and returning to large-scale data in biobanks and EHRs, Unlu et al. demonstrated a new approach in integrating biobanks for detecting associations between gene expression levels and ocular phenotypes and providing new insights on the comorbidity between ocular and vascular diseases.

As new knowledge emerges from the scientific community, EHR-linked genetic data can be repurposed to confirm associations, which can then be further explored in clinical and translational research. Future research can be expanded to take into account patient medication and response, surgery outcomes, and environmental factors, in combination with biobank data, to better guide personalized approaches to guiding treatment decision processes and disease prediction. In this regard, EHR-driven genomic research has opened up unprecedented avenues to study the pathogenesis of ocular disease to augment clinical care.

1.3 HEALTH INSURANCE DATABASES

1.3.1 What Are Health Insurance Databases?

Several countries, including the USA, Taiwan, and South Korea, have utilized their national health insurance database for research purposes (32). The national health insurance in these countries provides coverage for enrolled citizens, which usually accounts for the majority of the population, in private and/or public healthcare delivery systems. The 'real-time' nature of these databases renders them useful in providing large and up-to-date clinical data. Data acquisiton methods differ by country. In the USA, each existing health insurance database has its own unique method. For example, commercial platforms like OptumInsight retrieve their data by accessing a proprietary database that belongs to Optum's parent company (33). On the other hand, the Medicaid analytic extract database contains administrative files and claims data that have been formatted in a standardized way, from citizens enrolled in the Medicaid and Children's Health Insurance Program (34). In Taiwan, the Taiwanese Government has established a contractual agreement with healthcare facilities such that physicians have to keep track and upload each patient's data to the national health insurance database for each consultation (35). South Korea receives its data from the national health insurance service, which is mandatory and covers all citizens (36). Lastly, the SNIIR-AM (National Health Insurance Fund for Salaried Workers) database is the main healthcare claim system in France and data are acquired through the integration of de-identified reimbursed claims from multiple health insurance plans that focus on different sub-populations (37). This database covers over 98.8% of the French population and tracks all forms of healthcare from expenditure to diagnoses, and personal information (e.g., employment status) from birth to death (38).

1.3.2 Applications of Health Insurance Databases in Ophthalmology
1.3.2.1 USA

Currently, there are a few health insurance databases used for analytic purposes (Table 1.3). This includes Medicare with Medicaid, which is an assistance program that mainly focuses on coverage of low-income individuals, and individuals above 65 years old; and commercial

insurance databases, such as Clinformatics Data Mart database and Marketscan research databases, which cover diverse populations in therapeutic markets (39). These health insurance data have been used to increase the data size available for evaluating the risk factors of diseases, and also to evaluate the association between insurance types and standard of medical care provided (39–42).

For instance, Elam et al. utilized the Medicaid Analytic Extract database and the Clinformatics Data Mart database to evaluate the impact of health insurance types and racial disparities on the amount of glaucoma care/service received (39). The authors found that almost 50% of patients who were Medicaid-insured did not receive glaucoma testing compared to around 20% of commercially insured patients, suggesting a vast disparity in the standard of care received between the cohorts insured under Medicaid and private insurers (39). On the other hand, Stein et al. evaluated the impact of household income level on the diagnostic rates of common childhood ocular diseases. It was reported that lower detection rates of strabismus and amblyopia were observed in children from families with lower household net worth (40).

Other studies have utilized different insurance databases in the USA to increase the statistical power for analyzing the effect of drug types and risk factors associated with ocular diseases. For instance, Zheng et al. utilized the Truven Health MarketScan and the Medicare Supplemental Insurance databases to evaluate the associations between 2,186 types of systemic medications and primary open-angle glaucoma (POAG). This study observed that intake of selective serotonin reuptake inhibitors (e.g., citalopram) was associated with reduced risk of POAG. In contrast, intake of calcium channel blocker drugs (e.g., amlodipine) was associated with higher risk of POAG (41).

Next, Zhou et al. utilized the Truven Health MarketScan and Medicare's supplementary databases to evaluate risk factors for central

Table 1.3 Summary of the health insurance databases

Database	Country	Year of commencement
Clinformatics Data Mart Database (OptumInsight) (39)	USA	2001
MarketScan Research Database (IBM, Truven Health) (41)	USA	1995
Medicaid Analytic Extract (67)	USA	1999
National Health Insurance Research Database (35)	Taiwan	2002
National Health Insurance Service (68)	South Korea	2015
SNIIR-AM (National Health Insurance Fund for Salaried Workers) (37)	France	2003

serous retinopathy (CSR) (42). Both databases contributed a sample size of 35,492 newly diagnosed cases of CSR, which was substantially greater than conventional clinical or population-based studies. The authors found that middle-aged male patients on steroids, along with individuals who had diabetes mellitus, AMD, and diabetic macular edema were more likely to develop CSR. In contrast, factors such as hypertension and pregnancy were not significantly associated with CSR risk (42).

1.3.2.2 Taiwan

Studies that utilized the National Health Insurance Research Database in Taiwan mainly examined the risk factors for ocular diseases as well as the associations between different ocular diseases. For instance, Koh et al. performed a retrospective study to evaluate the epidemiology of keratitis in Taiwan (43). They examined the demographics and medical history of patients with different forms of ocular diseases and concluded that diabetes mellitus, eye trauma, and dry eye were the main risk factors for keratitis (43). On the other hand, Chang et al. analyzed the association between keratoconus and mitral valve prolapse (MVP). It was found that keratoconus patients aged 40 years old and older were 1.77 times likely to have MVP, while female keratoconus patients had a 1.48 times risk of getting MVP (44).

There were also other studies that utilized the National Health Insurance Research Database to evaluate utilization patterns of eyecare service. Leveraging on 6,341,266 of outpatient records from the database, Hsu et al. evaluated

the epidemiology landscape of ocular diseases in Taiwan (45). By integrating demographic factors such as age and sex as well as general information, including frequency of visits to ophthalmology outpatient services, the authors established the top ocular disease types within each age group (45). Cataract and glaucoma form the 'senile peaks' of common eye diseases among elderly population. The epidemiological insight provided by this study would be useful for primary practitioners, ophthalmologists, and policy makers. By understanding the trends in eyecare utilization, better care and more optimal public health policies could be designed and delivered.

1.3.2.3 South Korea

The majority of the studies that used Korea's National Health Insurance Database focused on the evaluation of ocular disease incidences and associated risk factors in the national population. Table 1.4 shows a brief summary of the findings derived from this database.

1.3.2.4 France

The SNIIR-AM database in France started in 2003. However, the usage of this database in ophthalmology is relatively new, and the data have mainly been used for the Epidemiology and Safety (EPISAFE) program in cataract surgery. Notable reports from this database included evaluation on incidence rates of cataract surgery between 2009 and 2012. It was observed that the incidence of cataract surgery increased from 9.86 to 11.08/1,000 person-years. The incidence of pseudophakic cystoid macular

Table 1.4 Brief summary of incidence rate studies using the Korea National Health Insurance Service Database

Ocular disease/condition	Incidence rate	Additional findings
Blindness (69)	34.2 in worse-seeing eye and 3.6 in better-seeing eye per 100,000 person-years	The incidence of blindness is greater in males than females and the incidence rate increases with age
Corneal transplantation (70)	1.69 per 100,000 person-years	Males were more likely to have repeated keratoplasty than females
Macular hole (71)	3.14 per 100,000 person-years	Females had a higher incidence rate than males and the incidence rates were the highest in patients aged 65–69
Primary congenital glaucoma (72)	11.0 per 100,000 births	Visual impairment and brain lesions were the most significant comorbidities present
Uveitis (73)	10.6 per 10,000 person-years	The incidence of uveitis increased with age, male sex, higher income, and in rural areas

edema was 0.95%. On the other hand, from 2005 to 2014, based on data derived from more than 6 million cataract surgeries, the incidence of endophthalmitis post-cataract surgery was recorded to decrease from 0.15 to 0.05% (46).

1.4 FUTURE OUTLOOK AND CHALLENGES

The concept of Big Data is gaining prominence exponentially in the healthcare field along with the focus on using AI to increase the efficiency of healthcare delivery. With the increasing adoption of EHR, escalation of data complexities, and advent of AI, it is crucial to also consider the challenges of expansion into Big Data and management systems like data registries for ophthalmology.

Currently, the application of AI to EHR data has been limited to four ocular diseases: cataract, glaucoma, DR, and AMD. While these diseases have shown certain successes in their applications in predictive diagnostic models, there is still room for improvement in terms of applying AI to EHR data, as shown in recent studies (47, 48). It is thus imperative to encourage continued adoption of EHRs in healthcare settings and to bring awareness to healthcare professionals regarding EHRs' role in data collection to derive more meaningful applications in research.

Other challenges that arise with the advent of Big Data sources include the need for complete data capture. Within ophthalmology EHRs, data heterogeneity exists in the forms of structured data, free-form texts within ocular examinations, images, and lab tests. To address the complexity surrounding clinical data extraction, increasing effort is devoted to developing and refining AI methods, such as phenotyping algorithms to accurately and efficiently extract clinical data (49–51). In addition, patients who receive treatment from different healthcare providers with varying EHR systems could also lead to decentralized and fragmented patient profiles due to the lack of standardized EHR systems. Data extraction strategies may also be further developed to allow linkage of EHR profiles across networks. More importantly, if Big Data is intended to be the game changer for research, promoting a collaborative system to integrate large-scale, complex ophthalmic data across different sources is critical to this field's development.

Lastly, central to the construction and maintenance of large-scale ophthalmic data is the safeguarding and responsible handling of patient data. Given that data registries contain demographic information and medical records of de-identified patients, it is imperative that cybersecurity development keeps pace with the growth of Big Data to best protect patient privacy and confidentiality. While the future of Big Data is dependent on data acquisition from patients of various sources, a balance between privacy protection and data accessibility is important.

1.5 CONCLUSION

In conclusion, research in ophthalmology has seen a recent surge in the utilization of Big Data, demonstrating enormous transformative potential in coming years. As Big Data is increasingly embedded into clinical care and its role continues to evolve, Big Data potentially exerts a growing influence over new scientific discoveries and healthcare delivery. With the expanding implementation of EHRs, disease registries, insurance databases, and other electronic platforms in medicine, it is essential for users, stakeholders, and patients to adapt to these emerging paradigms in health systems in a bid to maximally leverage this complex information for biomedical research and beyond.

REFERENCES

1. Lee CH, Yoon HJ. Medical big data: Promise and challenges. *Kidney Res Clin Pract*. 2017;36(1):311.

2. Cheng C-Y, Soh ZD, Majithia S, Thakur S, Rim TH, Tham YC, et al. Big data in ophthalmology. *Asia-Pacific J Ophthalmol*. 2020;9(4):291–8.

3. Elliott AF, Davidson A, Lum F, Chiang MF, Saaddine JB, Zhang X, et al. Use of electronic health records and administrative data for public health surveillance of eye health and vision-related conditions in the United States. *Am J Ophthalmol*. 2012;154(6 Suppl):S63–70.

4. Bailey IL, Bullimore MA, Raasch TW, Taylor HR. Clinical Grading and the effects of scaling. *Investig Ophthalmol Vis Sci*. 1991;32(2):422–32.

5. Ehrenstein VKH, Lehmann H, et al. Obtaining data from electronic health records. Tools and technologies for registry interoperability. In: Gliklich RE, Dreyer NA, Leavy MB (eds.), *Registries for Evaluating Patient Outcomes: A User's Guide*. Rockville (MD): Agency for Healthcare Research and Quality (US), 2019.

6. Christian J, Dasgupta N, Jordan M, Juneja M, Nilsen W, Reites J. Digital health and patient registries: Today, tomorrow, and the future. In: Gliklich RE, Dreyer NA, Leavy MB (eds.), *21st Century Patient Registries: Registries for Evaluating Patient Outcomes: A User's Guide: 3rd Edition, Addendum*. Rockville (MD): Agency for Healthcare Research and Quality (US), 2018.

7. Scanlon PH, Foy C, Malhotra R, Aldington SJ. The influence of age, duration of diabetes, cataract, and pupil size on image quality in digital photographic retinal screening. *Diabetes Care*. 2005;28(10):2448.

8. Kortüm K, Müller M, Kern C, Babenko A, Mayer W, Kampik A, et al. Using electronic health records to build an ophthalmologic data warehouse and visualize patients' data. *Am J Ophthalmol*. 2017;178.

9. Bommakanti NK, Zhou Y, Ehrlich JR, Elam AR, John D, Kamat SS, et al. Application of the sight outcomes research collaborative ophthalmology data repository for triaging patients with glaucoma and clinic

11

appointments during pandemics such as COVID-19. *JAMA Ophthalmol*. 2020;138(9):974–80.

10. Pershing S, Lum F, Hsu S, Kelly S, Chiang MF, Rich WL, 3rd, et al. Endophthalmitis after cataract surgery in the United States: A report from the Intelligent Research in Sight Registry, 2013–2017. *Ophthalmology*. 2020;127(2):151–8.

11. Mahr MA, Lum F, Fujino D, Kelly SP, Erie JC. Return to the operating room for removal of retained lens fragments after cataract surgery: IRIS Registry (Intelligent Research in Sight) analysis. *Ophthalmology*. 2020;127(5):698–9.

12. Cantrell RA, Lum F, Chia YF, Morse LS, Rich WL, Salman CA, et al. Treatment patterns for diabetic macular edema: An Intelligent Research in Sight (IRIS) registry analysis. *Ophthalmology*. 2020;127(3):427–9.

13. Repka MX. Amblyopia outcomes through clinical trials and practice measurement: room for improvement: The LXXVII Edward Jackson Memorial Lecture. *Am J Ophthalmol*. 2020;219:A1–A26.

14. Stein JD, Rahman M, Andrews C, Ehrlich JR, Kamat S, Shah M, et al. Evaluation of an algorithm for identifying ocular conditions in electronic health record data. *JAMA Ophthalmology*. 2019;137(5):491–7.

15. Cornish EE, Teo KY, Nguyen V, Squirrel D, Young S, Gillies MC, et al. Five-year incidence and visual acuity outcomes for intravitreal therapy in bilateral neovascular age-related macular degeneration: Fight Retinal Blindness! Project. *Retina*. 2021;41(1):118–24.

16. Chong Teo KY, Saxena N, Gan A, Wong TY, Gillies MC, Chakravarthy U, et al. Detrimental effect of delayed re-treatment of active disease on outcomes in neovascular age-related macular degeneration: The RAMPS study. *Ophthalmol Retina*. 2020;4(9):871–80.

17. Hebbring S. Genomic and phenomic research in the 21st Century. *Trends Genet*. 2019;35(1):29–41.

18. Abul-Husn NS, Kenny EE. Personalized medicine and the power of electronic health records. *Cell*. 2019;177(1):58–69.

19. Wolford BN, Willer CJ, Surakka I. Electronic health records: the next wave of complex disease genetics. *Hum Mol Genet*. 2018;27(R1):R14–21.

20. Roden DM, Xu H, Denny JC, Wilke RA. Electronic medical records as a tool in clinical pharmacology: Opportunities and challenges. *Clin Pharmacol Ther*. 2012;91(6):1083–6.

21. Denny JC, Ritchie MD, Crawford DC, Schildcrout JS, Ramirez AH, Pulley JM, et al. Identification of genomic predictors of atrioventricular conduction: using electronic medical records as a tool for genome science. *Circulation*. 2010;122(20):2016–21.

22. Denny JC, Bastarache L, Ritchie MD, Carroll RJ, Zink R, Mosley JD, et al. Systematic comparison of phenome-wide association study of electronic medical record data and genome-wide association study data. *Nat Biotechnol*. 2013;31(12):1102–10.

23. Shah NH. Mining the ultimate phenome repository. *Nat Biotechnol*. 2013;31(12):1095–7.

24. Roden DM. Phenome-wide association studies: A new method for functional genomics in humans. *J Physiol*. 2017;595(12):4109–15.

25. Zhao J, Cheng F, Jia P, Cox N, Denny JC, Zhao Z. An integrative functional genomics framework for effective identification of novel regulatory variants in genome-phenome studies. *Genome Med*. 2018;10(1):7.

26. Ritchie MD, Denny JC, Zuvich RL, Crawford DC, Schildcrout JS, Bastarache L, et al. Genome- and phenome-wide analyses of cardiac conduction identifies markers of arrhythmia risk. *Circulation*. 2013;127(13):1377–85.

27. Bastarache L, Hughey JJ, Hebbring S, Marlo J, Zhao W, Ho WT, et al. Phenotype risk scores identify patients with unrecognized Mendelian disease patterns. *Science*. 2018;359(6381):1233–9.

28. Li R, Chen Y, Ritchie MD, Moore JH. Electronic health records and polygenic risk scores for predicting disease risk. *Nat Rev Genet*. 2020;21(8):493–502.

29. Ritchie MD, Verma SS, Hall MA, Goodloe RJ, Berg RL, Carrell DS, et al. Electronic medical records and genomics (eMERGE) network exploration in cataract: Several new potential susceptibility loci. *Mol Vis*. 2014;20:1281–95.

30. Choquet H, Thai KK, Yin J, Hoffmann TJ, Kvale MN, Banda Y, et al. A large multi-ethnic genome-wide association study identifies novel genetic loci for intraocular pressure. *Nat Commun*. 2017;8(1):2108.

31. Unlu G, Gamazon ER, Qi X, Levic DS, Bastarache L, Denny JC, et al. *GRIK5* Genetically regulated expression associated with eye and vascular phenomes: discovery through iteration among biobanks, electronic health records, and zebrafish. *Am J Hum Genet*. 2019;104(3):503–19.

32. Ng JYS, Ramadani RV, Hendrawan D, Duc DT, Kiet PHT. National Health Insurance databases in Indonesia, Vietnam and the Philippines. *PharmacoEconomics - Open*. 2019;3(4):517–26.

33. OptumInsight. Available from: https://ldi.upenn.edu/ldi-health-services-research-data-center/optum insight.

34. Medicaid Analytic eXtract (MAX) General Information: CMS.gov. Available from: www.cms.gov/Research-Statistics-Data-and-Systems/Computer-Data-and-Systems/MedicaidDataSourcesGenInfo/MAXGeneralInformation#:~:text=Each%20state's%20Medicaid%20agency%20collects,Management%20Information%20System%20(MMIS).

35. Lin LY, Warren-Gash C, Smeeth L, Chen PC. Data resource profile: The National Health Insurance Research Database (NHIRD). *Epidemiol Health*. 2018;40:e2018062.

36. Bahk J, Kim YY, Kang HY, Lee J, Kim I, Lee J, et al. Using the National Health Information Database of the National Health Insurance Service in Korea for monitoring mortality and life expectancy at national and local levels. *J Korean Med Sci*. 2017;32(11):1764–70.

37. Moulis G, Lapeyre-Mestre M, Palmaro A, Pugnet G, Montastruc JL, Sailler L. French health insurance databases: What interest for medical research? *Rev Med Interne*. 2015;36(6):411–17.

38. Bezin J, Duong M, Lassalle R, Droz C, Pariente A, Blin P, et al. The national healthcare system claims databases in France, SNIIRAM and EGB: Powerful tools for pharmacoepidemiology. *Pharmacoepidemiol Drug Saf*. 2017;26(8):954–62.

39. Elam AR, Andrews C, Musch DC, Lee PP, Stein JD. Large disparities in receipt of glaucoma care between enrollees in Medicaid and those with commercial health insurance. *Ophthalmology*. 2017;124(10):1442–8.

40. Stein JD, Andrews C, Musch DC, Green C, Lee PP. Sight-threatening ocular diseases remain

underdiagnosed among children of less affluent families. *Health Aff (Millwood)*. 2016;35(8):1359–66.

41. Zheng W, Dryja TP, Wei Z, Song D, Tian H, Kahler KH, et al. Systemic medication associations with presumed advanced or uncontrolled primary open-angle glaucoma. *Ophthalmology*. 2018;125(7):984–93.

42. Zhou M, Bakri SJ, Pershing S. Risk factors for incident central serous retinopathy: Case-control analysis of a US national managed care population. *Br J Ophthalmol*. 2019;103(12):1784–8.

43. Koh YY, Sun CC, Hsiao CH. Epidemiology and the estimated burden of microbial keratitis on the health care system in Taiwan: A 14-year population-based study. *Am J Ophthalmol*. 2020;220:152–9.

44. Chang YS, Tai MC, Weng SF, Wang JJ, Tseng SH, Jan RL. Risk of mitral valve prolapse in patients with keratoconus in Taiwan: A population-based cohort study. *Int J Environ Res Public Health*. 2020;17(17).

45. Hsu CA, Hsiao SH, Hsu MH, Yen JC. Utilization of outpatient eye care services in Taiwan: A nationwide population study. *J Ophthalmol*. 2020;2020:2641683.

46. Daien V, Korobelnik JF, Delcourt C, Cougnard-Gregoire A, Delyfer MN, Bron AM, et al. French Medical-Administrative Database for Epidemiology and Safety in Ophthalmology (EPISAFE): The EPISAFE collaboration program in cataract surgery. *Ophthalmic Res*. 2017;58(2):67–73.

47. Lin W-C, Chen JS, Chiang MF, Hribar MR. Applications of artificial intelligence to electronic health record data in ophthalmology. *Transl Vis Sci Technol*. 2020;9(2):13.

48. Lin H, Long E, Ding X, Diao H, Chen Z, Liu R, et al. Prediction of myopia development among Chinese school-aged children using refraction data from electronic medical records: A retrospective, multicentre machine learning study. *PLoS Med*. 2018;15(11):e1002674-e.

49. Stein JD, Rahman M, Andrews C, Ehrlich JR, Kamat S, Shah M, et al. Evaluation of an algorithm for identifying ocular conditions in electronic health record data. *JAMA Ophthalmol*. 2019;137(5):491–7.

50. Lin WC, Chen JS, Chiang MF, Hribar MR. Applications of artificial intelligence to electronic health record data in ophthalmology. *Transl Vis Sci Technol*. 2020;9(2):13.

51. Mbagwu M, French DD, Gill M, Mitchell C, Jackson K, Kho A, et al. Creation of an accurate algorithm to detect Snellen best documented visual acuity from ophthalmology electronic health record notes. *JMIR Med Inform*. 2016;4(2):e14.

52. Bycroft C, Freeman C, Petkova D, Band G, Elliott LT, Sharp K, et al. The UK Biobank resource with deep phenotyping and genomic data. *Nature*. 2018;562(7726):203–9.

53. Denny JC, Rutter JL, Goldstein DB, Philippakis A, Smoller JW, et al. The "All of Us" research program. *N Engl J Med*. 2019;381(7):668–76.

54. Vanderbilt University Medical Center. BioVU. Department of Biomedical Informatics. Available from: www.vumc.org/dbmi/biovu.

55. Vanderbilt Institute for Clinical and Translational Research. What is BioVU? Available from: https://victr.vumc.org/what-is-biovu/.

56. Carey DJ, Fetterolf SN, Davis FD, Faucett WA, Kirchner HL, Mirshahi U, et al. The Geisinger MyCode community health initiative: An electronic health record-linked biobank for precision medicine research. *Genet Med*. 2016;18(9):906–13.

57. Kaiser Permanente Research Bank. Available from: https://researchbank.kaiserpermanente.org/faq/.

58. Gaziano JM, Concato J, Brophy M, Fiore L, Pyarajan S, Breeling J, et al. Million Veteran Program: A mega-biobank to study genetic influences on health and disease. *J Clin Epidemiol*. 2016;70:214–23.

59. deCODE genetics. Available from: www.decode.com/.

60. Leitsalu L, Alavere H, Tammesoo ML, Leego E, Metspalu A. Linking a population biobank with national health registries – The Estonian experience. *J Pers Med*. 2015;5(2):96–106.

61. Danish National Biobank. Available from: danishnationalbiobank.com.

62. FinnGen. Health registries. Available from: www.finngen.fi/en/health_registries.

63. Nagai A, Hirata M, Kamatani Y, Muto K, Matsuda K, Kiyohara Y, et al. Overview of the BioBank Japan Project: Study design and profile. *J Epidemiol*. 2017;27(3S):S2–S8.

64. Kubo M, Guest E. BioBank Japan project: Epidemiological study. *J Epidemiol*. 2017;27(3S):S1.

65. Chen Z, Chen J, Collins R, Guo Y, Peto R, Wu F, et al. China Kadoorie Biobank of 0.5 million people: Survey methods, baseline characteristics and long-term follow-up. *Int J Epidemiol*. 2011;40(6):1652–66.

66. Cho SY, Hong EJ, Nam JM, Han B, Chu C, Park O. Opening of the national biobank of Korea as the infrastructure of future biomedical science in Korea. *Osong Public Health Res Perspect*. 2012;3(3):177–84.

67. Gao X, Lin S, Wong TY. Automatic feature learning to grade nuclear cataracts based on deep learning. *IEEE Trans Bio-Med Eng*. 2015;62.

68. Greenspan H, Ginneken BV, Summers RM. Guest editorial: Deep learning in medical imaging: Overview and future promise of an exciting new technique. *IEEE Trans Med Imaging*. 2016;35(5):1153–9.

69. Rim TH, Kim DW, Chung EJ, Kim SS. Nationwide incidence of blindness in South Korea: A 12-year study from 2002 to 2013. *Clin Exp Ophthalmol*. 2017;45(8):773–8.

70. Shin KY, Lim DH, Han K, Chung TY. Higher incidence of penetrating keratoplasty having effects on repeated keratoplasty in South Korea: A nationwide population-based study. *PLoS One*. 2020;15(7):e0235233.

71. Cho SC, Park SJ, Byun SJ, Woo SJ, Park KH. Five-year nationwide incidence of macular hole requiring surgery in Korea. *Br J Ophthalmol*. 2019;103(11):1619–23.

72. Lee SJ, Kim S, Rim TH, Pak H, Kim DW, Park JW. Incidence, comorbidity, and mortality of primary congenital glaucoma in Korea from 2001 to 2015: A nationwide population-based study. *Korean J Ophthalmol*. 2020;34(4):316–21.

73. Rim TH, Kim SS, Ham DI, Yu SY, Chung EJ, Lee SC. Incidence and prevalence of uveitis in South Korea: A nationwide cohort study. *Br J Ophthalmol*. 2018;102(1):79–83.

2 Application of Mobile and Wearable Technology in Data Collection for Ophthalmology

Ashwin Venkatesh and Pradeep Ramulu

2.1 OVERVIEW OF GENERAL USE CASES OF REMOTE MONITORING

Remote monitoring of patients has expanded the capacity and ease with which clinicians manage and monitor the wellbeing of their patients. Moreover, in the setting of pandemics, where patients may not want to present to the clinic for evaluation and testing, this may become the only available method for monitoring patients. These systems involve the use of digital technologies by patients (or research study participants) to collect, in their native environment, data on behaviors relevant to health. These data are then, via direct download or a cloud-based system, electronically transmitted to the healthcare providers/research team members for assessment. Some devices (such as implanted biosensors or wearable technology) may be automated to record and transmit health data in real time, without any action from the patient. Other technologies may require patients to input their own health data through a secure interface, such as devices or applications that record serial images, log physiologic parameters, or remotely fill out questionnaires. When such systems are employed by patients, and the information is put in their hands, they become empowered to make independent assessments of their own wellbeing, gain additional health information, and ultimately make better-informed healthcare decisions. When researchers use these systems, they gain access to behavioral information and longer-term parameters that cannot be accessed in the clinical setting.

2.2 DOMAINS OF REMOTE MEASUREMENTS

There are several health/wellbeing domains in which remote monitoring can provide information. From an epidemiologic perspective, data gathered within these domains can serve as study outcomes (i.e., home visual testing), or important exposures which define novel risk factors for disease (i.e., physical activity as a risk factor for disease prevalence). Parameters such as disease outcomes, exposures, intervention efficacies, as well as spatiotemporal data can be analyzed using remote methods. We propose that the types of remote measurements made can be further classified into the following domains: physiological, functional, metabolic, behavioral, and patient-centered outcome

measures (Table 2.1). Whilst there are many uses for remote monitoring (e.g., chronic and progressive cardiovascular and metabolic diseases), this chapter will survey examples of established, novel, and potential uses of remote monitoring in these domains in the context of ophthalmology and vision research.

2.2.1 Physiological Measures

An example of a physiologic parameter in eye disease is intraocular pressure (IOP), which remains a principal risk factor for, and the only known method to slow or halt, the development and progression of glaucomatous disease.[1] Maintenance of a target IOP over time is therefore a critical physiological objective for follow-up assessment. Since IOP has been shown to undergo diurnal variation, isolated measurements in clinic may be inadequate and more extensive monitoring outside of the healthcare setting may be necessary.[2] However, work fully capturing the relevance of IOP patterns, particularly IOP patterns outside of clinical hours, to clinical outcomes such as glaucoma prevalence and progression, has been limited by the ability to measure these patterns. Moreover, the impact of various treatments on detailed 24-hour IOP patterns is limited.

Many methods are available for remote measurement of IOP, both through self-assessment in the home and through automated monitoring over different timescales (Table 2.2).

In the home setting, iCare Home has been developed as a commercially available self-tonometer. This device incorporates rebound technology, by which a magnetic probe is propelled on to the cornea from where it rebounds. IOP can be closely correlated to certain motion parameters of the probe, particularly deceleration time. This is a rapid method with minimal adverse complications, and without the need for anesthetic drops, and it has been shown to correlate closely with the standard Goldmann applanation tonometer (GAT) and with excellent repeatability and usability.[3] One limitation of the device is that, in the United States, the machine is approved to be used only under the guidance of a physician, and patients do not have immediate access to their IOP readings.

Continuous IOP monitoring over short durations has also been accomplished using wearable contact lens sensor devices such

DOI: 10.1201/9781315146737-3

Table 2.1 Novel classification of various types of remote measurements

Domain	Definition	Examples
Physiological	An internal parameter that is maintained around a target set-point in health and deranged in disease	Blood pressure, intraocular pressure
Functional	Parameters associated with a bodily system that have important effects on the responses of that system	Visual acuity, visual fields
Metabolic	Biologic processes where there is a transformation of a chemical substance	Blood glucose
Behavioral	Observable patterns of patient activity	Amount of physical activity, travel outside the home
Patient-centered outcome measure	Patient perceptions of their health and experiences, which are key to providing patient-centered care	Self-reports of mental, physical, and psychosocial symptoms and quality-of-life aspects

Table 2.2 Methods for remote monitoring of intraocular pressure

Type of device	Type of monitoring	Example
Self-tonometer	Periodic self-assessment	iCare Home
Wearable device: contact lens sensor	Continuous monitoring over short durations (e.g., <1 day)	Sensimed Triggerfish CLS
Implanted device: intraocular lens pressure transducer	Continuous monitoring over long durations (e.g., >1 day)	Implandata EyeMate

as the Sensimed Triggerfish CLS (Sensimed, Lausanne, Switzerland). This silicone contact lens has two strain gauges embedded within it that detect changes in corneal shape that are postulated to correlate with IOP changes.[4] Due to its automated nature, this type of device may offer a more convenient and user-friendly means of continuously measuring IOP, particularly for those familiar with contact lens application. This wearable contact lens sensor is further supported by evidence of its safety (Food and Drug Administration [FDA]-approved), tolerability, and reproducibility, but is limited in that it may only provide data on relative rather than absolute changes in IOP.

More long-term measures of continuous IOP monitoring are now available in the form of intraocular lens pressure transducers (e.g., Implandata EyeMate). Each pressure sensor is composed of two parallel plates: a thin flexible plate that indents with changes in IOP and a thicker rigid base plate. Distance comparisons between the plates can determine changes in IOP, generating a corresponding analog signal that is then converted to a digital signal to be transmitted externally by radiofrequency. The Implandata EyeMate lens has been trialed in the ARGOS-01 study recruiting patients undergoing cataract surgery, in whom the retinal sensor chip could be concurrently implanted.

This study found that glaucoma control was maintained in these patients, with minimal ensuing complications.[5] Future implementations are likely to involve further miniaturization of implantable intraocular sensors in order to allow safer and more minimally invasive implantation with fewer adverse postoperative complications (e.g., inflammation).[6] These developments have permitted precise long-term measurements of IOP, which may allow optimization of therapeutic regimens and reinforce adherence to them, thereby halting the progression of visual field loss due to glaucoma.

Other pertinent physiologic parameters such as tear osmolarity and retinal blood flow may also be interesting and important to monitor, yet their potential for remote measurement is limited and has to date been underexplored.

2.2.2 Functional Measures

Visual acuity (VA) remains a frequently measured visual parameter in clinical practice. VA is functionally important as it enables tasks such as reading text, interpreting and manipulating fine objects, and recognizing faces. VA is therefore a strong predictor of self-reported vision-related quality of life.[7] Given the importance of VA, clinical trials and other studies evaluating treatment outcomes in numerous disease states (cataract surgery, diabetic retinopathy

[DR], macular degeneration) frequently employ VA as a primary outcome measure.

One challenge faced by clinical trials looking to evaluate and compare changes in vision in response to therapy is that VA can only be evaluated during clinic visits, with each visit placing a burden on both the study participant and research staff. As such, significant improvements in trial design would be possible if more frequent VA could be acquired, especially if such measures did not require leaving the home.

Novel smartphone applications have been developed with important clinical promise for remote monitoring of VA. For instance, the Portable Eye Examination Kit (Peek) Acuity is a logMAR-style smartphone-based VA test which can be performed in the patient's native environment. The participant points in the direction they perceive the arms of the E to be pointing and the tester (who is masked to the presented optotype) uses the touch screen to swipe accordingly, translating the gestures from the patient. Peek Acuity has been tested on 233 Kenyan adults aged over 55 and the results were found to have greater precision and reliability (test–retest variability = ±0.033 logMAR) than standard Snellen charts.[8] Moreover, data can be stored and shared, and the record can be geotagged, which is helpful in resource-limited settings where addresses may not be available and patient follow-up is challenging. Another smartphone interface is the Sightbook app, which is paired with the Digisight network, and allows patients to reproducibly test VA (intraclass correlation coefficient >0.75), amongst a set of other quantitative near-vision tests, which can be remotely prescribed by ophthalmologists in appropriate intervals and sequences.[9] In addition to its testing capabilities, the SightBook app can also be used to log treatments and to keep track of upcoming appointments.

Studies using the modalities described here have thus far largely focused on screening for acuity impairments. Future studies should therefore seek to address their consistency and efficacy in judging the trajectory of disease progression or evaluation of treatment outcomes. A recent scoping review reviewed 42 e-health tools for the self-testing of VA.[10] The authors found that tools could assess near and distance vision, about half (n = 20) used bespoke optotypes, the majority (n = 25) presented optotypes one by one, and that four included a calibration procedure. Notably, only one tool was validated against gold-standard measures. This highlights a need for regulation of tools for the self-testing of VA to reduce potential risk or confusion to users.

There are a number of factors to take into account, and challenges to overcome, for remote VA measurements to be widely adopted. Firstly, a number of conditions must be standardized between each test: the viewing angle, viewing distance, and screen illuminance relative to ambient lighting. It is also important to consider how the collected data will be transmitted, whether through uploading into cloud storage or whether it will be locally downloaded. Some devices (e.g., SVOne and EyeNetra) have the capacity for automated refraction, which provides an objective measurement of a patient's refractive error validated against established methods.[11] Ultimately, all assessments should report test–retest variability for their reliable application. Further work is also required to integrate these remote measurement tools into clinical systems of care, while maintaining patient privacy.

Visual field damage is superior to VA with regard to diagnosing or judging the presence or progression of various optic nerve (i.e., glaucoma, non-arteritic anterior ischemic optic neuropathy) and retinal (i.e., retinitis pigmentosa) disease. Several devices recently have been developed that could allow visual field assessments away from clinical settings and potentially could be performed without the direct supervision of a trained clinician. These include tablet-based devices, head-mounted displays, and virtual reality (VR) goggle perimetry programs. The Visual Fields Easy app and Melbourne Rapid Fields app are both iPad-based applications that monitor visual field changes for a variety of conditions, with the latter now released as a commercially available product. The Wills Eye Glaucoma app is a free application dedicated for glaucoma patients, which includes educational videos, eye drop and appointment reminders, medical and ocular data storage, visual field tutorial, and IOP tracker. These features aim to increase patients' level of knowledge about glaucoma and improve their adherence to medication and follow-up appointment recommendations.

There are a number of factors to take into account and challenges to overcome for remote visual field measurements to be widely adopted (Table 2.3). Firstly, a number of conditions must be standardized between each test: the viewing angle, viewing distance, and screen illuminance relative to ambient lighting. Also, commercially available screens are often not bright enough to allow sufficient dimming to detect very mild defects. Additionally, devices would ideally track patient viewing distance over the course of the test, and also fixation, though the latter may not be a strong predictor of reliability in

Table 2.3 Factors/challenges influencing remote visual field measurements

Device	Variation	Standardized for ambient light?	Data storage	Size of visual field	Average duration of test	Are fixation losses measured?
Visual Fields Easy app	Poorly reproducible: ICC = 0.532	Yes	Cloud	30° horizontal; 24° vertical	3 minutes, 18 seconds	No
Melbourne Rapid Fields app	Highly reproducible: ICC = 0.98	Yes	Cloud	30° horizontal; 24° vertical	4 minutes	Yes

Abbreviation: ICC, intraclass correlation coefficient.

persons who have previously completed visual field testing, and that test–retest variability may be described.[12]

A novel solution overcoming the inability to control fixation and the distance from the eye to the screen is through the use of VR headsets. These employ adjustable fixation using gaze tracking such that no matter where the patient looks, the stimulus can be shown relative to fixation at that moment. Gyroscopes can account for head movement, and the immersive environment can improve user engagement. VR headsets can take advantage of smartphones and test individual eyes without one needing to be patched. There are multiple inexpensive, lightweight, mobile VR applications and software platforms that are either available or in development, such as Vivid Vision, BioFormatix's VirtualEye Perimeter, MicroMedical Devices' PalmScan VF2000, and Elisar's eCloud Perimeter. A high correlation was noted between the reliability of visual field testing using the VR testing system they developed and the conventional Humphrey test.[13]

Metamorphopsia is a perceived distortion of visual space, commonly seen in disorders of macular function. The ForeseeHome device (Notal Vision, Tel Aviv, Israel) uses preferential hyperacuity perimetry to measure visual distortions in age-related macular degeneration and is designed for unsupervised use by patients in their homes. The test involves 500 retinal data points over 14° of the patient's central visual field, collected in approximately 3 minutes, and allows quantitative monitoring of changes in macular function in metamorphopsia with greater sensitivity than the Amsler grid.[14] Results are automatically transmitted to Notal Vision's Monitoring Center, where they are logged with all previous tests from that patient. Patients who generate an alert on the ForeseeHome test trigger an immediate recall to their ophthalmologist's office for additional diagnostic testing and examination. The utility of this device is highlighted by the AREDS2-HOME clinical trial, which concluded that the ForeseeHome device enabled earlier detection of choroidal neovascularization in high-risk patients with age-related macular degeneration.[15]

Contrast sensitivity is a measure of the ability to detect differences in luminance (brightness) across borders. Poor contrast sensitivity deficits significantly affect overall quality of life, impair target identification, and are associated with an increased risk of falls.[7,16,17] Contrast sensitivity is impaired in a variety of ophthalmic and neurologic conditions, including age-related macular degeneration, amblyopia, dry eye, glare, glaucoma, myopia, ocular hypertension, cerebral lesions, and multiple sclerosis. Importantly, contrast sensitivity may be impaired in visual neuropathology that does not affect acuity. Remote monitoring of contrast sensitivity has been developed as both applications and web-based tests. For instance, the Spaeth/Richman contrast sensitivity test (SPARCS) is an internet-based test that features multiple answer choices and a bracketing technique, evaluating contrast sensitivity in both central and peripheral regions with high test–retest reliability and highly correlating with the conventional Pelli–Robson chart test.[18,19] iPad applications have also been developed which have shown similar repeatability and may be a rapid and convenient alternative to some existing measures.[20,21] This has thus far been implemented to screen for amblyopia in children and to monitor the development of vision in congenitally blind children and teenagers after cataract removal.[22,23] However, despite the use of a portable device, these studies involved supervision by a researcher and were not implemented for self-assessment in the home setting. This may be due to the concern that completely unsupervised settings hinder the robustness of their tests; for instance, different light conditions and glare might affect test results. Changes in viewing distance also change the retinal size of presented stimuli; however the front-facing camera of the iPad may be used to ensure viewing distance compliance. Thus, future studies could test the feasibility of home measurements of contrast sensitivity in these disease contexts.

2.2.3 Metabolic/Structural Measures

Regular screening and monitoring of risk factors, glycemic control, and prompt diagnosis form an important strategy to prevent or limit the progression of DR. The Diabetes Control and Complications Trial (DCCT) has shown that optimal glucose control in diabetes slows the onset and worsening of complications such as DR.[24] There is therefore a need for monitoring in the remote setting to measure and reinforce appropriate glycemic control. Traditional devices (e.g., Accu-Chek) involved pricking the finger with a lancet and placing a drop of blood on a disposable test strip that is read with a digital meter.

However, since glucose levels are fluctuant, continuous glucose monitoring (CGM) may provide a more accurate indicator of intra- and inter-day glycemic excursions. The Dexcom G5 (Dexcom), Medtronic Enlite (Medtronic), and FreeStyle Libre Flash systems are among the most common real-time CGM systems marketed. These novel needle-free devices sub-cutaneously measure interstitial glucose levels and provide real-time numerical and graphical information about the current glucose level, glucose trends, and trend arrows, which indi-cate the direction and velocity of changing glucose. Programmable alerts/alarms can be used to remind/warn patients of current and/or impending high or low glucose. Real-time alerts and alarms can be 'shared' with caregivers (currently available on the Dexcom G5 system). A large prospective study used a subcutaneous CGM system (Medtronic, Northridge, CA) to track participants' blood glucose for 3 days and correlated findings with fundus images. This study found that patients with more advanced DR had significantly less time in range (TIR), i.e., the time an individual spends within their target glucose range.[25] The company has now released the Guardian Connect CGM (Medtronic, Northridge, CA) for commercial use with FDA approval, designed for remote monitoring in those on insulin injections. The most recent real-time CGM system, Eversense (Senseonics), features the first implantable sensor, whose accuracy and safety has been validated in the PRECISE II and PRECISION clinical trials.[26] It is hoped that in the longer term, continuous monitoring studies will aid further evaluation of the progression and prevention of diabetic complications, including retinal complications such as retinopathy and macular edema.

The improvement in optical and sensory cap-abilities of smartphone cameras has allowed their use in serial fundus imaging to directly monitor retinal pathology. This is particularly useful in low-resource or remote settings and smartphones have been approved by the FDA for this purpose. In smartphone retinal imaging, the smartphone camera's coaxial flashlight in conjunction with a condensing lens create an indirect ophthalmoscopy-like optical system whilst placing an external LED light source closer to the smartphone camera can effectively transform it into a direct ophthalmoscope.[27,28] Other adaptors may be paired with smartphones to augment the quality of the captured image, offering mechanical stabilization of hardware along the pupillary axis with ideal light control through an external light source and reduction of ambient light pollution. Commercially available, FDA-approved examples include D-EYE and the Welch Allyn iExaminer System.[29] One difficulty is that most implementations require the image to be taken by someone other than the patient. However, technical training is much easier than the table-top fundus camera allowing non-specialists to examine, and now fundus 'selfie' techniques permit image capture by the patients themselves.[30] Another limitation is that most protocols involve pharmacologic dilation of the pupil to increase the field of view, but this is both difficult and inconvenient to perform remotely, and unnecessary if a smaller field of view is suf-ficient (e.g., visualizing the optic disc). Portable non-mydriatic retinal imaging cameras are now commercially available as separate devices (e.g., Zeiss Visuscout 100).

Following image capture, the image must be analyzed and compared to determine patho-logical deterioration or resolution. Earlier methods would involve interpretation by ophthalmologists, which is time-consuming and inefficient, but novel technologies have incorporated artificial intelligence software (e.g., EyeArt software) that can read images in real time and determine whether subsequent referral is required.[31] Whilst aimed at primary care doctors and clinics, it is conceivable that such technologies could be made more access-ible and available for patients at high risk, e.g., those with persistently deranged blood glucose levels, since specialized operator training is not required. Smartphone-based fundus photog-raphy devices may therefore provide a prom-ising, cost-effective, and portable alternative to screen and monitor for vision-threatening diseases.

2.2.4 Behavioral Measures

Individuals with visual impairments may have distinct activity patterns and interactions with the world around them. Whilst this may be a consequence of their reduced vision, it is important to appreciate that this may be a risk factor contributing to further visual decline. Hence, monitoring of patient activity patterns may be useful to highlight modifiable risk factors for disease onset or progression or limitations resulting from disease. For instance, accelerometers, location trackers, and step counters have become embedded within smartwatches and smartphone health applications and have been implemented in recent research. These studies have revealed that diminished VA and severity of visual field loss are associated with a lower daily step count and individuals who are more house-bound, and that increases in physical activity correlated with decreased rates of visual field loss.[32–35]

It is plausible that activity-monitoring technologies implemented in other fields could be transferrable for use in an ophthalmic context. For instance, the Center for Technology and Aging describes methods for remote monitoring of dementia patients who are at risk for falls – an issue that is also faced by visually impaired individuals.[36] In particular, those with glaucoma are more susceptible to falls at home than away from home, as adjudged by questionnaires, accelerometer and GPS recordings.[37] Sensors can be affixed to the individual or their assistive mobility devices, and monitor an individual's location, gait, linear acceleration, and angular velocity, and utilize a mathematical algorithm to predict the likelihood for falls, detect movement changes, and alert caregivers if the individual has fallen.[38] Furthermore, tracking capabilities via Wi-Fi, GPS, or radio frequency enables caregivers to locate wandering elders. However, this may not be feasible for those who do not have access to such connectivity services.

An additional aspect of behavior that can be captured through remote monitoring is medication adherence, which is a well-recognized challenge to successful treatment.[39] The reasons for non-adherence are multifactorial and can be either unintentional (e.g., reliance on others) or intentional. Smart technologies are being developed to address this issue remotely, either by monitoring adherence, or through acting as interventions directed at improving adherence. A recent systematic review identified three broad categories of adherence strategies: reminder, behavioral, and educational.[39]

Home devices are available that serve as monitors of patient adherence behaviors. There are also devices that monitor medication events, such as the Medication Event Monitoring System (MEMS SmartCap) and the Eye Drop Application Monitor (EDAM). These devices track the time and history of application. EDAM directly measures compliance through using a video monitoring system, enabling remote assessment of the patient's administration technique by the clinician. Wireless smart monitors are now in development for eye drops. For instance, the Kali drop device attaches to the body of an eye drop bottle and uses a combination of motion and tactile sensors to track eye drop usage.[40] The Devers drop device is a reusable, silicone monitor and alert system that couples to any eye drop bottle cap while permitting normal functioning of the bottle cap.[41] These appear sustainable methods of measuring and improving eye drop adherence.

The advent of the smartphone has bridged the gap between monitoring adherence and acting to improve adherence. Reminder modalities include alarms, push notifications, and SMS. One study utilized telecommunication-based reminders linked to personal health records, in which glaucoma patients using once-daily eye drops set up an automated telecommunication-based reminder system (call or text). It was found that the median adherence rate in the intervention group increased from 53% to 64% (and even higher, 73%, when comparing the participants who successfully completed the study after randomization), while there was no statistical change in the control group, thus validating this strategy.[42] More recent smartphone applications such as the Wills Eye Glaucoma, MyEyeDrops, EyeDROPS, RxmindME, and MEMOTEXT serve not only to act as automated dosing reminders, but also as electronic diaries that log adherence to treatment regimens. In addition, these apps can serve as information portals, offering instructive videos of proper administration techniques and/or knowledge summaries to educate patients regarding various disease aspects.

Whilst smartphone interventions are increasingly attractive owing to their widespread accessibility, their efficacy in enhancing adherence is contentious. A systematic review found that 65% of included studies encompassing a broad range of health conditions showed positive adherence outcomes for mobile interventions using SMS reminders.[43] The mixed benefit of smartphone interventions may reflect additional behavioral complexities, such as: presence of psychological problems, in particular depression; lack of primary support; occurrence of medication side effects; and if the treatment is focused on treating an asymptomatic disease. To holistically address non-adherence therefore, these various aspects of behavior should be simultaneously addressed by developers, and future high-quality studies should seek to demonstrate whether smartphone interventions effectively reduce the causes or consequences of non-adherence in ophthalmic contexts.

2.2.5 Patient-Centered Outcome Measures

Patient-centered outcome measures (PCOMs) encompass objective functional measures and subjective patient-reported outcome measures (PROMs) that are important determinants of a patient's quality of life. PCOMs are therefore valuable in the clinical decision-making process as they inform on patient priorities, whilst also providing advantages beyond clinic and research, such as in communicating in simple terms the impact of the disease to governments or policy makers.

Questionnaires have been helpful to remotely elucidate the patient's perspective of their mental, physical, and psychosocial status as well as quality-of-life aspects (PROMs). Generic ophthalmic questionnaires that assess the impact of visual impairment on vision-related quality of life have been validated (e.g., the Impact of Vision Impairment [IVI] scale).[44–46] More specific ophthalmic questionnaires have been prominently applied in the context of glaucoma, evaluating specific activity limitation, quality-of-life measures for patient and caregiver, medication adherence, and satisfaction with eye drops.[47–53] Remote implementation of questionnaires has been described in a bespoke web-based diary tool, wherein patients periodically complete a basic questionnaire and document their symptoms and the effect of their condition on their lives, allowing them to self-monitor their illness over time.[54] Whilst there is any abundance of ophthalmic questionnaires evaluating PCOMs, there is a lack of evidence of their remote usage in comparison to other chronic conditions, such as in cancer (Kræftværket app), frailty (FrailSurvey app), and arthritis, wherein questionnaires have been implemented in smartphone applications with push notifications.[55–57] Incorporating simple questionnaires evaluating ophthalmic PROMs in user-friendly smartphone applications may therefore be effective for self-monitoring purposes and empower patients in the clinical decision-making process. Ideally, such questionnaires could be specifically tailored to the degree of impairment for a given individual, and the domains which are most affected, using computerized adaptive testing (CAT) algorithms.[47]

Recent technological advances have seen a growth in VR headsets that allow users to experience and interact with artificially replicated dynamic three-dimensional environments, which can potentially be useful for functional visual assessment. For instance, the Virtual Reality-Glaucoma Visual Function Test (VR-GVFT) has been developed to assess visual function limitation in glaucoma using VR.[58] More novel portable brain–computer interfaces (e.g., nGoggle) can evaluate electrical brain responses (measured by wireless electroencephalography) associated with visual field stimulation and thus provide an objective assessment of visual field loss whilst the patient engages in the VR environment. In a research setting, nGoggle was able to reproducibly distinguish between healthy eyes and those with glaucomatous neuropathy.[59] Moreover, this device represents an advancement on the VR perimetry programs described earlier that required the subjective aspect of clicking to indicate when a visual stimulus is seen, since nGoggle can detect the response without direct patient input. By simulating real-world tasks, VR provides a novel method of safely investigating and reflecting the difficulties with day-to-day tasks experienced by each patient. These enhancements may facilitate more reliable and rapid monitoring of visual function without restriction to a healthcare setting.

2.3 CONCLUSION

Novel advancements in ophthalmology have enhanced our opportunities to collect clinical and/or research data relevant to ocular disease outside the clinical environment. These include technologies such as smartphone or tablet applications, internet-based tests, wearable devices, implanted biosensors, and even more specialist instruments commercialized and simplified for remote patient usage. For patients, these technologies facilitate access to care, which is particularly helpful in contexts where their mobility is restricted (e.g., disability or pandemic settings) or their native environments are remote. They also enable patients to actively assess and monitor their disease and wellbeing and evaluate their healthcare priorities and thereby empower them in clinical decision-making. Additionally, through these means, ophthalmologists and researchers are able to follow relevant physiological, functional, metabolic, behavioral, and patient-centered outcome parameters more closely and over a more prolonged period. This extends the possibilities for patient care and vision research, permitting optimal treatment regimens to be devised and adherence to them reinforced. Together, the foundation for remote technologies in ophthalmology is established, and the scope of its future potential remains to be further explored.

REFERENCES

1. Weinreb, R. N., Aung, T. & Medeiros, F. A. The pathophysiology and treatment of glaucoma: A review. *JAMA* **311**, 1901–1911 (2014).

2. Hughes, E., Spry, P., & Diamond, J. 24-hour monitoring of intraocular pressure in glaucoma management: A retrospective review. *J Glaucoma* 12, 232–236 (2003).

3. Cvenkel, B. A.-O. & Atanasovska Velkovska, M. Self-monitoring of intraocular pressure using Icare HOME tonometry in clinical practice. *Clin Ophthalmol* 13, 841–847 (2019).

4. Dunbar, G. E., Shen, B. Y. & Aref, A. A. The Sensimed Triggerfish contact lens sensor: Efficacy, safety, and patient perspectives. *Clin Ophthalmol* 11, 875–882 (2017).

5. Ittoop, S. M., SooHoo, J. R., Seibold, L. K., Mansouri, K. & Kahook, M. Y. Systematic review of current devices for 24-h intraocular pressure monitoring. *Adv Ther* 33, 1679–1690 (2016).

6. Lee, J. O. *et al.* A microscale optical implant for continuous in vivo monitoring of intraocular pressure. *Microsyst Nanoeng* 3, 17057–17057 (2017).

7. West, S. K. *et al.* How does visual impairment affect performance on tasks of everyday life? The SEE project. Salisbury Eye Evaluation. *Arch Ophthalmol* 120, 774–780 (2002).

8. Bastawrous, A. *et al.* Development and validation of a smartphone-based visual acuity test (PEEK acuity) for clinical practice and community-based fieldwork. *JAMA Ophthalmol* 133, 930–937 (2015).

9. Phung, L., Gregori, N. Z., Ortiz, A., Shi, W. & Schiffman, J. C. Reproducibility and comparison of visual acuity obtained with Sightbook mobile application to near card and Snellen chart. *Retina (Philadelphia, Pa.)* 36, 1009–1020 (2016).

10. Yeung, W. K. *et al.* eHealth tools for the self-testing of visual acuity: A scoping review. *npj Digit Med* 2, 1–7 (2019).

11. Ciuffreda, K. J. & Rosenfield, M. Evaluation of the SVOne: A handheld, smartphone-based autorefractor. *Optom Vis Sci* 92, 1133–1139 (2015).

12. Yohannan, J. *et al.* Evidence-based criteria for assessment of visual field reliability. *Ophthalmology* 124, 1612–1620 (2017).

13. Tsapakis, S. *et al.* Visual field examination method using virtual reality glasses compared with the Humphrey perimeter. *Clin Ophthalmol* 11, 1431–1443 (2017).

14. Loewenstein, A. Use of home device for early detection of neovascular age-related macular degeneration. *Ophthalmic Res.* 48 Suppl 1, 11–15 (2012).

15. Chew, E. Y. *et al.* Randomized trial of a home monitoring system for early detection of choroidal neovascularization Home Monitoring of the Eye (HOME) study. *Ophthalmology* 121, 535–544 (2014).

16. Lord, S. R. & Dayhew, J. Visual risk factors for falls in older people. *J Am Geriatr Soc* 49, 508–515 (2001).

17. Roh, M., Selivanova, A., Shin, H. J., Miller, J. W. & Jackson, M. L. Visual acuity and contrast sensitivity are two important factors affecting vision-related quality of life in advanced age-related macular degeneration. *PLoS ONE* 13, e0196481 (2018).

18. Richman, J. *et al.* The Spaeth/Richman contrast sensitivity test (SPARCS): Design, reproducibility and ability to identify patients with glaucoma. *Br J Ophthalmol* 99, 16–20 (2015).

19. Thakur, S., Ichhpujani, P., Kumar, S., Kaur, R. & Sood, S. Assessment of contrast sensitivity by Spaeth Richman contrast sensitivity test and Pelli Robson chart test in patients with varying severity of glaucoma. *Eye (Lond)* 32, 1392–1400 (2018).

20. Kollbaum, P. S., Jansen, M. E., Kollbaum, E. J., Bullimore, M. A. Validation of an iPad test of letter contrast sensitivity. *Optom Vis Sci.* 91, 291–296 (2014).

21. Dorr, M., Lesmes, L. A., Lu, Z.-L. & Bex, P. J. Rapid and reliable assessment of the contrast sensitivity function on an iPad. *Invest Ophthalmol Vis Sci* 54, 7266–7273 (2013).

22. Kwon, M. *et al.* Assessing binocular interaction in amblyopia and its clinical feasibility. *PLoS One* 9, e100156–e100156 (2014).

23. Kalia, A. *et al.* Development of pattern vision following early and extended blindness. *Proc Natl Acad Sci USA* 111, 2035–2039 (2014).

24. Nathan, D. M. & DCCT/EDIC Research Group. The Diabetes Control and Complications Trial/Epidemiology of Diabetes Interventions and Complications study at 30 years: Overview. *Diabetes Care* 37, 9–16 (2014).

25. Lu, J. *et al.* Association of time in range, as assessed by continuous glucose monitoring, with diabetic retinopathy in type 2 diabetes. *Diabetes Care* 41, 2370–2376 (2018).

26. Christiansen, M. P. *et al.* A prospective multicenter evaluation of the accuracy and safety of an implanted continuous glucose sensor: The PRECISION study. *Diabetes Technol Ther* 21, 231–237 (2019).

27. Nazari Khanamiri, H., Nakatsuka, A. & El-Annan, J. Smartphone fundus photography. *J Vis Exp* (2017) doi:10.3791/55958.

28. Shanmugam, M. P., Mishra, D. K. C., Rajesh, R. & Madhukumar, R. Unconventional techniques of fundus imaging: A review. *Indian J Ophthalmol* 63, 582–585 (2015).

29. Nagra, M. & Huntjens, B. Smartphone ophthalmoscopy: Patient and student practitioner perceptions. *J Med Syst* 44, 10 (2019).

30. T Stryjewski, S. M. The retina selfie: A techniques video demonstrating smartphone ophthalmoscopy. *Digit J Ophthalmol* (2016).

31. Rajalakshmi, R., Subashini, R., Anjana, R. M. & Mohan, V. Automated diabetic retinopathy detection in smartphone-based fundus photography using artificial intelligence. *Eye* 32, 1138–1144 (2018).

32. Kasneci, E., Black, A. & Wood, J. Eye-tracking as a tool to evaluate functional ability in everyday tasks in glaucoma. *J Ophthalmol* 2017 (2017).

33. Ramulu, P. Y. *et al.* Glaucomatous visual field loss associated with less travel from home. *Optom Vis Sci* 91, 187–193 (2014).

34. Lee, M. J. *et al.* Greater physical activity is associated with slower visual field loss in glaucoma. *Ophthalmology* 126, 958–964 (2019).

35. Willis, J. R., Jefferys, J. L., Vitale, S. & Ramulu, P. Y. Visual impairment, uncorrected refractive error, and accelerometer-defined physical activity in the United States. *Arch Ophthalmol* 130, 329–335 (2012).

36. Center for Technology and Aging. *mHealth Technologies: Applications to Benefit Older Adults.* (2011).

37. Ramulu, P. Y., Mihailovic, A., West, S. K., Gitlin, L. N. & Friedman, D. S. Predictors of falls per step and falls

per year at and away from home in glaucoma. *Am J Ophthalmol* **200**, 169–178 (2019).

38. Okeke, C. O. *et al.* Adherence with topical glaucoma medication monitored electronically the Travatan Dosing Aid study. *Ophthalmology* 116, 191–199 (2009).

39. Ahmed, I. *et al.* Medication adherence apps: Review and content analysis. *JMIR Mhealth Uhealth* **6**, e62–e62 (2018).

40. Gatwood, J. D., Johnson, J. & Jerkins, B. Comparisons of self-reported glaucoma medication adherence with a new wireless device: A pilot study. *J. Glaucoma* **26**, 1056–1061 (2017).

41. Kinast, R. M. & Mansberger, S. L. Glaucoma adherence – from Theriac to the future. *Am J Ophthalmol* **191**, xiii–xv (2018).

42. Boland, M. V. *et al.* Automated telecommunication-based reminders and adherence with once-daily glaucoma medication dosing: The Automated Dosing Reminder Study. *JAMA Ophthalmol* **132**, 845–850 (2014).

43. Anglada-Martinez, H. *et al.* Does mHealth increase adherence to medication? Results of a systematic review. *Int J Clin Pract* **69**, 9–32 (2015).

44. Weih, L. M., Hassell, J. B. & Keeffe, J. Assessment of the impact of vision impairment. *Invest Ophthalmol Vis Sci* **43**, 927–935 (2002).

45. Lamoureux, E. L., Pallant, J. F., Pesudovs, K., Hassell, J. B. & Keeffe, J. E. The impact of vision impairment questionnaire: An evaluation of its measurement properties using Rasch analysis. *Invest Ophthalmol Vis Sci* **47**, 4732–4741 (2006).

46. Lamoureux, E. L. *et al.* The impact of vision impairment questionnaire: An assessment of its domain structure using confirmatory factor analysis and Rasch analysis. *Invest Ophthalmol Vis Sci* **48**, 1001–1006 (2007).

47. Fenwick, E. K., Man, R. E., Aung, T., Ramulu, P. & Lamoureux, E. L. Beyond intraocular pressure: Optimizing patient-reported outcomes in glaucoma. *Prog Retin Eye Res* 100801 (2019) doi:10.1016/j.preteyeres.2019.100801.

48. Barber, B. L., Strahlman, E. R., Laibovitz, R., Guess, H. A. & Reines, S. A. Validation of a questionnaire for comparing the tolerability of ophthalmic medications. *Ophthalmology* **104**, 334–342 (1997).

49. Mansberger, S. L. *et al.* Psychometrics of a new questionnaire to assess glaucoma adherence: The Glaucoma Treatment Compliance Assessment Tool (an American Ophthalmological Society thesis). *Trans Am Ophthalmol Soc* **111**, 1–16 (2013).

50. Gothwal, V. K., Bharani, S. & Mandal, A. K. Quality of life of caregivers of children with congenital glaucoma: Development and validation of a novel questionnaire (CarCGQoL). *Invest Ophthalmol Vis Sci* **56**, 770–777 (2015).

51. Khadka, J. *et al.* Identifying content for the glaucoma-specific item bank to measure quality-of-life parameters. *J Glaucoma* **24**, 12–19 (2015).

52. Prior, M. *et al.* Theoretical and empirical dimensions of the Aberdeen Glaucoma Questionnaire: A cross sectional survey and principal component analysis. *BMC Ophthalmol* **13**, 72 (2013).

53. Béchetoille, A. *et al.* Measurement of health-related quality of life with glaucoma: Validation of the Glau-QoL 36-item questionnaire. *Acta Ophthalmol* **86**, 71–80 (2008).

54. McDonald, L., Glen, F. C., Taylor, D. J. & Crabb, D. A.-O. Self-monitoring symptoms in glaucoma: A feasibility study of a web-based diary tool. *J Ophthalmol* 2017, 8452840 (2017).

55. Braithwaite, T., Calvert, M., Gray, A., Pesudovs, K. & Denniston, A. K. The use of patient-reported outcome research in modern ophthalmology: Impact on clinical trials and routine clinical practice. *Patient Relat Outcome Meas* **10**, 9–24 (2019).

56. Elsbernd, A. *et al.* Cocreated smartphone app to improve the quality of life of adolescents and young adults with cancer (Kraeftvaerket): Protocol for a quantitative and qualitative evaluation. *JMIR Res Protocols* **7**, e10098 (2018).

57. Nishiguchi, S. *et al.* Self-assessment tool of disease activity of rheumatoid arthritis by using a smartphone application. *Telemed J e-Health*: **20**, 235–40 (2014).

58. Goh, R. L. Z. *et al.* Objective assessment of activity limitation in glaucoma with smartphone virtual reality goggles: A pilot study. *Translat Vis Sci Technol* **7**, 10–10 (2018).

59. Nakanishi, M. *et al.* Detecting glaucoma with a portable brain–computer interface for objective assessment of visual function loss. *JAMA Ophthalmol* **135**, 550–557 (2017).

3 Telemedicine in Ophthalmology

Jane Scheetz, Samantha Simkin, Zachary Tan, Shuan Dai, and Mingguang He

3.1 TELEMEDICINE

The literal meaning of *telemedicine* is 'healing at distance'. The advancement of information and communication technologies (ICTs) led to the creation of the term in the 1970s (1). Part of the difficulty in achieving equitable access to health care can be attributed to the need for clinicians and patients to be present in the same location at the same time. Telemedicine has enormous potential to address these barriers faced by both developed and developing countries that find it difficult to provide high-quality health care services that are accessible and cost-effective. The use of ICTs enables health care providers to overcome barriers relating to geography and is therefore able to increase access to essential medical services. The benefits of telemedicine are felt most in rural and underserved areas that traditionally suffer from poorer access to health care.

Telemedicine's overall goal is to improve health outcomes by providing clinical support using various types of ICTs, and to overcome barriers associated with geography to connect clinicians and patients who are in different locations. Services can range from diagnosis, treatment, prevention, education, and even research (2). Telemedicine has successfully been applied to many medical specialties that are highly image-driven, such as oncology, dermatology, radiology, and ophthalmology (3).

3.1.1 Teleophthalmology

An increase in overall life expectancy has amplified the need for eye care services and placed immense pressure on health care systems to provide equitable care in rural and remote settings (4). In the absence of appropriate interventions, the number of people who are blind is set to reach 76 million by 2020. The delivery of teleophthalmology services is considered an appropriate and cost-effective solution to provide eye care to everyone, no matter where they are located.

Teleophthalmology is a division of telemedicine that enables eye care to be delivered by using telecommunications technology and digital medical equipment. Over the last two decades, teleophthalmology has progressed from being a research concept to a fully functioning model of service delivery. As a speciality, ophthalmology has been a leader in telemedicine research and service delivery as imaging plays a significant role in the diagnosis of many ocular conditions.

Prior to the development of telemedicine, ophthalmology services were unavailable in many parts of the world. A future shortage in practicing clinicians is predicted, with the number of ophthalmologists increasing at half the rate of the global population over 60 years of age (5). Further to this, current statistics show there are 23 countries with less than one ophthalmologist per million people (5). With an aging global population, the incidence of eye disease is certain to rise along with the demand for eye care professionals. Many ophthalmic conditions require timely assessment and treatment, placing a significant burden on eye care providers. Innovative methods of delivering ophthalmology services will be critical to the provision of eye care in the future.

3.1.2 Teleophthalmology Scope and Delivery

The scope of teleophthalmology is broad and includes enabling access to specialist eye services for those who live in rural and remote settings; the screening, diagnosis, and management of ocular conditions; collaboration of research activities; and remote continuing education. Information obtained from teleophthalmology consultations can be transmitted in a variety of forms, such as text, audio, video, or still images.

Teleophthalmology can be delivered in two different ways and is categorized according to the time information is collected and delivered, and how personnel are required to interact. Interactions can be between two health professionals or between health professionals and patients (6).

The store-and-forward method is when patient data are exchanged between two or more individuals at different times. This is sometimes called the asynchronous method. For example, a patient's retinal images are transmitted to an ophthalmologist who later sends them back with a grading outcome for diabetic retinopathy (DR) and referral recommendations. In contrast, real-time, or synchronous teleophthalmology, requires involved personnel to be present concurrently. This form of telemedicine is historically performed in real time using video or teleconferencing technology and aims to mimic a traditional clinician–patient consultation. The use of real-time ophthalmology encourages discussion of ocular history and further exploration of examination findings between the patient, referrer, and attending clinician. Real-time teleophthalmology focuses on diagnosis,

DOI: 10.1201/9781315146737-4

management, and therapeutic intervention whereas store-and-forward is largely restricted to disease screening. The combination of store-and-forward and real-time teleophthalmology is referred to as the hybrid method. Lions Outback Vision has successfully implemented a hybrid teleophthalmology service in rural Western Australia (WA) (7, 8). The program is described below.

3.1.2.1 Hybrid Teleophthalmology: Lions Outback Vision in Rural Western Australia

Lions Outback Vision provides outreach ophthalmology care to people living in rural and remote regions of WA. The state of WA is vast, covering 2.646 million square kilometers (km). The closest community engaged in the program is 416 km and the furthest is 3,215 km away from the capital city of Perth.

A typical teleophthalmology consultation involves an optometrist, general practitioner (GP), or aboriginal health worker taking a patient's history and performing appropriate imaging based on symptoms and prior ocular history (Figure 3.1). The information is sent via a referral system to an ophthalmologist

situated in Perth. The treating ophthalmologist then participates in a real-time consultation with the health care provider and patient. This can happen either immediately or at another designated time.

A 12-month audit of the program revealed that a total of 709 patients were referred for teleconsultations and 683 were conducted (26 patients did not attend their real-time teleconsultation) (8). The most common diagnoses were cataract ($n = 287$), glaucoma ($n = 77$), age-related macular degeneration ($n = 30$), and DR ($n = 26$). Almost 50% of referrals had at least one of the following investigations performed: optical coherence tomography (OCT), fundus photography, visual fields, and slit-lamp photography. Because of the comprehensive nature of referrals received, only 3.4% of patients needed to be seen face to face by an ophthalmologist to determine a precise diagnosis. Recent analysis of cataract surgery interventions found that when optometrists performed preoperative consultations via teleophthalmology there was a statistically significant reduction in wait times (9). Those booked via teleophthalmology waited a median of 111 days

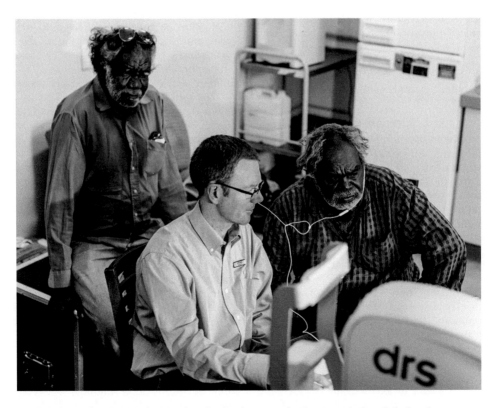

Figure 3.1 An optometrist from Lions Outback Vision facilitating a teleophthalmology consultation in the remote town of Jigalong in the Pilbara region. (Courtesy of Alan McDonald.)

compared to 201 days (9). Lions Outback Vision patient satisfaction is outstanding, with over 90% of patients indicating they were either satisfied or very satisfied with the service provided (7).

Financial incentive has been cited as a major barrier to the uptake of teleophthalmology services. The success of the program run by Lions Outback Vision led to the introduction of a Medicare Benefits Schedule (MBS) item number. An MBS item number indicates a medical service that is subsidized by the Australian Government. This MBS item number allowed for a reimbursement to optometrists for referrals for real-time teleophthalmology consultations. The introduction of the service is a testament to the valuable health service that Lions Outback Vision is providing to Australians living in rural and remote locations where ophthalmology services are not readily available.

3.1.3 Teleophthalmology Challenges

Teleophthalmology is underutilized across the globe despite its huge potential to improve delivery of eye care services to rural, remote, and urban populations. This can be caused by challenges facing the service provider, clinician, and patient. These may include:

- Building telecommunication infrastructure
- Initial costs for equipment
- Reimbursement for services
- Continual operational costs

- Recruitment of staff and training
- Legal liability
- Privacy and security

Although there are many benefits to performing teleophthalmology, there are medical, psychosocial, and economic factors that can act as barriers to the implementation and uptake of teleophthalmology services. These can include patient age, educational status, patient awareness, accessibility to services, the need for dilation, as well as time constraints for both patients and clinicians, including the burden and complexity of tasks required to be performed by a primary care physician (10–12). Understanding the barriers and facilitators of both patients and clinicians is important to the continued success of any teleophthalmology program. Table 3.1 highlights the barriers and facilitators to teleophthalmology in diabetic eye screening.

To ensure the success of teleophthalmology services it is imperative that program objectives are clearly identified, and careful planning is performed. This includes identifying technology and staff requirements, protocols and guidelines for service delivery, and validation of the service to align with the goals of the program. Successful and longstanding teleophthalmology programs across the world are often the product of meticulous planning, comprehensive management, sustainable funding, and staff who are well trained, engaged, and committed to providing exceptional health care.

Table 3.1 Barriers and facilitators to teleophthalmology use for diabetic eye screening

Patients	Barriers	■ Lack of familiarity with teleophthalmology ■ Misconceptions about eye screening ■ Time, transport, out-of-pocket costs ■ Anxiety about receiving a negative diagnosis
	Facilitators	■ Receiving a recommendation from a primary care provider ■ Convenience of teleophthalmology ■ Belief that eye screening is important for preventing vision loss ■ Teleophthalmology considered to be high-quality
Clinicians	Barriers	■ Difficulty determining which patients need to be screened ■ Lack of familiarity with teleophthalmology ■ Lack of time (competing clinical tasks) ■ Concerns about conflicts with local eye specialists
	Facilitators	■ Ease of referral process and results communication ■ Patient benefits ■ Improved patient adherence to screening guidelines ■ Organizational benefits

Source: Adapted from Liu Y, Zupan NJ, Swearingen R, et al. Identification of barriers, facilitators and system-based implementation strategies to increase teleophthalmology use for diabetic eye screening in a rural US primary care clinic: A qualitative study. *BMJ Open* 2019;9(2):e022594.

Along with the growing divide between the number of individuals suffering from ophthalmic disease and the number of ophthalmologists practicing, there is also an increased rate of prematurity, particularly in the United States. This is of concern as only 54% of eligible retinal or pediatric specialists are willing to manage conditions like retinopathy of prematurity (ROP) (13). Regarding screening for DR, up to 50% of those with diabetes do not adhere to recommended screening intervals (14). Recent literature reviews of teleophthalmology programs identify DR and ROP as the most common single disease-screening programs currently being delivered (4, 15, 16). Therefore, this chapter will focus on the implementation of teleophthalmology screening of DR and ROP.

3.2 DIABETIC RETINOPATHY BACKGROUND

Diabetes mellitus (DM) is one of the world's most rapidly growing chronic diseases, with the number of people diagnosed set to reach approximately 366 million by 2030 (17). DR is the most common complication of type 1 and type 2 DM and remains a leading cause of vision loss in working-aged adults (18). It is categorized as a microvascular disease and can be divided into two stages: non-proliferative DR (NPDR) and proliferative DR (PDR). Signs such as microaneurysms, hemorrhages, and hard exudates are commonly seen in those with NPDR, an earlier stage of the disease. At this time, many patients remain undiagnosed as they are asymptomatic. The more advanced stages, including PDR, can result in severe vision loss. This is due to the growth of new retinal vessels (neovascularization). These new and abnormal vessels are more susceptible to breakage which in turn can lead to vitreous hemorrhage or scarring and tractional retinal detachment. However, the most common cause of vision loss is due to diabetic macular edema (DME), and this can occur during any stage of DR. This is caused by increased permeability of the inner blood–retina barrier and decreased outflow of fluid across the retinal pigment epithelium (19). This process leads to a build-up of intraretinal fluid which causes swelling at the macula and reduced central vision (19). The global prevalence of any DR is estimated to be 34.6%, and 7% of this is considered vision-threatening DR (VTDR), which encompasses severe NPDR, PDR, and DME (18). The medical, social, and economic complications of DR are significant. Over 40 years of clinical evidence have proven that treatment for DR such as pan-retinal photocoagulation (PRP) is able to reduce the risk of severe visual loss by >50% in eyes with high-risk characteristics.

3.2.1 Justification for Implementation

The World Health Organization (WHO) recommends that the following should be considered before medical screening is implemented: (1) the disease in question is an important health problem with a recognizable symptomatic state; (2) the screening procedure in question is appropriate and acceptable to the public and health care professionals; (3) treatment is safe, effective, and universally accepted; and (4) the economic cost of early diagnosis is taken into consideration (20). Based on this, DM and its ocular complications provide an ideal model for teleophthalmology programs. This is because DR is a leading cause of vision loss and blindness in the community, it is classified based on distinct retinal lesions, individuals are impacted on a personal and economic level, and it can be treated if detected early enough. Teleophthalmology has the potential to deliver eye care to those with minimal access to ophthalmology services as well as facilitate the recruitment of clinical trial participants, create a link to clinical trial data, and offer continuing education to eye care professionals, patients, and community organizations.

Despite growing evidence of the effectiveness of routine assessment and early intervention, compliance with DR examination guidelines is suboptimal, with reports suggesting that less than 50% of diabetics have routine eye checks (14, 21). Screening using teleophthalmology offers great potential to improve access and quality of care to those with diabetes; however, programs should be planned and deployed in a safe and effective way. There must be guidelines and protocols in place to determine whether standards of care are being met. Whilst the assessment of high-quality retinal photographs by trained professionals is effective in identifying most clinically significant DR, a validated teleophthalmology DR screening is not a substitute for a comprehensive dilated fundus examination by an ophthalmologist or experienced optometrist.

3.2.2 Examination Frequency and Referral Recommendations

The guidelines presented here are taken from the *Guidelines for the Management of Diabetic Retinopathy* and *Patient Screening and Referral Pathway Guidelines for Diabetic Retinopathy*, published by the National Health and Medical Research Council in Australia (22) and the Royal Australian and New Zealand College of Ophthalmologists (23), respectively. These guidelines are designed to help health care practitioners make appropriate decisions about the care of patients with diabetes. Only those guidelines relevant to teleophthalmology screening for DR are presented.

The following guidelines should be followed when a patient initially presents for teleophthalmology screening:

1. All patients with diabetes should undergo screening for DR at the time of diagnosis of diabetes and then every 2 years if no retinopathy is present, provided that no other risk factors for DR or its progression are present.

2. Screen children with type 1 DM for DR when they reach puberty.

3. Pregnant women with a history of diabetes should be screened within the first trimester. Those who develop gestational diabetes do not require screening during pregnancy.

The level of DR identified during screening will dictate the timeline for follow-up and/or referral to an ophthalmologist. These guidelines are described in Table 3.2.

3.2.3 Screening Modalities for Detecting DR

Currently, the International Council of Ophthalmology (ICO) guidelines for DR screening advise that retinal examination be performed in one of two ways:

1. Direct or indirect ophthalmoscopy or slit-lamp biomicroscopy.

2. Mydriatic or non-mydriatic fundus imaging with $\geq 30°$ monoscopic or stereoscopic photography, with or without OCT.

There are many variables that will dictate which testing modality is used. These may include the number of available trained health care workers such as ophthalmologists, optometrists, endocrinologists, or GPs, geography, equipment, and the resources required to utilize these modalities. The gold standard in retinal examination and diagnosis is the use of binocular indirect ophthalmoscopy (BIO) by an ophthalmologist or seven field stereoscopic fundus images of each eye that are interpreted by highly experienced graders. In the case of teleophthalmology screening, one of the major aims is to overcome barriers associated with lack of access to clinicians, therefore, utilizing ophthalmologists in screening is unlikely to occur. Fundus imaging has the advantage of creating a permanent record, and for this reason, it is the preferred method for teleophthalmology DR assessment. However, the gold-standard Early Treatment Diabetic Retinopathy Study (ETDRS) seven 30° field stereoscopic slides are not time- or cost-effective for teleophthalmology purposes. Table 3.3 describes available instruments for DR assessment and their corresponding advantages and disadvantages (24).

Table 3.2 Guidelines for reviewing and referring diabetic patients post-screening

DR level	Referral
No DR	Repeat screening is recommended *bi-annually* In indigenous Australians or those of non-English speaking backgrounds, those with longer duration of diabetes, or patients with poor glycemic, hypertension, or blood lipid control, or with renal disease, *annual examinations* are recommended
Mild NPDR	Repeat screening in 12 months
Moderate NPDR	Referral to ophthalmologist within 12 weeks
Severe NPDR	Referral to ophthalmologist within 4 weeks
PDR	Refer to ophthalmologist within 1 week
Sudden severe visual loss (unexplained)	Refer to ophthalmologist on the same day
Non-center-involving DME	Referral to ophthalmologist within 12 weeks
Center-involving DME	Referral to ophthalmologist within 4 weeks

Abbreviations: DR, diabetic retinopathy; NPDR, non-proliferative DR; PDR, proliferative DR; DME, diabetic macular edema.
Source: Adapted from Mitchell P, Foran S. *Guidelines for the Management of Diabetic Retinopathy.* National Health and Medical Research Council; 2008.

Table 3.3 Assessment instruments and their advantages and disadvantages

Technique	Recommended setting	Advantages/disadvantages
Slit-lamp biomicroscopy	Core for management	Advantages ■ Large field Disadvantages ■ Requires pupil dilation ■ Immobile ■ Requires special lenses ■ No ability to retrospectively audit
Non-mydriatic retinal photography	Optional for screening and management	Advantages ■ Large field ■ Can be used by non-medically trained staff ■ No pupil dilation required in 80–90% of cases ■ Some are portable – can be transported to the community in mobile units ■ Can be linked to computers and images can be stored for the long term ■ Allows objective comparison of the same person, or between different groups of people, examined at different times or by different professionals ■ Can be used as a patient education tool, giving immediacy and personal relevance ■ Readily recalled for evaluation of screener performance and audit of grading Disadvantages ■ Relatively expensive ■ A dark space is required for maximum pupil dilation
Non-mydriatic retinal photography used with mydriasis	Optional for screening and management	Advantages ■ As above except pupils are dilated for better-quality photographs Disadvantages ■ As above ■ Requires pupil dilation
Mydriatic retinal photography (conventional fundus camera)	Optional for screening and management	Advantage ■ Large field Disadvantages ■ Requires pupil dilation ■ Expensive ■ Bright flash constricts the pupil for a long time
Fluorescein angiography	Not recommended for screening and optional for management	Advantage ■ Only method of assessing capillary circulation Disadvantages ■ Invasive and needs general health status assessment ■ Expensive ■ Dilatation needed. Cannot be used by non-medically trained staff
Optical coherence tomography (OCT)	Optional for screening and management	Advantages ■ One of the best ways to assess macular edema (retinal thickening and intraretinal edema) Disadvantages ■ Expensive ■ Dilatation needed ■ Cannot be used by non-medically trained staff

Source: Adapted from the International Council of Ophthalmology. ICO guidelines for diabetic eye care: available in English, Chinese, French, Portuguese, Serbian, Spanish, and Vietnamese. www.icoph.org/resources/309/ICO-Guidelines-for-Diabetic-Eye-Care-availablein-English-Chinese-French-Portuguese-Serbian-Spanish-andVietnamese.html.

3.2.4 DR Screening Personnel

The mode of delivery (store-and-forward or real-time) will determine the personnel that are required. As a minimum, personnel are required for retinal image acquisition, review and evaluation of images, supervision of results, patient care, and data storage.

3.2.4.1 Imager

Personnel at all levels can usually be trained to perform retinal imaging. This can include anyone from reception staff to nurses and doctors. New automated retinal cameras such as the Digital Retinography System (DRS) (Figure 3.2) are making it easier for untrained personnel to perform these tasks. The DRS is non-mydriatic, takes approximately 30 seconds to capture an image, and is approved for use in diabetic eye-screening programs. It typically takes less than 1 day of training for a nurse with no background in eye health care to become confident with set-up, acquisition, and storage of retinal images using the DRS camera.

3.2.4.2 Image Grader

To perform image-grading responsibilities, the individual must be specially trained in how to interpret retinal images for disease. Most commonly, ophthalmologists or optometrists are used in diabetic teleophthalmology programs; however, non-medical staff can also be trained to undertake this role. The quality and consistency of image grading are essential to the effectiveness of a teleophthalmology program. The UK National Health Service (NHS) DR screening program requires a minimum qualification to be qualified as an image grader (25). This includes undertaking a level 3 qualification

in DR screening and providing evidence of ongoing professional development such as monthly quality assurance tests that include grading a set of 20 random retinal images (25). Other retinal grading certification programs are available through the University of Wisconsin Fundus Photograph Reading Center and the Retinal Reading Program at the University of California. Various fundus photograph reading centers exist across the globe and have the capacity to grade not only for DR but other sight-threatening disease such as glaucoma and macular degeneration. For those cases that are not clear-cut, an adjudicating grader should be consulted. In many cases, this will be a highly specialized grader such as an ophthalmologist who specializes in retinal disease.

3.2.5 Validation of DR Teleophthalmology Programs

Compared to other ocular diseases that are screened using teleophthalmology, DR is far more developed in terms of program validation. Decades-worth of literature has provided a strong evidence base for diagnosing and treating DR, and teleophthalmology programs should follow these clinical standards when it comes to program performance and grading of DR. The American Telemedicine Association (ATA) recommends using the ETDRS 30°, stereo seven standard fields, color, 35-mm slides as the gold standard to compare against (26). However, it is recognized that alternatives other than the ETDRS are often used for grading DR. The program protocol should explicitly state the standards used for validation and datasets used for comparison. The ATA practice guidelines for DR have developed four categories for program

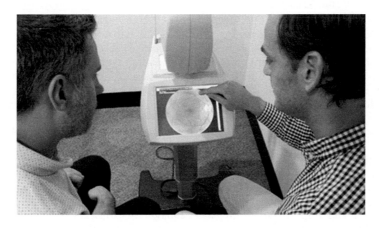

Figure 3.2 Personnel can be trained to use the non-mydriatic automated Digital Retinography System (DRS) camera after only one training session. Here, an examiner is showing a patient an image of the back of his eye using a DRS camera.

Table 3.4 Levels of validation for diabetic retinopathy teleophthalmology programs

	American Telemedicine Association clinical validation categories			
	Category 1	Category 2	Category 3	Category 4
Disease characterization	(a) No or minimal DR (b) Worse than minimal DR	(a) Any level of DME (b) Severe or worse NPDR, or PDR	(a) Mild, moderate, or severe NPDR (b) Early or high-risk PDR (c) DME (d) Comparable to clinical examination by dilated fundoscopy	Exceeds ability of ETDRS photos to determine all levels of DR and DME
Clinical value	Screening only	Screening and risk stratification	Screening, risk stratification, and treatment recommendations	Replaces ETDRS photos in clinical and research settings
Current validated DR programs	OPHDIAT (France) EyePacs (USA) Digiscope (USA)	EyeCheck (Netherlands) NHS Diabetic Eye Screening Program (UK)	Joslin Vision Network (USA) SiDRP (Singapore) University of Alberta (Canada)	None

Abbreviations: DR, diabetic retinopathy; DME, diabetic macular edema; NPDR, non-proliferative DR; PDR, proliferative DR; ETDRS, Early Treatment Diabetic Retinopathy Study.

Source: Adapted from Li HK, Horton M, Bursell S-E, et al. Telehealth practice recommendations for diabetic retinopathy. *Telemedicine and e-health* 2011;17(10):814–837.

validation using ETDRS as the gold standard. These four categories, their disease characterization, clinical value, and examples of well-known teleophthalmology DR screening programs are presented in Table 3.4. The Joslin Vision Network (JVN) is an example of a category 3 validated teleophthalmology program and is described below.

3.2.5.1 The Joslin Vision Network: A Category 3 Validated Teleophthalmology Program

The JVN diabetes eye care program in the United States was developed in 2000 in collaboration with the Joslin Diabetes Center, Veterans Health Administration, and the Department of Defense. Those who have a higher risk of developing visual impairment from DR are opportunistically screened in primary care settings, endocrinology clinics, or other medical offices.

The program uses non-mydriatic, color, stereo photos. Three 45° images are taken: (1) the optic disc and macula; (2) superior temporal to the optic disc; and (3) nasal to the optic disc. In addition, an external non-stereo image is taken of the anterior eye and adnexa. Patient images, along with additional data including blood pressure and average glucose levels, are transferred electronically to a secure JVN reading and evaluation center at the Joslin Diabetes

Center in Massachusetts. Images are graded by ophthalmologists, optometrists, and trained clinical staff. Staff grading images can designate specific levels of DR and provide guidance on the appropriate treatment for patients, as well as grade for pathology other than DR.

The JVN program has been extensively validated. The initial rationale for the use of three stereo fields instead of the standard seven fields was based on a study by Moss et al. (27) This study evaluated fundus photographs of 2,410 patients and found 91% agreement between three- and seven-field imaging when comparing against eight ETDRS levels for DR diagnosis. Specific validation of JVN images showed that the program was able to achieve a sensitivity of 98% and specificity of 100% within one ETDRS level and perfect agreement for the diagnosis of DME (28, 29). A further study using the JVN program has shown that Veterans Affairs patients enrolled in teleophthalmology were more likely to attend annual screening than those in traditional screening programs (30).

When compared to clinic-based ophthalmology, the use of JVN teleophthalmology has been shown to result in improved patient outcomes and greater cost-effectiveness (31). These outcomes included improved examination efficiency, shorter examination times, lower labor costs, and reduced travel time and expenses for patients.

3.2.6 Integration into Routine Clinical Practice

Not all teleophthalmology programs are implemented successfully. There are many aspects that need to be considered, such as how will the program fit into the current workflow? And do our personnel have the motivation, skills, and knowledge to perform related tasks? Whilst barriers such as technical problems are of concern, the greatest potential risk of program failure is caused by poor organizational structure and lack of human resources (15). Organizations must consult with their current workforce to determine the most appropriate way to deliver new models of teleophthalmology care without disrupting current workflow and ensuring patients with diabetes receive eye screening when necessary. There are several strategies that have been proposed to manage how these patients are identified and screened.

1. Scheduling appointment times for patients: This approach allows for planning around staff availability, especially if screening occurs on a particular day and time. However, asking patients to return for DR screening is likely to lead to higher non-attendance rates.

2. Integrating screening directly into current clinic flow: For this strategy to be successful there are situations that need to be considered. For example, how will patients who need screening be identified? How will clinicians refer for screening? And will new diabetics automatically be sent for screening?

3. Mass screening: There is opportunity to conduct screening at diabetes education events, seminars, or other community events. As this is outside of a medical setting, all patients should be screened for DR as self-reported compliance with eye screening or previous diagnoses can often be inconsistent.

3.2.7 Limitations

Efforts are being made by policy makers, researchers, and administrators to deliver telemedicine programs across the globe. Limitations associated with internet connectivity and storage space have been overcome in developed nations; however, developing nations are still lacking in these areas and this has led to slower uptake and acceptance of the technology. While there are many successful examples of telemedicine, there are just as many failures which can be attributed to many reasons. For example, there are large initial start-up costs to deploy ICTs, developing protocols, validating programs, expert image grading, and the outlay for equipment such as a retinal camera can cost upwards of US$10,000. Furthermore, there need to be champions such as nurses, photographers, technical personnel, and physicians who are passionate and dedicated to delivering the programs.

Many DR teleophthalmology programs utilize standard two-dimensional retinal photographs, and this has been shown to be accurate in comparison to ETDRS seven-field photography (27). However, without OCT the ability to accurately diagnose macular edema and vascular lesions in hemorrhagic forms of DR is dramatically reduced (32).

3.2.8 Future Directions

In the last decade artificial intelligence (AI) has come to the forefront of science, especially in highly image-driven specialties such as ophthalmology. A significant number of groups across the world are investigating the use of machine learning and deep learning techniques to classify referrable DR and DME (33–35). These systems have shown that they are able to classify images with high sensitivity, specificity, and accuracy, which is particularly important given the high number of diabetic patients requiring ophthalmological review. The ability to provide an immediate AI grading outcome for patients is an advantage over traditional store-and-forward teleophthalmology techniques given that it can be difficult to follow up certain cohorts of patients following initial screening. Whilst there are many algorithms in development, very few have been tested in real-world settings where inexperienced examiners are acquiring fundus images and providing grading outcomes. Future peer-reviewed literature in this area will provide us with a greater understanding of the clinical application of these AI technologies being used for DR screening.

3.3 RETINOPATHY OF PREMATURITY BACKGROUND

ROP is a multifactorial, vasoproliferative disorder affecting the retinas of premature infants and remains a significant cause of avoidable childhood blindness worldwide (36, 37). The incidence and severity of ROP are correlated with lower gestational age and birth weight (36). Whilst the majority of ROP is mild, up to 10% can progress to severe ROP, which can lead to retinal detachment and permanent blindness if not treated (36).

ROP was first observed in concurrence with the dramatically increased survival of premature infants in industrialized countries in the 1940s and 1950s due to exposure of infants to unmonitored supplemental oxygen; this was deemed the 'first epidemic' (38). Even with developments in oxygen monitoring, a 'second epidemic' occurred in the 1960s and 1970s with increasing survival of extremely premature and low-birth-weight infants (38). Rates of ROP are highly dependent on neonatal care and are therefore region- and country-dependent (38, 39). Low-income nations have the lowest incidence of ROP due to high infant mortality rates for premature infants (40). High-income nations report an increasing rate of ROP in extremely premature and low-birth-weight infants, as the result of increasing rates of survival of these at-risk infants (40), whilst middle-income nations, including China, India, and South American nations, are experiencing a significant increase in the incidence of ROP (40). Improved neonatal care in these countries has led to increased survival of premature infants without concomitant improvements in infrastructure for ROP detection and treatment (38). This current global increase in ROP disease burden is described as the 'third epidemic' (40). The latest estimates for global ROP incidences indicate 184,700 premature infants developed ROP of any stage (39). Of these infants over 30,000 became visually impaired or blind from ROP (39).

3.3.1 Screening for ROP

ROP is classified by the disease location and severity into four stages in accordance with the International Classification of Retinopathy of Prematurity (ICROP) guidelines (41). ICROP denotes the location (zone I–III), severity (stage 1–4), and vascular competence (presence of plus disease), characterized by retinal venous tortuosity and arterial dilatation in zone I or zone II. ROP stages and plus disease are illustrated in Figures 3.3 and 3.4. Recommendation for ROP treatment is based on the presence of type 1 ROP, which is defined as stage 3 ROP in zone I, or any stage of ROP in zone I or II with plus disease (42). Treatment of type 1 ROP is with peripheral retinal laser photocoagulation or with intravitreal injuection of anti-vascular endothelial growth factors (anti-VEGF), with early treatment of both modalities having demonstrated clear structural and functional efficacy (42, 43). However, early detection of type 1 ROP is challenging, often due to a lack of either ROP screening guidelines or an ophthalmologist able to perform ROP screening (39).

Joint American Academy of Ophthalmology (AAO) and American Academy of Pediatrics (AAP) guidelines recommend screening for all infants with a birth weight ≤1500 grams or a gestational age of ≤30 weeks (44). In Australia and New Zealand a more restrictive ROP screening guideline is followed where infants born with gestational age ≤31 weeks, or birthweight less than ≤1250 grams are screened for ROP (45). In contrast, in Karnataka, India, screening guidelines are for birth weight ≤2000 grams or ≤34 weeks' gestational age (46). This reflects the regional variation in the incidence of ROP and neonatal care. In many emerging economies the lack of region-specific ROP guidelines presents significant barriers to early ROP diagnosis (39).

3.3.2 Traditional ROP Screening

Screening examinations have traditionally been completed by an experienced specialized ophthalmologist conducting serial examinations using BIO. Screening for ROP typically has a low treatment yield of approximately 8% (42), meaning a large number of infants are screened to find the relative few requiring treatment. Screening with BIO requires extensive training, is labor-intensive, technically challenging, and can be a significant time burden. BIO examination needs pupil dilation, topical anesthetic, and an eyelid speculum to be inserted for reliable views. Invariably it requires scleral depression to adequately view the peripheral retina for ROP diagnosis and this is associated with increased blood pressure and a decrease in oxygen saturation, indicating infant stress (47). BIO examination results are then documented via hand-drawn annotations. Significant subjectivity and inconsistency have been shown, with several studies showing poor inter- and intra-expert agreement for the diagnosis of plus disease (48–50). Analog documentation and significant variability in ROP diagnosis have led to a high medico-legal risk associated with this traditional ROP screening practice (51–53).

Specialist ophthalmologists experienced in ROP screening are clustered in large centers; this has either required the ophthalmologist traveling to remote centers, or infants need to be transferred for repeated ROP screening examinations. Transfers increase the risk of infant morbidity and mortality (54), with a recent Australian analysis calculating that the average cost, per eye, per screening examination for transferred infants was A$5,110 (55). Despite increasing ROP incidence and demand for screening (56), these complex clinical, logistical, and medico-legal factors have led to a decrease in the number of clinicians who are willing to carry out ROP screening.

3.3.3 Wide-Field Digital Retinal Imaging

The advent of wide-field digital retinal imaging (WFDRI) technology for infants addressed some of the challenges experienced with traditional BIO screening. RetCam (Clarity Medical Systems, Pleasanton, CA, USA) uses a wide-angle contact

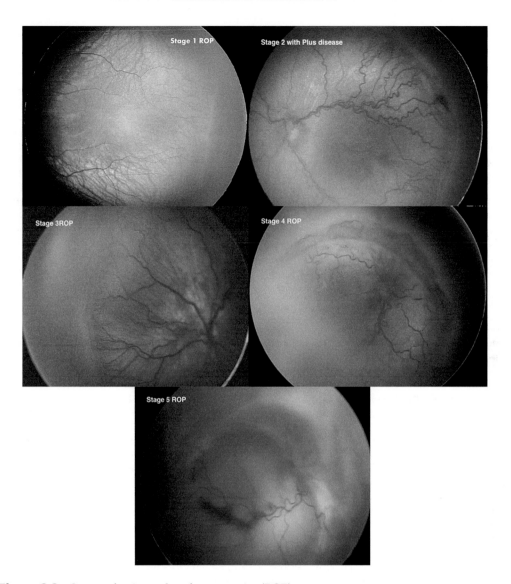

Figure 3.3 Stages of retinopathy of prematurity (ROP).

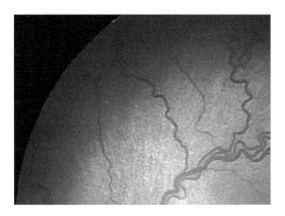

Figure 3.4 Retinal photograph displaying the presence of plus disease.

camera to capture fundal images at a standard 130° field of view. Like BIO screening, pupil dilatation, topical ocular anesthetic, and an eyelid speculum are required. A viscous gel couples the camera lens to the ocular surface while the images are captured. Appropriate close cardiac and respiratory status monitoring should be in place in the neonatal intensive care unit (NICU), although image capture via WFDRI has been shown to carry less risk of cardiorespiratory stress compared to traditional BIO screening (57). The minimum number of images captured per eye varies depending on implementation and local guidelines ranging from three – posterior pole, nasal retina, and temporal retina (45) – to six, including five images of the retina (one posterior pole, four of each peripheral aspect) and one non-contact image of the anterior segment (58, 59). The AAO and others have confirmed WFDRI to be equally accurate to BIO for ROP diagnosis (60, 61).

WFDRI has many advantages over traditional BIO. WFDRI allows objective photographic documentation and this mitigates the medico-legal risk associated with traditionally subjective methods of ROP grading and documentation (60). In addition, serial retinal imaging offers more accurate disease classification and monitoring of ROP progression, as well as the ease of seeking a second opinion. Images can also be used for education and training to improve ROP management. WFDRI can be used in a teleophthalmology model, potentially providing an answer to some of the serious challenges in ROP screening.

3.3.4 Teleophthalmology

Teleophthalmology addresses the current challenges, by providing an effective alternative model to traditional ROP screening. Images can be captured at one location, with grading of images and management decisions by an ophthalmologist occurring at a different location. Early implementations which evaluated the safety and efficacy of teleophthalmology versus traditional BIO employed the use of trained ophthalmologists to capture images (59, 62–66). As these screening models have matured, implementations typically now employ trained neonatal nurses (45, 58, 67), ophthalmic photographers (68, 69), and trained technicians (46, 70, 71).

The use of trained non-ophthalmologists has many advantages, primarily releasing ophthalmologists from the time taken to screen, allowing them to focus their time on grading images and treatment decision making. Non-ophthalmologist image acquirers may also acquire images in units or regions where ROP screening may not have previously been

available, limiting the need for infant transfer and addressing the access issues which were one of the key constraints on traditional screening models of care.

Screening images can be reviewed in different ways. Images can either be directly interpreted at the bedside, or more typically, a 'store-and-forward' model is used, which involves transmission of the image electronically for evaluation by an expert grader based remotely (72). The expert grader is typically a specialized ophthalmologist experienced in ROP care. Novel models in settings in which access to expert grading is limited, and images are evaluated by appropriately trained non-physician technicians, are also showing promise (46, 73, 74).

Images may be captured across several different NICUs, and images transmitted to a central reading and treatment center for evaluation (45). Images should be transmitted via a secure electronic server or electronic health record, and if possible, be accompanied with any relevant patient demographic and clinical information to assist the grader's evaluation.

Reporting of disease should follow the ICROP revised guidelines (41), or any local ROP screening guidelines. The frequency of follow-up imaging examinations should be carried out by the recommended schedule outlined in the joint AAO/AAP, which range from 1 to 3 weeks dependent on ROP disease severity or should follow local ROP screening guidelines (44, 61). Infants should be followed until they meet the ROP screening examination termination criteria set out in the same joint guidelines, or the appropriate local guidelines.

3.3.5 Current Implementations and Efficacy

Implementations of teleophthalmology models for ROP screening may improve both quality and accessibility of care. Successful implementations have been carried out in several real-world settings, including the Auckland Regional Telemedicine Retinopathy of Prematurity (ART-ROP) network in New Zealand (45, 67, 75), Stanford University Network for Diagnosis of Retinopathy of Prematurity (SUNDROP) in Northern California (58, 76), the KID-ROP (46, 73), ROPE-SOS (70), and Vittala ROP networks in South India (77), Montana (78), and the Bavarian ROP-Telemedicine Project in Germany (59). The ART-ROP screening network program is described below.

3.3.5.1 The Auckland Regional Telemedicine Retinopathy of Prematurity Screening Network

Auckland, the most populated region in New Zealand, with approximately 1.5 million individuals, has four geographically separated NICUs, all requiring ROP screening services, and ophthalmologists who were required to spend excessive time traveling between locations or at-risk infants who were required to undergo costly and potentially health-impacting transfers between hospitals (79). With the introduction of WFDRI with the RetCam (80), the ART-ROP was established in 2006 with three NICUs and expanded to include the fourth NICU in 2010. ART-ROP utilizes non-ophthalmologists, a specially trained nurse specialist who is supported by a medical photographer, to capture retinal images of infants deemed at risk of ROP (81). A minimum of three images from each eye are required for telemedicine review: the posterior pole, the nasal retina, and the temporal retina (Figure 3.5) (45). Images are captured through dilated pupils with a speculum in place. Dilating drops are instilled in advance by NICU staff, whilst the anesthetic is instilled by the nurse specialist just prior to speculum insertion. Images are reviewed by the trained nurse specialist to determine if they are clear and gradable and images are retaken if required. Captured images are stored on the secure ART-ROP network server in an uncompressed and encrypted format. These can then be accessed by the consultant pediatric ophthalmologist for assessment and reporting, with the resultant report and images uploaded and incorporated into the infant's electronic medical record. This results in the outcome of screening being automatically sent to the infant's NICU together with the management plan for follow-up, treatment, or discharge. The ART-ROP network exclusively uses WFDRI and telemedicine for ROP screening, diagnosis, and discharge, and thus represents a real-world ROP telemedicine screening program (45).

A recent comprehensive review of the ART-ROP service from 2006 to 2015 indicated the efficacy of the program (45). A total of 1,181 infants were screened across this time period with a mean of four screening sessions per infant. Treatment-requiring ROP was detected in 83 infants, who all received treatment for their ROP (45). The total number of infants requiring screening significantly increased over the decade (R^2 = 0.7993); however, the proportion of infants requiring treatment significantly decreased (R^2 = 0.9205) (45). A reduction in the number of infants transferred between NICUs in the Auckland region was observed during the implementation of the ART-ROP network and again during its expansion to include the fourth NICU. The reduction of infant transfers is of great importance to the well-being of those infants undergoing ROP screening, as well as having the additional benefit of reducing service costs (55, 79). ART-ROP demonstrates an effective, real-world model of telemedicine screening for ROP which decreased time pressure in the challenging ophthalmologist workflow conundrum with the goal of increasing access to ROP screening for at-risk infants (45).

Several studies have evaluated the accuracy and safety of teleophthalmology for ROP. For the diagnosis of any ROP, including mild or worse

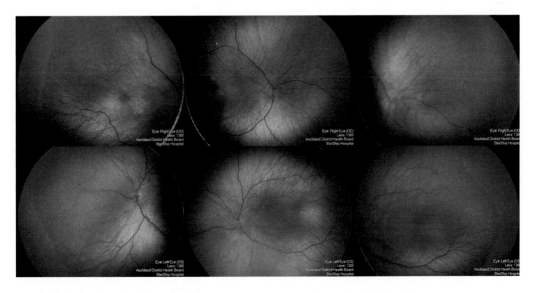

Figure 3.5 The standard images captured as part of the Auckland Regional Telemedicine Retinopathy of Prematurity (ART-ROP) screening network. Three high-quality images are captured per eye: the posterior pole with the optic nerve centered, nasal and temporal retina.

disease, teleophthalmology has been shown in a systematic review to have a sensitivity of 0.82–0.86 and specificity of 0.91–0.96, when compared to a reference standard of dilated ophthalmoscopy carried out by expert ophthalmologist graders (72). Lower sensitivity in reviewed studies has been attributed to missed cases of mild peripheral ROP that were not captured during retinal imaging. Further studies have shown a higher accuracy for detecting ROP in infants at later post-menstrual ages (82, 83). Increased age has been attributed to improved image quality and acquisition due to larger palpebral fissures, larger eyes, and less corneal and vitreous haze.

For the diagnosis of pre-threshold or worse ROP, sensitivities of 0.72–1.00 and specificities of 0.90–0.98 have been reported (72, 83–85). Two prospective studies which assessed the accuracy of teleophthalmology versus traditional ophthalmoscopy in the detection of moderate to severe ROP showed sensitivities of 0.92–1.00 and specificities of 0.37–0.96 (63, 65). The sensitivity for detecting moderate to severe ROP, in particular in infants with plus disease or those with treatment-requiring type 1 ROP, appears to be higher than the detection of early or very peripheral disease. AAO has confirmed WFDRI to be equally accurate to BIO for ROP diagnosis (86).

For teleophthalmology to be sustainable in the long term, the health economics must be considered. Teleophthalmology may require a significant upfront capital outlay, particularly to purchase WFRDI equipment and train appropriate clinical personnel. However, the ongoing application of teleophthalmology has been shown to be cost-effective when measured in quality-adjusted life years (QALYs) (87). In the United States reimbursement setting, substantial cost savings can be achieved with teleophthalmology, with $3,193 per QALY gained using this screening practice versus $5,617 per QALY gained for traditional ophthalmoscopy (87). An early study from the United Kingdom showed that teleophthalmology models using image capture by visiting nurses and grading by visiting nurses or remote ophthalmologists (£172 and £201 respectively per infant examined) were cost-effective compared to traditional bedside ophthalmoscopy (£321) (88).

3.3.6 Limitations

Several technical limitations remain for teleophthalmology which need to be considered before implementation. The quality of images captured may at times be inadequate. Several studies have reported that up to 8–21% images captured may be difficult to interpret (65, 75, 85). Adequate-quality images may be particularly difficult to capture for infants with dark fundi and small palpebral fissures, which limit adequate contact between the RetCam lens and the corneal surface. These challenges however appear to be improved with newer, updated versions of the RetCam device and appropriate training of staff capturing images to assess for image quality.

Further, significant initial capital outlay is required to purchase imaging equipment and to adequately train clinical staff for screening. Initial costs, estimated to be up to US$125,000 (70), may limit the uptake of teleophthalmology programs, particularly in middle-income countries where the current burden of disease is at its highest. The emergence of new retinal cameras will likely significantly decrease these costs.

Compared to BIO, WFDRI has decreased magnification and lacks stereopsis. Further, the field of view may not always be able to capture the full retina up to the ora serrata unless scleral indentation is applied. Though this may not influence the diagnosis of treatment requiring ROP (45), it may restrict the ability to capture very peripheral disease, reflected in decreased sensitivity in the diagnosis of mild to moderate ROP seen in early studies (72).

3.3.7 Future Directions

Various studies have shown that current real-world implementations of teleophthalmology for ROP screening are effective, particularly for the detection of moderate to severe disease. A number of outstanding questions remain, which have the potential to improve quality and access to ROP screening care.

Firstly, the role of traditional BIO in teleophthalmology-led models of ROP remains unclear. Early validation and real-world implementation studies of teleophthalmology included at least one or more instances of ophthalmoscopy examination prior to the discharge of the infant from screening and follow-up (76). More recent studies, including the ART-ROP case study, have demonstrated that teleophthalmology exclusive models which do not include ophthalmoscopy prior to discharge from screening are safe and effective (45). Future implementations of the ART-ROP model which do not require ophthalmoscopy may further reduce the cost, and improve the accessibility of screening (45).

Access to experts who can grade fundal images remains another bottleneck limiting broader access to ROP care. Several teleophthalmology education initiatives are now under way, including the GEN-ROP and KID-ROP programs, which are developing a non-physician workforce to grade images (73, 74). Non-physician readers have been shown to offer similar accuracy in detecting treatment-requiring ROP (73), and may be particularly effective in developing countries, including Mongolia, Nepal, and India, where screening demand is immense relative to current numbers of expert physician image graders.

Lastly, several groups are now evaluating the role of computer-based image analysis and AI systems for the automated diagnosis of fundal images (89). These systems have been able to diagnose plus disease with high sensitivity, negative predictive value, and accuracy, which is particularly important in a disease detection context. This may have several translational clinical applications, including providing point-of-care diagnosis, and reducing the amount of time required for image interpretation in 'store-and-forward' teleophthalmology implementations. Further, automated diagnosis with a high sensitivity and negative predictive value may significantly reduce the number of images which have to be reviewed by expert clinicians, particularly given the low treatment yield of ROP screening and the limited number of qualified graders. Significant research is ongoing in developing automated systems which may objectively quantify the degree of pathology present in the image beyond current discrete categories of diagnosis, which may have clinical application in disease and post-treatment monitoring and reducing inter-clinician variability in diagnosis.

3.4 CONCLUSION

With an aging population and increased rates of prematurity there is a need to deliver innovative health care services. The introduction of teleophthalmology has the ability to improve the accessibility, cost, quality, safety, and reliability of these essential services.

REFERENCES

1. Strehle EM, Shabde N. One hundred years of telemedicine: Does this new technology have a place in paediatrics? *Archives of Disease in Childhood.* 2006;91(12):956–9.

2. Morse A. Telemedicine in ophthalmology: Promise and pitfalls. *Ophthalmology.* 2014;121(4):809–11.

3. Newton MJ. The promise of telemedicine. *Survey of Ophthalmology.* 2014;59(5):559–67.

4. Labiris G, Panagiotopoulou E-K, Kozobolis VP. A systematic review of teleophthalmological studies in Europe. *International Journal of Ophthalmology.* 2018;11(2):314.

5. Resnikoff S, Felch W, Gauthier T-M, Spivey B. The number of ophthalmologists in practice and training worldwide: A growing gap despite more than 200 000 practitioners. *British Journal of Ophthalmology* 2012;96(6):783–787.

6. Craig J, Petterson V. Introduction to the practice of telemedicine. *Journal of Telemedicine.* 2005;11(1):3–9.

7. Host BKJ, Turner AW, Muir J. Real-time teleophthalmology video consultation: An analysis of patient satisfaction in rural Western Australia. *Clinical and Experimental Optometry.* 2018;101(1):129–34.

8. Bartnik SE, Copeland SP, Aicken AJ, Turner AW. Optometry-facilitated teleophthalmology: An audit of the first year in Western Australia. *Clinical and Experimental Optometry.* 2018;101(5):700–3.

9. McGlacken-Byrne A, Turner AW, Drinkwater J. Review of cataract surgery in rural north Western Australia with the Lions Outback Vision. *Clinical & Experimental Ophthalmology.* 2019;47(6):802–3.

10. Mukamel BD, Bresnick HG, Wang Q, Dickey FC. Barriers to compliance with screening guidelines for diabetic retinopathy. *Ophthalmic Epidemiology.* 1999;6(1):61–72.

11. Gower EW, Silverman E, Cassard SD, Williams SK, Baldonado K, Friedman DS. Barriers to attending an eye examination after vision screening referral within a vulnerable population. *Journal of Health Care for the Poor and Underserved.* 2013;24 (3):1042–52.

12. Liu Y, Swearingen R. Diabetic eye screening: Knowledge and perspectives from providers and patients. *Current Diabetes Reports.* 2017;17(10):94.

13. Richter GM, Williams SL, Starren J, Flynn JT, Chiang MF. Telemedicine for retinopathy of prematurity diagnosis: Evaluation and challenges. *Survey of Ophthalmology.* 2009;54(6):671–85.

14. Keel S, Xie J, Foreman J, Van Wijngaarden P, Taylor HR, Dirani M. The prevalence of diabetic retinopathy in Australian adults with self-reported diabetes: The National Eye Health Survey. *Ophthalmology.* 2017;124(7):977–84.

15. Caffery LJ, Taylor M, Gole G, Smith AC. Models of care in tele-ophthalmology: A scoping review. *Journal of Telemedicine and Telecare.* 2019;25(2):106–22.

16. Bahaadinbeigy K, Yogesan K. *A literature review of teleophthalmology projects from around the globe.* In: Yogesan K, Goldschmidt L, Cuadros J (eds.) *Digital Teleretinal Screening.* Berlin: Springer; 2012. pp. 3–10.

17. Wild S, Roglic G, Green A, Sicree R, King H. Global prevalence of diabetes: Estimates for the year 2000 and projections for 2030. *Diabetes Care.* 2004;27(5):1047–53.

18. Yau JW, Rogers SL, Kawasaki R, Lamoureux EL, Kowalski JW, Bek T, et al. Global prevalence and major risk factors of diabetic retinopathy. *Diabetes Care* 2012;35(3):556–64.

19. Schaal S, Kaplan HJ. *Cystoid Macular Edema: Medical and Surgical Management.* Springer; 2016.

20. Wilson JMG, Jungner G. *Principles and Practice of Screening for Disease.* Geneva: World Health Organization; 1968.

21. Tapp RJ, Shaw JE, Harper CA, De Courten MP, Balkau B, McCarty DJ, et al. The prevalence of and factors associated with diabetic retinopathy in the Australian population. *Diabetes Care.* 2003;26(6):1731–7.

22. Mitchell P, Foran S. *Guidelines for the Management of Diabetic Retinopathy.* National Health and Medical Research Council; 2008.

23. Royal Australian and New Zealand College of Ophthalmologists. Patient Screening and Referral

Pathway Guidelines for Diabetic Retinopathy 2019. Available from: https://ranzco.edu/policies_and_guideli/clinical-notes-for-ranzco-screening-and-referral-pathway-for-diabetic-retinopathy-in-australia-2019/.

24. International Council of Ophthalmology. ICO Guidelines for Diabetic Eye Care 2017. Available from: www.icoph.org/downloads/ICOGuidelinesforDiabeticEyeCare.pdf.

25. Scanlon PH. The English National Screening Programme for diabetic retinopathy 2003–2016. *Acta Diabetologica* 2017;54(6):515–25.

26. Li HK, Horton M, Bursell S-E, Cavallerano J, Zimmer-Galler I, Tennant M, et al. Telehealth practice recommendations for diabetic retinopathy. *Telemedicine and e-health.* 2011;17(10):814–37.

27. Moss SE, Meuer SM, Klein R, Hubbard LD, Brothers RJ, Klein BE. Are seven standard photographic fields necessary for classification of diabetic retinopathy? *Investigative Ophthalmology & Visual Science.* 1989;30(5):823–8.

28. Cavallerano AA, Cavallerano JD, Katalinic P, Tolson AM, Aiello LP, Aiello LM. Use of Joslin Vision Network digital-video nonmydriatic retinal imaging to assess diabetic retinopathy in a clinical program. *Retina.* 2003;23(2):215–23.

29. Ahmed J, Ward TP, Bursell S-E, Aiello LM, Cavallerano JD, Vigersky RA. The sensitivity and specificity of nonmydriatic digital stereoscopic retinal imaging in detecting diabetic retinopathy. *Diabetes Care.* 2006;29(10):2205–9.

30. Conlin PR, Fisch BM, Cavallerano AA, Cavallerano JD. Nonmydriatic teleretinal imaging improves adherence to annual eye examinations in patients with diabetes. *Journal of Rehabilitation Research and Development.* 2006;43(6):733.

31. Whited JD, Datta SK, Aiello LM, Aiello LP, Cavallerano JD, Conlin PR, et al. A modeled economic analysis of a digital teleophthalmology system as used by three federal healthcare agencies for detecting proliferative diabetic retinopathy. *Telemedicine Journal & E-Health.* 2005;11(6):641–51.

32. Gómez-Ulla F, Fernandez MI, Gonzalez F, Rey P, Rodriguez M, Rodriguez-Cid MJ, et al. Digital retinal images and teleophthalmology for detecting and grading diabetic retinopathy. *Diabetes Care* 2002;25(8):1384–9.

33. Keel S, Lee PY, Scheetz J, Li Z, Kotowicz MA, MacIsaac RJ, et al. Feasibility and patient acceptability of a novel artificial intelligence-based screening model for diabetic retinopathy at endocrinology outpatient services: A pilot study. *Scientific Report.* 2018;8(1):4330.

34. Li Z, Keel S, Liu C, He Y, Meng W, Scheetz J, et al. An automated grading system for detection of vision-threatening referable diabetic retinopathy on the basis of color fundus photographs. *Diabetes Care.* 2018;41(12):2509–16.

35. Bellemo V, Lim G, Rim TH, Tan GSW, Cheung CY, Sadda S, et al. Artificial intelligence screening for diabetic retinopathy: The real-world emerging application. *Current Diabetes Report.* 2019;19(9):72.

36. Fielder AR, Shaw DE, Robinson J, Ng YK. Natural history of retinopathy of prematurity: A prospective study. *Eye.* 1992;6(3):233–42.

37. Gilbert C, Foster A. Childhood blindness in the context of VISION 2020: The right to sight. *Bulletin of the World Health Organization.* 2001;79(3):227–32.

38. Gilbert C. Retinopathy of prematurity: A global perspective of the epidemics, population of babies at risk and implications for control. *Early Human Development.* 2008;84(2):77–82.

39. Blencowe H, Lawn JE, Vazquez T, Fielder A, Gilbert C. Preterm-associated visual impairment and estimates of retinopathy of prematurity at regional and global levels for 2010. *Pediatric Research.* 2013;74(S1):35–49.

40. Gilbert C, Fielder A, Gordillo L, Quinn G, Semiglia R, Visintin P, et al. Characteristics of infants with severe retinopathy of prematurity in countries with low, moderate, and high levels of development: Implications for screening programs. *Pediatrics.* 2005;115(5):e51–e525.

41. International Committee for the Classification of Retinopathy of Prematurity. The international classification of retinopathy of prematurity revisited. *Archives of Ophthalmology.* 2005;123(7):991.

42. Good WV, on behalf of the Early Treatment for Retinopathy of Prematurity Cooperative Group. Final results of the Early Treatment for Retinopathy of Prematurity (ETROP) randomized trial. *Transactions of the American Ophthalmological Society.* 2004;102:233.

43. Mintz-Hittner HA, Kennedy KA, Chuang AZ. Efficacy of intravitreal bevacizumab for stage 3 retinopathy of prematurity. *New England Journal of Medicine.* 2011;364(7):603–15.

44. Section on Ophthalmology American Academy of Pediatrics, American Academy of Ophthalmology, American Association for Pediatric Ophthalmology, Strabismus. Screening examination of premature infants for retinopathy of prematurity. *Pediatrics.* 2006;117(2):572–6.

45. Simkin SK, Misra SL, Han JV, McGhee CNJ, Dai S. Auckland regional telemedicine retinopathy of prematurity screening network: A ten year review. *Clinical & Experimental Ophthalmology.* 2019.

46. Vinekar A, Jayadev C, Mangalesh S, Shetty B, Vidyasagar D, eds. Role of tele-medicine in retinopathy of prematurity scre\ening in rural outreach centers in India – A report of 20,214 imaging sessions in the KIDROP program. *Seminars in Fetal and Neonatal Medicine;* 2015: Elsevier.

47. Laws DE, Morton C, Weindling M, Clark D. Systemic effects of screening for retinopathy of prematurity. *British Journal of Ophthalmology.* 1996;80(5):425–8.

48. Campbell JP, Kalpathy-Cramer J, Erdogmus D, Tian P, Kedarisetti D, Moleta C, et al. Plus disease in retinopathy of prematurity: A continuous spectrum of vascular abnormality as a basis of diagnostic variability. *Ophthalmology.* 2016;123(11):2338–44.

49. Gschließer A, Stifter E, Neumayer T, Moser E, Papp A, Pircher N, et al. Inter-expert and intra-expert agreement on the diagnosis and treatment of retinopathy of prematurity. *American Journal of Ophthalmology.* 2015;160(3):55–560. e3.

50. Chiang MF, Jiang L, Gelman R, Du YE, Flynn JT. Interexpert agreement of plus disease diagnosis in retinopathy of prematurity. *Archives of Ophthalmology.* 2007;125(7):875–80.

51. Demorest BH. Retinopathy of prematurity requires diligent follow-up care. *Survey of Ophthalmology.* 1996;41(2):175–8.

52. Sekeroglu MA, Hekimoglu E, Sekeroglu HT, Arslan U. Retinopathy of prematurity: A nationwide survey to evaluate current practices and preferences of ophthalmologists. *European Journal of Ophthalmology.* 2013;23(4):546–52.

53. Mills MD. Retinopathy of prematurity malpractice claims. *Archives of Ophthalmology.* 2009;127(6):803–4.

54. Towers CV, Bonebrake R, Padilla G, Rumney P. The effect of transport on the rate of severe intraventricular hemorrhage in very low birth weight infants. *Obstetrics and Gynecology.* 2000;291–5.

55. Yu TY, Donovan T, Armfield N, Gole GA. Retinopathy of prematurity: The high cost of screening regional and remote infants. *Clinical & Experimental Ophthalmology.* 2018;46(6):645–51.

56. Tan Z, Chong C, Darlow B, Dai S. Visual impairment due to retinopathy of prematurity (ROP) in New Zealand: A 22-year review. *British Journal of Ophthalmology.* 2015;99(6):801–6.

57. Mukherjee AN, Watts P, Al-Madfai H, Manoj B, Roberts D. Impact of retinopathy of prematurity screening examination on cardiorespiratory indices: A comparison of indirect ophthalmoscopy and retcam imaging. *Ophthalmology.* 2006;113(9):1547–52.

58. Fijalkowski N, Zheng LL, Henderson MT, Wallenstein MB, Leng T, Moshfeghi DM. Stanford University Network for Diagnosis of Retinopathy of Prematurity (SUNDROP): Four years of screening with telemedicine. *Current Eye Research.* 2013;38(2):283–91.

59. Lorenz B, Spasovska K, Elflein H, Schneider N. Wide-field digital imaging based telemedicine for screening for acute retinopathy of prematurity (ROP). Six-year results of a multicentre field study. *Graefe's Archive for Clinical and Experimental Ophthalmology.* 2009;247(9):1251–62.

60. Chiang MF, Melia M, Buffenn AN, Lambert SR, Recchia FM, Simpson JL, et al. Detection of clinically significant retinopathy of prematurity using wide-angle digital retinal photography: A report by the American Academy of Ophthalmology. *Ophthalmology.* 2012;119(6):1272–80.

61. Dai S, Austin N, Darlow B, New Zealand Paediatric Ophthalmology Interest Group; Newborn Network; Fetus and Newborn Special Interest Group; Paediatric Society of New Zealand. Retinopathy of prematurity: New Zealand recommendations for case detection and treatment. *Journal of Paediatrics and Child Health.* 2015;51:955–959.

62. Schwartz SD, Harrison SA, Ferrone PJ, Trese MT. Telemedical evaluation and management of retinopathy of prematurity using a fiberoptic digital fundus camera. *Ophthalmology.* 2000;107(1):25–8.

63. Ells AL, Holmes JM, Astle WF, Williams G, Leske DA, Fielden M, et al. Telemedicine approach to screening for severe retinopathy of prematurity: A pilot study. *Ophthalmology.* 2003;110(11):2113–17.

64. Shah PK, Narendran V, Saravanan VR, Raghuram A, Chattopadhyay A, Kashyap M. Screening for retinopathy of prematurity – A comparison between binocular indirect ophthalmoscopy and RetCam 120. *Indian Journal of Ophthalmology.* 2006;54(1).

65. Photographic Screening for Retinopathy of Prematurity Cooperative Group. The photographic screening for retinopathy of prematurity study (Photo-ROP): Primary outcomes. *Retina.* 2008; 28(3):S47–S54.

66. Dhaliwal C, Wright E, Graham C, McIntosh N, Fleck BW. Wide-field digital retinal imaging versus binocular indirect ophthalmoscopy for retinopathy of prematurity screening: A two-observer prospective, randomised comparison. *British Journal of Ophthalmology.* 2009;93(3):355–9.

67. Shah SP, Wu Z, Iverson S, Dai S. Specialist nurse screening for retinopathy of prematurity – A pilot study. *The Asia-Pacific Journal of Ophthalmology.* 2013;2(5):300–4.

68. Morrison D, Bothun ED, Ying G-S, Daniel E, Baumritter A, Quinn G. Impact of number and quality of retinal images in a telemedicine screening program for ROP: Results from the e-ROP study. *Journal of the American Association for Pediatric Ophthalmology and Strabismus.* 2016;20(6):481–5.

69. Quinn GE, Ying G-S, Daniel E, Hildebrand PL, Ells A, Baumritter A, et al. Validity of a telemedicine system for the evaluation of acute-phase retinopathy of prematurity. *JAMA Ophthalmology.* 2014;132(10):1178–84.

70. Shah PK, Narendran V, Kalpana N. Evolution of ROP screening at Aravind Eye Hospital, Coimbatore – Lessons learnt and the way ahead. *Community Eye Health.* 2018;31(101):S23.

71. Shah PK, Ramya A, Narendran V. Telemedicine for ROP. *Asia-Pacific Journal of Ophthalmology (Philadelphia, Pa).* 2018;7(1):52–5.

72. Richter GM, Williams SL, Starren J, Flynn JT, Chiang MF. Telemedicine for retinopathy of prematurity diagnosis: Evaluation and challenges. *Survey of Ophthalmology.* 2009;54(6):671–85.

73. Vinekar A, Gilbert C, Dogra M, Kurian M, Shainesh G, Shetty B, et al. The KIDROP model of combining strategies for providing retinopathy of prematurity screening in underserved areas in India using wide-field imaging, tele-medicine, non-physician graders and smart phone reporting. *Indian Journal of Ophthalmology.* 2014;62(1):41.

74. Chan RVP, Patel SN, Ryan MC, Jonas KE, Ostmo S, Port AD, et al. The Global Education Network for Retinopathy of Prematurity (Gen-Rop): Development, implementation, and evaluation of a novel tele-education system (an American Ophthalmological Society thesis). *Transactions of the American Ophthalmological Society.* 2015;113.

75. Dai S, Chow K, Vincent A. Efficacy of wide-field digital retinal imaging for retinopathy of prematurity screening. *Clinical & Experimental Ophthalmology.* 2011;39(1):23–9.

76. Wang SK, Callaway NF, Wallenstein MB, Henderson MT, Leng T, Moshfeghi DM. SUNDROP: Six years of screening for retinopathy of prematurity with telemedicine. *Canadian Journal of Ophthalmology.* 2015;50(2):101–6.

77. Murthy KR, Murthy PR, Shah DA, Nandan MR, Niranjan HS, Benakappa N. Comparison of profile of retinopathy of prematurity in semiurban/rural and urban NICUs in Karnataka, India. *British Journal of Ophthalmology.* 2013;97(6):687–9.

78. Weaver DT, Murdock TJ. Telemedicine detection of type 1 ROP in a distant neonatal intensive care unit. *Journal of American Association for Pediatric Ophthalmology and Strabismus*. 2012;16(3):229–33.

79. Towers CV, Bonebrake R, Padilla G, Rumney P. The effect of transport on the rate of severe intraventricular hemorrhage in very low birth weight infants. *Obstetrics & Gynecology*. 2000;95(2):291–5.

80. Chiang MF, Melia M, Buffenn AN, Lambert SR, Recchia FM, Simpson JL, et al. Detection of clinically significant retinopathy of prematurity using wide-a ngle digital retinal photography: A report by the American Academy of Ophthalmology. *Ophthalmology*. 2012;119(6):1272–80.

81. Shah SP, Wu Z, Iverson S, Dai S. Specialist nurse screening for retinopathy of prematurity – a pilot study. *The Asia-Pacific Journal of Ophthalmology*. 2013;2(5):300–4.

82. Yen KG, Hess D, Burke B, Johnson RA, Feuer WJ, Flynn JT. Telephotoscreening to detect retinopathy of prematurity: Preliminary study of the optimum time to employ digital fundus camera imaging to detect ROP. *Journal of the American Association for Pediatric Ophthalmology and Strabismus*. 2002;6(2):64–70.

83. Chiang MF, Keenan JD, Starren J, Du YE, Schiff WM, Barile GR, et al. Accuracy and reliability of remote retinopathy of prematurity diagnosis. *Archives of Ophthalmology*. 2006;124(3):322–7.

84. Chiang MF, Wang L, Busuioc M, Du YE, Chan P, Kane SA, et al. Telemedical retinopathy of prematurity diagnosis: Accuracy, reliability, and image quality. *Archives of Ophthalmology*. 2007;125(11):1531–8.

85. Wu C, Petersen RA, VanderVeen DK. RetCam imaging for retinopathy of prematurity screening. *Journal of American Association for Pediatric Ophthalmology and Strabismus*. 2006;10(2):107–11.

86. Fierson WM, American Academy of Pediatrics Section on Ophthalmology, American Academy of Ophthalmology, American Association for Pediatric Ophthalmology, Strabismus, American Association of Certified Orthoptists. Screening examination of premature infants for retinopathy of prematurity. *Pediatrics*. 2013;131(1):189–95.

87. Jackson KM, Scott KE, Zivin JG, Bateman DA, Flynn JT, Keenan JD, et al. Cost-utility analysis of telemedicine and ophthalmoscopy for retinopathy of prematurity management. *Archives of Ophthalmology*. 2008;126(4):493–9.

88. Castillo-Riquelme MC, Lord J, Moseley MJ, Fielder AR, Haines L. Cost-effectiveness of digital photographic screening for retinopathy of prematurity in the United Kingdom. *International Journal of Technology Assessment in Health Care*. 2004;20(2):201–13.

89. Wallace DK, Zhao Z, Freedman SF. A pilot study using "ROPtool" to quantify plus disease in retinopathy of prematurity. *Journal of the American Association for Pediatric Ophthalmology and Strabismus*. 2007;11(4):381–7.

4 Biochemical Markers in Ophthalmology

Abdus Samad Ansari and Pirro G. Hysi

4.1 INTRODUCTION

In living organisms, health is maintained through complex homeostatic biological processes, involving hundreds of thousands of proteins, enzymatic and metabolic pathways processing various organic compounds, nutrients, and energy. These processes are partly genetically determined but may vary widely as a result of both DNA sequence diversity and the surrounding environment which interacts with the genome. Impairment of these processes leads to quantitative or qualitative changes in the levels of biochemical compounds in specific cells, tissues, or body compartments, which may ultimately result in disease. Measuring the levels of specific biochemical compounds in cells and body tissues may often be a superior method to monitor health and disease than early clinical symptoms or other objective findings.

Biological markers ("biomarkers") are characteristics that are "objectively measured and evaluated as an indicator of normal biological processes, pathogenic processes, or pharmacologic responses to a therapeutic intervention" [1]. They can be used to evaluate the risk of developing a health condition, as diagnostic or disease-stratifying tools, indicators of disease prognosis, and to monitor response to treatment.

Biomarkers can be of any nature (products of imaging techniques, biochemicals etc.); however, in this chapter we focus on biochemical markers within the human body. This class of biomarkers is often measured by dedicated high-throughput methods and, within this context, they are referred to as "omics" (Figure 4.1). Each "omics" platform targets specific classes of biochemicals located at the main biological stages of the living cell: genomics target variations of the DNA sequence, epigenetics and transcriptomics target different aspects of gene expression regulation, and proteomics and metabolomics assess the availability of different proteins and intermediate small molecules, respectively. Additionally, "microbiomics," or the objective assessment of the microbial flora that lives in human hosts, have increasingly become of clinical interest, driven by the important role microorganisms play in our body's immune response and metabolism.

This chapter will describe the use of omics biomarkers in ophthalmology, the opportunities associated with them, and future challenges.

4.2 GENOMIC MARKERS IN OPHTHALMOLOGY

Initial attempts to identify genomic sequence variations that predispose humans to specific phenotypic traits made in the second half of the 20th century were met with mixed results. However, the completion of the sequencing of the human genome, soon after the dawn of the new century [2, 3], was a truly momentous achievement, marking the birth of genomic medicine. Human DNA is composed of over three billion nucleotide base-pairs distributed across 22 pairs of autosomal chromosomes and two sex chromosomes. In each human DNA sequence position only one nucleotide (adenine, cytosine, guanine, or thymidine) may be present at a time and their succession determines the properties of protein-coding mRNA transcripts. Across the world, the DNA sequence is almost identical and genomic positions that have polymorphic values (variance of nucleotides seen in that position in different individuals) is less than 1% of the genome length [4]. Most sequence polymorphisms are believed to be functionally neutral, but many have downstream consequences that result in the expression of unusual phenotypic traits.

All common ocular diseases are contributed to, in large parts, by genetic predisposition caused by sequence polymorphisms [5]. Different platforms that measure DNA variation can be used to identify polymorphic genomic markers of a disease. Typically, these platforms fall in one of three categories: microsatellite-based, high-throughput arrays that simultaneously target up to millions of polymorphisms, especially single-nucleotide polymorphisms (SNPs), and sequencing technologies that individually identify each nucleotide in the sequence of the entire genome or smaller regions of interest. Each platform suits the circumstances of the trait under study and makes a compromise between assay costs and information resolution. Microsatellites were often used in linkage analyses of multigenerational pedigrees to identify broad regions harboring polymorphisms

DOI: 10.1201/9781315146737-5

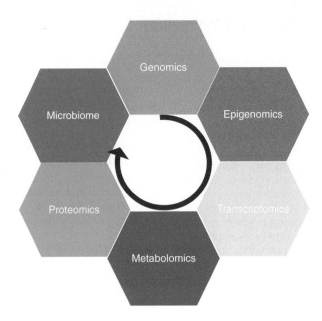

Figure 4.1 Common "omics" biomarkers used in current research in ophthalmology.

conferring high relative risks that are often causative of rare diseases, whilst SNP arrays and genome sequencing are best suited to larger cross-sectional association studies [6]. Due to their low cost per unit of information, SNP arrays have become particularly popular and have driven the growth of genetic knowledge in the field of ophthalmology and other fields, by enabling the introduction and massive adaptation of designs such as genome-wide association studies (GWAS) [7].

4.2.1 Basic Notions, Disease Heritability, and Polygenicity of Phenotypes

In complex organisms, all traits or phenotypes are determined by a combination of heritable genetic factors and environmental exposures. The relative contribution of these components varies. Short-term variations in the living environment in which the organism operates, including diet, exposure to physical or chemical agents, and cultural practices, can limit or expand the role of less changeable heritable factors. For example, smoking and unhealthy diet would change the risk of cardiovascular disease, regardless of the presence or absence of specific genetic variants [8]. The genetic contribution to a phenotype varies at an individual level (a risk to a particular disease will be proportional to the amount of genetic risk inherited from the parents) but remains constant in a population over short periods of time. Mutations of the genomic sequence, some of which affect phenotypic expressions, typically take several generations to reach a sufficiently

high frequency to significantly alter the disease susceptibility in a population.

In most cases, disentangling contributions arising from the genetic versus environmental components is difficult, because any given population shares the environmental risks present in the same geographical location and similar living conditions. Twin studies [9] can discriminate between environmental and genetic risk factors. They take advantage of the fact that monozygotic (identical) twins, arising from the division of the same fertilized egg, have inherited the same genetic material from both parents. Dizygotic, or fraternal, twins inherit on average half of their genetic material from each parent, and like any other siblings, share a 50% genetic identity. Assuming that twins, whether identical or fraternal, share the living environmental conditions at the same measure [10], differences in phenotypic expression between monozygotic and dizygotic twins are attributable to the 50% difference in genetic identity. This logic is often further extended to other familial relationships and heritability can be modeled as a function of genetic similarity in parent–sibling trios, multi-generational families, or even individuals who share very little genetic material from some remote common ancestor [11].

Heritability studies of eye phenotypes have confirmed that, like for most other human traits, genetic factors have a significant influence. A meta-analysis of several twin and family-based studies concluded that the heritability for most common eye phenotypes varies between

0.37 (optic disc rim area) and 0.85 (central corneal thickness) [5], with slight variations caused by the demographic specificities of each population, such as age structure, ethnicity, and different environmental exposures [12].

The distribution across the genome, phenotypic effects arising from each individual polymorphism, and their modalities of action vary and give each disease a distinct architecture [13]. They form a spectrum, at one end of which are diseases caused by a small number of variations, with powerful deterministic effects, located in one or two functionally linked genes. Due to their deleterious effects over fitness and the slow but steady acting effects of natural selection, these diseases, like the genetic variants causing them, usually are of low frequency in the population. Examples include congenital glaucoma [14] and a host of other rare inborn or developmental diseases. Microsatellite-based linkage analysis of selected pedigrees, followed up by association-based fine mapping, is often the method of choice for the identification of genetic variants causing rare diseases.

The genetic architecture of common traits and disorders is more complex. These traits and disorders tend to have a more elaborate genetic architecture, where a large number of common variants located over the entire genome, each with individually small effects, tend to collectively explain the majority of the phenotypic heritability [15]. Although phenotypically powerful rare variants may contribute to common disorders [16], their contribution at the general population level is often modest.

4.2.2 Genomic Biomarkers and Age-Related Macular Degeneration

One of the landmark achievements in the field of genomic research was in the field of ophthalmology. The first successful GWAS led to the identification of associations between polymorphisms within the complement factor H (*CFH*) and AMD [17], symbolically marking the transition of genetics into the era of 21st-century genomic research. Although the study used a small number of cases and controls and a low-resolution SNP array, its success was sealed because the SNP rs1061170, coding for a tyrosine to histidine amino acid change in the complement factor H protein, conferred an unusually high risk of AMD (odds ratio [OR] = 7.4).

Like any other statistical method, the power of the GWAS improves as the sample sizes increase. Successive attempts at identifying DNA polymorphisms affecting susceptibility to AMD have, at the time of writing, culminated in a study of 16,144 patients and 17,832 controls from 27 international centers participating in the International Age-related Macular Degeneration Genomics Consortium (IAMDGC) [18]. The IAMDGC study identified 52 SNPs in 34 genomic regions (or "locus", plural "loci") associated with altered susceptibility to AMD. In addition to the CFH genomic locus, strong associations have also been identified elsewhere, such as at loci near the *ARMS2-HTRA1* genes and near the complement factor B (*CFB*) gene. These two SNPs alone explain more than half of the AMD genetic predisposition. Together, all 52 genomic markers are used to make predictions of AMD risk at birth (area under the curve [AUC] = 0.74–76) [18].

The discovery of genomic biomarkers for AMD has also improved knowledge on the pathophysiological processes underlying the disease. Enrichment for functional gene properties suggests that genetically determined impairment of the alternative complement activation pathway, high-density lipoprotein (HDL) transport, and extracellular matrix organization are important in the pathogenesis of AMD [18]. These biomarkers are capable of better phenotyping and stratifying, therefore contributing to the application of precision medicine in the context of AMD. For example, variants in the *CFH* gene may play a greater role in the development of incuticular drusen, drusenoid pigment epithelial detachments, and type I choroidal neovascular membranes [19–21]. Reticular pseudodrusen and geographic atrophy have strong associations with the *ARMS2-HTRA1* alleles [22].

Other biomarkers, not associated with AMD risk in the population, may also influence disease progression; for example, polymorphisms within the vascular endothelial growth factor receptor (VEGFR) alter the risk of exudative AMD [23]. Similarly, the same variants that are associated with AMD risk appear to confer differential response to anti-VEGF treatment in patients, with some of the variants associated with better visual outcomes after 1 year; need for retreatment was also higher for carriers of AMD risk alleles in the *ARMS2-HTRA1* and *CFH* loci, compared to other patients.

Alongside environmental and dietary factors, AMD-associated variants are associated with speed of disease progression [24]. Generally, alleles that increase AMD susceptibility also lead to a faster rate of progression [25], seen for example in carriers of variants within the *CFH* gene and those in the *ARMS2-HTRA1* loci.

Research on disease progression and pharmacogenomics of AMD is still in its early stages. Much of this work still lacks sufficient statistical power, requiring longitudinal analyses and multiple follow-up examinations so that changes in the disease status and visual performance of the patients can be assessed. Future and statistically more empowered work will enlighten us on the complex genetic control of disease, outlook, and management.

4.2.3 Genomic Biomarkers Associated with Primary Open-Angle Glaucoma and Its Related Endophenotypes

POAG is the most common form of glaucoma observed in the general population. It is a progressive and degenerative disease of the optic nerve [26], and is characterized by loss of retinal ganglion cells and optic disc cupping. Although disc cupping is the hallmark of all forms of glaucoma [27], its origin is not entirely clear. From Albert von Graefe and his co-workers [28] and more contemporary research, we know that elevated intraocular pressure (IOP) causes optic disc excavations. IOP is associated with both POAG incidence and prevalence [29, 30], and its effect is incremental [29, 31, 32].

The investigation of the genomic biomarkers associated with POAG risk has the potential to elucidate the pathogenetic mechanisms involved. Given the clear importance of IOP and individual propensity to optic disc cupping towards POAG risk, significant efforts have also been made towards identifying genetic polymorphisms that are associated with variation in IOP and cup-to-disc ratio variation in the general population, even in individuals without any clinical signs of glaucoma.

4.2.3.1 Linkage-Based Identification of Genomic Biomarkers for Glaucoma

The first successful identification of a glaucoma-causing genetic locus was conducted through family-based linkage studies. An early study located a disease risk locus on chromosome 1 in a family with autosomal-dominant juvenile glaucoma, presenting with extremely high IOP [33]. Further fine-mapping follow-up analyses identified several variants within the protein-coding portion of the *MYOC* gene as the source of the linkage signal and strongly causative of glaucoma [34]. These variants predominantly cause high-pressure glaucoma and, although rare, may be responsible for up to 4.3% of the POAG cases in the population [35].

Another early genetic risk factor identified through family-based linkage studies was located on the short arm of chromosome 10 in a single large multigeneration British family [36]. Subsequent fine-mapping analyses found that a missense mutation in the optineurin (*OPTN*) gene was the source of the linkage signal. This and other rare variants within the *OPTN* gene may be responsible for up to 17% of familial

cases of glaucoma [37] and contribute a sizable number of POAG cases in the general population [38–40]. Unlike *MYOC* gene variants, the *OPTN* one almost invariably leads to low- and normal-pressure POAG cases [41, 42], highlighting the importance of both IOP and disc-related mechanisms underlying disease.

4.2.3.2 Genome-Wide Association Studies for POAG Endophenotypes

Endophenotypes are, by definition, correlated with the risk of developing a discrete disease phenotype. They may cause disease either directly (e.g., IOP causing glaucoma) or are closely related proxies (e.g., education attainment in relation to myopia). They are always quantitatively distributed across the general population, with values near distribution extremities seen in individuals at significantly altered risk. The disease is most likely to happen if these endophenotypes cross a certain physiological threshold, which is known as the "liability threshold" model [43].

In parallel, this applies to the genetic risk alleles contributing to endophenotype variation. There is therefore a good rationale to study genetic contribution to endophenotypes in the context of discrete clinical diseases, such as POAG. Variants associated with endophenotypes contribute to the development of diseases, but they also present advantages in terms of statistical power. Subjects enrolled from general populations, unselected for any particular disease characteristic, but assessed purely with respect to the value of the endophenotype they express, are much easier to ascertain and enrol in genetic studies, as part of multi-purpose population-wide cohorts and biobanks. Endophenotype GWAS throughout the years have greatly contributed to our understanding of POAG pathophysiology and selection of powerful genomic markers of the disease. Several endophenotypes are known to be correlated to POAG risk [44], of which two, IOP and vertical cup-to-disc ratio (VCDR), will be described in most detail below.

4.2.3.2.1 GWAS on Intraocular Pressure

The genetic exploration of IOP started in earnest during second decade of the 21st century when the genotypes from a Dutch and multinational cohort of fewer than 20,000 volunteers were analyzed. Genetic variants at two gene loci, *TMCO1* and *GAS7*, were significantly associated with IOP [45]. Consistent with the "common variant – common disease" hypothesis [15], these variants were common and conferred modest effect sizes in the population (an increase of 0.19–0.28 mmHg IOP for each additional risk allele in the *GAS7* and *TMCO1* loci respectively).

The GWAS discoveries grow exponentially with statistical power, which is a function of the size of samples assessed in the study, and characteristics of the risk loci such as strength of their effects and frequency of risk alleles. An increase in sample size allows discoveries of genetic risk factors that are of ever weaker effect, but which because of their frequent presence in the population continue to be important to POAG development [46]. Subsequent studies added additional power to IOP GWAS, through the rise of international collaborations and academic consortia. These collaborative efforts soon showed their true potential and the discovery of novel POAG risk factors and biomarkers, which has been led by the genetic investigation of endophenotypes such as IOP [47, 48].

At the time of writing, the most powerful and therefore informative GWAS involved data from the UK Biobank [49, 50]. These studies have identified over a hundred variants associated with elevated IOP and high POAG risk. Interestingly, these markers showed considerable associations and were also predictive of normal or low-tension glaucoma [49]. This suggests that existing disc susceptibility in certain individuals may progress towards clinical POAG even in the presence of moderate IOP.

4.2.3.2.2 GWAS on Disc Size Parameters

Several groups and international academic consortia have reported results of the GWAS discovery of genetic markers associated with several optic disc morphology parameters, of which the VCDR is of primary interest [51–53]. However, the advent of big biobank availability in genomics research has brought about huge changes in the study of optic nerve morphology. The availability of fundus imaging through the UK Biobank created immense opportunities in terms of statistical power, but also application of novel methodologies, such as the diagnostic and phenotyping using artificial intelligence.

In one published study, UK Biobank information was acquired though human marking of over 67,000 gradable fundus images. For each participant, the VCDR values were obtained from one of the eyes and, following quality assurance and control procedures, they were compared with the genotypes at over 20 million polymorphic loci across the genome. Following a traditional phenotyping approach, due to the immense improvement in power, a total of 66 genomic regions, three-quarters for the first time, were associated with VCDR and POAG risk [54].

A team of scientists led by Google followed a slightly different approach. They initially used thousands of fundus images to fine-tune a deep convolutional neural network that was later applied to both eyes (whenever gradable) of all gradable UK Biobank fundus images [55]. The advantages of this approach were two-fold. A well-performing artificial intelligence algorithm is applied consistently across large datasets, removing human subjectivity and error. This approach is also easily scalable and obtains information from both eyes of the same subject, which can further reduce measurement error. As expected, the algorithmic scoring of the VCDR in the same UK Biobank subjects identified twice as many loci (123) as the expert-labeled VCDR study. These loci consistently explained higher proportions of both VCDR and POAG variance in independent test populations compared to the manual approach and outperformed manual approaches in terms of glaucoma prediction (see section 4.2.3.5).

4.2.3.3 Genome-Wide Association Studies of POAG

Endophenotypes represent notable advantages in terms of power, as they can be studied in larger numbers of subjects and, because of the objectivity of measurements, they are robust to misclassification. Yet the relationship of individual genetic components with disease phenotypes is not always linear and exceptions or products of bias may occasionally arise. Central corneal thickness may induce an upward bias in IOP measurement, without changing the POAG risk [56], and constitutional disc morphological characteristics caused by some genes can similarly affect VCDR but not glaucoma [57]. Although endophenotypes are almost always more powerful than case–control study designs, analyses of clinical samples are irreplaceable, as they fully clarify the contribution of individual genetic loci in disease mechanisms and more objectively assess the magnitude of the disease-causing risk associated with their alleles.

Several GWAS studies that took place between 2010 and 2020 identified several genomic regions that altered susceptibility to POAG [58–61]. Using well-selected clinically diagnosed POAG samples and comparing their genotypes with healthy controls, these studies identified genetic loci that are associated with the highest risk to POAG in general populations. The pathogenetic mechanisms were almost always clear, as the same loci tended to show strong association with glaucoma endophenotypes such as IOP (e.g., *TMCO1*, *CAV1,2,* and *GAS7* loci) or optic nerve head morphology (*CDKN2B-AS1*).

As previously discussed, international academic cooperation with the participation of powerful national biobanks has led to unprecedented power which exponentially improves knowledge on disease biomarkers. In 2021, members of the International Glaucoma Genetics Consortium, with the addition of population biobank information and privately owned clinical datasets, published a landmark meta-analysis of POAG [62]. This study led to the discovery of previously unknown markers, located in 44 genomic loci, as well as the replication and confirmation of many loci that were discovered in prior GWAS on POAG or its phenotypes.

4.2.3.4 Learning About Mechanisms Underlying POAG from Genetic Analyses

Disease-associated genes often share basic functional properties, whose study can inform about disease mechanisms. There are many functional gene sets that are statistically enriched among the GWAS-identified POAG genes. One very enriched set of functional properties among POAG-associated genes is the cell cycle, cell division, inhibition, and apoptosis [53, 63]. These genes tend to be associated with endophenotypes underlying optic disc morphology features, such as VCDR, disc and rim areas. This seems to suggest that retinal ganglion cell vitality may be a mechanism leading to glaucoma. The presence of such a strong link between cell division inhibition and POAG points to potentially new and transformative pharmacological POAG treatments that will aim to boost cells' regenerative capabilities and resilience. This is interesting, as to date there is only one available therapeutical option with neuroprotective properties (brimonidine). Experimental intervention aimed at inhibiting cyclin-dependent kinases, a protein family, which also included the CDKN2B protein, whose production and activity are under strong genetic regulation in POAG, have shown neuroprotection and improved clinical outcomes [64, 65]. Extending these studies to human glaucoma patients may lead to the development of novel treatments against the disease.

Enrichment analyses suggest that lipid binding and transportation including apolipoprotein binding and negative regulation of lipid storage are also important mechanisms underlying glaucoma [66]. Genes exhibiting these properties are mostly associated with elevated IOP [47, 49, 50]. Interestingly, statins, a pharmaceutical class that interferes with lipid metabolism, were shown to reduce POAG risk in some [67], although not all, studies [68].

Other genes also show a statistically significant enrichment for properties involving angiogenesis and lymphangiogenesis [62]. Traditionally, functional dysfunction of the trabecular meshwork has been postulated as one of the main mechanisms of IOP elevation and increased glaucoma risk. A lymphatic element in the pathogenesis of POAG suggests first-hand involvement of the Schlemm's canal, which could change the way this disease is understood and managed.

4.2.3.5 Predicting POAG Using Genetic Biomarkers

One key aspect of genomic biomarkers is their ability to predict lifelong risk to disease. At the time of writing, the best predictive models rely on discoveries of genomic biomarkers for common eye diseases using data from large national biobanks, such as the UK Biobank [69], in partnership with academic consortia or commercially generated datasets.

Most GWAS on ocular traits and diseases have relied on samples of similar sizes. They have, unsurprisingly, identified genomic biomarkers which explain similar proportions of disease variability. The markers identified from these studies explain up to 17% of IOP variability [49] and 18% of spherical equivalent heritability [70], and 44–52% of AMD heritability (depending on the AMD form).

DNA polymorphisms associated with IOP are already predictive of POAG [49], both high-tension (AUC = 0.76) and, to a surprisingly high degree, the normal-tension form of POAG (AUC = 0.70). SNPs associated with VCDR only also enable strongly predictive models for POAG [55], especially normal-tension glaucoma (AUC = 0.76). An effective combination of markers identified through the most recent endophenotype analyses and POAG [62] has not yet been attempted at the time of writing, but they will almost certainly improve the previous predictive performance (AUC = 0.73) observed in previous, less-powered studies [54].

4.2.4 Genomic Biomarkers in Complex Eye Disease: The Near Future

We are now entering an era in which genomic research has finally reached its maturity. More powerful datasets are being used in combination of ever-improving bioinformatic tools to produce findings that can be further enhanced and better interpreted because of knowledge accrued from research in related disciplines and from other omics, partly described in the following sections [71]. Although current genetic prediction models are not yet at the levels required for medical screening [72], the pace of the progress made inspires confidence that in the near future we will have the ability to better understand the genomic architecture of common eye diseases, explain ever bigger proportions of their heritability, and considerably improve our ability to predict lifelong disease risk at birth.

The encouraging performances of genetic prediction models may overstate our ability to estimate disease risk among all groups and patient subpopulations. Risk-predicting biomarkers are biased in favour of European and native populations from other high-income countries, that are not representative of the world population, or the multicultural and multiethnic societies in Europe and the United States. These biomarkers contribute knowledge on pathogenetic mechanisms across all ethnic groups, but their disease-predicting value among individuals of non-European ancestries or of ethnically mixed background, a particularly rising demographic in many societies [73, 74], will be significantly reduced.

It will however not be possible to make fully accurate disease risk predictions based on genomic information alone. Non-heritable, environmental factors are responsible for about half of the disease risk and classic epidemiological investigation need to elucidate the nature and modalities of their involvement. Genomics knowledge may additionally contribute to research that has traditionally been the preserve of classic epidemiology, by supporting causal inference tools, such as Mendelian randomization [75], which are outside the scope of this chapter, but which can be of great value for the identification and understanding of non-heritable nature involved in ocular disease.

4.3 EPIGENETIC AND TRANSCRIPTION REGULATION BIOMARKERS AND OCULAR DISEASE PHENOTYPES

4.3.1 Epigenetic Control of Transcription and Phenotype Expression

Barring rare mutational events introduced during subsequent cell divisions and DNA replication during mitoses, all cells in an organism share the same genome. Yet their expression profiles vary, depending on the development stage, germline tissue characteristics, or in response to environmental stimuli. Often phenotypic expression variations occur even in individuals who are genetically identical, such as monozygotic siblings [76, 77].

Epigenetics is the term that describes modifications of the genome which do not affect the DNA sequence. The notion of "epigenetic landscape" was first introduced in the 1940s [78] to describe the environmentally driven modifications of the phenotypic expression of the genes. Several epigenetic mechanisms are important to transcription control, but this chapter will specifically focus on DNA methylation as one of the best-characterized and understood regulators of gene expression in humans.

DNA methylation (DNAm) is an attachment of a methyl group to the cytosine residue in the DNA. Somewhat reductively, we distinguish three separate molecular mechanisms involved in DNAm. The first, mediated primarily by DNMT3A and DNMT3B enzymes [79], methylates cytosine residues in previously unmethylated DNA. This process is of particular importance during early developmental stages and germline cell differentiation. This process causes cells to gradually lose their embryonic pluripotency and acquire methylation profiles that are characteristic of a specific line, organ, and tissue, distinct from other cell lines and tissues. Pluripotency and loss thereof, during cell differentiation processes, is controlled by not yet fully understood mechanisms and involves a small number of transcription factors. Among those, four transcription factors (Oct3/4, Sox2, Klf4, and Myc), the so-called Yamanaka factors [80], appear to act as master regulators. Tissue specificity arising since the earliest embryonic stages is a main feature of DNAm and is conserved across the different species [81].

Promoter methylation is usually associated with transcription inhibition [82], although in some cases, it may inhibit elements that naturally inhibit transcription, therefore resulting in enhanced transcriptions [83, 84]. DNAm needs to be maintained within a specific range and especially preserved from dilution in subsequent cycles of cell mitotic divisions. DNAm is maintained primarily through the involvement of the methylation maintenance (DNMT1) and the E3 ubiquitin-protein ligase UHRF1 enzymes [85, 86]. Promoter methylation is not irreversible and often varies to dynamically respond to stimuli emanating from the environment [87]. DNA de-methylation is therefore the third and last component participating in normal DNAm and is normally carried out by TET methylcytosine dioxygenase enzymes [88, 89].

DNAm shows considerable intra-individual variation in a population. It is under significant genetic control [90–92], although most methylation changes accumulating throughout life are caused by non-heritable factors and are environmentally driven [93].

Many of the common ocular diseases are age-related. Changes in DNAm that occur as a result of cell aging are of particular relevance in ophthalmology. Typically, aging DNA shows patterns of global hypomethylation, with more localized focal points of hypermethylation compared to younger ages. This is driven by several factors, including DNAm dilution that accumulates through consecutive cell divisions [94] and decreased capability of senescent cells to maintain methylation [95].

A large proportion of the age-related epigenetic changes are related to the constant adaptive

DNAm changes in response to exposure to a variety of environmental stimuli during the life course [96]. The cumulative methylation changes observed with age have led to the notion of the "epigenetic clock," in which the epigenetic age of the DNA is correlated with both chronological and biological age. Accelerated age, i.e., when the epigenetic age is higher than the chronological one, is associated with risk for several diseases [97] and decreased longevity [98]. However, not even age-related changes are completely irreversible and the cell preserves a pluripotency memory and age of somatic cells can be reprogrammed or fully reset, through manipulation of the expression of the Yamanaka factors [99, 100].

4.3.1.1 DNA Methylation Biomarkers and Ocular Disease

There are several experimental approaches to profiling genome-wide methylation, ranging from probe-based to sequencing-based methodologies [101]. A detailed description of these methodologies is outside the scope of this review, but similarly to platforms used for the assessment of genomic markers, each represents a particular compromise between resolution and costs and there are differences in their resolution and performance [102].

Another important consideration is that DNAm profiles are very specific to their cell line and developmental stage. Methylation changes in some cases may transcend strict tissue specificity, but the evaluation of DNAm in the tissue and at the time most relevant to a disease is important and remains a challenge in ophthalmic research. Unlike genomic markers which can be obtained from any tissue, including easily accessible epithelial and blood cells available in large population-based biobanks, epigenetic study designs in ophthalmology invariably have to balance the tissue-specific information that may be obtained from difficult-to-obtain eye tissues (typically acquired post-mortem or during operating procedures) and the statistical power from large sample sizes that can be generated from more conveniently obtained peripheral tissues.

Variations in DNAm caused by heritable factors (i.e., increased or decreased methylation of a genomic region due to the presence of *cis*-regulatory SNPs) are significantly less tissue-specific [92]. It is therefore possible to use DNAm information from a large number of samples acquired from peripheral tissues to investigate mechanisms through which genomic markers associated with certain phenotypic traits exert their effect and produce clinical phenotypes. There are several bioinformatic tools that can assess if certain GWAS associations to a phenotype are mediated through changes of methylation levels at a particular locus, even if these changes occur much earlier in life and before the disease manifests clinically. For example, a recent GWAS has identified several polymorphisms of the genomic DNA sequence that are associated with keratoconus, many of which appear to affect cell differentiation. A causal inference analysis correlated the observed association of these SNPs with keratoconus with the level of association of the same SNPs with methylation changes observed in the peripheral blood of other, independent samples. The results suggested that SNPs located in certain regions associated with keratoconus caused changes in the methylation levels of the *KLF4* and *KLF5* gene promoters and enhancers, whose altered activity contributed to the development of keratoconus [103].

In specific circumstances, studying peripheral blood tissues may be scientifically motivated and optimal, when blood cell methylation changes are expected to best capture the range of environmental exposures influencing phenotypic expression. For example, early-life exposures and events are associated with refractive error and other visual outcomes [104]. Elusive intrauterine factors that influence subsequent risk of refractive error were studied in an elegant work which focused on DNA methylation levels observed in umbilical cord tissues in 519 Singaporean children. Methylation levels were modeled against the risk of early myopia, defined through cycloplegic autorefraction at the age of 3. Although the statistical power was relatively modest, variations of DNA methylation at several locations were significantly associated with the development of early refractive errors in infants [105].

Age-related ocular disease may also be amenable to epigenetic assays in easily accessible peripheral blood tissues. Many age-related changes in DNAm are also ubiquitous, such as those involving the *ELOVL2* gene locus [106]. Age-related *ELOVL2* promoter methylation changes are also seen in the retina as in peripheral tissues, and in experimental animals have been shown to be associated with visual function decline and other phenotypic changes similar to those observed in AMD [107]. No large-scale work conducted in humans has yet attempted at replicating these findings. However, a relatively small study that compared peripheral blood genome-wide methylation variation of AMD cases with age- and sex-matched controls found evidence of differential methylation at several loci, notably the *ARMS2* gene promoter [108].

A conceptually similar study conducted on POAG, another age-related disease, compared

DNA methylation levels in the peripheral blood of 178 individuals with normal-tension glaucoma with those of 202 matched controls. It found evidence of statistically significant differential methylation in the promoter of the *CDKN2B* gene [109], a locus previously associated with optic disc morphology and POAG in previous GWAS [59]. This locus also shows gradual but consistent hypermethylation with age [110], which may be one of the possible reasons why individuals carrying genetic susceptibility to POAG typically start to develop symptoms in the later decades of their lives.

4.3.1.1.1 Potential Use of Epigenetic Biomarker Knowledge for the Treatment of Eye Disease

As previously mentioned, methylation changes are dynamically regulated and reversible. Unlike genomic biomarkers, they can be experimentally and potentially therapeutically altered to induce specific beneficial phenotypic outcomes.

Recently published work has evaluated the ability of the Yamanaka factors to reset aging signatures and restore vision *in vivo* [111]. In several animal models, they found that retinal ganglion cells obtained from animal models of glaucoma reverted to a significantly younger cellular age and recovered from severe injury when three of the four Yamanaka factors were ectopically expressed. Crucially, these factors enhanced axon regeneration in human cells, and also, more importantly, fully restored vision in mice in which glaucoma had been experimentally induced through sustained increases of IOP and subsequent optic disc damage. Significant improvements were also observed in older eyes, which raises the possibility that similar techniques could be fine-tuned for use in real-life elderly human glaucoma patients.

With improved understanding of epigenetic regulation of aging and other pathogenetic processes, better treatment targets are likely to become available. For example, the Yamanaka factors, used in the previously described experiment, are master regulators of aging and cell differentiation. Identification of lower-tier, perhaps retina-specific epigenetic biomarkers may facilitate intervention options that can have higher efficacy and fewer unwanted side effects if applied to humans.

4.3.1.2 Genetic Control of Transcriptional Activity

Epigenetic and specifically DNA methylation are among the mechanisms that control mRNA production and the transcriptional profile of each cell. Transcriptomics is the field of science that aims at studies and characterizes transcription in healthy physiological states as well as in relation to human disease.

Similar to the epigenetic profiles, mRNA expression is controlled by a combination of influences arising from heritable factors such as SNPs, but also the developmental stage, cell lineage, and environmental exposures. Therefore, the balance between tissue specificity and accessibility is as important in the field of transcriptomics as in epigenomic research.

Despite the parallels, transcriptomic research is currently benefiting from a wealth of tissue-specific data not yet available in the field of epigenetic research. This information has been primarily generated as part of the Genotype-Tissue Expression (GTEx) project [16]. While still ongoing, this project has so far generated volumes of data on tissue expression of all known human mRNA transcripts in over 50 different body tissues, from several hundred donors. Both genotypic and phenotypic information is available for the samples, which has enabled the identification of thousands of genetic markers that are associated with tissue-specific transcription regulation.

GTEx data are routinely used for the purposes of improving the power of GWAS studies through integration of genomic and expression information, but also to functionally explore mechanisms through which SNPs associated with a phenotype ultimately lead to disease. Several bioinformatic methodologies are able to generalize smaller-scale observations of SNP–transcript associations in GTEx project samples and predict the expected levels of gene transcripts in the same tissues of independent subjects based on SNP information alone. Transcriptome-wide association studies [112] are currently conducted without any actual measurement of mRNA levels, and were successfully used to improve the power of GWAS and enhance biomarker discovery in the context of many ocular diseases [49, 50, 62].

Large-scale transcriptomic data analysis in ocular tissues is relatively recent but significantly picking up speed. Data from the transcriptomic profiling of 453 unrelated AMD cases and matched controls [113] form a great example of the benefits of large-scale generation of transcriptomic data from difficult-to-access ocular tissues. This study successfully identified additional biomarkers for AMD development and disease stratification. But perhaps even more importantly, it has provided the members of the scientific community with tools that will allow the investigation of disease mechanisms involving changes in mRNA transcription that are specific to the retina.

4.4 SMALL MOLECULES AND PROTEINS IN OPHTHALMOLOGY

In addition to genomic, epigenetic, and transcription biomarkers, the last decades have seen the emergence of newer technologies that enable detection and analyses of markers that are located closer to the cell sites where diseases develop. Newer platforms can evaluate impairment of cell metabolism as well as changes in the protein composition that may be involved in disease development and progression. These techniques are less known, therefore the subsequent sections aim at giving a more detailed account of their underlying principles, technological implementations, and a wider range of examples of their adaptation in the field of ophthalmology.

4.4.1 Introduction to Metabolomics

Metabolites are small molecules or compounds that are either the end or by-product of biochemical reactions in the living cell. Metabolomics is a newly emerging field that extensively analyzes the presence of metabolites in a biological specimen. Although originally metabolites were used to diagnose complex metabolic disease and monogenic disorders such as inborn errors of metabolism [114], it has evolved well beyond the scope of basic clinical chemistry techniques, to include the parallel "quantitative measurement of the dynamic multiparametric metabolic response of living systems to pathophysiological stimuli or genetic modifications" [115]. Metabolomics allows for the accurate analysis of hundreds of metabolites, permitting the characterization of metabolic phenotypes, metabolic derangements that inspire disease, the identification of innovative therapeutic targets, and the detection of biomarkers that may guide treatment and monitor disease progression [116].

Targeted metabolomics involves the precise analysis of a pre-defined set of specific small molecule metabolites that have a well-established chemical structure and biological role [117]. The compounds of interest are subsequently measured using one specific analytical technique of best performance. Conversely, untargeted metabolomics compares the metabolome of control and experimental groups. This allows for the identification of variances that may reflect specific biological conditions as well as hypothesis generation and biomarker discovery [118].

4.4.1.1 Available Technologies

To date, there is no single investigative methodology or platform that allows for the reporting of the entire metabolome. This is due to the complexity and physiochemical variability of the

structures involved. Additionally, it is important to note the presence of exogenous metabolites from external factors such as medications, food, and environmental pollutants, coupled with the fact that many metabolites have specific tissue or biofluid localization [117]. Currently, two major analytical platforms have been applied to metabolomic studies. Nuclear magnetic resonance (NMR) spectroscopy quantifies and measures the behavior of a nuclei of atoms when they are subjected to a magnetic field. The excitation and subsequent relaxation of these atoms generate radiofrequency signals that are expressed as frequency spectral lines. NMR spectroscopy can be used for the qualitative and quantitative analysis of molecules and mixtures, even if the compound is unknown. During this process, the peak pattern that is generated by each metabolite is used for its identification, whilst peak areas are used to quantify metabolites within the sample [119]. NMR spectroscopy can be applied to various samples, irrespective of the state they are collected (liquid, gas, tissue, etc.), requiring minimal sample preparation and preservation of samples. It is however not as sensitive as mass spectrometry (MS).

MS allows for identifying metabolites based on their mass-to-charge (m/x) ratio. This process involves the ionization of atoms and molecules prior to them being accelerated to have the same kinetic energy. A magnetic field then deflects these particles. The amount of "deflection" is directly related to their masses and their positive charges. The most widely used technique that separates the compounds is ultra-high-performance liquid chromatography. It performs well on a wider range of metabolites. Accessible instruments, and vast open-source processing software availability, give MS a high sensitivity and ability to detect a larger number of metabolites [120].

4.4.2 Metabolomics in Ophthalmology

The role of metabolomic profiling in ophthalmic research is vast. The prospective of biomarker discovery has led to a variety of anterior- and posterior-segment diseases being evaluated in recent years.

4.4.2.1 Glaucoma

Neurodegeneration, elevated IOP, and oxidative stress are among the factors leading to disease development and progression. Metabolomic studies have looked to evaluate how we can better identify metabolic changes in these patients. Markers for oxidative stress have been found in both serum and aqueous samples. These include 2-mercaptoethanesulfonic acid,

D-erythronolactone, dehydroascorbic acid, galactose, mannose, pelargonic acid, ribitol, N-acetyl-L-leucine, RAC-glycerol 1-myristate, arginine, 1-oleoyl-RAC-glycerol, and cystathionine [121, 122]. One systematic review identified malonyldialdehyde as one of the best biomarkers for oxidative stress in serum for patients with glaucoma [123]. Other studies have indicated that spermine and spermidine may play a metabolic role in individuals with POAG [122], potentially affecting mitochondrial membrane potential, thus influencing a degree of neuroprotection on the optic nerve. More recently a metabolome-wide association study employing machine learning and Mendelian randomization found that levels of O-methylascorbate, a circulating product of vitamin C metabolism, significantly lowered IOP in subjects from the general population [124].

4.4.2.2 Dry-Eye Disease

Targeted metabolomic assays have been used to analyze tear samples, conjunctival epithelial cells, and serum of patients with dry-eye disease (DED), evaluating metabolite differences in varied environments [125, 126]. Commonly found tear metabolites include neutral lipids, cholesterol, lactate, glutamate, glucose, cholesterol, amino butyrate, and choline [127]. Studies have shown that oral supplementation of certain antioxidants in patients with DED and healthy controls showed a varied level of tear metabolites, including choline/acetylcholine ratio, increased glucose, and lactate results which are directly correlated to the severity of DED [125]. Other studies have been able to identify more than 150 common metabolites whose levels were altered in the tears of patients with DED, directing towards metabolites linked to inflammatory processes, gluconeogenesis, and amino acid metabolism as potential agents involved in this disease [128].

Finally, another study found associations between DED and decreased serum androgens, suggesting that sex hormones may have a potential role in the disease and may be suitable therapeutic targets in the future [129].

4.4.2.3 Age-Related Macular Degeneration and Retinal Disease

Metabolomics have also been used to evaluate several retinal diseases, including AMD [130], diabetic retinopathy (DR) [131], rhegmatogenous retinal detachment [132], and proliferative vitreoretinopathy (PVR) [133]. Significant differences in plasma metabolites have been seen in patients with AMD compared to controls, varying with severity of disease.

This most noticeable include variability in certain amino acids, lipid, and nucleotide profiles, with pathway analysis identifying clear changes in glycerophospholipid, purine, taurine and hypotaurine, and nitrogen metabolism [134]. Other metabolites associated with disease include N-acetyl-L-alanine, L-tyrosine, L-phenylalanine, L-methionine, and L-arginine. It is believed that many of these variances are linked to oxidative stress and amino acid metabolism. Other differences identified include that of glutamate and glutamine which are associated with neurotransmitter supply within the retina. One study comparing urinary metabolomic signatures in patients with different stages of AMD to those of controls found depletion of certain amino acids and citrate was associated with disease [135].

4.4.2.4 Diabetic Eye Disease

Metabolomic studies in diabetes have identified altered levels of several biomarkers. This includes cytidine, which has been thought to have the highest sensitivity and specificity of those investigated potential metabolites. One study that analyzed vitreous samples from patients with diabetes and proliferative disease revealed dysregulation of arginine, proline, citrulline, methionine, allantoin, and octanoylcarnitine in patients with proliferative diabetic retinopathy [136]. In the retina, arginine is metabolized by the arginase pathway to ornithine and urea and by nitric oxide synthase to citrulline and nitric oxide. It is possible that hyperactivity of the arginase pathway may result in reduced nitric oxide availability, impaired vasodilation, endothelial dysfunction, increased generation of oxygen and nitrogen reactive species, characteristic for DR [117].

4.4.2.5 Retinal Detachment

Untargeted metabolomic analyses of vitreous tissue of patients with rhegmatogenous retinal detachment have found a varied level of metabolites in patients with choroidal detachment [137]. Over 20 different metabolites were identified in one study, predominantly those participating in the urea and tricarboxylic acid cycles, including uric acid, succinate, lactate, and phenylpyruvate. These differences are thought to be associated with variance in inflammation, proliferation, and energy consumption. For instance, L-carnitine has been found to be significantly reduced in patients with retinal detachments in comparison to patients with PVR [133]. Conversely, in PVR samples there is an increase in ascorbate and valine levels while the urea is decreased, suggesting more active fibroblast proliferation.

4.5 PROTEOMICS

The term proteomics relates to the analysis of the entire protein complement of a cell, tissue, or organism under a specified set of defined conditions [138]. Proteomics is the process by which different proteins are studied to determine how they interact with each other and the role they play within an organism [139]. Proteomics has facilitated the reporting of an ever-increasing number of proteins and encompasses the investigation of proteomes from the overall level of protein activity, composition, and structure.

Although information regarding protein expression can be indirectly collected by studying mRNA expression, these levels do not always correlate well with protein expression levels [140]. This indirect evaluation also does not account for post-translational modifications, cleavage, complex formation, and localization, which are essential for protein function. Proteomics technologies have enabled critical advancements in early disease recognition, progression, prognosis, and also drug development by characterizing the structure, function, interaction, and modifications of proteins at different stages during the process of disease [141].

4.5.1 Proteomics Techniques

Several conventional low-throughput methods can be utilized in proteomics. Antibody-based methods such as enzyme-linked immunosorbent assay (ELISA) and western blotting depend on the availability of antibodies targeted toward specific proteins or epitopes [142]. Gel-based methods include two-dimensional gel electrophoresis and differential gel electrophoresis. These utilize electric current to separate proteins, before further analysis is completed using alternate testing such as MS [143]. Chromatography-based methods can separate proteins from biological mixtures through various modalities such as ion exchange, size exclusion, and affinity chromatography. Other gel-free chromatographic techniques include gas chromatography and liquid chromatography [144].

High-throughput methods include protein microarrays [145]. This process involves the application of small amounts of sample to a "chip" for analysis. Antibodies are subsequently fixated to the chip surface and used to capture target proteins in a complex model. This process is often referred to as analytical protein microarray [145]. Functional microarrays allow for the characterization of protein functions, including enzyme substrate turnover and protein–RNA interactions [146]. Reverse-phase protein microarray involves the process of using both healthy and diseased tissue bound to a chip, which is subsequently probed with antibodies against

target proteins. MS-based proteomics is also a form of complex gel-free methods of separating proteins. This includes isotope-coded affinity tag, stable isotope labeling with amino acids in culture, and isobaric tags [147].

The ultimate downstream MS workflow comprises several common steps, including ionization of peptides and their separation according to their mass charge ratio. Top-down proteomics separates proteins in a sample prior to them being ionized and bottom-up proteomics digests proteins into a complex mixture of peptides first [148, 149].

4.5.2 Proteomics in Ophthalmology

Proteomics can play an invaluable role in generating knowledge and insight into the pathogenesis, treatment, and diagnosis of eye disease. In 2013 the Human Eye Proteome Project was founded, an open initiative aiming to establish a standard for ocular proteome research, identifying and quantifying proteins within the eye. Since its inception, nearly 10,000 non-redundant proteins have been identified, correlating to several different structures within the human eye [150].

4.5.2.1 Proteomics Application in Glaucoma Research

Several studies have looked at various biofluids within the eye to better evaluate this, including tears [151], aqueous humor [152], optic nerve [153], and vitreous [154]. Significant variation after glaucoma surgery was observed in aqueous humor concentrations of 718 unique proteins, splice variants, and isoform in patients who underwent tube shunt surgery compared to trabeculectomy [155], which may also explain risk variance for corneal decompensation following surgical intervention [155].

Characterization of protein patterns in tears in individuals with pseudoexfoliative glaucoma and POAG has identified altered levels of lysozyme C, lipocalin-1, protein S100, immunoglobulins, and prolactin-inducible protein [156].

Proteomic analysis of retinal and vitreous tissue has also shown 122 identified proteins linked with the pathophysiology of Alzheimer's disease. A pathway analysis of these differentially regulated proteins highlighted the possibility of defects in mitochondrial oxidative phosphorylation [154]. Proteomics analyses have also implicated peptidyl arginine deiminase 2 (PAD2) and optic nerve citrullination as pressure-related proteins [153].

4.5.2.2 Proteomics of Dry-Eye Disease

The assessment of human tear proteome has been particularly successful in the study of

DED [157, 158]. Several studies seem to suggest that downregulation of protective antibacterial proteins, including lactoferrin, lysozyme, and immunoglobulin A (IgA)-alpha, is pathogenetically related to DED. Proteomic studies may also be useful to stratify DED into different subforms that may show unique pattern variation in protein expression, including Sjögren's syndrome [157]. Machine learning analyses of high-dimension proteomic datasets can distinguish between patients with DED and healthy controls with a specificity and sensitivity of 90% [158].

4.5.2.3 Age-Related Macular Degeneration

Various proteomic techniques have studied AMD. Given screening limitations in detecting early forms of the disease, proteomic work potentially holds a gateway to understanding a set of optimal biomarkers, accessible from body fluids, that may allow for a reliable way to monitor disease and response to treatment. The tear film is easily accessible and non-invasive, with one tear proteomic study identifying a total of 342 proteins concerning AMD. This includes Shootin-1, histatin-3, fidgetin-like protein 1, SRC kinase signaling inhibitor, Graves' disease carrier protein, actin cytoplasmic 1, prolactin-inducible protein 1, and protein S100-A7A, all of which were shown to be upregulated in tear samples from patients with AMD [159].

Better proteomic understanding also holds an improved understanding of the progression of AMD. Studies have shown varied proteome make-up of the macular and peripheral neurosensory retina at distinctive phases of AMD. One study was able to identify 26 proteins that exhibited change at disease onset, progression, and end-stage disease. Proteins were found to be involved in critical functional pathways, including protection from stress-induced protein unfolding and microtubule regulation. The proteomic variation between different regions of the retina suggests that both the macula and peripheral retina are affected in this disease [160].

Non-exudative AMD remains a clinical challenge for clinicians to manage, given the difficulty in monitoring progression and lack of effective treatment. Proteomic studies have detected a moderate subclinical leakage of the blood–retinal barrier in this form of disease, suggesting that potentially harmful plasma components, including complement or iron, could enter the retina in AMD patients before advanced disease [161]. Therefore, therapies that stabilize the blood–retinal barrier might play a pivotal role in the future management of this disease.

4.5.2.4 Proteomics Application to Other Retinal Disorders

This desire to develop optimal treatment strategies for ocular conditions has also led to large-scale protein studies using proteomic techniques for various other ocular diseases. Retinal vein occlusion (RVO), for example, is thought to be the most common retinal vascular disorder after diabetic retinopathy, resulting in increasing levels of VEGF and a multitude of inflammatory markers. Proteome changes have identified the downregulation of fibroblast growth factor 4 precursor, hepatoma-derived growth factor isoform a, and α-crystallin A. A comparison of vitreous samples of 30 treatment-naive RVO patients with 16 controls found that levels of clusterin, complement C3, Ig lambda-like polypeptide 5, and vitronectin were drastically upregulated, while opticin levels was considerably downregulated [162].

Proteomics using animal RVO models have also provided a wealth of information on the disease. One study noted increased levels of proteins involved in the integrin signaling pathway [163], suggesting a potential role of anti-integrin therapies (currently being developed for the treatment of diabetic macular edema) in the treatment of this disorder [164].

Similarly, proteomic analyses have improved our understanding of the various stages of DR [165–167]. Proteomic work has identified anhydrase-I as a cause of retinal permeability, suggesting that inhibitors of carbonic anhydrase-I theoretically may play a role in future treatment modalities. After a significant upregulation of vitreous carbonic anhydrase-I was noted in patients with proliferative disease, a subsequent trial of injection of purified human carbonic anhydrase-I into the vitreous of rat models amplified retinal vascular permeability, with the co-injection of acetazolamide or methazolamide inhibiting this vascular permeability [168].

4.5.3 Proteomics in Ophthalmology: A Look into the Future

With the poor prognosis of certain ocular ailments and limited treatment strategies, proteomic studies may improve the understanding of disease mechanisms and drive translational work on novel therapies. Proteomics applications have a huge potential that may materialize after its methodologies are fully deployed for research on ocular diseases. Conditions such as retinal artery occlusion, or the proteomic effects seen in eyes after certain treatment modalities such as intravitreal dexamethasone, are currently underexplored but may benefit enormously from application of proteomics toolkits.

The proteome is highly dynamic, with complexities driven by the regulatory systems that control the expression of these proteins. Tremendous technological advances are being introduced at pace, much of which has never been seen before, improving the reproducibility and performance of results and subsequently our understanding of the human eye.

4.6 MICROBIOME AND HUMAN DISEASE

The human microbiome consists of trillions of symbiotic microbial cells which are harbored by individual people. It comprises various communities of bacteria, viruses, and fungi. In humans there are several distinct microbial floras, including those living in the digestive tract, skin, lungs, and mouth [169].

Recent advances in genome-sequencing technologies and metagenomic analysis have created a new platform to further understand the link between microbiomes and disease [170]. Large-scale metagenomic projects such as the Human Genome Project and the European Metagenomics Programme have reported a huge diversity in microbial presence in humans, with more than 3 million unique protein-encoding genes, providing information on reference genomes and descriptive data on the microbiota of healthy humans. Such studies have been able to highlight the function of the normal gut flora and underline the vital homeostatic mechanisms behind its influence, including enhanced metabolism [171], resistance to infection and inflammation [172], prevention of autoimmunity [173], and even the synthesis of vitamins [174].

4.6.1 Methods Utilized in Microbiome Analysis

Recent advances and reduced costs associated with sequencing have made it possible to identify specific microbial taxa found within the human body [170]. Current techniques can generate millions of bacterial sequences per biological sample, providing the ability to assess differences in microbial colonies and allow the application of powerful computational tools to analyze the vast amount of data generated.

Structural microbiome studies employ amplicon-based analysis as a standard approach. This involves targeted sequencing including 16s rRNA sequencing for bacteria [175], 18s rRNA for fungi and other eukaryotes [176], and internal transcribed space (ITS) region sequencing [177]. Depending on the question being asked, a single component or the microbiome in its entirety can be studied.

Conversely, functional studies utilize a whole-genome shotgun (WGS) metagenomics approach when looking at the human microbiome [178].

These metagenomics studies offer a more complete picture of the microbiome by also providing taxonomic and functional profiling information. The main benefit of this WGS-based metagenomics is the ability to capture genetic information from all available organisms present within a sample, including those that are unknown or that are not amenable to standard culturing protocols. A number of tools can subsequently be utilized for analysis including mothur [179], W.A.T.E.R.S [180], Ribosomal Database Project (RDP) pyrosequencing [181], and QIIME [182]. Data generated from targeted analysis allow for the assignment of an organism to a specific taxonomy and count the frequency of a group of organisms.

4.6.2 Microbiome and Ophthalmology

Study of the human microbiome gives an insight to how microbial metabolites and other by-products contribute to host biology and may eventually allow us to apply this knowledge to clinical practice, including disease monitoring, screening, and potential therapeutics in the future. As our knowledge regarding the way various microbiotas regulate immune and metabolic homeostasis across the human body increases, several studies have looked at the relationships between ocular disease and the microbiota of the digestive tract, oral cavity, and ocular surface.

4.6.2.1 Microbiome Research in AMD

Much research has recently been done looking at the potential influence of extraocular microbiome of AMD. Inflammation is assumed to be an important pathogenic mechanism underlying this disease, as inflammatory molecules such as prothrombin and complement proteins were detected in early AMD drusen [24, 183]. Gut microbiome is also considered to be involved in the development and maturity of the immune system. For example, a state of systemic low-grade inflammation and metabolic endotoxemia may activate the proinflammatory signaling pathways, inducing ocular inflammation [184, 185]. Although our knowledge in this domain is still scant, many potentially interesting associations have already been observed in the literature. Current evidence has shown significant differences in the taxonomical and functional profiles of patients with AMD and controls. Patients with wet AMD have gut microbiotas enriched with *Anaerotruncus* spp., *Prevotella* spp., *Ruminococcus torques*, and *Eubacterium ventriosum*, while microbiota of healthy controls were enriched for *Bacteroides eggerthi* and *Rikenellacea* [186]. It is possible that the correlation between certain microbiome profiles and

AMD may indeed be linked to dietary intake that is also known to influence AMD risk and progression [183]. There is evidence to suggest that a high-fat or high-glycemic diet adversely affects disease progression [187]. Alternative explanations that may link the gut microbiome to the pathophysiology of AMD may include alterations in the levels of activated microglia and macrophages seen in the exudative stage of AMD [188].

4.6.2.2 Microbiome Research in Glaucoma

Several studies have attempted to evaluate the potential impact of the oral microbiota on patients with POAG. One such study noted different bacterial 16s rRNA levels in oral samples from POAG patients [189]. Dental studies have also hinted at a possible relationship between glaucoma and tooth loss, severe periodontal disease, or number of natural teeth [190, 191].

More recently, increased levels of streptococci 16 rRNA in saliva of POAG cases compared to controls supported a role of oral microbiota in the pathogenesis of glaucoma [190]. Gut microbiota may also influence the production of neuroprotective factors which may encourage the survival of retinal ganglion cells [192]. Several studies have noted a possible relationship between glaucoma and *Helicobacter pylori* [193, 194]. For example, intraocular colonization of *H. pylori* of trabeculectomy specimens has previously been reported in one study [195]. Eradication of *H. pylori* may be associated with a reduction in IOP and visual field measurements in patients [196]. A meta-analysis also found a significant association between *H. pylori* and risk of POAG and normal-tension glaucoma [197].

4.6.2.3 The Microbiome of the Ocular Surface

Microbiota are dynamic communities, which inevitably evolve depending on a range of environmental factors. Studies have shown alterations in ocular surface microbiota with the use of contact lenses [198] and increased abundance of genera such as *Pseudomonas*, *Methylobacterium*, and *Acinetobacter* in contact lens wearers compared to non-wearers [199]. Contact lens use was also reportedly associated with a reduction in genera typical of a healthy ocular surface, although it is still unclear if this variation in microbiota occurs at the time of contact lens insertion or after a period of extended wear [200].

Recent studies evaluating culture and molecular-based swabs of the ocular surface have revealed the presence of a microbiome different from the surrounding skin. One study was able to show Th17 cells to be vulnerable to change in microbiome in experimental DED, evoking the possibility that increased microbial abundance may encourage the development of DED by altering the T-cell subpopulation on the surface of the eye [201].

4.6.3 Microbiomes in Ophthalmology

The number of ocular diseases in which microbiome research is being introduced is growing at a rapid pace and currently includes autoimmune uveitis [202, 203], Sjögren's syndrome [204], blepharitis [205], and retinal conditions such as diabetic retinopathy [206].

Microbiome research is emerging as a potential tool that holds the promise to bring about diagnostic and treatment improvements. Much work remains be done in the future to fully establish this technology alongside others in ophthalmology.

REFERENCES

[1] Biomarkers Definitions Working Group, "Biomarkers and surrogate endpoints: preferred definitions and conceptual framework," *Clin Pharmacol Ther*, vol. 69, no. 3, pp. 89–95, Mar 2001.

[2] E. S. Lander *et al.*, "Initial sequencing and analysis of the human genome," *Nature*, vol. 409, no. 6822, pp. 860–921, Feb 15 2001.

[3] J. C. Venter *et al.*, "The sequence of the human genome," *Science*, vol. 291, no. 5507, pp. 1304–51, Feb 16 2001.

[4] S. A. Tishkoff and K. K. Kidd, "Implications of biogeography of human populations for 'race' and medicine," *Nat Genet*, vol. 36, no. 11 Suppl, pp. S21–7, Nov 2004.

[5] P. G. Sanfilippo, A. W. Hewitt, C. J. Hammond, and D. A. Mackey, "The heritability of ocular traits," *Surv Ophthalmol*, vol. 55, no. 6, pp. 561–83, Nov-Dec 2010.

[6] J. Nsengimana and D. T. Bishop, "Design considerations for genetic linkage and association studies," *Methods Mol Biol*, vol. 1666, pp. 257–281, 2017.

[7] J. MacArthur *et al.*, "The new NHGRI-EBI Catalog of published genome-wide association studies (GWAS Catalog)," *Nucleic Acids Res*, vol. 45, no. D1, pp. D896–D901, Jan 4 2017.

[8] J. D. Berry *et al.*, "Lifetime risks of cardiovascular disease," *N Engl J Med*, vol. 366, no. 4, pp. 321–9, Jan 26 2012.

[9] D. Boomsma, A. Busjahn, and L. Peltonen, "Classical twin studies and beyond," *Nat Rev Genet*, vol. 3, no. 11, pp. 872–82, Nov 2002.

[10] J. Felson, "What can we learn from twin studies? A comprehensive evaluation of the equal environments assumption," *Soc Sci Res*, vol. 43, pp. 184–99, Jan 2014.

[11] J. Yang *et al.*, "Common SNPs explain a large proportion of the heritability for human height," *Nat Genet*, vol. 42, no. 7, pp. 565–9, Jul 2010.

[12] N. G. Asefa, A. Neustaeter, N. M. Jansonius, and H. Snieder, "Heritability of glaucoma and glaucoma-related endophenotypes: systematic review and meta-analysis," *Surv Ophthalmol*, vol. 64, no. 6, pp. 835–851, Nov–Dec 2019.

[13] T. A. Manolio et al., "Finding the missing heritability of complex diseases," *Nature,* vol. 461, no. 7265, pp. 747–53, Oct 8 2009.

[14] C. J. Lewis, A. Hedberg-Buenz, A. P. DeLuca, E. M. Stone, W. L. M. Alward, and J. H. Fingert, "Primary congenital and developmental glaucomas," *Hum Mol Genet,* vol. 26, no. R1, pp. R28–R36, Aug 1 2017.

[15] D. E. Reich and E. S. Lander, "On the allelic spectrum of human disease," *Trends Genet,* vol. 17, no. 9, pp. 502–10, Sep 2001.

[16] GTEx Consortium, "Human genomics. The Genotype-Tissue Expression (GTEx) pilot analysis: multitissue gene regulation in humans," *Science,* vol. 348, no. 6235, pp. 648–60, May 8 2015.

[17] R. J. Klein et al., "Complement factor H polymorphism in age-related macular degeneration," *Science,* vol. 308, no. 5720, pp. 385–9, Apr 15 2005.

[18] L. G. Fritsche et al., "A large genome-wide association study of age-related macular degeneration highlights contributions of rare and common variants," *Nat Genet,* vol. 48, no. 2, pp. 134–43, Feb 2016.

[19] M. R. Duvvari et al., "Analysis of rare variants in the CFH gene in patients with the cuticular drusen subtype of age-related macular degeneration," *Mol Vis,* vol. 21, pp. 285–92, 2015.

[20] C. Delcourt et al., "Associations of complement factor H and smoking with early age-related macular degeneration: the ALIENOR study," *Invest Ophthalmol Vis Sci,* vol. 52, no. 8, pp. 5955–62, Jul 29 2011.

[21] K. Mori et al., "Phenotype and genotype characteristics of age-related macular degeneration in a Japanese population," *Ophthalmology,* vol. 117, no. 5, pp. 928–38, May 2010.

[22] R. P. Finger et al., "Reticular pseudodrusen: a risk factor for geographic atrophy in fellow eyes of individuals with unilateral choroidal neovascularization," *Ophthalmology,* vol. 121, no. 6, pp. 1252–6, Jun 2014.

[23] J. M. Lin et al., "Vascular endothelial growth factor gene polymorphisms in age-related macular degeneration," *Am J Ophthalmol,* vol. 145, no. 6, pp. 1045–1051, Jun 2008.

[24] T. J. Heesterbeek, L. Lores-Motta, C. B. Hoyng, Y. T. E. Lechanteur, and A. I. den Hollander, "Risk factors for progression of age-related macular degeneration," *Ophthalmic Physiol Opt,* vol. 40, no. 2, pp. 140–70, Mar 2020.

[25] T. J. Heesterbeek et al., "Genetic risk score has added value over initial clinical grading stage in predicting disease progression in age-related macular degeneration," *Sci Rep,* vol. 9, no. 1, p. 6611, Apr 29 2019.

[26] R. N. Weinreb, T. Aung, and F. A. Medeiros, "The pathophysiology and treatment of glaucoma: a review," *JAMA,* vol. 311, no. 18, pp. 1901–11, May 14 2014.

[27] M. O. Gordon et al., "The Ocular Hypertension Treatment Study: baseline factors that predict the onset of primary open-angle glaucoma," *Arch Ophthalmol,* vol. 120, no. 6, pp. 714–20; discussion 829–30, Jun 2002.

[28] A. Weber, "Ein Fall von partieller Hyperämie der Chorioidea bei einem Kaninchen," *Arch Ophthalmol,* vol. 1, no. 1, pp. 133–157, 1855.

[29] X. Jiang et al., "Baseline risk factors that predict the development of open-angle glaucoma in a population: the Los Angeles Latino Eye Study," *Ophthalmology,* vol. 119, no. 11, pp. 2245–53, Nov 2012.

[30] A. Le, B. N. Mukesh, C. A. McCarty, and H. R. Taylor, "Risk factors associated with the incidence of open-angle glaucoma: the visual impairment project," *Invest Ophthalmol Vis Sci,* vol. 44, no. 9, pp. 3783–9, Sep 2003.

[31] M. C. Leske, S. Y. Wu, A. Hennis, R. Honkanen, B. Nemesure, and Barbados Eye Studies Group, "Risk factors for incident open-angle glaucoma: the Barbados Eye Studies," *Ophthalmology,* vol. 115, no. 1, pp. 85–93, Jan 2008.

[32] A. Sommer et al., "Relationship between intraocular pressure and primary open angle glaucoma among white and black Americans. The Baltimore Eye Survey," *Arch Ophthalmol,* vol. 109, no. 8, pp. 1090–5, Aug 1991.

[33] A. T. Johnson, A. V. Drack, A. E. Kwitek, R. L. Cannon, E. M. Stone, and W. L. Alward, "Clinical features and linkage analysis of a family with autosomal dominant juvenile glaucoma," *Ophthalmology,* vol. 100, no. 4, pp. 524–9, Apr 1993.

[34] E. M. Stone et al., "Identification of a gene that causes primary open angle glaucoma," *Science,* vol. 275, no. 5300, pp. 668–70, Jan 31 1997.

[35] J. H. Fingert et al., "Analysis of myocilin mutations in 1703 glaucoma patients from five different populations," *Hum Mol Genet,* vol. 8, no. 5, pp. 899–905, May 1999.

[36] M. Sarfarazi et al., "Localization of the fourth locus (GLC1E) for adult-onset primary open-angle glaucoma to the 10p15-p14 region," *Am J Hum Genet,* vol. 62, no. 3, pp. 641–52, Mar 1998.

[37] T. Rezaie et al., "Adult-onset primary open-angle glaucoma caused by mutations in optineurin," *Science,* vol. 295, no. 5557, pp. 1077–9, Feb 8 2002.

[38] Y. F. Leung et al., "Different optineurin mutation pattern in primary open-angle glaucoma," *Invest Ophthalmol Vis Sci,* vol. 44, no. 9, pp. 3880–4, Sep 2003.

[39] N. Fuse et al., "Molecular genetic analysis of optineurin gene for primary open-angle and normal tension glaucoma in the Japanese population," *J Glaucoma,* vol. 13, no. 4, pp. 299–303, Aug 2004.

[40] J. Zhou et al., "Tissue-specific DNA methylation is conserved across human, mouse, and rat, and driven by primary sequence conservation," *BMC Genomics,* vol. 18, no. 1, p. 724, Sep 12 2017.

[41] W. L. Alward et al., "Evaluation of optineurin sequence variations in 1,048 patients with open-angle glaucoma," *Am J Ophthalmol,* vol. 136, no. 5, pp. 904–10, Nov 2003.

[42] T. Aung et al., "Clinical features and course of patients with glaucoma with the E50K mutation in the optineurin gene," *Invest Ophthalmol Vis Sci,* vol. 46, no. 8, pp. 2816–22, Aug 2005.

[43] P. M. Visscher and N. R. Wray, "Concepts and misconceptions about the polygenic additive model applied to disease," *Hum Hered,* vol. 80, no. 4, pp. 165–70, 2015.

[44] V. Laville et al., "Genetic correlations between diabetes and glaucoma: an analysis of continuous and dichotomous phenotypes," *Am J Ophthalmol,* vol. 206, pp. 245–55, Oct 2019.

[45] L. M. van Koolwijk et al., "Common genetic determinants of intraocular pressure and primary open-angle glaucoma," *PLoS Genet,* vol. 8, no. 5, p. e1002611, 2012.

[46] P. Ojha, J. L. Wiggs, and L. R. Pasquale, "The genetics of intraocular pressure," *Semin Ophthalmol*, vol. 28, no. 5–6, pp. 301–5, Sep-Nov 2013.

[47] P. G. Hysi *et al.*, "Genome-wide analysis of multi-ancestry cohorts identifies new loci influencing intraocular pressure and susceptibility to glaucoma," *Nat Genet*, vol. 46, no. 10, pp. 1126–30, Oct 2014.

[48] H. Choquet *et al.*, "A large multi-ethnic genome-wide association study identifies novel genetic loci for intraocular pressure," *Nat Commun*, vol. 8, no. 1, p. 2108, Dec 13 2017.

[49] A. P. Khawaja *et al.*, "Genome-wide analyses identify 68 new loci associated with intraocular pressure and improve risk prediction for primary open-angle glaucoma," *Nat Genet*, vol. 50, no. 6, pp. 778–82, Jun 2018.

[50] S. MacGregor *et al.*, "Genome-wide association study of intraocular pressure uncovers new pathways to glaucoma," *Nat Genet*, vol. 50, no. 8, pp. 1067–71, Aug 2018.

[51] W. D. Ramdas *et al.*, "A genome-wide association study of optic disc parameters," *PLoS Genet*, vol. 6, no. 6, p. e1000978, Jun 10 2010.

[52] D. R. Nannini *et al.*, "A genome-wide association study of vertical cup-disc ratio in a Latino population," *Invest Ophthalmol Vis Sci*, vol. 58, no. 1, pp. 87–95, Jan 1 2017.

[53] H. Springelkamp *et al.*, "New insights into the genetics of primary open-angle glaucoma based on meta-analyses of intraocular pressure and optic disc characteristics," *Hum Mol Genet*, vol. 26, no. 2, pp. 438–53, Jan 15 2017.

[54] J. E. Craig *et al.*, "Multitrait analysis of glaucoma identifies new risk loci and enables polygenic prediction of disease susceptibility and progression," *Nat Genet*, vol. 52, no. 2, pp. 160–6, Feb 2020.

[55] B. Alipanahi *et al.*, "Large-scale machine learning-based phenotyping significantly improves genomic discovery for optic nerve head morphology," *arXiv preprint arXiv:2011.13012*, 2020.

[56] A. P. Khawaja *et al.*, "Associations with intraocular pressure across Europe: the European Eye Epidemiology (E(3)) Consortium," *Eur J Epidemiol*, vol. 31, no. 11, pp. 1101–11, Nov 2016.

[57] C. Venturini *et al.*, "Clarifying the role of ATOH7 in glaucoma endophenotypes," *Br J Ophthalmol*, vol. 98, no. 4, pp. 562–6, Apr 2014.

[58] G. Thorleifsson *et al.*, "Common variants near CAV1 and CAV2 are associated with primary open-angle glaucoma," *Nat Genet*, vol. 42, no. 10, pp. 906–9, Oct 2010.

[59] K. P. Burdon *et al.*, "Genome-wide association study identifies susceptibility loci for open angle glaucoma at TMCO1 and CDKN2B-AS1," *Nat Genet*, vol. 43, no. 6, pp. 574–8, Jun 2011.

[60] J. N. Bailey *et al.*, "Genome-wide association analysis identifies TXNRD2, ATXN2 and FOXC1 as susceptibility loci for primary open-angle glaucoma," *Nat Genet*, vol. 48, no. 2, pp. 189–94, Feb 2016.

[61] Y. Shiga *et al.*, "Genome-wide association study identifies seven novel susceptibility loci for primary open-angle glaucoma," *Hum Mol Genet*, vol. 27, no. 8, pp. 1486–96, Apr 15 2018.

[62] P. Gharahkhani *et al.*, "Genome-wide meta-analysis identifies 127 open-angle glaucoma loci with consistent effect across ancestries," *Nat Commun*, vol. 12, no. 1, p. 1258, Feb 24 2021.

[63] J. L. Wiggs, "Glaucoma genes and mechanisms," *Prog Mol Biol Transl Sci*, vol. 134, pp. 315–42, 2015.

[64] Q. Marlier *et al.*, "Genetic and pharmacological inhibition of Cdk1 provides neuroprotection towards ischemic neuronal death," *Cell Death Discov*, vol. 4, p. 43, 2018.

[65] D. J. Loane, B. A. Stoica, and A. I. Faden, "Neuroprotection for traumatic brain injury," *Handb Clin Neurol*, vol. 127, pp. 343–66, 2015.

[66] Y. Liu and R. R. Allingham, "Major review: molecular genetics of primary open-angle glaucoma," *Exp Eye Res*, vol. 160, pp. 62–84, Jul 2017.

[67] J. D. Stein, P. A. Newman-Casey, N. Talwar, B. Nan, J. E. Richards, and D. C. Musch, "The relationship between statin use and open-angle glaucoma," *Ophthalmology*, vol. 119, no. 10, pp. 2074–81, Oct 2012.

[68] B. Whigham *et al.*, "The influence of oral statin medications on progression of glaucomatous visual field loss: a propensity score analysis," *Ophthalmic Epidemiol*, vol. 25, no. 3, pp. 207–14, Jun 2018.

[69] C. Bycroft *et al.*, "The UK Biobank resource with deep phenotyping and genomic data," *Nature*, vol. 562, no. 7726, pp. 203–9, Oct 2018.

[70] P. G. Hysi *et al.*, "Meta-analysis of 542,934 subjects of European ancestry identifies new genes and mechanisms predisposing to refractive error and myopia," *Nat Genet*, vol. 52, no. 4, pp. 401–7, Apr 2020.

[71] X. Han, P. Gharahkhani, P. Mitchell, G. Liew, A. W. Hewitt, and S. MacGregor, "Genome-wide meta-analysis identifies novel loci associated with age-related macular degeneration," *J Hum Genet*, vol. 65, no. 8, pp. 657–65, Aug 2020.

[72] K. Hajian-Tilaki, "Receiver operating characteristic (ROC) curve analysis for medical diagnostic test evaluation," *Caspian J Intern Med*, vol. 4, no. 2, pp. 627–35, Spring 2013.

[73] P. Rees, P. Wohland, P. Norman, and P. Boden, "A local analysis of ethnic group population trends and projections for the UK," *J Popul Res*, vol. 28, no. 2–3, pp. 149–83, 2011.

[74] D. Coleman, "Projections of the ethnic minority populations of the United Kingdom 2006–2056," *Popul Dev Rev*, vol. 36, no. 3, pp. 441–86, 2010.

[75] G. D. Smith and S. Ebrahim, "Mendelian randomization: prospects, potentials, and limitations," *Int J Epidemiol*, vol. 33, no. 1, pp. 30–42, Feb 2004.

[76] M. F. Fraga *et al.*, "Epigenetic differences arise during the lifetime of monozygotic twins," *Proc Natl Acad Sci U S A*, vol. 102, no. 30, pp. 10604–9, Jul 26 2005.

[77] A. H. Wong, Gottesman, II, and A. Petronis, "Phenotypic differences in genetically identical organisms: the epigenetic perspective," *Hum Mol Genet*, vol. 14 Spec No 1, pp. R11–18, Apr 15 2005.

[78] C. H. Waddington, "Organisers and genes," *Organisers and Genes*. Cambridge: Cambridge Biological Studies University Press, 1940.

[79] M. Okano, D. W. Bell, D. A. Haber, and E. Li, "DNA methyltransferases Dnmt3a and Dnmt3b are essential for de novo methylation and mammalian development," *Cell*, vol. 99, no. 3, pp. 247–57, Oct 29 1999.

[80] K. Takahashi and S. Yamanaka, "Induction of pluripotent stem cells from mouse embryonic and adult fibroblast cultures by defined factors," *Cell*, vol. 126, no. 4, pp. 663–76, Aug 25 2006.

[81] T. Zhou *et al.*, "Contribution of mutations in known mendelian glaucoma genes to advanced early-onset primary open-angle glaucoma," *Invest Ophthalmol Vis Sci*, vol. 58, no. 3, pp. 1537–44, Mar 1 2017.

[82] M. Weber *et al.*, "Distribution, silencing potential and evolutionary impact of promoter DNA methylation in the human genome," *Nat Genet*, vol. 39, no. 4, pp. 457–66, Apr 2007.

[83] S. Domcke, A. F. Bardet, P. Adrian Ginno, D. Hartl, L. Burger, and D. Schubeler, "Competition between DNA methylation and transcription factors determines binding of NRF1," *Nature*, vol. 528, no. 7583, pp. 575–9, Dec 24 2015.

[84] Y. Yin *et al.*, "Impact of cytosine methylation on DNA binding specificities of human transcription factors," *Science*, vol. 356, no. 6337, May 5 2017.

[85] M. Bostick, J. K. Kim, P. O. Esteve, A. Clark, S. Pradhan, and S. E. Jacobsen, "UHRF1 plays a role in maintaining DNA methylation in mammalian cells," *Science*, vol. 317, no. 5845, pp. 1760–4, Sep 21 2007.

[86] S. Ishiyama *et al.*, "Structure of the Dnmt1 reader module complexed with a unique two-mono-ubiquitin mark on histone H3 reveals the basis for DNA methylation maintenance," *Mol Cell*, vol. 68, no. 2, pp. 350–60 e7, Oct 19 2017.

[87] F. Marasca, B. Bodega, and V. Orlando, "How polycomb-mediated cell memory deals with a changing environment: variations in PcG complexes and proteins assortment convey plasticity to epigenetic regulation as a response to environment," *Bioessays*, vol. 40, no. 4, p. e1700137, Apr 2018.

[88] J. A. Hackett *et al.*, "Germline DNA demethylation dynamics and imprint erasure through 5-hydroxymethylcytosine," *Science*, vol. 339, no. 6118, pp. 448–52, Jan 25 2013.

[89] S. Yamaguchi, L. Shen, Y. Liu, D. Sendler, and Y. Zhang, "Role of Tet1 in erasure of genomic imprinting," *Nature*, vol. 504, no. 7480, pp. 460–4, Dec 19 2013.

[90] L. C. Schalkwyk *et al.*, "Allelic skewing of DNA methylation is widespread across the genome," *Am J Hum Genet*, vol. 86, no. 2, pp. 196–212, Feb 12 2010.

[91] D. Zhang *et al.*, "Genetic control of individual differences in gene-specific methylation in human brain," *Am J Hum Genet*, vol. 86, no. 3, pp. 411–19, Mar 12 2010.

[92] A. K. Smith *et al.*, "Methylation quantitative trait loci (meQTLs) are consistently detected across ancestry, developmental stage, and tissue type," *BMC Genomics*, vol. 15, p. 145, Feb 21 2014.

[93] J. van Dongen *et al.*, "Genetic and environmental influences interact with age and sex in shaping the human methylome," *Nat Commun*, vol. 7, p. 11115, Apr 7 2016.

[94] W. Zhou *et al.*, "DNA methylation loss in late-replicating domains is linked to mitotic cell division," *Nat Genet*, vol. 50, no. 4, pp. 591–602, Apr 2018.

[95] H. A. Cruickshanks *et al.*, "Senescent cells harbour features of the cancer epigenome," *Nat Cell Biol*, vol. 15, no. 12, pp. 1495–506, Dec 2013.

[96] D. Martino *et al.*, "Longitudinal, genome-scale analysis of DNA methylation in twins from birth to 18 months of age reveals rapid epigenetic change in early life and pair-specific effects of discordance," *Genome Biol*, vol. 14, no. 5, p. R42, May 22 2013.

[97] L. Perna, Y. Zhang, U. Mons, B. Holleczek, K. U. Saum, and H. Brenner, "Epigenetic age acceleration predicts cancer, cardiovascular, and all-cause mortality in a German case cohort," *Clin Epigenetics*, vol. 8, p. 64, 2016.

[98] L. Christiansen *et al.*, "DNA methylation age is associated with mortality in a longitudinal Danish twin study," *Aging Cell*, vol. 15, no. 1, pp. 149–54, Feb 2016.

[99] C. Sheng *et al.*, "A stably self-renewing adult blood-derived induced neural stem cell exhibiting patternability and epigenetic rejuvenation," *Nat Commun*, vol. 9, no. 1, p. 4047, Oct 2 2018.

[100] N. Olova, D. J. Simpson, R. E. Marioni, and T. Chandra, "Partial reprogramming induces a steady decline in epigenetic age before loss of somatic identity," *Aging Cell*, vol. 18, no. 1, p. e12877, Feb 2019.

[101] W. S. Yong, F. M. Hsu, and P. Y. Chen, "Profiling genome-wide DNA methylation," *Epigenetics Chromatin*, vol. 9, p. 26, 2016.

[102] BLUEPRINT Consortium, "Quantitative comparison of DNA methylation assays for biomarker development and clinical applications," *Nat Biotechnol*, vol. 34, no. 7, pp. 726–37, Jul 2016.

[103] A. J. Hardcastle *et al.*, "A multi-ethnic genome-wide association study implicates collagen matrix integrity and cell differentiation pathways in keratoconus," *Commun Biol*, vol. 4, no. 1, p. 266, Mar 1 2021.

[104] J. S. Rahi, P. M. Cumberland, and C. S. Peckham, "Myopia over the lifecourse: prevalence and early life influences in the 1958 British birth cohort," *Ophthalmology*, vol. 118, no. 5, pp. 797–804, May 2011.

[105] W. J. Seow *et al.*, "In-utero epigenetic factors are associated with early-onset myopia in young children," *PLoS One*, vol. 14, no. 5, p. e0214791, 2019.

[106] Q. Zhang *et al.*, "Improved precision of epigenetic clock estimates across tissues and its implication for biological ageing," *Genome Med*, vol. 11, no. 1, p. 54, Aug 23 2019.

[107] D. Chen *et al.*, "The lipid elongation enzyme ELOVL2 is a molecular regulator of aging in the retina," *Aging Cell*, vol. 19, no. 2, p. e13100, Feb 2020.

[108] V. F. Oliver *et al.*, "Differential DNA methylation identified in the blood and retina of AMD patients," *Epigenetics*, vol. 10, no. 8, pp. 698–707, 2015.

[109] K. P. Burdon *et al.*, "DNA methylation at the 9p21 glaucoma susceptibility locus is associated with normal-tension glaucoma," *Ophthalmic Genet*, vol. 39, no. 2, pp. 221–7, Apr 2018.

[110] C. G. Bell *et al.*, "Novel regional age-associated DNA methylation changes within human common disease-associated loci," *Genome Biol*, vol. 17, no. 1, p. 193, Sep 23 2016.

[111] Y. Lu *et al.*, "Reprogramming to recover youthful epigenetic information and restore vision," *Nature*, vol. 588, no. 7836, pp. 124–9, Dec 2020.

[112] A. Gusev *et al.*, "Integrative approaches for large-scale transcriptome-wide association studies," *Nat Genet*, vol. 48, no. 3, pp. 245–52, Mar 2016.

[113] R. Ratnapriya *et al.*, "Author correction: Retinal transcriptome and eQTL analyses identify genes associated with age-related macular degeneration," *Nat Genet*, vol. 51, no. 6, p. 1067, Jun 2019.

[114] C. B. Clish, "Metabolomics: an emerging but powerful tool for precision medicine," *Cold Spring Harbor Mol Case Studies*, vol. 1, no. 1, p. a000588, 2015.

[115] S. Nalbantoglu, "Metabolomics: basic principles and strategies," *Mol Med*, 2019.

[116] F. J. Blanco and C. Ruiz-Romero, "Osteoarthritis: metabolomic characterization of metabolic phenotypes in OA," *Nat Rev Rheumatol*, vol. 8, no. 3, pp. 130–2, Feb 7 2012.

[117] N. Nazifova-Tasinova, M. Radeva, B. Galunska, and C. Grupcheva, "Metabolomic analysis in ophthalmology," *Biomed Pap Med Fac Univ Palacky Olomouc Czech Repub*, vol. 164, no. 3, pp. 236–46, Sep 2020.

[118] M. Vinaixa, E. L. Schymanski, S. Neumann, M. Navarro, R. M. Salek, and O. Yanes, "Mass spectral databases for LC/MS-and GC/MS-based metabolomics: state of the field and future prospects," *TrAC Trends Analyt Chem*, vol. 78, pp. 23–35, 2016.

[119] A. Emwas *et al.*, "NMR spectroscopy for metabolomics research," *Metabolites*, 9 (7), p. 123, 2019.

[120] C. S. Clendinen, C. Pasquel, R. Ajredini, and A. S. Edison, "13C NMR metabolomics: INADEQUATE network analysis," *Anal Chem*, vol. 87, no. 11, pp. 5698–706, 2015.

[121] C.-W. Pan *et al.*, "Differential metabolic markers associated with primary open-angle glaucoma and cataract in human aqueous humor," *BMC Ophthalmol*, vol. 20, pp. 1–8, 2020.

[122] A. Buisset *et al.*, "Metabolomic profiling of aqueous humor in glaucoma points to taurine and spermine deficiency: findings from the eye-D study," *J Proteome Res*, vol. 18, no. 3, pp. 1307–15, 2019.

[123] C. Benoist d'Azy, B. Pereira, F. Chiambaretta, and F. Dutheil, "Oxidative and anti-oxidative stress markers in chronic glaucoma: a systematic review and meta-analysis," *PLoS One*, vol. 11, no. 12, p. e0166915, 2016.

[124] P. G. Hysi *et al.*, "Ascorbic acid metabolites are involved in intraocular pressure control in the general population," *Redox Biol*, vol. 20, pp. 349–53, Jan 2019.

[125] C. Galbis-Estrada, M. D. Pinazo-Durán, S. Martínez-Castillo, J. M. Morales, D. Monleón, and V. Zanon-Moreno, "A metabolomic approach to dry eye disorders. The role of oral supplements with antioxidants and omega 3 fatty acids," *Mol Vision*, vol. 21, p. 555, 2015.

[126] A. M. Munoz-Hernandez, C. Galbis-Estrada, E. Santos-Bueso, R. Cuiña-Sardiña, D. Díaz-Valle, J. A. Gegúndez-Fernández, M. D. Pinazo-Durán, J. M. Benítez-del-Castillo, "Human tear metabolome," *Arch Soc Espanola Oftalmol*, vol. 91, no. 4, pp. 157–9, 2016.

[127] M. Yazdani, K. B. P. Elgstøen, H. Rootwelt, A. Shahdadfar, Ø. A. Utheim, and T. P. Utheim, "Tear metabolomics in dry eye disease: a review," *Int J Mol Sci*, vol. 20, no. 15, p. 3755, 2019.

[128] X. Chen *et al.*, "Integrated tear proteome and metabolome reveal panels of inflammatory-related molecules via key regulatory pathways in dry eye syndrome," *J Proteome Res*, vol. 18, no. 5, pp. 2321–30, 2019.

[129] J. Vehof, P. G. Hysi, and C. J. Hammond, "A metabolome-wide study of dry eye disease reveals serum androgens as biomarkers," *Ophthalmology*, vol. 124, no. 4, pp. 505–11, 2017.

[130] C. N. Brown, B. D. Green, R. B. Thompson, A. I. den Hollander, I. Lengyel, and EYE-RISK Consortium, "Metabolomics and age-related macular degeneration," *Metabolites*, vol. 9, no. 1, Dec 27 2018.

[131] G. Liew *et al.*, "Metabolomics of diabetic retinopathy," *Curr Diabetes Rep*, vol. 17, no. 11, pp. 1–6, 2017.

[132] N. R. Haines, N. Manoharan, J. L. Olson, A. D'Alessandro, and J. A. Reisz, "Metabolomics analysis of human vitreous in diabetic retinopathy and rhegmatogenous retinal detachment," *J Proteome Res*, vol. 17, no. 7, pp. 2421–7, 2018.

[133] M. Li, H. Li, P. Jiang, X. Liu, D. Xu, and F. Wang, "Investigating the pathological processes of rhegmatogenous retinal detachment and proliferative vitreoretinopathy with metabolomics analysis," *Mol BioSystems*, vol. 10, no. 5, pp. 1055–62, 2014.

[134] I. Lains *et al.*, "Human plasma metabolomics in age-related macular degeneration (AMD) using nuclear magnetic resonance spectroscopy," *PLoS One*, vol. 12, no. 5, p. e0177749, 2017.

[135] I. Lains *et al.*, "Urine nuclear magnetic resonance (NMR) metabolomics in age-related macular degeneration," *J Proteome Res*, vol. 18, no. 3, pp. 1278–88, Mar 1 2019.

[136] L. Chen *et al.*, "Plasma metabonomic profiling of diabetic retinopathy," *Diabetes*, vol. 65, no. 4, pp. 1099–108, 2016.

[137] M. Yu, Z. Wu, Z. Zhang, X. Huang, and Q. Zhang, "Metabolomic analysis of human vitreous in rhegmatogenous retinal detachment associated with choroidal detachment," *Investig Ophthalmol Vis Sci*, vol. 56, no. 9, pp. 5706–13, 2015.

[138] W. P. Blackstock and M. P. Weir, "Proteomics: quantitative and physical mapping of cellular proteins," *Trends Biotechnol*, vol. 17, no. 3, pp. 121–7, 1999.

[139] M. Vaudel *et al.*, "Exploring the potential of public proteomics data," *Proteomics*, vol. 16, no. 2, pp. 214–25, 2016.

[140] J. Renaut, J. F. Hausman, and M. E. Wisniewski, "Proteomics and low-temperature studies: bridging the gap between gene expression and metabolism," *Physiologia Plantarum*, vol. 126, no. 1, pp. 97–109, 2006.

[141] M. Frantzi, A. Latosinska, and H. Mischak, "Proteomics in drug development: the dawn of a new era?," *Proteomics – Clin Appl*, vol. 13, no. 2, p. 1800087, 2019.

[142] R. A. Alharbi, "Proteomics approach and techniques in identification of reliable biomarkers for diseases," *Saudi J Biol Sci*, vol. 27, no. 3, pp. 968–74, 2020.

[143] P. Y. Lee, N. Saraygord-Afshari, and T. Y. Low, "The evolution of two-dimensional gel electrophoresis – from proteomics to emerging alternative applications," *J Chromatogr A,* vol. 1615, p. 460763, 2020.

[144] B. Aslam, M. Basit, M. A. Nisar, M. Khurshid, and M. H. Rasool, "Proteomics: technologies and their applications," *J Chromatogr Sci,* vol. 55, no. 2, pp. 182–96, 2017.

[145] J. G. Duarte and J. M. Blackburn, "Advances in the development of human protein microarrays," *Exp Rev Proteomics,* vol. 14, no. 7, pp. 627–41, 2017.

[146] J. Soria et al., "Tear proteome analysis in ocular surface diseases using label-ree LC-MS/MS and multiplexed-microarray biomarker validation," *Sci Rep,* vol. 7, no. 1, pp. 1–15, 2017.

[147] A. Swiatly, A. Horala, J. Matysiak, J. Hajduk, E. Nowak-Markwitz, and Z. J. Kokot, "Understanding ovarian cancer: iTRAQ-based proteomics for biomarker discovery," *Int J Mol Sci,* vol. 19, no. 8, p. 2240, 2018.

[148] B. Chen, K. A. Brown, Z. Lin, and Y. Ge, "Top-down proteomics: ready for prime time?," *Anal Chem,* vol. 90, no. 1, pp. 110–27, 2017.

[149] N. P. Manes and A. Nita-Lazar, "Application of targeted mass spectrometry in bottom-up proteomics for systems biology research," *J Proteomics,* vol. 189, pp. 75–90, 2018.

[150] M. T. Ahmad, P. Zhang, C. Dufresne, L. Ferrucci, and R. D. Semba, "The Human Eye Proteome Project: updates on an emerging proteome," *Proteomics,* vol. 18, no. 5–6, p. e1700394, Mar 2018.

[151] C. Rossi et al., "Multi-omics approach for studying tears in treatment-naive glaucoma patients," *Int J Mol Sci,* vol. 20, no. 16, Aug 18 2019.

[152] A. Anshu et al., "Alterations in the aqueous humor proteome in patients with a glaucoma shunt device," *Mol Vis,* vol. 17, p. 1891, 2011.

[153] S. K. Bhattacharya, J. S. Crabb, V. L. Bonilha, X. Gu, H. Takahara, and J. W. Crabb, "Proteomics implicates peptidyl arginine deiminase 2 and optic nerve citrullination in glaucoma pathogenesis," *Invest Ophthalmol Vis Sci,* vol. 47, no. 6, pp. 2508–14, Jun 2006.

[154] M. Mirzaei et al., "Age-related neurodegenerative disease associated pathways identified in retinal and vitreous proteome from human glaucoma eyes," *Sci Rep,* vol. 7, no. 1, p. 12685, Oct 4 2017.

[155] C. Rosenfeld, M. O. Price, X. Lai, F. A. Witzmann, and F. W. Price, Jr., "Distinctive and pervasive alterations in aqueous humor protein composition following different types of glaucoma surgery," *Mol Vis,* vol. 21, pp. 911–18, 2015.

[156] D. Pieragostino et al., "Differential protein expression in tears of patients with primary open angle and pseudoexfoliative glaucoma," *Mol Biosyst,* vol. 8, no. 4, pp. 1017–28, Apr 2012.

[157] N. Tomosugi, K. Kitagawa, N. Takahashi, S. Sugai, and I. Ishikawa, "Diagnostic potential of tear proteomic patterns in Sjögren's syndrome," *J Proteome Res,* vol. 4, no. 3, pp. 820–5, May–Jun 2005.

[158] F. H. Grus et al., "SELDI–TOF–MS ProteinChip array profiling of tears from patients with dry eye," *Invest Ophthalmol Vis Sci,* vol. 46, no. 3, pp. 863–76, Mar 2005.

[159] M. Winiarczyk, K. Kaarniranta, S. Winiarczyk, Ł. Adaszek, D. Winiarczyk, and J. Mackiewicz, "Tear film proteome in age-related macular degeneration," *Graefes Arch Clin Exp Ophthalmol,* vol. 256, no. 6, pp. 1127–39, Jun 2018.

[160] C. M. Ethen, C. Reilly, X. Feng, T. W. Olsen, and D. A. Ferrington, "The proteome of central and peripheral retina with progression of age-related macular degeneration," *Invest Ophthalmol Vis Sci,* vol. 47, no. 6, pp. 2280–90, Jun 2006.

[161] H. Schultz et al., "Increased serum proteins in non-exudative AMD retinas," *Exp Eye Res,* vol. 186, p. 107686, Sep 2019.

[162] M. Reich et al., "Proteomic analysis of vitreous humor in retinal vein occlusion," *PLoS One,* vol. 11, no. 6, p. e0158001, 2016.

[163] L. J. Cehofski, A. Kruse, B. Kjærgaard, A. Stensballe, B. Honoré, and H. Vorum, "Proteins involved in focal adhesion signaling pathways are differentially regulated in experimental branch retinal vein occlusion," *Exp Eye Res,* vol. 138, pp. 87–95, Sep 2015.

[164] M. T. Bolinger and D. A. Antonetti, "Moving past Anti–VEGF: novel therapies for treating diabetic retinopathy," *Int J Mol Sci,* vol. 17, no. 9, p. 1498, 2016.

[165] H. Wang, L. Feng, J. Hu, C. Xie, and F. Wang, "Differentiating vitreous proteomes in proliferative diabetic retinopathy using high-performance liquid chromatography coupled to tandem mass spectrometry," *Exp Eye Res,* vol. 108, pp. 110–19, Mar 2013.

[166] T. Shitama et al., "Proteome profiling of vitreoretinal diseases by cluster analysis," *Proteomics Clin Appl,* vol. 2, no. 9, pp. 1265–80, Sep 2008.

[167] M. Ouchi, K. West, J. W. Crabb, S. Kinoshita, and M. Kamei, "Proteomic analysis of vitreous from diabetic macular edema," *Exp Eye Res,* vol. 81, no. 2, pp. 176–82, Aug 2005.

[168] B. B. Gao et al., "Extracellular carbonic anhydrase mediates hemorrhagic retinal and cerebral vascular permeability through prekallikrein activation," *Nat Med,* vol. 13, no. 2, pp. 181–8, Feb 2007.

[169] P. Amon and I. Sanderson, "What is the microbiome?," *Arch Dis Child – Education Amp Pract Ed,* vol. 102, no. 5, pp. 257–60, 2017.

[170] L. K. Ursell, J. L. Metcalf, L. W. Parfrey, and R. Knight, "Defining the human microbiome," *Nutr Rev,* vol. 70 Suppl 1, pp. S38–44, 2012.

[171] M. Nieuwdorp, P. W. Gilijamse, N. Pai, and L. M. Kaplan, "Role of the microbiome in energy regulation and metabolism," *Gastroenterology,* vol. 146, no. 6, pp. 1525–33, 2014.

[172] Y. Taur and E. G. Pamer, "Microbiome mediation of infections in the cancer setting," *Genome Med,* vol. 8, no. 1, pp. 1–7, 2016.

[173] A. D. Proal, P. J. Albert, and T. G. Marshall, "The human microbiome and autoimmunity," *Curr Opin Rheumatol,* vol. 25, no. 2, pp. 234–40, 2013.

[174] R. E. Steinert, Y.–K. Lee, and W. Sybesma, "Vitamins for the gut microbiome," *Trends Mol Med,* vol. 26, no. 2, pp. 137–40, 2020.

[175] T. Větrovský and P. Baldrian, "The variability of the 16S rRNA gene in bacterial genomes and its consequences for bacterial community analyses," *PLoS One,* vol. 8, no. 2, p. e57923, 2013.

[176] S. Banos, G. Lentendu, A. Kopf, T. Wubet, F. O. Glöckner, and M. Reich, "A comprehensive fungi-specific 18S rRNA gene sequence primer toolkit suited for diverse research issues and sequencing platforms," *BMC Microbiol*, vol. 18, no. 1, p. 190, Nov 20 2018.

[177] J. R. White, C. Maddox, O. White, S. V. Angiuoli, and W. F. Fricke, "CloVR–ITS: automated internal transcribed spacer amplicon sequence analysis pipeline for the characterization of fungal micro-biota," *Microbiome*, vol. 1, no. 1, pp. 1–11, 2013.

[178] R. Ranjan, A. Rani, A. Metwally, H. S. McGee, and D. L. Perkins, "Analysis of the microbiome: advantages of whole genome shotgun versus 16S amplicon sequencing," *Biochem Biophys Res Commun*, vol. 469, no. 4, pp. 967–77, 2016.

[179] P. D. Schloss *et al.*, "Introducing mothur: open-source, platform-independent, community-supported software for describing and comparing microbial communities," *Appl Environ Microbiol*, vol. 75, no. 23, pp. 7537–41, Dec 2009.

[180] A. L. Hartman, S. Riddle, T. McPhillips, B. Ludäscher, and J. A. Eisen, "Introducing W.A.T.E.R.S.: a work-flow for the alignment, taxonomy, and ecology of ribosomal sequences," *BMC Bioinformatics*, vol. 11, p. 317, Jun 12 2010.

[181] J. R. Cole *et al.*, "The Ribosomal Database Project: improved alignments and new tools for rRNA ana-lysis," *Nucleic Acids Res*, vol. 37, Database issue, pp. D141–5, Jan 2009.

[182] J. G. Caporaso *et al.*, "QIIME allows analysis of high-throughput community sequencing data," *Nat Methods*, vol. 7, no. 5, pp. 335–6, May 2010.

[183] A. Zisimopoulos, O. Klavdianou, P. Theodossiadis, and I. Chatziralli, "The role of the microbiome in age-related macular degeneration: a review of the literature," *Ophthalmologica*, 2021.

[184] M. Chen and H. Xu, "Parainflammation, chronic inflammation, and age-related macular degener-ation," *J Leukoc Biol*, vol. 98, no. 5, pp. 713–25, Nov 2015.

[185] N. Chaiwiang and T. Poyomtip, "Microbial dysbiosis and microbiota–gut–retina axis: the lesson from brain neurodegenerative diseases to primary open-angle glaucoma pathogenesis of autoimmunity," *Acta Microbiol Immunol Hung*, vol. 66, no. 4, pp. 541–58, Dec 1 2019.

[186] M. S. Zinkernagel *et al.*, "Association of the intestinal microbiome with the development of neovascular age-related macular degeneration," *Sci Rep*, vol. 7, p. 40826, Jan 17 2017.

[187] E. M. Andriessen *et al.*, "Gut microbiota influences pathological angiogenesis in obesity-driven chor-oidal neovascularization," *EMBO Mol Med*, vol. 8, no. 12, pp. 1366–79, Dec 2016.

[188] M. K. Adams *et al.*, "Abdominal obesity and age-related macular degeneration," *Am J Epidemiol*, vol. 173, no. 11, pp. 1246–55, Jun 1 2011.

[189] K. Astafurov *et al.*, "Oral microbiome link to neurodegeneration in glaucoma," *PLoS One*, vol. 9, no. 9, p. e104416, 2014.

[190] L. R. Pasquale *et al.*, "Prospective study of oral health and risk of primary open-angle glaucoma in men: data from the health professionals follow-up study," *Ophthalmology*, vol. 123, no. 11, pp. 2318–27, Nov 2016.

[191] D. Polla, K. Astafurov, E. Hawy, L. Hyman, W. Hou, and J. Danias, "A pilot study to evaluate the oral microbiome and dental health in primary open-angle glaucoma," *J Glaucoma*, vol. 26, no. 4, pp. 320–7, Apr 2017.

[192] A. Gupta, "Harnessing the microbiome in glaucoma and uveitis," *Med Hypotheses*, vol. 85, no. 5, pp. 699–700, Nov 2015.

[193] S. C. Saccà, A. Vagge, A. Pulliero, and A. Izzotti, "*Helicobacter pylori* infection and eye diseases: a sys-tematic review," *Medicine (Baltimore)*, vol. 93, no. 28, p. e216, Dec 2014.

[194] A. Zullo, L. Ridola, C. Hassan, V. Bruzzese, F. Papini, and D. Vaira, "Glaucoma and *Helicobacter pylori*: eyes wide shut?," *Dig Liver Dis*, vol. 44, no. 8, pp. 627–8, Aug 2012.

[195] C. Zavos, J. Kountouras, G. Sakkias, I. Venizelos, G. Deretzi, and S. Arapoglou, "Histological presence of *Helicobacter pylori* bacteria in the trabeculum and iris of patients with primary open-angle glaucoma," *Ophthalmic Res*, vol. 47, no. 3, pp. 150–6, 2012.

[196] J. Kountouras *et al.*, "Eradication of *Helicobacter pylori* may be beneficial in the management of chronic open-angle glaucoma," *Arch Intern Med*, vol. 162, no. 11, pp. 1237–44, Jun 10 2002.

[197] J. Zeng, H. Liu, X. Liu, and C. Ding, "The relation-ship between *Helicobacter pylori* infection and open-angle glaucoma: a meta-analysis," *Invest Ophthalmol Vis Sci*, vol. 56, no. 9, pp. 5238–45, Aug 2015.

[198] F. Stapleton, M. D. Willcox, C. M. Fleming, S. Hickson, D. F. Sweeney, and B. A. Holden, "Changes to the ocular biota with time in extended- and daily-wear disposable contact lens use," *Infect Immun*, vol. 63, no. 11, pp. 4501–5, Nov 1995.

[199] M. Boost, P. Cho, and Z. Wang, "Disturbing the balance: effect of contact lens use on the ocular proteome and microbiome," *Clin Exp Optom*, vol. 100, no. 5, pp. 459–72, Sep 2017.

[200] H. Shin, K. Price, L. Albert, J. Dodick, L. Park, and M. G. Dominguez-Bello, "Changes in the eye micro-biota associated with contact lens wearing," *mBio*, vol. 7, no. 2, p. e00198, Mar 22 2016.

[201] K. A. Willis *et al.*, "The closed eye harbours a unique microbiome in dry eye disease," *Sci Rep*, vol. 10, no. 1, p. 12035, Jul 21 2020.

[202] P. Lin *et al.*, "HLA-B27 and human β2-microglobulin affect the gut microbiota of transgenic rats," *PLoS One*, vol. 9, no. 8, p. e105684, 2014.

[203] J. T. Rosenbaum, P. Lin, and M. Asquith, "The microbiome, HLA, and the pathogenesis of uveitis," *Jpn J Ophthalmol*, vol. 60, no. 1, pp. 1–6, Jan 2016.

[204] C. S. de Paiva *et al.*, "Altered mucosal microbiome diversity and disease severity in Sjögren syndrome," *Sci Rep*, vol. 6, p. 23561, Apr 18 2016.

[205] S. C. Saccà *et al.*, "Prevalence and treatment of *Helicobacter pylori* in patients with blepharitis," *Invest Ophthalmol Vis Sci*, vol. 47, no. 2, pp. 501–8, Feb 2006.

[206] S. Rowan and A. Taylor, "The role of microbiota in retinal disease," *Adv Exp Med Biol*, vol. 1074, pp. 429–35, 2018.

5 Statistical Methods for Big Data

Emmanuel Kemel, Alexandre Thiery, and Simon Nusinovici

5.1 INTRODUCTION

Big data are widely used in ophthalmology and many different techniques are available, ranging from traditional statistical models to artificial intelligence (AI), including machine (ML) and deep learning (DL). This chapter presents commonly used techniques and their main characteristics, with examples from the literature. The objective is to provide a synthetic overview of this fast-developing field, accessible to non-specialists, as well as key references pointing to more formal and complete presentations.

5.1.1 What Are the Big Data in Healthcare?

Big data can be defined as "large volumes of high velocity, complex, and variable data that require advanced techniques and technologies to enable the capture, storage, distribution, management and analysis of the information" (1). Big data in healthcare refer to a wide variety of data, including physician's written notes and prescriptions, medical imaging, laboratory, pharmacy (possibly all combined in electronic health records [EHRs]); omics data (e.g., genomic, transcriptomic, proteomic, and metabolomics); insurance and other administrative data; and machine-generated/sensor data. These data can be unstructured, like the notes or images of a physician, or structured, like omics data. Big data can either refer to the large number of samples (n), or the large number of variables (p), or both. We will call variables interchangeably "predictors" or "features." The variable denoting the outcome of interest is the outcome variable.

5.1.2 Hypothesis-Driven versus Data-Driven Analysis

Classical statistical modeling (such as regression models or survival analysis) uses the hypothetico-deductive approach that consists in collecting data to test an a priori hypothesis. Big data modify this paradigm as analysts have access to large amounts of data. The analysis of big data is generally referred to as a data-driven approach. This does not mean that there is no hypothesis, but instead of starting with a specific hypothesis (e.g., an increase in glucose blood level is associated with an increased risk of diabetic retinopathy [DR]), data-driven approaches often start with a broad hypothesis (e.g., people with and without DR have different

blood metabolic profiles) and use a large amount of data representing complex biologic systems to explore this hypothesis. The results can be used to generate more specific hypotheses that can be further tested (2).

5.2 FUNDAMENTAL NOTIONS OF STATISTICAL MODELING

5.2.1 Inference and Prediction

As for classical epidemiological data, such as cross-sectional or cohort studies, analyses involving big data can have two different objectives: estimation and/or prediction. In the first case, the analyst wants to quantify the relationships between a set of predictors and an outcome (and test it if using inferential methods). More specifically, the analyst may want to investigate which predictors influence the outcome, or what is the relationship between the outcome and each predictors. In the second case, the analyst may only want to predict the outcome given a set of possible predictors.

If the objective is estimation without predictive purposes, a classical hypothesis-driven model may be preferred (section 5.3.1). If the objective is prediction, the choice of the method may depend on the characteristics of the data. If there are more observations than predictors with a reasonable number of predictors, then a simple model such as logistic regression may perform well (3). If the data are big and complex, then more advanced and flexible data-driven methods may be preferred (section 5.3.2). In this case, the level of complexity of the model may be carefully evaluated (section 5.2.4) using appropriate procedures (section 5.2.6).

5.2.2 Classification versus Regression

A model links a set of predictors to an outcome variable using a mathematical function. When the outcome is a continuous variable (e.g., body mass index), we refer to a regression problem. When the outcome is categorical, with two (e.g., disease cases vs. non-cases) or more classes (e.g., if accounting for disease severity stages), we refer to a classification problem. We focus in this chapter on classification problems with a binary outcome, typical in epidemiology. In classification, the objective is to find the boundaries that separate the two classes of the outcome. Figure 5.1A illustrates this concept of linear and

DOI: 10.1201/9781315146737-6

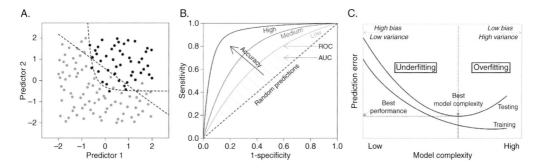

Figure 5.1 (A) Linear/non-linear boundaries for a classification problem with two classes. (B) Receiver operating characteristic (ROC) curves. (C) Plot of training and testing prediction error against model complexity illustrating the trade-off bias variance. AUC, area under the curve.

non-linear boundaries between cases (dark-blue dots) and non-cases (light-blue dots).

5.2.3 Model Evaluation

The performance of a model needs to be assessed. This implies measuring its errors, and this can be done via a comparison of the predicted values with the observed values. In order to estimate the generalizable predictive error, different data are preferably used for model development and testing. There are several metrics that highlight different aspects of the predictive performance: classification, discrimination, and calibration (4, 5).

- *Classification*: The main classification metrics are accuracy (Acc), sensitivity (Se), and specificity (Sp). Acc reflects the overall agreement between the observed and predicted classes (binary prediction: case versus non-case). While its interpretation is straightforward, its use is limited since it does not distinguish between the different types of errors. Se and Sp measure how well the model classifies cases and non-cases. Se corresponds to the proportion of cases correctly predicted as cases among true cases (true-positive rate). Sp corresponds to the proportion of correctly predicted non-cases among true non-cases (true-negative rate).

- *Discrimination*: The area under the receiver operating characteristic (ROC) curve is a widely used measure of discrimination. The ROC curve allows the balance to be captured between Se and Sp by plotting Se along the vertical axis (true-positive rate) and one minus Sp along the horizontal axis (false-positive rate) (Figure 5.1B). The area under that ROC curve (AUC) corresponds to the probability that the model predicts a higher probability for a case than for a non-case.

- *Calibration*: This measure reflects the agreement between observed outcomes and predictions from the model (probability of being a case). Both discrimination and calibration should be reported because a model can perfectly discriminate between cases and non-cases but yet be very poorly calibrated. Calibration is generally reported graphically using a calibration plot.

Because predictive models are used for risk management and medical decision making, assessment of their predictive performance and proper evaluation are crucial.

5.2.4 Variance–Bias Trade-Off

A key aspect of modeling consists in finding a compromise between complexity and predictive performance. A model should be flexible enough to capture the relationships between the predictors and the outcome. On the one hand, failure to extract relevant information (not enough complexity) is called underfitting and corresponds to an increase in bias (Figure 5.1C). The bias consists in systematic prediction errors. On the other hand, a model with too much flexibility may achieve very good performance in one dataset but would not generalize well with unseen data. A very flexible model would likely capture random variation of the sample (or noise), and therefore over-emphasize patterns that are not reproducible. This is called overfitting and corresponds to an increase in prediction variance, leading to poor generalization performance. As a general rule, more flexible models are associated with an increase in variance and a decrease in bias. Simultaneously achieving low variance and low bias allows us to minimize the error of the model (maximize the performance) when used on unseen data.

63

5.2.5 Training and Testing Performances

When using the same data for fitting a model and estimating its performance, the predictive error, called training (or apparent) error, always decreases when the complexity of the model increases (Figure 5.1C). To assess the generalization properties of a model, it needs to be trained and tested on separate datasets. Datasets are generally split into a training dataset used to fit the model, and a testing dataset used to estimate predictive performance. This splitting is crucial to avoid overfitting. The splitting process can be repeated to create multiple splits to train and test the model. The testing performances are then aggregated, allowing us to get more stable estimates of performance.

5.2.6 Resampling Techniques

Instead of splitting the data, resampling methods, such as cross-validation or bootstrapping, can be used to produce appropriate estimates of model performance. These approaches are especially useful when the sample size is not large. Resampling methods typically allow estimation of the generalizable predictive error more reliably than if a single test set was used (6). The overall idea of resampling methods consists in repeatedly fitting the model on a subset of the data and in evaluating its performance on the remaining part of the data.

- *Cross-validation*: In k-fold cross-validation, the samples are randomly partitioned into k (generally 5 or 10) subsets, the folds, of equal size. The model is fitted on all the sample except one fold. Then predictions are made on this fold in order to estimate performance. This procedure is repeated for each fold, and the corresponding k estimates of performance are then summarized. Repeating the k-fold cross-validation process can be used to increase the precision of the estimates.

- *Bootstrapping*: A bootstrap sample is a random sample of the data with replacement (7). Some individuals can be selected several times and others never. The non-selected individuals are referred to as the out-of-bag sample. For each iteration of the bootstrap, a model is built on the selected samples and used to predict the out-of-bag samples. Then, the estimates of performance are summarized.

5.2.7 Tuning Parameters

Some of the models presented in the following sections are extremely flexible and can consequently easily overfit. To control the model complexity, and therefore the bias–variance trade-off, these models have tuning parameters. Classically, these parameters are optimized using resampling methods. The objective is to identify model parameters that yield the best and more realistic predictive performance. A common study design when different models are compared consists in splitting the data in 70% for training and 30% for testing (or 80%/20%). The training dataset is used to train and tune different models, compare their performance, and choose a final one using resampling methods. The testing dataset is used to assess the model's performance. In the specific case of image analyses using DL, where the number of parameters is generally in the order of the millions, overfitting issues are particularly important. Proper resampling methods are therefore crucial and large datasets are also required to be trained reliably.

5.3 THE MAIN MACHINE LEARNING MODELS

ML refers here to a set of methods, including classical hypothesis-based models, as well as extensions and alternative methods that offer greater flexibility to capture patterns in the data (data-driven models). Typically, hypothesis-based models rely on hypothesis and are explanatory. On the other hand, data-driven models do not rely on specific a priori hypotheses and are more exploratory. Both types of model can be used for predictions. Hypothesis-based models have advantages over data-driven models in terms of interpretation and inference, i.e., they estimate coefficients with confidence intervals and p-values. However, they have in return limitations that notably affect their predictive power. First, they rely on equations that imply making assumptions about the relationships between the predictors and the outcome. Second, these equations can lead to a lack of flexibility, which may fail to extract the relevant information from the features. Unless non-linear relationships and interactions are explicitly specified, these models produce linear boundaries between cases and non-cases.

It is important to note that neither ML nor big data solve the fundamental problems of causality in observational data (8). Although they can increase predictive abilities, they only capture associations among variables (even if these associations are complex). Therefore, the risk of spurious associations remains. In the case of DL, the extreme flexibility of the models makes them especially vulnerable to this risk (9).

5.3.1 Hypothesis-Based Models
5.3.1.1 Logistic Model

To model the relationships between an outcome variable Y and predictor X, the logistic model uses a sigmoid transformation (or logit function) that can be written as $\log(p(Y)/(1 - p(Y)) = \alpha + \beta X$. A positive (negative) coefficient β corresponds to a positive (negative) association between the predictors and the outcome. The exponential of the coefficients can be interpreted as the odds ratios. The interpretability of odds ratios is the main advantage of the logistic model. Standard errors of the coefficients are also estimated, which allows confidence intervals to be calculated and a hypothesis to be tested. Additionally, non-linear effects and interactions can be added. Indeed, the linearity assumption can be relaxed using different methods (10), such as polynomial components, smoothing splines, or generalized additive models (GAM). The last option provides a general framework for extending linear modeling by allowing non-linear functions of each variable (11) (Figure 5.2A).

When the number of predictors is larger than the number of individuals, the coefficients of the logistic model cannot be accurately estimated.

One way to limit the number of predictors is to perform a stepwise selection (12). When using stepwise selection, the selection of the predictors to be included in the final model should be based on the Akaike Information Criteria (AIC) (12) rather than on the p-values (13). Another way to limit the number of predictors is to perform dimension reduction on the predictors using principal component analysis (PCA). This approach extracts information by performing a linear combination of predictors into a reduced number of components. These components can then be used as predictors to fit a logistic model. This approach is particularly relevant if the predictors are highly correlated. Correlation among predictors, called multicollinearity, can causes inferential problems (unstable models).

Furthermore, testing many predictors can lead to multiple testing issues. The repeated hypothesis testing is likely to result in a high number of false positives. Two methods are commonly used to correct for that issue by applying a form

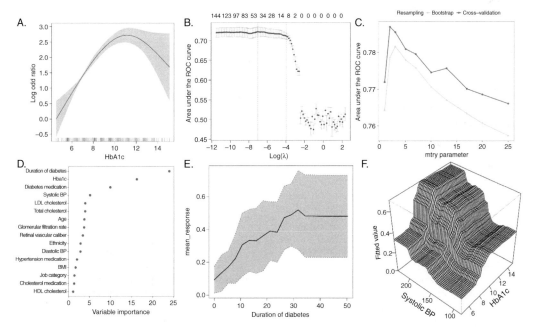

Figure 5.2 (A) Non-linear relationship between glycated hemoglobin (HbA1c) and the risk of diabetic retinopathy (expressed in log odds ratio) estimated using generalized additive models (GAM). (B) Feature selection using least absolute shrinkage and selection operator (LASSO). The lower the value of the penalty (x-axis), the higher the number of predictors selected (on the top of the figure), based on the area under the receiver operating characteristic (ROC) curve. (C) Tuning of the "mtry" parameter (number of randomly selected variables at each split) for a random forest model using bootstrapping and 10-fold cross-validation. (D) Variable importance corresponding to the random forest model with mtry = 3. (E) Partial dependence plot corresponding to the relationship between duration of diabetes and probability of diabetic retinopathy (DR) using a gradient-boosting machine model. (F) Interaction between HbA1c and systolic blood pressure (BP) with the risk of diabetic retinopathy using the gradient-boosting machine model.

of *p*-value correction: Bonferroni correction or the false discovery rate (FDR) (14). Moreover, increasing the number of predictors increases the risk of multicollinearity.

5.3.1.2 Penalized Model

Instead of reducing the number of predictors, penalized models investigate all the predictors simultaneously, even when the number of observations is small. The two most popular techniques are ridge model and least absolute shrinkage and selection operator (LASSO) (15). In the ridge model, the coefficients are shrunk towards zero, which reduces model variance, thereby increasing predictive performance. In LASSO, some of the coefficient estimates are forced to be exactly zero, which leads to variable selection and models that are generally much easier to interpret (Figure 5.2B). Note, however, that the substantial reduction in the variance of predictions comes at the expense of a slight increase in bias. The tuning parameter is the penalty size. The two approaches can be combined if the two penalties are included simultaneously (elastic net) (16). This approach is particularly efficient when the number of predictors is bigger than the number of observations and when the predictors are correlated.

5.3.1.3 Linear Discriminant Analysis and (Orthogonal) Partial Least Square Discriminant Analysis

Linear discriminant analysis (LDA) is another popular model used for classification problems (17, 18). Bayes' rule is used to produce prediction probabilities. LDA may be preferred to the logistic model when *n* is small, when the outcome has more than two classes, and when predictors are correlated. Noticeable disadvantages are that LDA relies on the restrictive assumption of normal distribution of the predictors, and involves parameters that cannot be interpreted in terms of effect size or odds ratios.

When there are more predictors than observations, or when the predictors are extremely correlated, it is recommended to use partial least square (or projection to latent structure) discriminant analysis (PLSDA). The PLSDA runs a partial least square (PLS) before the discriminant analysis. PLS involves reduction of the number of predictors by extracting latent components. PLS finds latent components that simultaneously reduce predictor dimensions and maximize correlation with the outcome. The tuning parameter of PLSDA is the number of latent components retained. Orthogonal partial least square (OPLSDA) is a variant of PLSDA using a different decomposition of variations that can improve the interpretability of the model.

5.3.2 Data-Driven Models

The previous section describes hypothesis-based models that are intrinsically linear, unless non-linear functions are explicitly specified. When the number of predictors is large, it becomes very tedious to add non-linear and interaction terms. Alternatively, data-driven models are non-linear and can learn more complex patterns. The cost of this higher flexibility is that they are overall less interpretable and are more prone to overfitting. These models therefore need to be tuned carefully.

5.3.2.1 K-Nearest Neighbors

The *k*-nearest neighbors (KNN) approach is very intuitive: KNN predicts a new sample using the *k*-closest observations. The prediction corresponds to the most common class among these closest observations. Closeness is determined by a distance metric (e.g., Euclidean, Minkowski). The number of neighbors is the only tuning parameter.

5.3.2.2 Single-Layer Neural Networks

In neural networks, the outcome is modeled by an intermediary set of latent linear combinations of the original predictors, called hidden units. These combinations are transformed by non-linear (logistic) functions. Another linear combination, also non-linearly transformed, connects the hidden units to the outcome. The model derives its name from the analogy with neurons that can be either activated or not. The prediction is made from an integration of the combination of activated neurons. The number of parameters to estimate can become very large; consequently, neural networks tend to overfit. Two tuning parameters control for this issue: weight decay (a penalization method to regularize the model) and the number of hidden units.

5.3.2.3 Multivariate Adaptive Regression Splines

Multivariate adaptive regression splines (MARS) automatically capture non-linear relationships. It uses step functions that break the range of predictors into bins and fit simple constants in each (19). A full set of knots is first identified (potentially highly non-linear). Then, knots not contributing significantly to predictive accuracy are removed using resampling. This process allows us to find the optimal number of knots and the corresponding number of terms to retain in the model. This model also identifies potential interactions between predictors. The two tuning parameters are number of terms retained and the maximum degree of interactions. By tuning the number of terms, MARS performs automated feature selection.

5.3.2.4 Support Vector Machines

A support vector machine (SVM) considers a margin around the classification boundary. It finds the boundary that provides the largest margin between the classes. Because the model relies only on several points close to the boundary, it is robust to outliers. SVM allows some points to be on the wrong side of the margin, and that amount of overlap is the main tuning parameter (called cost). By tuning this parameter, the model finds an optimal trade-off between maximizing the margin and minimizing errors, and thus imposes limits on the model complexity. SVM can also produce very flexible non-linear boundaries by adding non-linear transformation (kernel) of the predictors. Several kernel functions exist, such as radial basis or polynomial, with additional tuning parameters.

5.3.2.5 Tree-Based Methods

Tree-based methods constitute a diverse and popular family of modeling techniques. The most basic one, a decision tree, is highly interpretable and easy to implement. Decision trees split the data into smaller groups that are homogeneous regarding outcome. A widely used decision tree is the classification and regression trees (CART) (20). Trees are very flexible and can capture interactions and non-linear effects. The cost complexity tuning parameter allows optimal tree depth and complexity to be found. However, trees generally have poor predictive performance (high variance).

In order to reduce the variance of predictions, a bootstrap aggregation, called bagging, has been introduced (21). The idea is to combine many trees into a single procedure. Each individual tree has high variance but low bias. Averaging (bagging) these trees reduces the variance and leads to a great improvement in accuracy. However, a limitation of bagged trees is that all the trees are similar and give correlated predictions (tree correlation), which does not allow an optimal variance reduction. Random forests (RFs) overcome this problem by forcing each split to consider only a subset of randomly selected predictors (22). That process reduces tree correlation and produces a more diverse set of trees. The main tuning parameter is the number of randomly selected variables at each split (Figure 5.2C). Boosting is another approach for improving the predictions resulting from a decision tree (23). Shallow trees (weak learners) are grown sequentially: each tree is grown using errors (residuals) made by the previous tree as the outcome. Therefore, each iteration learns a different aspect of the data, focusing on observations that are difficult to classify. The main tuning parameters are: (1) the number of trees; (2) the shrinkage parameter (controls the learning rate); and (3) the interaction depth (corresponding to the number of splits in each tree and controls the complexity). Tree-based models are robust to outliers.

5.3.3 Deep Learning

DL is a subfield of ML. It has emerged over the last decade as a leading methodology for extracting insights from unstructured data such as images, volumetric data, text corpora, or audio signals. The flexibility of DL approaches makes them especially powerful at identifying patterns. These reasons have led to the rapid adoption of DL techniques within the medical imaging community. DL methods are designed to automatically extract features through the learning of successive layers of representations of the data. Automated hierarchical learning is used to extract high-level and complex data representations. Importantly, this circumvents partially the reliance on domain expertise to structure the data. In practice, these DL algorithms are implemented by stacking neural network layers. The "depth" of the algorithm corresponds to the number of these layers of feature extractions. At the time of writing, standard deep neural networks routinely involve tens or hundreds of successive layers. Although artificial neural networks were developed in the 1950s, they were only recently widely adopted. This can be explained by the combination of the development of powerful hardware, the availability of large datasets, and the creation of high-level and user-friendly programming frameworks.

5.3.3.1 DL for Images: CNNs and RNNs

There are several wide classes of neural network architectures that are used in practice. The analysis of ophthalmic images and volumetric data mainly relies on convolutional neural networks (CNNs). In this class of model, each neuron in a given neural layer is connected to only a small region of the previous layer, its "receptive field." Different neurons are specialized to detect and process particular local patterns or textures. Furthermore, these local connectivity patterns greatly reduce the number of parameters necessary to be learned. Each layer can be thought of as a more abstract representation of the previous layer. Figure 5.3 depicts the so-called "U-net" architecture, a particular instance of a CNN, widely used for analyzing medical images.

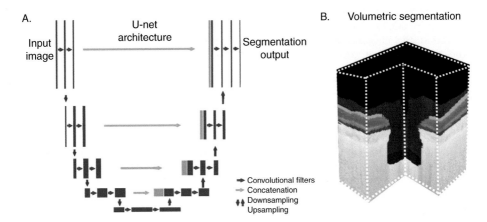

Figure 5.3 (A) "U-net" architecture for segmentation of medical scans and volumetric data. (B) Automated segmentation of a volumetric optical coherence tomography scan of the optic nerve head.

5.3.3.2 DL for Text: RNNs and LSTMs

For the extraction of information contained in text corpora such as medical reports, recurrent neural network (RNNs) architectures such as long short-term memory (LSTMs) (24) and gated recurrent units (GRUs) (25) are tools of choice. These architectures are designed to analyze sequential data and extract long-range dependencies. For example, when used to extract insights from text data, i.e., natural language processing (NLP), words are processed sequentially and the output of the network is fed back into its own input at each consecutive iteration. Consequently, the input of an RNN depends on the current word being processed, but also on all of the information contained in the words previously processed.

5.3.3.3 Calibration Issues

Unlike other methods such as logistic or ML models, deep neural networks often produce predictions that are poorly calibrated: the probabilistic predictions typically do not reflect the observations. Although this important drawback is well known by practitioners, few reliable solutions exist to this day. Methods such as dropout techniques (26), Bayesian methods (27), and ensembling approaches (28) can, at least partly, mitigate these fundamental calibration issues.

5.3.4 Summary of the Main Characteristics of the Models Reviewed

Models have more or less complex and flexible structures, different estimation procedures, and different levels of interpretability. Hypothesis-based models involving coefficients (e.g., logistic model and its penalized versions) and decision trees are the most interpretable models (Figure 5.4). Hypothesis-based models however can lack flexibility. Inversely, data-driven models such as KNN, SVM, and neural networks are the least interpretable (often called "black box" models). The lack of interpretability is the price to pay for the flexibility that leads to improved predictive performance.

An important characteristic when working with big data is the ability of the model to handle a very large number of predictors. In these cases, models performing automatic variable selection can be of interest, such as LASSO, MARS, or some tree-based methods (Figure 5.4). When the number of predictors is higher than the number of observations, specific methods using dimension reduction (PLSDA or OPLSDA) are appropriate. Models like SVM or neural network can also be considered; however, they can be affected by the amount of non-informative predictors (12, 29). An interesting approach can be to use models that can handle very large datasets to explore new patterns and generate new hypotheses. These hypotheses can then be tested using inference from classical models in a setting with fewer predictors.

The following points may be considered to guide which model to choose:

- First and foremost, the choice depends on the objective.

  - If the objective is to test a specific hypothesis, there are clear advantages of using simple and interpretable models, with *p*-value correction for multiple testing if needed.

  - If the objective is to identify possible biomarkers among hundreds or thousands

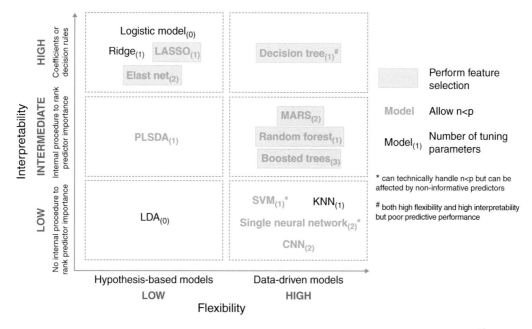

Figure 5.4 Summary of the main characteristics of some selected models. Tuning parameters: logistic model: none; ridge and LASSO models: one penalty; elast net: one penalty and one mixing parameter. LDA: none; PLSDA: number of latent components; KNN: number of neighbors; single-layer neural network: weight decay, number of hidden units; MARS: number of terms, maximum degree of interactions; SVM: cost; decision tree: cost complexity; random forest: number of randomly selected variables; boosted trees: number of trees, learning rate, interaction depth; CNN: number of layers, filter size; LASSO, least absolute shrinkage and selection operator; LDA, linear discriminant analysis; PLSDA, partial least square discriminant analysis; KNN, k-nearest neighbor; MARS, multivariate adaptive regression splines; SVM, support vector machine; CNN, convolutional neural network.

of variables, then models that perform feature selection can be suitable.

- If the objective is only prediction, the lack of interpretability is not an issue and more flexible models may be preferred.

- Moreover, the choice should be made according to the characteristics of the data.

  - If we expect complex data with many non-linear effects and interactions, then tree-based can be relevant.

  - If the number of predictors is higher than the number of observations, then specific methods can be used such as dimension reduction methods (PLSDA or OPLSDA), as well as SVM or neural network.

  - If the data are unstructured, such as images or free text, then DL should be used.

An overall strategy can consist in selecting several models based on these considerations and comparing their performance to choose the most accurate. Nowadays, many user-friendly

software and packages make it possible to compare the performance of a wide range of models without an excessive amount of coding (30).

5.3.5 Interpretability

Interpretability is a key to increasing the acceptance of ML models by the medical community and patients. There is an active area of research for making ML more interpretable (31). For some models, it is possible to calculate a metric called variable importance (VI) (Figure 5.2D), that ranks the predictors in terms of strength or relevance with regard to the outcome. This metric is calculated differently according to the method: using z-statistics for logistic model or using the sum of the reduction in errors across all splits, aggregated across all trees for tree-based methods. Among those presented here, PLSDA, MARS, and penalized models also have their measures of variable importance (Figure 5.4). However, some models like SVM do not have such metrics. Alternatively, model-agnostic metrics can be used like permutation feature importance measurement. This metric measures a feature's importance by calculating the increase in prediction error after randomly permuting the predictors. Another approach to understand how the model makes a prediction is partial dependence, corresponding to the marginal effect of a predictor on the predicted outcome. This allows an understanding of how the outcome changes when a predictor changes while accounting for the average effect of all the other predictors (Figure 5.2E). Furthermore, some methods investigate possible interactions between predictors and plot the corresponding synergetic effect (Figure 5.2F). Finally, some methods help to understand which predictor influences the outcome for a given observation (local interpretable model-agnostic explanations or LIMEs).

Regarding DL, "features visualization" approaches such as saliency maps attempt to make the learned features explicit (32, 33). This type of tool allows an understanding of which features in the images have been leveraged by the model during the prediction process. Standard practices consist in highlighting these crucial features on a heatmap superposed on the input image.

5.4 EXAMPLES OF STATISTICAL METHODS IN BIG DATA

Many ML models are used in ophthalmology (34). We now give examples of studies using omics data, EHR, retinal fundus images, and administrative databases.

5.4.1 Omics Data

Several methods can be used to analyze omics data, ranging from logistic model corrected for multiple testing (35) to more advanced ML models such as SVM, neural networks or tree-based methods (36). We report two examples, one regarding the genetic variants of age-related macular degeneration (AMD) and one regarding the metabolomics signature of primary open-angle glaucoma (POAG). The first study is a genome-wide association study (GWAS) that aimed to identify genetic variants associated with AMD among >12 million rare and common variants in 16,144 advanced AMD cases and 17,832 controls (37). The analyses mainly consisted in the following two steps. First, in order to identify independently associated variants, single-variant associations for each of the >12 million variants were computed, followed by a sequential forward selection approach. A low threshold for p-values was considered to correct for multiple testing ($p \leq 5 \times 10^{-8}$). The 52 variants identified are presented in a Manhattan plot (Figure 5.5A).

Second, in order to estimate independent effect sizes for all identified variants, a logistic model including all identified variants was computed, and a weighted genetic risk score based on these effect sizes was calculated for each individual. From these analyses, the authors concluded that the 52 variants explain 27.2% of disease variability. Moreover, individuals in the highest decile of genetic risk have 44-fold increased risk of developing advanced AMD in comparison to those in the lowest decile (Figure 5.5B).

The second example concerns a study investigating the differential metabolomics signature of 34 patients with POAG compared to 30 age- and gender-matched controls, using liquid chromatography coupled to high-resolution mass spectrometry (160 metabolites in total) (38). In order to identify a relevant metabolomics signature, the authors performed four different approaches and compared the results obtained. First, a univariate analysis was performed using hypothesis testing (Wilcoxon non-parametric test) with FDR correction (threshold at 5%). Second, an OPLSDA was performed (Figure 5.5C) and the variable importance in the projection (VIP) was calculated. Third, an iterative algorithm based on three ML models run in parallel (PLSDA, RF, and SVM) was used to assess the importance of the metabolites. Fourth, a LASSO model was performed using a repeated random splitting scheme ($n = 1,000$) into training (~2/3) and testing (~1/3). The results corresponding to the different methods are presented in a Venn diagram (Figure 5.5D). One metabolite, nicotinamide, was identified by all the methods and was further validated in a replication cohort of 35 individuals, highlighting a potential interest for glaucoma treatment.

5.4.2 Electronic Health Records

EHRs can be seen as multimodal datasets combining structured data such as demographic information or laboratory tests, and unstructured data such as text notes or images. ML applied to EHR has been used to improve ocular disease diagnosis, risk assessment, and disease progression (39). Many different models are used, such as logistic model, decision tree, RF, SVM, boosting, LASSO, DL techniques, and NLP. NLP was for example used to extract information from free-text documents and showed good performance in identifying cataract subjects (positive predictive values >95%) (40). The complexity and heterogeneity of EHR data make them appropriate for DL applications and many DL models have been developed for that purpose (41). Rajkomar et al. have applied DL models on the entire EHR and show that

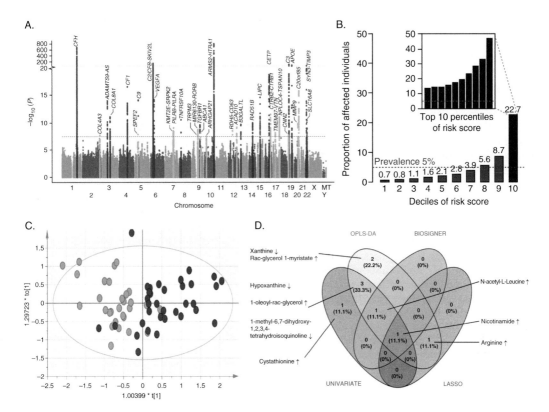

Figure 5.5 (A) Manhattan plot corresponding to a genome-wide single-variant association analysis in 16,144 patients with advanced age-related macular degeneration (AMD) versus 17,832 controls. Genetic variants with p-values $<5 \times 10^{-8}$ (genome-wide significance, horizontal lines in red) are highlighted in green (new AMD loci) and blue (known AMD loci). (B) Proportion of affected individuals based on the 52 identified variants by genetic risk score intervals (deciles and top ten percentiles in embedded bar plot). (C) Score plot for the orthogonal partial least squares discriminant analysis (OPLSDA) model based on the most significant metabolites with control samples in green circles and cases in blue circles. (D) Venn diagram illustrating the global primary open-angle glaucoma (POAG) signature. (Reproduced with permission from Fritsche LG, Igl W, Bailey JNC, Grassmann F, Sengupta S, Bragg-Gresham JL, et al. A large genome-wide association study of age-related macular degeneration highlights contributions of rare and common variants. *Nat Genet*. 2016 Feb;48(2):134–43.)

they can be efficient to predict important clinical outcomes (42). They built a generic data-processing pipeline that can take raw EHR (including clinical notes) as input. Using 216,221 hospitalizations involving 114,003 patients, this system achieved high accuracy for predicting in-hospital mortality (AUC across sites 0.93–0.94), 30-day (AUC 0.75–0.76) or prolonged (AUC 0.85–0.86) readmission, and final discharge diagnosis (AUC 0.90).

5.4.3 Retinal Fundus Images

Several studies have shown that DL systems can accurately detect several eye diseases such as DR, glaucoma, and AMD, as well as

identifying cardiovascular risk factors and diseases (43). For example, the performance of a CNN was evaluated in detecting DR, possible glaucoma, and AMD using 494,661 retinal images from multi-ethnic cohorts of patients with diabetes (44). The authors trained and tuned the DL system for DR detection in a first dataset with images collected in 2010–2013 (76,370 images), performed a primary validation (testing) on the same dataset with images collected in 2014–2015 (71,896 images), and further evaluated it with ten external datasets (40,752 images). The AUC for referable DR was 0.936 (95% confidence interval [CI] 0.925–0.943) in the primary validation dataset, and ranged between 0.889 and 0.983 in the external datasets. Another study used DL on fundus images to predict cardiovascular risk factors (45). The authors trained their CNN model on data from 284,335 patients, and validated (tested) on two independent datasets of 12,026 and 999 patients. They were able to predict age (within 3.26 years), gender (AUC = 0.97), and systolic blood pressure (within 11.23 mmHg). Finally, using heatmaps, they showed that the model used distinct aspects of the anatomy, such as optic disc or blood vessels, to generate each prediction.

5.4.4 Administrative Databases

Administrative data, although not primarily designed for research purposes, can be very useful because of their national coverage. These data offer interesting opportunities for pharmacoepidemiology. For example, South Korea and France have National Health Insurance Services that include almost the entire populations (>97%). However, in such non-randomized studies, the effect of treatment on outcomes can be subject to treatment selection bias in which treated subjects systematically differ from non-treated individuals. In such an observation framework, propensity score (PS) methods are used to reduce bias, i.e., to balance the observed characteristics between the treated and non-treated groups and therefore mimic randomized design (46). For example, the Korean insurance database has been used to investigate whether the long-term regular use of low-dose aspirin is associated with an increased risk of neovascular AMD (47). The authors estimated the PS based on sociodemographic factors and a comorbidity index using a logistic model. This score corresponded to the probability to receive aspirin treatment. Then this score was used: (1) as an adjustment variable in a Cox survival model performed in the entire cohort ($n = 482,613$); and (2) to match treated and non-treated subjects based on their PS (5:1 ratio) and then a Cox survival model was performed in this matched cohort ($n = 74,196$). While the incidence of neovascular AMD was higher among regular aspirin users in the entire cohort, the PS-matched analysis showed no association, suggesting the safety of aspirin use in the development of neovascular AMD.

5.5 CONCLUSION

Many methods have been developed during the past decades to analyze big and complex data commonly generated in clinical practice. There is no single model that performs well in every

situation and these methods form a continuum with traditional methods. All the models have their own advantages and limitations and can be seen as complementary. A good practice consists in selecting several models based on the research question and the characteristics of the data, and comparing their performance to choose the most accurate or relevant. ML models can handle very large datasets and are thus very powerful to explore complex data, find new patterns, and thereby generate hypotheses. The analysis of unstructured data such as images or free text using DL has led to very promising systems for accurate disease detection. However, more research is needed to increase their interpretability and help in their acceptance by physicians and patients. Finally, future research is crucial to evaluate the clinical deployment and cost-effectiveness of AI-based systems in clinical practice.

REFERENCES

1. Raghupathi W, Raghupathi V. Big data analytics in healthcare: promise and potential. *Health Inf Sci Syst*. 2014 Dec [cited 2020 Jun 27];2(1). Available from: http://link.springer.com/10.1186/2047-2501-2-3

2. McCue ME, McCoy AM. The scope of big data in one medicine: unprecedented opportunities and challenges. *Front Vet Sci*. 2017 Nov 16 [cited 2020 Jun 24];4. Available from: http://journal.frontiersin.org/article/10.3389/fvets.2017.00194/full

3. Nusinovici S, Tham YC, Chak Yan MY, Wei Ting DS, Li J, Sabanayagam C, et al. Logistic regression was as good as machine learning for predicting major chronic diseases. *J Clin Epidemiol*. 2020 Jun;122:56–69.

4. Steyerberg EW, Vickers AJ, Cook NR, Gerds T, Gonen M, Obuchowski N, et al. Assessing the performance of prediction models: a framework for traditional and novel measures. *Epidemiol Camb Mass*. 2010 Jan;21(1):128–38.

5. Moons KGM, Altman DG, Reitsma JB, Ioannidis JPA, Macaskill P, Steyerberg EW, et al. Transparent Reporting of a multivariable prediction model for Individual Prognosis or Diagnosis (TRIPOD): explanation and elaboration. *Ann Intern Med*. 2015 Jan 6;162(1):W1–73.

6. Kuhn M, Johnson K. Over-fitting and model tuning. In: *Applied Predictive Modeling*. New York: Springer New York; 2013 [cited 2019 Jul 25]. pp. 61–92. Available from: http://link.springer.com/10.1007/978-1-4614-6849-3_4

7. Efron B, Tibshirani R. Bootstrap methods for standard errors, confidence intervals, and other measures of statistical accuracy. *Stat Sci*. 1986;1(1):54–75.

8. Obermeyer Z, Emanuel EJ. Predicting the future — big data, machine learning, and clinical medicine. *N Engl J Med*. 2016 Sep 29;375(13):1216–19.

9. Lapuschkin S, Wäldchen S, Binder A, Montavon G, Samek W, Müller K-R. Unmasking Clever Hans predictors and assessing what machines really learn. *Nat Commun*. 2019 11;10(1):1096.

10. James G, Witten D, Hastie T, Tibshirani R. Moving beyond linearity. In: *An Introduction to Statistical Learning*. New York: Springer New York; 2013 [cited 2020 Jul 3]. pp. 265–301. Available from: http://link.springer.com/10.1007/978-1-4614-7138-7_7

11. Hastie T, Tibshirani R. Generalized additive models. *Statist Sci*. 1986;1(3):297–318.

12. Kuhn M, Johnson K. An introduction to feature selection. In: *Applied Predictive Modeling*. New York: Springer New York; 2013 [cited 2020 Jun 25]. pp. 487–519. Available from: http://link.springer.com/10.1007/978-1-4614-6849-3_19

13. Harell F. *Regression Modeling Strategies: With Applications to Linear Models, Logistic Regression, and Survival Analysis*. New York: Springer; 2001.

14. Glickman ME, Rao SR, Schultz MR. False discovery rate control is a recommended alternative to Bonferroni-type adjustments in health studies. *J Clin Epidemiol*. 2014 Aug;67(8):850–7.

15. Tibshirani R. Regression shrinkage and selection via the lasso. *J R Stat Soc Ser B Methodol*. 1996 Jan;58(1):267–88.

16. Zou H, Hastie T. Regularization and variable selection via the elastic net. *J R Stat Soc Ser B Methodol*. 2005;67:301–20.

17. Fisher R. The use of multiple measurements in taxonomic problems. *Ann Eugen*. 1936;7(2):179–88.

18. Welch B. Note on discriminant functions. *Biometrika*. 1939;31:218–20.

19. Friedman JH. Multivariate adaptive regression splines. *Ann Stat*. 1991;19(1):1–67.

20. Breiman L, Friedman J, Olshen R, Stone C. *Classification and Regression Trees*. New York: Chapman and Hall; 1984.

21. Breiman L. Bagging predictors. *Mach Learn*. 1996;24:123–40.

22. Breiman L. Random forests. *Mach Learn*. 2001;45(1):5–32.

23. Friedman J, Hastie T, Tibshirani R. Additive logistic regression: a statistical view of boosting. *Ann Stat*. 2000;38:337–74.

24. Gers FA, Schmidhuber J, Cummins F. Learning to forget: continual prediction with LSTM. *Neural Comput*. 2000 Oct;12(10):2451–71.

25. Cho K, van Merriënboer B, Gulcehre C, Bahdanau D, Bougares F, Schwenk H, et al. Learning phrase representations using RNN encoder-decoder for statistical machine translation. *Proc 2014 Conf Empir Methods Nat Lang Process EMNLP*. 2014;1724–34.

26. Gal Y, Ghahramani Z. Dropout as a bayesian approximation: representing model uncertainty in deep learning. *Int Conf Mach Learn*. 2016;1050–9.

27. MacKay D. *Information Theory, Inference and Learning Algorithms*. Cambridge: Cambridge University Press, 2006.

28. Dietterich T. Ensemble methods in machine learning. In *International Workshop on Multiple Classifier Systems*. Berlin: Springer, 2000;1–15.

29. Kuhn M, Johnson K. Nonlinear classification models. In: *Applied Predictive Modeling*. New York: Springer; 2013 [cited 2020 Jun 29]. pp. 329–67. Available from: http://link.springer.com/10.1007/978-1-4614-6849-3_13

30. Kuhn, M. Building predictive models in R using the caret package. *J Stat Softw*. 2008;28(5).

31. Boehmke B, Greenwell B. Interpretable machine learning. In: *Hands-On Machine Learning with R*. New York: Chapman and Hall/CRC; 2019. pp. 305–42.

32. Selvaraju R, Cogswell M, Das A, Vedantam R, Parikh D, Batra D. Grad-cam: visual explanations from deep networks via gradient-based localization. *Proc IEEE Int Conf Comput Vis*. 2017;618–26.

33. Gilpin L, Bau D, Yuan B, Bajwa A, Specter M, Kagal L. Explaining explanations: an overview of interpretability of machine learning. 2018 IEEE 5th *Int Conf Data Sci Adv Anal DSAA*. 2018;80–9.

34. Caixinha M, Nunes S. Machine learning techniques in clinical vision sciences. *Curr Eye Res*. 2017 Jan 2;42(1):1–15.

35. Dunkler D, Sánchez-Cabo F, Heinze G. Statistical analysis principles for omics data. In: Mayer B, editor. *Bioinformatics for Omics Data*. Totowa, NJ: Humana Press; 2011 [cited 2020 Jun 24]. pp. 113–31. Available from: http://link.springer.com/10.1007/978-1-61779-027-0_5

36. McDermott JE, Wang J, Mitchell H, Webb-Robertson B-J, Hafen R, Ramey J, et al. Challenges in biomarker discovery: combining expert insights with statistical analysis of complex omics data. *Expert Opin Med Diagn*. 2013 Jan;7(1):37–51.

37. Fritsche LG, Igl W, Bailey JNC, Grassmann F, Sengupta S, Bragg-Gresham JL, et al. A large genome-wide association study of age-related macular degeneration highlights contributions of rare and common variants. *Nat Genet*. 2016 Feb;48(2):134–43.

38. Kouassi Nzoughet J, Guehlouz K, Leruez S, Gohier P, Bocca C, Muller J, et al. A data mining metabolomics exploration of glaucoma. *Metabolites*. 2020 Jan 28;10(2):49.

39. Lin W-C, Chen JS, Chiang MF, Hribar MR. Applications of artificial intelligence to electronic health record data in ophthalmology. *Transl Vis Sci Technol*. 2020 Feb 27;9(2):13.

40. Peissig PL, Rasmussen LV, Berg RL, Linneman JG, McCarty CA, Waudby C, et al. Importance of multimodal approaches to effectively identify cataract cases from electronic health records. *J Am Med Inform Assoc*. 2012 Mar;19(2):225–34.

41. Shickel B, Tighe PJ, Bihorac A, Rashidi P. Deep EHR: a survey of recent advances in deep learning techniques for electronic health record (EHR) analysis. *IEEE J Biomed Health Inform*. 2018 Sep;22(5):1589–604.

42. Rajkomar A, Oren E, Chen K, Dai AM, Hajaj N, Hardt M, et al. Scalable and accurate deep learning with electronic health records. *Npj Digit Med [Internet]*. 2018 Dec [cited 2020 Jun 24];1(1). Available from: www.nature.com/articles/s41746-018-0029-1

43. Ting DSW, Peng L, Varadarajan AV, Keane PA, Burlina PM, Chiang MF, et al. Deep learning in ophthalmology: The technical and clinical considerations. *Prog Retin Eye Res*. 2019;72:100759.

44. Ting DSW, Cheung CY-L, Lim G, Tan GSW, Quang ND, Gan A, et al. Development and validation of a deep learning system for diabetic retinopathy and related eye diseases using retinal images from multiethnic populations with diabetes. *JAMA*. 2017 Dec 12;318(22):2211.

73

45. Poplin R, Varadarajan AV, Blumer K, Liu Y, McConnell MV, Corrado GS, et al. Prediction of cardiovascular risk factors from retinal fundus photographs via deep learning. *Nat Biomed Eng.* 2018;2(3):158–64.

46. Austin PC. An introduction to propensity score methods for reducing the effects of confounding in observational studies. *Multivar Behav Res.* 2011 May 31;46(3):399–424.

47. Rim TH, Yoo TK, Kwak J, Lee JS, Kim SH, Kim DW, et al. Long-term regular use of low-dose aspirin and neovascular age-related macular degeneration. *Ophthalmology.* 2019 Feb;126(2):274–82.

6 Common Statistical Issues in Ophthalmic Research

Catey Bunce and Gabriela Czanner

6.1 INTRODUCTION

Ophthalmology is a specialty within medicine which is quick to embrace innovation. Innovation within medicine is becoming increasingly multi-professional, bringing together clinicians, scientists – laboratory and computer, statisticians, epidemiologists, and those working within industry such as the pharmaceutical companies and device manufacturers. Increasingly also patients and the public are invited to collaborate in recognition of the fact that medical research places those it seeks to help at the heart of its endeavors. Multi-professional collaboration ensures that the work delivered embraces innovation whilst maintaining scientific and academic rigor so that the public receives optimal benefit, and so that patients are not harmed, their health improves, and resources are used appropriately.

6.1.1 Is Misuse of Statistics Common in Ophthalmic Research?

Whilst multi-professional collaboration offers huge potential and indeed delivers this, on occasion it also presents challenges that need to be acknowledged and overcome. Perhaps the most prevailing challenge is due to professionals having the habit of developing their own terminology. This speeds up communication within the profession but can present difficulties when trying to work across professions [1]. Terms such as correlation and significance may mean one thing to a clinician yet something completely different to a medical statistician. This can result in misunderstanding and indeed errors within the interpretation of data analysis results. Whilst many researchers in the UK are familiar with the phrase "lies, damned lies, and statistics," statistical errors in medicine and healthcare have the potential to lead to patient harm. Professor Doug Altman within the UK has championed the message that "Misuse of statistics in medicine is unethical" since the 1980s [2]. Medical statisticians have felt it their duty to highlight errors but perhaps have not illustrated clearly how these errors can impact upon healthcare. Many mistakes are likely to be made simply as a result of a lack of training. Within medicine there can be a desire to go alone rather than work alongside someone who has spent many years learning how to analyze data and learning what assumptions are necessary for results to be robust. Medical statisticians can instantly see the potential error, as was the case when the paper by Wakefield and colleagues was first published in the *Lancet* [3]. But what was evident (or perhaps predictable logically) to the statistical community was not immediately evident to others because their focus was on different messages from that paper. Many of the issues identified within this chapter might become less common with better communication between different professional disciplines and an acknowledgment that those different professionals may think very differently to each other, which itself presents challenges [4].

To our knowledge there is no evidence to indicate that statistical errors are more common in ophthalmic research than in other areas of medicine. There are particular challenges that the unwary researcher may face when analyzing ophthalmic data but in reality these issues present in other specialties too [5]. Unit of analysis issues feature also in nephrology, dentistry, and research into hearing health problems, for example. Reviews of statistical practice have been conducted within ophthalmic research and these have identified common areas of inappropriate use of statistics [6–8]. This may not mean, however, that ophthalmic research is full of people who cannot do statistics; it merely reflects the fact that applied medical statisticians who care passionately about the appropriate use of statistics just happen to have found themselves working in research in eyes and vision and they are working together to improve the accuracy and reporting of analyses.

It is important to acknowledge that this chapter reflects the current state of play in ophthalmic research. Statistical methodology, like all science, evolves over time and over time issues in translation from statistical theory to applied medicine become evident. Particular methods become fashionable in research; currently we see, for example, Mendelian randomization and propensity score analysis. With increasing use, misuse starts to become evident and then collaborative efforts may be made to stem such errors. An area within medicine which has seen much activity and attempts to reduce misuse of statistical methods is that of method agreement [9].

We have written this chapter based upon what we have seen during our time in ophthalmic research (between 5 and 25 years) but there are new issues arising in the area of big data where computer scientists are introducing artificial intelligence and computer programming which challenge some fundamental statistical

DOI: 10.1201/9781315146737-7

75

tenets. It is essential for the benefit of science not to get angry with each other when seeing our discipline misused but to communicate areas of concern – perhaps highlighting more clearly the potential impact upon people and always to listen – properly!

6.2 WHAT IS STATISTICS AND WHY DO WE USE IT?

We live in a world surrounded by data and there is an enormous push to learn as much and as fast as we can from the data. Whilst when we say or hear the word data we might think of variables captured within a research study (intraocular pressure, retinal thickness, eye color), almost anything that is measured and stored can be viewed as data – the number of times our heart beats, whether we feel better or worse after treatment, the constellation of stars in the sky. In recent years there has been an explosion in the volume of data that we deal with. Whilst genetic analyses, for example, used to focus upon whether or not individuals had particular genes, the unlocking of the human genome has allowed focus to shift to particular mutations within genes. Genome-wide association studies consider many thousands of genes and analyses are now conducted at the protein level [10]. This recent explosion of data highlights the importance of statistics and its two pillars: statistical design of studies and statistical data analysis methods.

Statistical design is about making sure that the data are measured and stored in a meaningful way. Data by itself can be meaningless. Researchers or clinicians will have research questions that they are seeking answers to using the data. They may conduct experiments or observe people and record measurements on people but it is statistical analyses that enable them to convert their data into knowledge that may answer their questions [11]. One needs to be careful when collecting data that the research question can be answered with such data. This means that the design of the study and the methods of measuring the variables must be chosen wisely and with the research question and data analysis methods in mind; otherwise the data may be meaningless.

Different research questions require different study designs and statistical methods in exactly the same way that different conditions require different treatment and different surgical techniques are needed for different ophthalmic conditions. Within this chapter we focus upon the use and misuse of statistical methods but it is important to comment that sometimes errors or issues arise because of imprecise study design and for this we would always advise early discussions with statistical colleagues.

Statistical analysis methods should be agreed at the study design stage. For clinical trials it is now good practice to write a statistical analysis plan in advance of analyzing the data. Typically the first analyses conducted by statisticians when looking at a new dataset will consist of descriptive methods. If an experiment has gathered retinal nerve fiber measures on both eyes of 100 patients the researcher will seek to summarize this information rather than listing all observations. Summarizing data typically involves reporting a measure of central location (the mean or median) and a measure of variability (such as the standard deviation or perhaps the range). Typically, after exploring and describing data, statisticians move to a second type of statistical method – the *inferential* statistical methods where statistical tests of hypotheses (t-tests, Chi-square tests, Wilcoxon signed rank test) and confidence intervals are employed. Such methods convert observations into probabilistic statements that researchers then may use to make diagnostic decisions – this is described in more detail later on in this chapter. Many statistical analyses will involve application of both descriptive and inferential techniques – method agreement studies (where one method of measuring an ocular parameter is compared against another method of measuring the same ocular parameter), meta-analyses (where results from different studies are "pooled") are examples of this.

Predictive (discriminatory, or prognostic) statistical methods are perhaps relatively new methods in use in vision and eye research. These methods are used to make statements about individual patients or eyes rather than groups of individuals. An example would be determining the likelihood that a patient with diabetic eye disease and a particular level of glucose and age will lose sight within 2 years.

Behind each statistical test is robust statistical methodology built on the grounds of mathematics and probability. Each statistical test was created by assuming that data have been captured in a particular fashion (sample size, independence, randomness, representativeness) and that such data follow a characteristic distribution (Gaussian, bimodal, etc.). If the assumed data collection and distribution are satisfied, then we can trust the results of the statistical test. The properties of the statistical test can be further studied to see whether the test is robust to some violations of the assumptions [12].

Whilst it may be seen as desirable, it is not essential to understand the underpinning statistical theory in order to be able to apply and interpret results from statistical tests. It is however, in our opinion, essential to be aware of the assumptions made by statistical tests so that assessment against adherence to such assumptions can be made. If a statistical test assumes that the data follow a particular distribution, an assessment that this is indeed the case is needed. If the data violate the assumption it is possible that the answers provided by the analysis will be incorrect. An assumption that is particularly challenging within ophthalmology is that of independence. Many tests assume independence of observations. The independence of two observations means that the knowledge of one cannot in any way influence knowledge of another. Fellow eyes are never truly independent and so analysis on fellow eyes should not make this assumption [13].

Statistics practice is not black and white in the same way that mathematics is. In mathematics there is often a correct way of doing things and an incorrect way of doing things. In statistical analyses whilst there can indeed be correct and incorrect ways of doing things, sometimes whether one method is correct is based upon a decision as to whether an assumption is adhered to and sometimes this decision is not that clear cut. There may be several ways of approaching a particular data analysis and the result may be the same even though very different methods have been used. The fact that different statisticians use different statistical methods to address a particular research question is often interpreted by other professionals as statisticians disagreeing with each other. In reality there may be no disagreement, just a preference for one approach against another. Sometimes a statistician can fervently believe that their approach is the correct method whilst that taken by another statistician is incorrect. As with all science there can be fierce debate amongst brilliant statisticians but in reality if the answer drawn by these different approaches is the same, does it actually matter?

An area where there has been much debate over time between medical statisticians is in the field of meta-analyses with a choice of fixed or random effects. Random effect modeling has received much criticism from statisticians such as Peto [14] and Petitti [15]. Use of the fixed-effect approach however often leads to spuriously tight confidence intervals and associated lower levels of significance, which merits concern [16]. Many of us lack the theoretical statistical knowledge to truly engage in this debate but equally many of us may feel that if the answer given by two approaches is the same (which, in the absence of heterogeneity, it will be), we may not mind.

As with any subject, the more you know, the more you realize you don't know. What perhaps matters most within medical research is whether the approach that has been taken is sufficiently

statistically correct for the answer to be trusted for clinical decisions.

6.3 COMMON ISSUES IN INFERENTIAL STATISTICAL METHODS

There is evidence of statistical errors in medical research [17]. This is deeply concerning given that the use of statistics in medicine can affect whether people live or die, whether their health is protected or harmed [18]. Having worked for many years in ophthalmic research we have encountered many statistical errors. It is essential to realize, however, that whilst it is important to avoid all statistical errors, some may be viewed as less important and it is helpful therefore when identifying an error to think hard as to whether in making this error the wrong result is reached with an analysis. It is important to realize that simply because you as a statistician might have approached an analysis in a particular manner and that that manner was not the method used within a report made by others, this does not mean that the authors have necessarily made an error. Simply there may be two or more legitimate ways to analyze the data. As commented on earlier, sometimes different statistical approaches are adopted by different statisticians but the result drawn from the analysis is the same. What matters most when considering an error or misuse is to think whether this could lead to a false conclusion. Statistical errors can however result in patients being given an ineffective treatment or not being given a treatment that does work and statistical errors may result in medical science being side-tracked.

6.3.1 Method Agreement

One of the most common issues that we and other statisticians working in ophthalmic research meet is misuse of the correlation coefficient in method agreement studies, i.e., in studies where we investigate if methods of measurements agree with each other or equivalently whether one method of measurement can be changed to another without impacting upon the clinical measurement [19, 20].

Ophthalmic research involves many different measurement techniques and is an area of medicine that has seen huge advances in imaging. Companies rapidly refine their technology and so methods are updated over time. Whilst these amendments may have huge value to researchers, clinicians, and patients, it is important not to overlook the fact that such amendments may be associated with the introduction of measurement error, that is, a difference between the actual value and the measured value. For example, testing a patient with optical coherence tomography using one piece of equipment might yield a different measurement to testing a patient with optical coherence tomography using a different piece of equipment. It may be that one method of measurement yields results which showed reduced variability (because it perhaps averages a greater number of images) but we simply never know this because this would involve being able to measure with complete precision and accuracy and in the real world there are many sources of error or variability – variability introduced by the patient, by the temperature, by the lighting, or by the observer [21].

Whenever making a measurement in medicine and research it is important to think very hard as to whether you are looking at values with high precision and accuracy or values with measurement error. Because there is such high use of technology within medicine and because technology is always evolving, many studies conducted in medicine either seek to establish whether a method of measurement is reliable or to see if one method yields a result that is agreeable with another measurement method. To deliver useful results that have impact, such studies really require collaboration between the physicists who have created the equipment, the clinicians who can determine whether or not differences have clinical relevance, the statistician to quantitatively examine agreement or reliability, the computer scientist who may know how the image has been processed, and others. As stated earlier, such inter-professional collaboration may be challenging since each profession is likely to have developed its own technical jargon and unfortunately the same word may have different meanings within different professions [22]. Physicists may describe measurement error as noise and view it as something to be reduced if possible by perhaps applying Gaussian filters. Statisticians may view the exact same thing as biological variability and seek to identify reasons for this, which might be helpful in learning about why measurement is different in different patients. When a medic speaks of correlation they may be speaking of a general association between two variables but when a statistician speaks of correlation they may be referring to a formal mathematical relationship quantified by a particular statistical parameter. Because of the overlap of language mistakes happen. Correlation coefficients have no place in method agreement studies, and yet many papers in ophthalmic research assume agreement based upon high correlations [23, 24]. Another statistic frequently seen within these studies is the intraclass correlation coefficient (ICC). Different equations exist for the ICC depending on the design of the study and hence they do not yield the same answer on the same dataset. A method might yield a high ICC simply because of large variability between subjects and because of this one cannot reliably infer reliability even with an ICC close to 1 [25]. The most appropriate method to use here is limits of agreement and these, like all other methods, require assessing adherence to assumptions – for this the Bland–Altman plot is inspected [26].

6.3.2 Significance Testing – Clinical Significance Is Not the Same as Statistical Significance

Research in ophthalmology is heavily populated by P-values. Whilst there have been concerted efforts to shift researchers away from the use of P-values towards adoption of confidence intervals, P-values have been here for a long time and are likely to remain [27]. P-values are generated by tests of significance and there are many different types of significance tests. The tests work in a similar fashion and may also be described as hypothesis tests because they operate in a framework which involves declaring the current belief or null hypothesis and an alternative belief or hypothesis. The test computes a test statistic based upon the observed data and then determines by reference to a specific statistical distribution (different for different tests) a P-value – the probability of observing as or more extreme data as that observed under the null hypothesis by chance alone. If the P-value is less than a certain threshold (often set at 0.05), researchers may declare statistical significance and if not, they may describe their results as not being statistically significant at that threshold. In making such a declaration however it is important to acknowledge that one of two mistakes may be made:

1. A type I error where a statistically significant difference is declared whereas in reality there is no difference

2. A type II error where a researcher declares the difference to be not statistically significant whereas in reality there is a difference

The chance of making a type I error is called alpha and this is the threshold of significance. If statistical significance is declared at a P-value of 0.05, the chance of making a type I error is 5%.

The chance of making a type II error is called beta and this depends on the effect and sample size. The effect size is the value that is used to indicate difference between groups – for example, in a study looking at treatments for glaucoma with a primary outcome of intraocular pressure, the effect size may be the mean difference in intraocular pressure between treated and untreated patients at 12 months after randomization. A trial comparing treatments for age-related macular degeneration may look at the number of patients who gain vision and the effect size may be the odds ratio comparing the odds of sight gain in a treated group versus that in an untreated group. The sample size is the number of patients (or eyes, dependent on the unit of analysis) in the analysis. Because of the dependence of the P-value on sample size, when analyzing large datasets even very small effect sizes may be declared statistically significant and similarly, if analyzing a very small dataset, statistical significance is unlikely to be achieved even where there is a large effect size. Some effect sizes matter clinically, while others do not; for example, a difference between groups in intraocular pressure of 1 mmHg may not matter clinically whilst one of 10 mmHg may do. It is important therefore to clearly distinguish statistical significance from clinical significance and yet in ophthalmic research this is not always done. The mantra is that *statistical significance is not the same as clinical significance.*

6.3.3 Absence of Evidence Does Not Mean Evidence of Absence

A non-significant P-value does not mean that there is not a clinically relevant difference. A non-significant P-value may be a result of an underpowered study because the probability of not rejecting the null hypothesis when it is true, beta, depends also on sample size. 1-beta is called the power of a test and whenever declaring non-significance it is important to consider the power of the study to detect a difference of a magnitude that has clinical importance. A common statistical issue in ophthalmic research is declaring that there is no difference between treatments when in reality the study simply lacked the power to detect a difference. This issue was highlighted within a paper by Altman and Bland: "absence of evidence is not evidence of absence" [28]. It was repeated with ophthalmic examples by Bunce et al. [29].

If a study declares non-significance, researchers are asked to identify the research question, identify the null hypothesis, compute the effect size with a 95% confidence interval, then consider the implications of changing practice if in reality the truth is the upper or lower bound of the confidence interval. An example of this might be a trial exploring whether or not posturing is needed for patients undergoing vitrectomy surgery. The null hypothesis here would be that there is no difference between the risk of failure in patients posturing face down after surgery and the risk of failure in patients not posturing after surgery. Suppose a clinical trial is then conducted with 200 patients in each arm of the study. In the face-down group, 1 patient requires additional surgery because their macular hole reopens. In the non-posturing group, 2 patients require repeat surgery. The odds ratio for this would be 2.02, with a confidence interval of 0.18–22.3. The P-value would be 0.999. This is a non-statistically significant result but does that mean that there is no requirement for patients to posture after surgery? There were twice as many patients in the non-posturing group who required repeat surgery and if we look at the confidence interval we see that although the data are consistent with there being no difference in risk between trial arms, there is much uncertainty attached to the estimate and the risk of failure in the non-posturing arm might actually be as much as 22 times greater than in the posturing arm.

6.3.4 Multiplicity

Earlier within this chapter it was stated that when a test of significance at the conventional 5% significance level is conducted, there is a 1 in 20 chance (or 0.05 probability) of concluding that there is significance when there is no real difference and a $1 - 0.05$ or 0.95 chance of being non-significant. If two tests of significance are conducted, the probability that neither is significant is $0.95 \times 0.95 = 0.90$. If 14 independent tests of significance were to be conducted, the probability that none is statistically significant would be $0.95^{14} = 0.49$ and the probability that at least one is significant is $1 - 0.49 = 0.51$. What we are demonstrating here is that if many tests of significance are conducted it is highly likely that there will be a spurious statistically significant result. This is called the multiplicity issue (or multiple test, or multiple comparison issue) and is discussed with ophthalmic examples by Cipriani et al. [30]. There are statistical adjustments that can be applied to deal with this. The one perhaps most widely known is the Bonferroni test, which simply divides the P-value of the significance test by the number of tests conducted. This adjustment has disadvantages in that it overcorrects if there are a large number of statistical tests or if these tests are related to each other.

It is not mandatory to always adjust for multiple testing. If the presented research work is clearly stated as exploratory and an acknowledgment is made that the research is being conducted in order to generate a hypothesis for further testing, then multiple test corrections may not be needed. It is best however to avoid multiple testing. Multiplicity is very commonly seen in genome-wide association studies where a very large number of genetic markers are tested. Here strict adjustment has become standard practice and a genome-wide significance level of

5×10^{-8} is often adopted. In bio-informatics studies more sophisticated multiple correction adjustments are made which allow for the non-independence of tests with specific software developed, such as Myriads, to cope with this issue [31].

6.3.5 Missingness

Whilst mistakes are often made in analyzing data, missing data have the real potential to skew findings and result in incorrect conclusions being drawn. Missing data occur in a variety of ways in ophthalmic research. Validated questionnaires may be used where a scoring algorithm is provided based upon answers to each question. Unfortunately, patients do not always provide answers to every question that they are asked. They may be embarrassed or misunderstand the question. They may view the information being asked as personal and not wish to share this with researchers. For a variety of reasons, they may leave a question blank. Researchers' hand-writing may be impossible to read so that even though an attempt has been made to answer a question, the data entry clerk is unable to trans-late the paper answer to an electronic answer and thus it is missing from the analysis. There may be a computer error which overwrites an answer or if electronic tablets are being used for data capture an error in the mobile network may result in lost data. In a clinical trial there may be a plan to do many different measurements on patients using sophisticated imaging equipment. No technology is immune from failure and there may be times during a trial when the imaging kit is not working and so subjects are unable to have these assessments made at the correct timing, thus leading to missing data.

All data on a particular patient may be absent at the final follow-up for a clinical trial – perhaps because the patient has moved to a different country or perhaps because the patient has suffered a serious adverse reaction to the drug being tested. This missing-data example is one which can cause huge issues within ophthalmic research. Suppose, for example, a trial was being conducted to compare two drugs which aim to decrease central retinal thickness in patients with diabetic eye disease. Suppose that 300 patients were included in such a trial – 150 are randomly allocated to treatment A and 150 are randomly allocated to treatment B. The primary outcome measure is assessed at 6 months after randomiza-tion. Data are available for 147 patients treated with drug A and 145 patients treated with drug B and show that retinal thickness is statistic-ally significantly lower with drug B. Suppose, however, that the 3 patients who were lost to follow-up on drug A had simply moved away

but all 5 patients on drug B had suffered side effects. If attention is placed solely on the avail-able data a recommendation to adopt treatment B may be made. Additional information on the subjects who originally did not provide data has changed the likelihood of treatment B being recommended. This issue is explored in greater detail by Bunce et al. [32].

Clinical trials are often analyzed according to an intention to treat (ITT) principle. In full this means that all patients are analyzed in the groups to which they were randomized even if they do not take the medication to which they have been randomized (perhaps because of harm). An ITT analysis is conducted so that the trial provides an estimate of effectiveness rather than efficacy. We may wish to know whether prescribing a particular treatment will have a particular result but if patients do not comply within the confines of a clinical trial it is highly unlikely that they would comply within the real world. By ana-lyzing patients in the groups to which they were randomized we get a more robust esti-mate of real-world effectiveness. Note, however, that the definition of ITT states that all patients randomized are analyzed. All patients are needed to ensure that balance provided by ran-domization is preserved at the point of analysis. If patients have been lost to follow-up we can no longer be sure that the groups are balanced in the way that they would be if we were to have all patients. Because of this, statistical methods have been introduced to impute data. In effect this may be viewed as "making up" data but the making up is based upon stringent statistical methodology aimed to ensure that there is little bias attached. Each method of imputation will be based upon assumptions and it is essential to state what assumptions are being made so that readers can assess whether they believe these to be credible.

Whilst missing data are being given stringent attention within clinical trials, it is important to remember their potential effect on studies of other design also. Epidemiological studies such as a case–control study may provide an incorrect answer if there is a systematic reason for missing data. Consider. for example, a case–control study where the cases examined within the study were "survivors." Individual cases who had perhaps smoked a lot had died. If one were only to use available case data here one might conclude that smoking was good for you.

If the fact that an observation is missing is unrelated to the observed and unobserved data, the data are said to be missing completely at random (MCAR). If data are MCAR then an ana-lysis of the available data will not yield an incor-rect answer, merely one which has less precision than if all the data were to be used. This might however be the difference between a finding that is statistically significant and one which is not [33].

Missingness is important also within big data analytics. Often such studies commence with the promise of bringing together very large and unique datasets – linking microbiome data with bioinformatic datasets with biobank datasets with clinical phenotype data that have been captured as part of electronic patient records. In practice however often the different databases may have captured data in very different ways. Consider, for example, the case where visual field has been captured in several databases. One of the databases has captured this as mean deviation whilst the other has captured it as a categorical variable classifying subjects as having lost central visual field, peripheral visual field, or having a full visual field. Whilst both datasets have captured variables that relate to visual field assessment, they do not have the same data and so merging is not possible unless someone transforms data, which can be hugely time consuming or require considerable programming. Datasets are often initiated at different time points so that although each may be very large indeed, the number of patients who have data common to all is small. As a result, whilst at the outset it appeared that there would be a huge volume of data, the analysis is actually conducted on a much smaller subset. Whilst this may be mentioned within a manuscript it is rare to find the potential impact of this missingness considered in full detail. If it is not, then the answers delivered by such analyses may be incorrect and erroneous.

6.3.6 Unit of Analysis

Perhaps the most obvious statistical issue within ophthalmic research is the non-independence of fellow eyes [34]. For a variety of reasons, including stereoscopic vision and greater visual field, humans have evolved with two eyes. Whilst having two eyes offers advantages for humanity, it presents challenges to researchers in ophthalmology who, unlike their colleagues in cardiology, will routinely face unit of analysis issues. Many statistical tests, for example the t-test, linear regression, and analysis of variance, make an assumption of independence of observations. Clearly however observations on fellow eyes are not independent of each other. If an analysis includes both eyes of any individual it needs to account for this non-independence. That said, having two eyes offers the opportunity for a paired study design – where one eye is treated in one manner and the fellow eye is treated in another manner. Use of the paired design may result in fewer patients needing to be recruited to a study because fellow eyes will be more similar genetically and environmentally to each other, allowing an analysis of treatment without adjusting for such genetic and environmental confounders as such confounders are adjusted for by the paired design. It is however very important to think hard as to whether a paired design will work in practice. If treatment is given to one eye, might it nevertheless impact upon outcome in the fellow eye either by leaking into the circulatory system or as a result of some systemic response to change in one eye?

Fortunately for researchers, statistical methods which allow for non-independence or make use of pairing are now more commonly available. There is evidence however that these methods are not being adopted [35]. Clearly if a study is being conducted within ophthalmology, the primary outcome is not always measured at the level of the eye. Quality-of-life scores, measured by validated questionnaires, are becoming more common and these are for obvious reasons measured at the patient level. Clearly in such studies it makes no sense to treat one eye in one manner and the fellow eye in another. Whilst some conditions are typically bilateral (glaucoma, macular degeneration), others are typically unilateral (trauma, ocular melanoma).

Sometimes it is obvious why one eye has been affected and not the other (e.g., trauma) but sometimes it is not obvious. Why, if fellow eyes are so similar in relation to genetics and environment, does one eye develop pathology but not the other? Why does glaucoma occur first in one eye and then in another [36]? These questions challenge our understanding of the similarity between eyes but it is possible that a genetic mutation has occurred within one eye that protects against a particular condition. The blood flow to fellow eyes may not be identical or even if it is, perhaps a clot has developed within the blood supply to one eye but not the other. Whenever reviewing or designing a study in eyes and vision it is important to identify whether or not one eye per patient will be used (this would present a loss of information) or both eyes of all patients and some patients contributing one eye and others contributing both eyes (this can make analysis more challenging). It is important to ensure that the analysis used reflects the design that has been adopted. For example, if a study has randomized one eye to one treatment and the fellow eye to another treatment, the analysis comparing outcome between the two must allow for the pairing of data. Cluster methods are used when both eyes are included and treated in the same manner because clearly fellow eyes are supplying less information about variability amongst patients than two eyes from two different people.

If reviewing an abstract or a manuscript it should be explicit how many eyes have been analyzed and how many patients these eyes have come from. It is important because this can impact upon the analysis, and this can impact upon the results and therefore the interpretation.

6.3.7 Reliance upon Statistical Testing to Establish Normality

There are statistical tests that can be used to examine whether or not there is evidence of departure from normality for a particular variable. Some researchers place absolute trust in such tests without remembering the need to consider the amount of data when interpreting statistical significance. If you have a very large dataset, these tests of significance may indicate evidence of non-normality but it may not be of a magnitude that will impact upon the statistical methods used because many are robust to non-normality, especially in large sample sizes. If the dataset is small, running such tests may be problematic because they are likely to be non-statistically significant, which is interpreted as no evidence of non-normality when actually the data skewed (the test simply lacks power because there are insufficient data). This is why many statisticians advise use of histograms to make a decision as to whether or not data follow a normal distribution (if it is normal the histogram will show an approximate bell-shaped distribution). One way to identify whether data are normal or not is to compute the standard deviation (SD) and the mean. If the data can only take positive values – duration of symptoms, intraocular pressure, central retinal thickness – none of these can be negative, as would be inferred by an interval that spans mean – 1.96 SD to the mean + 1.96 SD, so if the mean is less than SD/2, it can be deduced that data are skewed and it is not OK to use the mean and SD.

6.4 COMMON ISSUES IN DESCRIPTIVE STATISTICAL METHODS

6.4.1 Use of the Mean with Skewed Data

If a histogram of the data is constructed and that histogram is skewed to the right or left (i.e., a few very large or very small values), the mean will be pulled towards these few outlying values and because of this the median would be a better measure of central location. An example of this might be the time between a minor ocular trauma and the person afflicted seeking medical attention. Whilst many people might seek help very rapidly there may be some patients who

resist seeking medical care unless symptoms persist or get worse. If the injury occurred whilst someone was doing something that they might wish not to disclose they may wait a considerable time before seeking help. If the mean is reported as the measure of central location of the population time to seeking medical attention, it will not reflect the typical time value because it is drawn towards the outlier (the patient wishing to keep the nature of their injury private). Because of this pull towards the outlier, the mean time would actually be larger than most of the time data that have been observed. In such a situation the median would be a more appropriate measure.

6.4.2 Use of the Standard Error Instead of the Standard Deviation

A measure of variability that is frequently used when describing data is the *standard deviation*. This is typically abbreviated to SD. Standard deviations are often used because continuous data often follow a normal distribution and if this is the case then statistical theory can be used to demonstrate that 95% of the data will lie between the mean – 1.96*SD and the mean + 1.96*SD. A value which sounds similar to the SD is the standard error, which may be abbreviated to SE. The standard error is *not* the same as the standard deviation. The standard error is used to reflect the uncertainty about a population parameter (such as the mean) and its dependency on the sample size whilst the standard deviation informs us about the spread of data. One of the reasons that the standard error might be chosen is that it is always smaller than the standard deviation – its use might therefore suggest less variability amongst measurements. If previous researchers have reported the SE then adopting the SD for your paper might suggest to reviewers who are unaware of the misuse of standard errors that your data have more variability and hence are less robust. A particular challenge is faced when researchers have inadvertently labeled standard errors standard deviations because they simply assume that error is another term for deviation and that the two are identical. This is an example of the challenges presented when terms have a special meaning within statistics that they may not have outside of statistics.

6.4.3 Use of the Term ± When Reporting a Standard Deviation

Data from a normal distribution are often summarized using the parameters of the normal distribution – the mean and SD. Many ophthalmic papers will report the mean and SD using the notation mean ± SD. This causes issues in interpretation since there is nothing special about the interval of a mean – SD to the mean +SD (it simply covers 68% of the data, which has little intuitive meaning). Because of this, authors are encouraged to use the notation mean (SD). Some journals (such as the *British Medical Journal*) may insist on such notation. Many do not. Whilst we would advocate reporting data using the terminology mean (SD), we would advise that use of the term ± is not incorrect – it is merely misleading. If therefore you are (wrongly ☺) advised that you must use it by researchers more senior than you or indeed journal editors, it is worth reassuring yourself of this.

6.4.4 Too Many Decimal Places

If a device measures to the nearest mmHg it is questionable whether it makes sense to report results which are not rounded up or down to the nearest mmHg. Similarly, when researchers report mean number of tablets taken by patients and provide results to the third decimal place, it is important to question the logic in doing this. Whilst it might be possible to halve a tablet, cutting it into hundredths seems unlikely and thus researchers are always encouraged to think hard about whether what they are presenting is grounded in reality. Spurious precision adds little to a paper and in fact detracts from its readability and so should be discouraged.

6.5 SUMMARY

This is absolutely not a comprehensive guide to every statistical issue that might arise in ophthalmic research. As indicated at the start of this chapter, statistics, just like medicine, is an evolving science. New tests are developed, perhaps because methodologists identify weaknesses in a test that is in current use or because someone develops a novel way of using data better. Issues in use become evident over time – perhaps in the same way that rare side effects are identified over time by large phase IV clinical trials. Fewer issues would be likely to arise if only those with formal statistical training used such methods; however it is not always easy to identify a colleague with the necessary skills and there are many training courses available on the internet which might allow people to feel that they do indeed have appropriate training. Whenever using a statistical test, check that the assumptions necessary for its use are adhered to – in the same way that you would check that medicines are applied to the right patient. If a test is used with scant regard to assumptions, then incorrect answers may arise and such answers might impact upon patients and the public.

Remember that whenever making a decision based upon a *P*-value you may be making a type I error – you may get statistical significance where there is none – or a type II error – you may not get statistical significance when in reality there is a true difference between groups or a true relationship between variables. Remember too that clinical significance is not the same as statistical significance.

Everyone makes mistakes. Indeed, "To err is human" is the title of the report from the Institute of Medicine on medical errors [37]. Fortunately, many mistakes leave no lasting impact and we learn from the experience. Statistical errors in medicine can and do on occasion result in harm to patients – a message most eloquently championed by Professor Doug Altman [2]. Despite attention being drawn to this in the 1980s, statistical errors continue to occur in the medical literature [38]. Professor Altman died in June 2018 and this has left a huge gap in the applied statistical community. His legacy remains however and we can demonstrate support for him by checking assumptions, reading his statistical notes in the *British Medical Journal*, and speaking out, politely, when we see misuse of statistics in medicine.

REFERENCES

1. Mankoff SP, Brander C, Ferrone S, Marincola FM. Lost in translation: obstacles to translational medicine. *J Transl Med.* 2004 May 18;2(1):14.
2. Altman DG. Statistics and ethics in medical research. Misuse of statistics is unethical. *Br Med J.* 1980 Nov 1;281(6249):1182–4.
3. Wakefield AJ, Murch SH, Anthony A, Linnell J, Casson DM, Malik M, Berelowitz M, Dhillon AP, Thomson MA, Harvey P, Valentine A, Davies SE, Walker-Smith JA. Ileal-lymphoid-nodular hyperplasia, non-specific colitis, and pervasive developmental disorder in children. *Lancet.* 1998 Feb 28;351(9103):637–41.
4. Greenfield T. Communicating statistics, *JR Stat Soc (A)* 1993;156, Part 2:287–97.
5. Coleman AL. The role of statistics in ophthalmology. *Am J Ophthalmol.* 2009 Mar;147(3):387–8.
6. Lee CF, Cheng ACO, Fong DYT. Eyes or subjects: are ophthalmic randomized controlled trials properly designed and analysed? *Ophthalmology.* 2012 Apr;119(4):869–72.
7. Karakosta A, Vassilaki M, Plainis S, Elfadl NH, Tsilimbaris M, Moschandreas J. Choice of analytic approach for eye-specific outcomes: one eye or two? *Am J Ophthalmol.* 2012 Mar;153(3):571–9.
8. Murdoch IE, Morris SS, Cousens S. People and eyes: statistical approaches in ophthalmology. *Br J Ophthalmol.* 1998 Aug;82(8):971–3.
9. Bunce C. Correlation, agreement and Bland Altman analysis – statistical analysis of method comparison studies. *Am J Ophthalmol.* 2009 Jul;148(1):4–6.
10. Baek JH, Lim D, Park KH, Chae JB, Jang H, Lee J, Chung H. Quantitative proteomic analysis of aqueous humor from patients with drusen and reticular pseudodrusen in age-related macular degeneration. *BMC Ophthalmol.* 2018 Nov 7;18(1):289.

11. Pocock JL, Kerry SM, Galise RR. *Presenting Medical Statistics from Proposal to Publication* (2nd edition). Oxford: Oxford University Press, 2017.

12. Wasserman LA. 2004. *All of Statistics: A Concise Course in Statistical Inference*. New York: Springer Science+ Business Media,

13. Bunce C, Patel KV, Xing W, Freemantle N, Doré CJ, Ophthalmic Statistics Group. Ophthalmic statistics note 1: unit of analysis. *Br J Ophthalmol.* 2014 Mar;98(3):408–12.

14. Peto R. Why do we need systematic overviews of randomized trials? *Stat Med* 1987;6:233–240.

15. Petitti DB. *Meta-Analysis Decision Analysis and Cost-Effectiveness Analysis. Methods for Quantitative Synthesis in Medicine*. New York: Oxford University Press, 1994.

16. Ntzani EE, Rizos EC, Ioannidis JP. Genetic effects versus bias for candidate polymorphisms in myocardial infarction: case study and overview of large-scale evidence. *Am J Epidemiol* 2007;165:973–84.

17. Strasak AM, Zaman Q, Pfeiffer KP, Göbel G, Ulmer H. Statistical errors in medical research – a review of common pitfalls. *Swiss Med Wkly.* 2007 Jan 27;137(3–4):44–9.

18. Gardenier JS, Resnik DB. The misuse of statistics: concepts, tools, and a research agenda. *Account Res.* 2002 Apr-Jun;9(2):65–74.

19. Patton N, Aslam T, Murray G. Statistical strategies to assess reliability in ophthalmology. *Eye (Lond).* 2006 Jul;20(7):749–54.

20. Bunce C. Correlation, agreement and Bland Altman analysis – statistical analysis of method comparison studies. *Am J Ophthalmol.* 2009 Jul;148(1):4–6.

21. Fujimoto JG, Pitris C, Boppart SA, Brezinsk ME. Optical coherence tomography: an emerging technology for biomedical imaging and optical biopsy. *Neoplasia.* 2000 Jan; 2(1–2): 9–25.

22. Gardenier JS. Recommendations for describing statistical studies and results in general readership science and engineering journals. *Sci Eng Ethics.* 2012 Dec;18(4):651–62.

23. Altman DG, Bland JM. Measurement in medicine: the analysis of method comparison studies. *Statistician* 1983. 32; 307–12.

24. Dewitte K, Fierens C, Stockl D, Thienpont LM. Application of the Bland–Altman plot for interpretation of method comparison studies: a critical investigation of its practice. *Clin Chem.* 2002 May;48:799–801.

25. Bruton A, Conway JH, Holgate ST. Reliability: what is it, and how is it measured? *Physiotherapy.* 2000;86:94–9.

26. Bland JM, Altman DG. Statistical methods for assessing agreement between two methods of clinical measurement. *Lancet.* 1986;i:307–10.

27. Wasserstein RL, Lazar NA. The ASA's statement on p-values: context, process, and purpose. *Am Statist.* 2016;70(2):129–33.

28. Altman DG, Bland JM. Absence of evidence is not evidence of absence. *BMJ.* 1995 Aug 19;311(7003):485.

29. Bunce C, Patel KV, Xing W, Freemantle N, Doré CJ, Ophthalmic Statistics Group. Ophthalmic statistics note 2: absence of evidence is not evidence of absence. *Br J Ophthalmol.* 2014 May;98(5):703–5.

30. Cipriani V, Quartilho A, Bunce C, Freemantle N, Doré CJ, Ophthalmic Statistics Group. Ophthalmic statistics note 7: multiple hypothesis testing—to adjust or not to adjust. *Br J Ophthalmol.* 2015 Sep;99(9):1155–7.

31. Carvajal-Rodríguez A. Myriads: P-value-based multiple testing correction. *Bioinformatics.* 2018 Mar 15;34(6):1043–5.

32. Bunce C, Quartilho A, Freemantle N, Doré CJ, Ophthalmic Statistics Group. Ophthalmic statistics note 8: missing data—exploring the unknown. *Br J Ophthalmol.* 2016 Mar;100(3):291–4.

33. Bell ML, Fairclough DL. Practical and statistical issues in missing data for longitudinal patient-reported outcomes. *Stat Methods Med Res.* 2014;23:440–59.

34. Bunce C, Patel KV, Xing W, Freemantle N, Doré CJ, Ophthalmic Statistics Group. Ophthalmic statistics note 1: unit of analysis. *Br J Ophthalmol.* 2014 Mar;98(3):408–12.

35. Zhang HG, Ying G. Statistical approaches in published ophthalmic clinical science papers: a comparison to statistical practice two decades ago. *Br J Opthalmol* 2018 Sept 102(9) 1188–91.

36. Poinoosawmy D, Fontana L, Wu JX, Bunce CV, Hitchings RA. Frequency of asymmetric visual field defects in normal-tension and high-tension glaucoma. *Ophthalmology.* 1998 Jun;105(6):988–91.

37. Institute of Medicine. *To Err is Human: Building a Safer Health System*. Washington, DC: National Academy of Sciences, 1999.

38. Diong J, Butler AA, Gandevia SC, Héroux ME. Poor statistical reporting, inadequate data presentation and spin persist despite editorial advice. *PLoS One.* 2018 Aug 15;13(8):e0202121.

PART II
UPDATES ON EPIDEMIOLOGY OF EYE DISEASES

7 Refractive Errors, Myopia, and Presbyopia

Ka Wai Kam, Chi Pui Pang, and Jason C. S. Yam

7.1 INTRODUCTION

Refractive errors are a group of ophthalmic disorders that individually or in combination affect individuals of all ages and ethnicities in both sexes. When the optical system in an eye fails to bring incoming light into focus on the retina, the resultant image perceived by the individual becomes blurred. Refractive errors can be classified into three main types: myopia, astigmatism, and hyperopia. There is also presbyopia, which literally means aging vision, and affects people at a later stage in life, usually in the fifth decade. It is sometimes included as a fourth type of refractive error, although it may be regarded not as an error of refraction because it is due to the loss of accommodation by the lens.

Untreated or under-corrected refractive errors during visual development may lead to amblyopia and strabismus. Furthermore, myopia poses one of the greatest challenges in public health as its prevalence has surged among children and young adults, particularly in East Asian countries in recent years. Myopia, especially high myopia that exerts the highest risk to permanent visual impairment, is associated with serious ophthalmic complications, including myopic macular degeneration (MMD), retinal detachment (RD), open-angle glaucoma (OAG), and cataracts.[1-3] As myopia afflicts people with these complications during their working age, it poses a heavy burden for both individuals and society in health and finance, creating enormous personal and societal impacts across the world. This chapter reviews the epidemiology of refractive errors globally, including a discussion on the reasons for their increased prevalence, risk factors, and prevention strategies.

7.2 MYOPIA

Myopia is the most common ocular disorder worldwide.[4] It is commonly defined as a spherical equivalent refraction (SER) of −0.50 D or less in either eye. High myopia is further defined as a SER of −6.00 D or less. Axial myopia is associated with excessive axial elongation of the globe. Notably, globe elongation, especially in high myopia, leads to vision-threatening complications, including MMD, RD, OAG, and cataracts.[2, 3, 5] A recent meta-analysis reveals that low, moderate, and high myopia are all associated with increased risks of ophthalmic complications at various degrees, including MMD (odds ratio [OR] = 13.57, 72.74, and 845.08

respectively), RD (OR = 3.15, 8.74, and 12.62), posterior subcapsular cataract (OR = 1.56, 2.55, and 4.55), nuclear cataract, and OAG (OR = 1.59 and 2.92 in low and moderate to high myopia respectively).[3]

7.2.1 Prevalence of Myopia
7.2.1.1 Prevalence of Myopia in Children
Myopia prevalence in preschool children, usually 6 years of age or younger in most societies, is in general lower than that of older children (Table 7.1). Among Chinese children it was 6.32% for 2–6-year-olds in Hong Kong in 2007[6] and 6.4% for 5–6-year-olds in Singapore in 2010.[7] Notably, the prevalence was lower in two Chinese cities according to more recent reports, 1.3% in Shenzhen in 2017[8] and 3.5% in Shanghai in 2016,[9] both for children aged 5 years. In the western population, it was 1.1% among those aged between 6 months and 6 years in Baltimore, USA, in 2009.[10] In the Multi-Ethnic Pediatric Eye Disease Study (MEPEDS) reported in 2013, myopia prevalence was 1.2% in non-Hispanic whites, 3.7% in Hispanics, 3.98% in Asians, and 6.6% in African Americans.[11]

Myopia prevalence starts to increase in children after they enter primary school at around 6 years of age, with regional and ethnic variations (Table 7.1). In 2020, the Hong Kong Children Eye Study (HKCES) reported a myopia prevalence of 12.7% at 6 years of age, 24.4% at 7 years, and 36.1% at 8 years.[12] In the Singapore SCORM study reported in 2002, the myopia rates were 29.0% at 7 years, 34.7% at 8 years, and 53.1% at 9 years.[13] In another city, Taipei, in Taiwan, the population-based Myopia Investigation Study revealed a myopia rate of 36.4% in 2016 among children aged 7 years (second-graders in primary school).[14]

In rural areas, myopia prevalence is lower. In Chinese children, it was[15] 7.7% for 7-year-olds in Guangzhou (urban)[15] and 14.3% in Shanghai (urban),[9] compared with only 3.9% in Anyang (rural).[16] Among teenagers aged 15 years, it was 78.4% in Guangzhou (urban),[17] and lower at 43.0% in Yangxi (rural).[17] Similarly, in India, it was higher in the city of Delhi (urban) at 15.3%,[18] compared with 6.72% in Mahabubnagar (rural).[19] A systemic review reported the myopia rate of Indian children younger than 15 years as 5.3%, breaking down to 10.8% in urban dwellings and 3.5% in a rural environment.[20] Overall, myopia prevalence is lower in less densely populated

DOI: 10.1201/9781315146737-9

Table 7.1 Myopia prevalence of children and adolescents in epidemiology studies based on cycloplegic refraction

Location of study	Study year	Ethnicity	Age (years)	Sample size	Definition of myopia	Prevalence	Age-specified prevalence
Hong Kong[6]	1997;2007	Chinese	2–6	1424	≤–1.0 D	2.33% in 1997; 6.32% in 2007	N/A
Hong Kong[184]	1999	Chinese	5–16	7560	≤–0.50 D	36.70%	<7y 17%; 7y 28.9%; 8y 37.5%; 9y 43.1%; 10y 48.2%; ≥11y 23.1%
Hong Kong (HKCES)[12]	2015–2018	Chinese	6–8	4257	≤–0.50 D	25.00%	6y 12.7%; 7y 24.4%; 8y 36.1%
Shunyi, China (rural) (RESC)[185]	1995	Chinese	5–15	5884	≤–0.50 D	21.60%	5–7y 2.6%; 14–15y 14.9%
Guangzhou, China (urban) (RESC)[15]	2000	Chinese	5–15	4364	≤–0.50 D	38.10%	5y 5.7%; 6y 5.9%; 7y 7.7%; 8y 14%; 9y 25.9%; 10y 30.1%; 11y 41.7%; 12y 49.7%; 13y 57.4%; 14y 65.5%; 15y 78.4%
Yangxi, China (rural) (RESC)[17]	2005	Chinese	13–17	2454	≤–0.50 D	42.40%	13y 36.8%; 14y 38.8%; 15y 43%; 16y 46.8%; 17y 53.9%
Anyang, China (rural) (ACES)[16]	2010	Chinese	7 (grade 1); 12 (grade 7)	7y: 2893; 12y: 2267	≤–0.50 D	7y: 3.9%; 12y: 67.3%	7y 3.9%; 12y 67.3%
Heilongjiang, China, China[186]	2010	Chinese	5–18	1700	≤–0.50D	5.00%	5–9y 0.9%; 10–14y 4.5%; 15–18y 8.2%
Handan, China (HOMS)[187]	2006–2007	Chinese	6–18	878	≤–0.50 D	23.50%	6–11y 14.4%; 12–18y 41.1%
Ejina, Gobi Desert of China[188]	2015	Chinese and Mongolian	6–21	1565	≤–0.50 D	60.00%	N/A
Shanghai, China[9]	2013	Chinese	3–10	8398	≤–0.50 D	20.10%	3y 1.8%; 4y 2.3%; 5y 3.5%; 6y 5.2%; 7y 14.3%; 8y 30.8%; 9y 41.4%; 10y 52.2%

Study	Year	Ethnicity	Age	n	Definition	Prevalence	Age-specific prevalence
Shenzhen, China[8]	2012	Chinese	3–6	1127	≤ −0.5 D	1.30%	3y 0; 4y 0.8%; 5y 1.3%; 6y 3.7%
Taiwan[189]	1995	Chinese	6–18	11178	≤ −0.25 D	Males: 50%; Females: 58%	7y 12%; 12y 56%; 15y 76%; 16–18y 84%
Taiwan[190]	2000	Chinese	7–18	10889	≤ −0.50 D	Males: 64%; Females: 59%	7y 20%; 12y 61%; 15y 81%
Taiwan (MIT)[14]	2013	Chinese	7.49 (grade 2)	11590	≤ −0.50 D	36.40%	N/A
Singapore (SCORM)[13]	2001	Chinese	7–9	1453	≤ −0.50 D	36.60%	7y 29.0%; 8y 34.7%; 9y 53.1%
Singapore (STARS)[7]	2009	Chinese	0.5–6	3009	≤ −0.50 D	11.40%	6–11.9m 15.8%; 12–23.9m 14.9%; 24–35.9m 20.2%; 36–47.9m 8.6%; 48–59.9m 7.6%; 60–72m 6.4%
Gombak, Malaysia (RESC)[21]	2003	Malay, Chinese and Indian	7–15	4634	≤ −0.50D	All: 20.7% Malay: 15.4%; Chinese: 46.4%; Indian: 16.2%	7y 10%; 8y 14%; 9y 16.3%; 10y 16.2%; 11y 22.6%; 12y 24.8%; 13y 25.3%; 14y 32.5%; 15y 32.5%
Andhra Pradesh, India (rural)[19]	2000	Indian	7–15	5067	≤ −0.50 D	4.10%	7y 2.8%; 8y 2.83%; 9y 3.9%; 10y 4.0%; 11y 2.73%; 12y 4.79%; 13y 5.43%; 14y 6.74%; 15y 6.72%
New Delhi, India (urban) (RESC)[191]	1999	Indian	5–15	6447	≤ −0.50 D	7.40%	5y 4.68%; 6y 5.87%; 7y 2.8%; 8y 2.83%; 9y 3.9%; 10y 4.0%; 11y 2.73%; 12y 4.79%; 13y 5.43%; 14y 6.74%; 15y 6.72%
Delhi, India (urban) (NIM Study)[18]		Indian	5–15	9884	≤ −0.50 D	13.10%	5–10y 8.4%; 11–13y 15.3%; 14–15y 15.3%

(continued)

Table 7.1 (continued)

Location of study	Study year	Ethnicity	Age (years)	Sample size	Definition of myopia	Prevalence	Age-specified prevalence
Mechi, Nepal (RESC)[23]	1998	Aryan, Mongol, and Tibetan	5–15	5067	≤ –0.50 D	1.20%	N/A
Jhapa, Nepal (RESC)[192]	2006	Aryan, Mongol and Tibetan	10–15	4282	≤ –0.50 D	19.00%	10y 10.9%; 11y 13.8%; 12y 16.5%; 13y 19.4%; 14y 23.3%; 15y 27.3%
Al Hassa, Saudi Arabia (RESC)[193]			6–14	2002	≤ –0.75 D	9.00%	6–8y 23.0%; 9–11y 19.3%; 12–14y 23.4%
Sydney, Australia (SMS)[194]	2004	Caucasian, Middle Eastern, East Asian, Middle Eastern and South Asian	12	2353	≤ –0.50D	11.90%	N/A
Sydney, Australia (SMS)[195]	2004	Caucasian, Middle Eastern, East Asian, Middle Eastern, and South Asian	6	1765	≤ –0.50 D	1.43%	N/A
America (BPEDS)[10]	2003–2007	White and African	0.5–6	3990	≤ –1.0 D	White: 1.1%; African: 9.6%	N/A

Study	Year	Ethnicity	Age	N	Definition	Prevalence	Age-specific prevalence
America (MEPEDS)[196]	2003-2007	African, Asian, Hispanic and non-Hispanic White	0.5–6	6024	≤ –1.0 D	Hispanic: 3.7%; African: 6.6%	N/A
Santiago, Chile (RESC)[25]	1998	Chilean	5–15	5293	≤ –0.50 D	7.30%	N/A
Durban, South Africa (RESC)[24]	2002	Asian, white, mixed-race, and African	5–15	4890	≤ –0.50D	4.00%	5y 3.2%; 6y 4.6%; 7y 2.5%; 8y 2.9%; 9y 3.1%; 10y 1.9%
Rotterdam, Netherlands[197]	6	European	6	5711	≤ –0.50 D	2.40%	N/A

Abbreviations: HKCES, Hong Kong Children Eye Study; RESC, Refractive Error Study in Children; ACES, Anyang Children Eye Study; HOMS, Handan Offspring Myopia Study; MIT, Myopic Investigation study in Taipei; SCORM, Singapore Cohort Study of the Risk Factors for Myopia; STARS, Strabismus, Amblyopia and Refraction Study; NIM, North India Myopia Study; SMS, Sydney Myopia Study; BPEDS, Baltimore Pediatric Eye Disease Study; MEPEDS, Multi-Ethnic Pediatric Eye Diseases Study.

areas with more open spaces. In Malaysia, it was 15.4% for Malay children between 7 and 15 years old.[21] In Iran, it was 3.64% in children younger than 15 years.[22] Among children aged 5–15 years, it was 1.2% in Nepal,[23] 4.0% in Durban, South Africa,[24] and 7.3% in Chile.[25]

7.2.1.2 Prevalence of Myopia in Adults

Ophthalmic complications in adult myopia and high myopia in adults affect vision of the working-age group. We reported in early 2020 an extremely high myopia prevalence at 72.2% among Chinese adults aged between 25 and 50 years in Hong Kong.[12] The Singapore Tanjong Pagar Study reported in 2000 myopia prevalence of Chinese only at 38.7%, whilst among males it was 45.2% for those aged 40–50 years and lower at 29.9% for the more elderly group of 60–70 years.[26] In Shihpai, Taiwan, it was 19.4% among adults, including both males and females older than 65 years.[27] But this was reported in 2003 and could not represent the current prevalence of adult myopia in Taiwan as the prevalence of school myopia has kept rising over the past two decades.[14] In mainland China, it was 32.3% among adults aged over 50 years in Guangzhou,[28] 22.9% among those older than 40 years in Beijing,[29] and 26.7% for those older than 30 years in Handan.[30] For other Asian populations, Singapore studies reported a prevalence of 30.70% in Malay adults from 2004 to 2006,[31] and 28.0% in Indian adults in Singapore over 40 years of age from 2007 to 2009.[32] In Japan, the prevalence of adults aged 40 years and older was 41.8%.[33] In Tamil Nadu in southern India, 50.6% of adults over 39 were myopes.[34] Across the entire country of India, the Andhra Pradesh Eye Disease Study reported 34.6% among those over 40 years of age.[35] As for other Asian regions, myopia prevalence was 36.5% for Pakistan,[36] 26.1% for Indonesia,[37] 22.1% for Bangladesh,[38] and 17.2% for Mongolia.[39] (Table 7.2). Most of these studies were reported more than a decade ago. Myopia in children keeps increasing in Asia. Current myopia prevalence in the adult populations in these different geographical regions and ethnicities in Asia may be closer to the very high 72.2% we reported for adult Chinese in the highly urbanized city of Hong Kong in January 2020.

In the USA, myopia prevalence was 26.2% among whites in Beaver Dam,[40] 28.1% among whites and 19.4% among blacks in the inner city of Baltimore.[41] These were data from more than 20 years ago. Later, in 2006, it was 16.8% among Latino adults in Los Angeles,[42] and 33.1% among adults nationwide as per the National Health and Nutrition Examination Survey in 2008.[43] More recently, in 2017, a myopia prevalence of 35.1% was reported among Chinese Americans in California,[44] which notably was comparable with the national rate. In Australia in 1999, the Blue Mountains Eye Study (BMES) reported a prevalence of 15% in adults aged over 49 years[45] and the Visual Impairment Project (VIP) reported 17.0% for Victoria, Australia.[46] In Barbados, the prevalence in 2005 was 21.9% in adults of African descent.[47] In Norway, the prevalence of young (20–25 years old) and middle-aged adults (40–45 years old) was found to be 35% and 30.3%, respectively, in 2002.[48] In Spain, the Segovia Study reported the prevalence of myopia to be 25.4% among adults aged 40–79.[49] In the United Kingdom, 49% of 44-year-old adults were myopic.[50] In a more recent report of 2015 from France, the prevalence was 39.1% among adults.[51] Along with the global trend of an increase in myopia in children over the past two decades, current adult myopia among European ethnic groups is expected to be higher than reported.

7.2.1.3 Prevalence of High Myopia

In Hong Kong Chinese, the current prevalence of high myopia was 13.5% among a sample of 5,880 adults aged 25–50.[12] This is the highest prevalence globally. For Chinese, it was 2.4% among adults over 65 years of age in the Shinpai Eye Study in Taiwan,[27] 2.6% in adults aged 40 and older in Beijing,[29] and 1.8% of 6,491 adults aged more than 30 years in Handan, China.[30] For Japanese, it was 8.2% in 3,021 adults over 40 years of age in Tajimi.[33]

High myopia is more prevalent in teenagers and individuals in their early 20s. In Shanghai, a cross-sectional study of young Chinese adults aged 20 years showed that 19.5% had high myopia.[52] In Fenghua, a population-based study of 43,858 high school students revealed that high myopia prevalence increased from 7.9% to 16.6% over a 15-year period.[53] In Singapore, the overall high myopia prevalence in a sample of 28,906 young males aged 16–25 increased from 13.1% in 1996–1997 to 14.7% in 2009–2010.[54] In South Korea, the prevalence of high myopia as indicated by cycloplegia was 21.6% among 23,616 males aged 19 years, who were conscripts, in the city of Seoul.[55] Very interestingly, from the rural area of Jeju, cycloplegic high myopia occurred in only 6.8% of 2,805 male conscripts also aged 19 years.[56] Outside East Asia, the prevalence of high myopia is lower. In Israel, the prevalence of high myopia increased only slightly from 1.7% in 1990 to 2.05% in 2002.[57] In Australia, high myopia was present in 1.9% of 17-year-old young adults in 2013.[58] In Denmark, the prevalence was only 0.3%, as reported in 2007.[59]

In summary, myopia is more prevalent among both children and adults in East Asians, i.e.,

Japanese, Koreans, and Chinese, than in other populations, while South Asians like Indians and Malays are more myopic than Caucasians. Nevertheless, there are cautions in interpretations of reported data. First, there are age and cohort effects. Second, the prevalence of high myopia was higher in teenagers than adults mostly in cross-sectional studies conducted in different periods. High prevalence of myopia or high myopia in teenagers indicates that the myopia boom will arrive later in the working age. Third, many studies reported non-cycloplegic refraction, which may lead to over-estimations, as cycloplegic refraction should be the gold standard, especially among children. Fourth, both axial length and cornea curvature should be reported. The ratio of axial length to corneal radius of curvature (AL/CR), which is highly correlated to spherical equivalent but not affected by cycloplegia, is an important parameter, especially in studies without cycloplegic refraction.

7.2.1.4 Prevalence of Pathologic Myopia

The definition of pathologic myopia has not been standardized for early studies. In 2015, the META-analysis for Pathologic Myopia (META-PM) study group proposed a classification.[60] Pathologic myopia was defined as myopic chorioretinal atrophy – either equal to or more serious than diffuse atrophy – and/or the presence of posterior staphylomas.[61] In China, the Beijing Eye Study showed a prevalence of pathologic myopia of 3.1% among 4,319 Chinese subjects over 40 years.[62] The Handan Eye Study showed a much lower rate of 0.9% among 6,603 Chinese subjects over 30 years.[30] Beijing is an urbanized city and Handan is more rural. Notably, both studies defined pathological myopia as myopic chorioretinal atrophy, staphyloma, lacquer cracks, or Fuchs spot. In Taiwan, the Shihpai Eye Study reported a prevalence of myopic maculopathy with posterior staphyloma at 3% among 1,058 adults over 65 years.[63] In Japan, the Hisayama study reported a prevalence of pathological myopia at 1.7% among 1,892 adults aged 40 years and older.[64] The Central India Eye and Medical Study reported a prevalence of 0.2% among 4,561 adults aged 30 years and older.[65] For Australian whites, the BMES reported a prevalence of 1.2% among 3,583 adults aged 49 years and older.[66] There is no obvious regional or ethnic discrimination in the occurrence of pathologic myopia.

7.2.2 Possible Causes for the Epidemic of Myopia

Epidemiological studies in both children and adults consistently show increasing trends of prevalence of myopia, high myopia, and pathological myopia globally. While genetic factors do play a role, changing environments and lifestyles in the past few decades may be the primary causes.

7.2.2.1 Myopia Genetics

During the past two decades, linkage analyses, candidate gene studies, genome-wide association studies (GWAS), whole-exome sequencing (WES), and next-generation sequencing (NGS) studies have remarkably advanced our understanding of the genetic architecture of myopia. At present, 26 chromosomal loci (MYP1–MYP27) are linked to non-syndromic high myopia (www.omim.org/). NGS has identified mutations in 13 genes associated with high myopia: ZNF644,[67] CCDC111,[68] NDUFAF7,[69] P4HA2,[70, 71] SCO2,[72] UNC5D,[73] BSG,[74] ARR3,[75] LOXL3,[76] SLC39A5,[77] LRPAP1,[78] CTSH,[78] and CPSF1.[79] GWAS has identified many susceptible genes for refractive errors, including 11q24.1,[80] 4q25, 13q12.12 (MIPEP),[81] and 5p15 (CTNND2),[82] MYP10 at 8p23 and MYP15 at 10p21.1,[83] ZC3H11B on 1q41,[84] VIPR2, SNTB1,[85] and ZFHX1B,[86] ZC3H11B,[84] GJD2,[87] RASGRF1,[88] HIVEP3, NFASC/CNTN2, CNTN4/CNTN6, FRMD4B, LINC02418, and AKAP13.[89] In 2018, a large-scale meta-GWAS of European ancestry replicated 37 genes and reported 104 novel susceptibility loci, but these loci are estimated to account for less than 8% of the phenotypic variance of refractive error.[90]

Current knowledge about the genetic architecture of myopia is still limited. Larger-scale genomic studies are warranted to identify more genes associated with myopia among different populations. Subsequent in-depth sequence analyses of the detected associated genes are needed to identify the causal variants for association signals. As sequencing technology becomes more advanced and less costly, whole-genome sequencing (WGS) analysis in large samples has become feasible to empower the discovery of genomic variants in human diseases. Moreover, gene–gene and gene–environment interaction analyses will enrich the growing understanding of the genetic architecture of myopia, whereas refined genotype–phenotype correlation analyses will unravel the clinical implications of genetic variants in the disorder. Furthermore, functional analyses are needed to elucidate the biological roles of those genes and loci in the pathogeneses of myopia to pave the way for identifying new intervention targets.

7.2.2.2 Environmental and Lifestyle Factors

Identifying the environmental and lifestyle factors associated with the development of

Table 7.2 Myopia prevalence of adults in epidemiology studies

Location of study	Study year	Ethnicity	Age	Sample size	Definition (SER)	Prevalence
Beijing, China (Beijing Eye Study)[29]	2001	Chinese	≥40	4319	M: < –0.50 D HM: < –6 D	M: 22.90% HM: 2.6%
Liwan, China (Liwan Eye Study)[28]	2003	Chinese	≥50	1269	M: < –0.50 D	M: 32.3%
Handan, China (Handan Eye Study)[30]	2006–2007	Chinese	≥30	7557	M: < –0.50D HM: < –50D	M: 26.7% HM: 1.8%
Shanghai, China[52]	2009	Chinese	20	5083	M: < –0.50D HM: <–6D	M: 95.5% HM: 19.50%
Fenghua, China[53]	2001–2015	Chinese	18	2932	M: ≤ –0.50 D HM: ≤ –6.0 D	M: 87.7% HM: 16.6%
Hong Kong (HKCES)[12]	2015–2018	Chinese	24–73	5880	≤ –0.50 D	M: 72.20%
Taipei, Taiwan (Shihpai Eye Study)[27]	1999	Chinese	≥ 65	2038	< –0.50 D	M: 19.40%
California, USA[44]	2010	Chinese	≥50	4144	< –0.50 D	M: 35.10%
Singapore (TPS)[26]	1997–1998	Chinese	40–79	1232	< –0.50 D	M: 38.70%
Singapore (SiMES)[31]	2004–2006	Malay	40–80	2974	< –0.50D	M: 30.70%
Singapore (SLAS)[198]		Chinese, Malays and Indians	55–85	1835	M: ≤ –0.50 D HM: < –6 D	M: 30.0% HM:3.1%
Singapore (SEEDS)[199]	2004–2011	Chinese, Malays and Indians	≥40	8772	M: < –0.50 D HM: <–5 D	M: 38.90% HM: 8.4%
South India (rural)[34]	2001–2003	Indian	> 39	2508	M: < –0.50 D HM: < –5 D	M: 50.60% HM:3.7%
Andhra Pradesh, India (APEDS)[35]	1996–2000	Indian	≥40	3642	M: < –0.50 D HM: –5 D	M: 36.5% HM: 4.8%
Singapore (SINDI)[32]	2007–2009	Indian	40–80	3400	< –0.50 D	M: 28.00%
Tajimi, Japan[33]	2000–2001	Japanese	>40	3021	< –5 D	M: 45.7 % HM:8.2%
Pakistan[36]	2002–2003	Pakistani	≥30	16507	M: < -0.50D HM: <-5D	M: 36.50% HM: 4.6%
Sumatra, Indonesia[37]	2001	Indonesian	≥21	1043	≤ -0.50D	M: 26.10%

Age-specified prevalence

N/A

50–59y	60–69y	70–79y	80–93y	
37.7%	31.1%	31.3%	46.7%	

<50y	50–59y	60–69y	70–79y	≥80y
44.8%	21.9%	27.2%	67.6%	87.8%

N/A

N/A

≤35y	36–40y	41–45y	46–50y	>50y
77.5%	74.5%	73.6%	66.6%	56.4%

65–69y	70–74y	75–79y	≥80y
12.8%	19.4%	26.5%	23.3%

50–59y	60–69y	70–79y	≥80y
36.1%	36.6%	28.8%	22.2%

Male				Female			
40–49y	50–59y	60–69y	70–79y	40–49y	50–59y	60–69y	70–79y
45.2%	25.2%	29.9%	31.7%	51.7%	27.1%	30.0%	40.3%

40–49y	50–59y	60–69y	≥70y
22.0%	16.8%	16.0%	36.9%

55–64y	65–74y	≥75y
32.0%	26.4%	32.6%

40–49y	50–59y	60–69y	70–80y
47.4%	35.9%	30.1%	32.7%

40–49y	50–59y	60–69y	≥70y
15.66%	33.82%	57.62%	67.19%

40–49y	50–59y	60–69y	≥70y
19.2%	38.3%	56.0%	54.1%

40–49y	50–59y	60–69y	70–80y
33.3%	23.8%	20.3%	26.9%

Male

40–49y	50–59y	60–69y	70–79y	≥80y
M: 70.3%	M: 49.6%	M: 20.8%	M: 13.5%	M: 21.6%
HM: 17.7%	HM: 8.7%	HM: 3.0%	HM: 0%	HM: 0%

Female

40–49y	50–59y	60–69y	70–79y	≥80y
M: 67.8%	M: 42.4%	M: 22.1%	M: 18.6%	M: 24.6%
HM: 15.0%	HM: 7.1%	HM: 4.4%	HM: 3.0%	HM: 4.3%

N/A

21–29y	30–39y	40–49y	≥50y
61.6%	50.6%	28.8%	39.7%

(continued)

Table 7.2 (continued)

Location of study	Study year	Ethnicity	Age	Sample size	Definition (SER)	Prevalence
Bangladesh[38]	1999	Bangladeshi	≥30	11624	≤ -0.50D	M: 22.10%
Hövsgöl and Ömnögobi, Mongolia[39]	1995	Mongolia	≥40	1617	< -0.50D	M: 17.20%
Wisconsin, USA (BDES)[40]	1987–1988	White	43 to 84	4926	< -0.50D	M: 26.20%
USA[41]	1988	White and Black	≥40	5308	< -0.50D	M: White: 28.1%; M: Black: 19.4%
Los Angeles, USA (LALES)[42]	2003	Latino	≥40	6357	≤ -1.00D	M: 16.80%
USA (NHANES)[43]	1999–2004	White, Black and Mexican	≥20	12010	≤ -1.00D	M: 33.10%
Sydney, Australia (BMES)[45]	1992–1993	White	≥49	3654	< -0.50D	M: 15%
Victoria, Australia (VIP)[46]	1986	White	≥40	4744	< -0.50D	M: 17%
Barbados[47]	1987–1992	Black	40–84	4709	< –0.50 D	M: 21.90%
Nord-Trøndelag, Norway[48]	1996–1997	White	20–25, 40–45	66000	≤ –0.50 D	M: 20–25y: 35.0%, M: 40–45y: 30.3%
Segovia, Spain[49]		European	40–79	510	≤ –0.50 D	M: 25.40%
UK[50]	1958 birth cohort	White	44	2847	≤ –0.75 D	M: 49%
Paris, Lyon and Bordeaux, France[51]	2012–2013	White	38.5	100429	M: ≤ –0.50 D	M: 39.1%

Abbreviations: SER, spherical equivalent refraction; HKCES, Hong Kong Children Eye Study; TPS, Tanjong Pagar Study; SiMES, the Singapore Malay Eye Survey; SLAS, Singapore Longitudinal Aging Study; SEEDS, Singapore Epidemiology of Eye Diseases Study; APEDS, The Andhra Pradesh Eye Disease Study; SINDI, Singapore Indian Eye Study; BDES, Beaver Dam Eye Study; LALES, Los Angeles Latino Eye Study; NHANES, National Health and Nutrition Examination Survey; BMES, Blue Mountains Eye Study; VIP, Visual Impairment Project; M, myopia; HM, high myopia.

Age-specified prevalence

Male

30–39y	40–49y	50–59y	60–69y	≥70y
19.7%	14.5%	25%	44.9%	69.9%

Female

30–39y	40–49y	50–59y	60–69y	≥70y
15.8%	10.4%	19.6%	40.1%	57.6%

40–49y	50–59y	60–69y	≥70y
15.6%	12.5%	21.4%	26.5%

43–54y	55–64y	65–74y	≥75y
42.9%	25.1%	14.8%	14.4%

40–49y	50–59y	60–69y	70–79y	≥80y
Black: 30.7%	Black: 20.9%	Black: 14.6%	Black: 12.6%	Black: 21.2%
White: 40.9%	White: 24.9%	White: 18.2%	White: 18.8%	White: 12.8%

Male					Female				
40–44y	45–49y	50–54y	55–59y	60–64y	40–44y	45–49y	50–54y	55–59y	60–64y
19.7%	14.5%	25%	44.9%	69.9%	19.5%	19.0%	16.9%	13.1%	14.1%
65–69y	70–74y	75–79y	≥80y		65–69y	70–74y	75–79y	≥80y	
15.8%	10.4%	19.6%	40.1%		15.7%	18.9%	20.0%	23.8%	

20–39y	40–59y	≥60y
36.2%	37.6%	20.5%

49–54y	55–64y	65–74y	75–84y	≥85y
25.4%	14.4%	11%	11.5%	10.3%

40–49y	50–59y	60–69y	70–79y	≥80y
23.6%	16.3%	12.4%	11.9%	16.8%

40–49y	50–59y	60–69y	70–79y	≥80y
17%	11.1%	20.7%	41.8%	55.1%

20–25y	40–45y
35.0%	30.3%

40–49y	50–59y	60–69y	70–79y
25%	54%	21%	61%

N/A

0–9y	10–19y	20–29y	30–39y	40–49y	50–59y
32.8%	59.9%	68.9%	65.1%	47.7%	41.7%

60–69y	70–79y	≥80y
37.1%	34.1%	40.0%

myopia in childhood is crucial to establishing prevention strategies. There are three major factors: education, near work, and outdoor time.

7.2.2.2.1 School Education

There is a consistent association between higher levels of school education with myopia development, as demonstrated in a study of 4,658 adults aged 35–74 years in Germany.[91] In a study of 67,798 adults in England, Wales, and Scotland based on the UK Biobank and designed to determine whether more years spent in education was a causal risk factor for myopia, every additional year of education was associated with a more myopic refractive error of –0.18 D/year.[92] Thus, a greater number of years in education contributes to the rising prevalence of myopia.[92]

7.2.2.2.2 Near Work

Near work such as reading and writing has long been taken as the mediator linking education with myopia progression. Back in 1989 the American National Sciences already stated near work is a risk for myopia.[93] However, with vigorous research conducted over the years in different parts of the world, the association between near work and myopia has not been consistent.[94, 95] In 2,103 children, the Sydney Adolescent Vascular and Eye Study reported that myopic children performed significantly more near work.[96] Both the time spent on near work activities and the dioptre-hours (Dh) of near work were much higher in myopes than that in non-myopes.[97] Urban Chinese children spent more time on near work of reading and writing than rural children.[98] In another Australian Chinese study, children who read continuously for more than 30 minutes were more likely to develop myopia compared to those who read for less than that duration.[99] Moreover, children who performed near work at a distance of less than 30 cm had a 2.5-fold of risk of developing myopia compared to those who worked at a longer distance.[99] A recent study in Taiwan on 1,958 children aged 7–12 years found that children attending private classes for 2 hours or more had an increased risk of incident myopia.[100] However, some studies did not find an association between near work and myopia. In 1,892 rural Chinese children, myopia was not associated with time and Dh spent on near activities.[101] Similar conclusions were reached in two later studies in Taiwan.[102, 103] A meta-analysis and systematic review in 2016 that synthesized all reported studies on near work showed that the odds of myopia increased by 2% for every Dh more of near work per week.[104]

7.2.2.2.3 Outdoor Time as a Protective Factor

Studies in different geographic locations and different populations provided consistent evidence for time outdoors as a protective factor against myopia onset and development.[96, 105, 106] In Australian children, spending about 2 hours a day outdoors could eliminate the additional risks associated with more near work.[107] A meta-analysis showed that children with normal vision or hyperopia spent on average 3.7 more hours per week outdoors than those with myopia.[106] In a population-based cohort study of 7–15-year-old British children, increased outdoor time was associated with a lower risk of developing myopia.[108] A population-based cohort study of 6- and 12-year-old Australian children revealed that moderate level of outdoor activity was linked with greater odds of developing myopia when compared to greater levels of outdoor activity, as observed in both younger and older cohorts.[96]

One challenge in studying near work together with outdoor time is that until now, the majority of studies have been conducted through parents completing questionnaires, a methodology known for potential recall or reporting bias. In future, there should be more objective measurements by devices such as wearable sensors, together with a standardized methodology to quantify both near work and outdoor time.

7.2.2.3 Parental Myopia

Parental myopia has long been known to affect childhood myopia and has been used as a predictor for childhood myopia.[109–111] Heredity of myopia from parents can be through genes. In theory direct and vertical transmission is possible if there are myopia-causative genes, and this is still to be confirmed. Parental influence can be exerted through a myogenic environment of limited outdoor activities, intensive reading, or frequently engaging in other forms of near work. Gene effects can be indirect through susceptibility to risk factors such as near work.[95] But the effects can be individual and therefore there are siblings growing up essentially in the same living environment sharing a similar lifestyle but who have developed various degrees of myopia or other types of refractive errors. Parental myopia is both a genetic and lifestyle factor.

Recently, in a population-based study of 2,055 family trios with cycloplegic refraction in children and non-cycloplegic refraction in both parents, we have shown that parental myopia confers, in a dose-related manner, the strongest independent effect on childhood myopia. Mild parental myopia did not increase the child's risk of myopia, but the risk increased to 11.2-fold when both parents were highly myopic.[109] These data show that it is possible to identify children who are at higher risk of developing myopia and provide early prevention based on their parental myopia status.[110]

7.2.3 Prevention Strategies

Myopia is a global health threat that also creates socioeconomic burdens. For prevention, it has to start from early childhood, and it requires efforts from family, school, and healthcare providers. There are currently three main approaches for prevention: lifestyle, optical, and pharmacological.

7.2.3.1 Lifestyle Intervention: Increasing Outdoor Time and Lessening Near Work

Protection of outdoor time against myopia development in schoolchildren is evident. Randomized controlled trials have been conducted to determine the optimal and practically possible outdoor time in the school curriculum. In a randomized study involving 16 schools in Taiwan, children were arranged to leave the classroom for outdoor activities after classes.[111] Myopia progression and axial elongation were significantly reduced in the intervention group compared to the control group (−0.35 D vs. −0.47 D and +0.28 mm vs. +0.33 mm, respectively). A previous study by the same research team compared two neighboring schools and found a significantly lower rate of myopia onset in the intervention group (8.41% vs. 17.65%).[112] Intermittent outdoor time of 80 minutes per day during recess decreased myopia onset by up to 9% in just 1 year.[112] A randomized trial of 952 schoolchildren in the city of Guangzhou in mainland China showed that an intervention of 40 minutes per day outdoors decreased myopia onset by 9% after 3 years.[113] Children have been advised to spend at least 2 hours per day outdoors, in addition to avoiding excessive near work. In Taiwan, policy interventions to promote increased time outdoors to 2 hours per day in schools were followed by a reversal of the long-term trend toward increased low visual acuity in schoolchildren.[114] The school-based approach to increasing children's time outdoors should be advocated in all parts of the world.

7.2.3.2 Optical Methods: Orthokeratology, Defocus Spectacles, and Contact Lenses

Orthokeratology or peripheral defocus spectacles are commonly used optical methods for myopia control, especially in Asia. The Retardation of Myopia in Orthokeratology (ROMIO) study in Hong Kong demonstrated significantly slower growth in axial length among the orthokeratology group compared to

single-vision glasses over 2 years.[115] A meta-analysis on orthokeratology in myopia control, which included three randomized controlled trials and six cohort studies, also indicated slowing of axial elongation.[116] Notably, the risk of infectious keratitis associated with orthokeratology lenses remains. Regarding peripheral retinal defocus, randomized controlled trials in Hong Kong demonstrated that, compared with single-vision lenses, both peripheral defocus contact lenses[117] and spectacles[118] can reduce myopic progression and axial elongation.

7.2.3.3 Pharmacologic Treatment: Low-Concentration Atropine Eye Drops

Atropine eye drops have long been used for myopia control. Current evidence suggests that 1% atropine is effective for myopia control, but associated side effects such as blurred near vision and photophobia limit its widespread use.[119] The Atropine for the Treatment on Myopia 2 (ATOM2) study evaluated the use of 0.5%, 0.1%, and 0.01% atropine on 400 myopic children, suggesting 0.01% as the optimal concentration with good efficacy and minimal side effects.[120] Since then, the use of atropine eye drops has transitioned from high- to low-concentration doses worldwide. In 2018, the Low-concentration Atropine for Myopia Progression (LAMP) study from Hong Kong evaluated the use of 0.05%, 0.025%, and 0.01% atropine eye drops and placebo group among 438 myopic children.[121] The study first provided placebo-compared evidence of low-concentration atropine eye drops in myopia control. Both efficacy and side effects followed a concentration-dependent response within the range of 0.01–0.05% atropine. The best efficacy and safety were achieved by 0.05% atropine.[122] Low-concentration atropine had no effect on both the cornea and lens power, instead acting mainly on reducing axial length.[123] Low-concentration atropine for young children is effective for myopia prevention.

7.3 ASTIGMATISM

Another global health burden, astigmatism is the second most common refractive error.[124] It occurs when light coming in from two different meridians is bent differently and focuses on to two points rather than a single point, resulting in blurred images. One dioptric difference in refractive powers at two meridians constitutes 1 D of astigmatism, which is sufficient to cause meridional amblyopia in children.[125] Although other thresholds such as −0.5 D and −0.75 D exist in defining astigmatism, −1.0 D remains clinically relevant as a guide for prescribing spectacle corrections.[126] Astigmatism can be categorized into simple myopic, compound myopic, hyperopic, or mixed astigmatism. Astigmatism in an eye is essentially determined by the curvatures of the cornea. Corneal astigmatism refers to the difference in dioptric refraction between the flattest and steepest curvatures of the cornea, whereas overall astigmatism of the eye is further influenced by the shapes of the lens, vitreous humor, and retina. When the axis is located near the horizontal meridian, it is classified as with-the-rule astigmatism, which constitutes the majority of astigmatism phenotypes observed in children. In people aged above 50 years, the axis shifts to around 90°, and this condition is known as against-the-rule astigmatism.

7.3.1 Prevalence of Astigmatism

Astigmatism is much more prevalent in adults than in children (Table 7.3). A recent meta-analysis estimated its global pooled prevalence at 14.9% among children and 40.4% among adults.[127] In the HKCES 22.1% of children and 30.9% of adults had at least 1.0 D of refractive astigmatism. Interestingly, 63.7% of children and 39.5% of adults had at least 1.0 D of corneal astigmatism, much higher than refractive astigmatism (unpublished data). This discrepancy may be related to the differences in internal compensation of astigmatism in a child's eye compared to an adult's eye.

Astigmatism prevalence has regional and ethnic variations. A higher prevalence was found among children of Asian descent compared to those of Caucasian descent.[128] The reported prevalence of at least 1.0 D of overall astigmatism in Chinese children was 19.2% in Singapore,[129] 13.0% for Taiwan,[130] 12.7% for Guangxi province in China,[131] and 17.8–21.1% in Hong Kong.[132, 133] But it was low at 4.8% for Australian whites.[134] Among adults, there is a wide range too in prevalence of overall astigmatism, from 73% in Chinese in Taiwan,[135] 53.4% among Chinese in the USA,[43] to 13% for Germans in Germany[136] (Table 7.4). Astigmatism is more prevalent in Asians, likely due to the shape of the cornea in relation to a narrower palpebral fissure.

7.3.2 Genetics of Astigmatism

In 2011, a meta-GWAS consisting mainly of Asian populations discovered *PDGFRA* (platelet-derived growth factor receptor alpha) on chromosome 4q12 as a susceptibility locus for corneal astigmatism.[137] This was later replicated and confirmed by the Consortium for Refractive Error and Myopia (CREAM). In addition, three candidate genes – *CLDN7* (chromosome 11), *ACP2* (chromosome 17), and *TNFAIP8L3* (chromosome 15) – were identified

through gene-based analysis.[138] The UK Biobank conducted the largest GWAS on astigmatism to date, involving more than 150,000 white middle-aged British adults.[139] Four novel genome-wide significant loci were identified (*ZC3H11B* on chromosome 1q41, *NPLOC4* on chromosome 17q25.3, *LINC00340* on chromosome 6p22.3, and *HERC2* on chromosome 15q13.1) for corneal astigmatism; all except *ZC3H11B* were also novel loci for refractive astigmatism. Notably, all loci except *HERC2* had an association with myopic ocular traits.[139]

7.3.3 Relationship Between Astigmatism and Myopia

Astigmatism is associated with myopia and myopic progression.[140, 141] Back in 1982, Fulton et al. observed that myopic SER in children was greater in astigmatic eyes and hypothesized that myopia development was initiated by visual blurring from astigmatism.[141] In Chinese children a higher degree of astigmatism at an initial examination was associated with a greater amount of myopic shift and axial length growth 5 years later.[132] These studies suggested that, besides genetic co-susceptibility, myopia and astigmatism may share lifestyle or environmental risk factors, such as increase in near work and lack of outdoor activities.[142, 143] Data from the HKCES of more than 9,000 children and parents showed a strong association between all types of astigmatism and myopic parameters, including axial length and SER (unpublished data).

7.4 HYPEROPIA

Hyperopia (or hypermetropia) refers to the condition where lights are focused behind the retina. Thus distant objects can be seen more easily but light rays emerging from near objects cannot be converged sufficiently on to the retina. People with hyperopia therefore often complain about difficulties with near visual tasks and require additional converging lenses as a refractive correction. Hyperopia, defined as a SER of ≥+ 2.0 D, is common during infancy and childhood. While neonates are born with hyperopia, from 3 months of age onwards, most infants display a progressive change in mean refraction from +2.0 D to approximately +0.75 D, a process of emmetropization. Some high hyperopes may fail to emmetropize and slowly evolve towards low hyperopia. In particular, moderate to high hyperopia (≥+4.0 D) is known to reduce visual function, including visual acuity, stereoacuity, and accommodative response,[144] and increase the risk of esotropia.[145, 146]

Table 7.3 Prevalence of refractive astigmatism in children and adults

Location of study	Year of publication	Sample size	Age range (years)	Prevalence (dioptre in absolute value)	Cylindrical power across age	Cylindrical power across gender	Phenotypes across age
Children							
Singapore[129]	2002	1,028	7–9	≥ 1.0 D: 19.2%	Stable	No difference	WTR predominant
Canada[200]	2004	129	3–5	≥ 1.0 D: 22.5%	N/A	N/A	WTR predominant
Taiwan[130]	2004	10,878	7–18	≥ 1.0–2.0 D: 13.0% > 3.0 D: 1.8%	N/A	No difference	WTR predominant > ATR > OBL
Hong Kong[132]	2004	522	2–6	≥ 0.5 D: 55.8% ≥ 1.0 D: 21.1% ≥ 2.0 D: 2.2%	Stable	No difference	WTR predominant > ATR > OBL
Australia[134]	2006	1,765	6–7	≥ 0.5 D: 22.6% ≥ 1.0 D: 4.8%	N/A	N/A	OBL predominant > WTR > ATR
Hong Kong[133]	2012	382	3–10	≥ 1.0 D: 17.8%	Stable	No difference	WTR predominant
China[131]	2014	2,304	3–6	≥ 1.25 D: 12.7%	Stable	No difference	WTR predominant > ATR > OBL
Hong Kong	2020	4,058	5.5–10	≥ 0.5 D: 63.5% ≥ 1.0 D: 22.1% ≥ 2.0 D: 6.29%	Stable	No difference	WTR predominant > OBL > ATR
Adults							
USA[43]	2008	14,213	20–60	≥ 1.0 D: 36.2%	Increases	M > F	N/A
Taiwan[135]	2011	1,360	>65	≥ 0.75 D: 73%	Increases	N/A	ATR shift with increasing age
Singapore[201]	2011	3,400	40–83	≥ 0.5 D: 54.9% ≥ 1.0 D: 21.3% ≥ 1.5 D: 10.2%	Increases	No difference	ATR shift with increasing age
Hong Kong[133]	2012	2,377	11–60	≥ 1.0 D: 28.4%	Stable	No difference	ATR shift with increasing age
USA[202]	2013	6,000	45–84	≥ 1.0 D: Chinese: 53.4% White: 45.6% Black: 43.0% Hispanic: 42.4%	Increases	M > F	N/A
Germany[136]	2017	13,558	35–74	≥ 1.0 D: 13.0%	Increases	No difference	ATR shift with increasing age
Hong Kong	2020	5,577	24–72	≥ 0.5 D: 71.6% ≥ 1.0 D: 33.6% ≥ 2.0 D: 7.47%	Stable	No difference	WTR predominant ATR shift with increasing age

Abbreviations: WTR, with-the-rule astigmatism; ATR, against-the-rule astigmatism; OBL, oblique astigmatism; M, male; F, female.

Table 7.4 Prevalence of corneal astigmatism in children and adults

Location of study	Year of publication	Age range (years)	Sample size	Prevalence (dioptre in absolute value)	Cylindrical power across age	Cylindrical power across gender	Phenotypes across age
Children							
Australia[134]	2006	6–7	1,765	≥ 0.5 D: 74.9% ≥ 1.0 D: 27.7%	N/A	N/A	N/A
USA[203]	2011	0.5–8	1,235	≥ 1.0 D: 78.3%	N/A	N/A	WTR predominant > OBL > ATR
Hong Kong[133]	2012	3–10	382	N/A	N/A	N/A	WTR predominant
Iran[204]	2014	4–6	3,701	≥ 1.0 D: 16.3% ≥ 2.0 D: 3.6% ≥ 3.0 D: 1.1%	Stable	No difference	WTR predominant
Australia[205]	2015	5–10	180	≥ 1.0 D: 27.5% ≥ 2.0 D: 9.2%	Stable	No difference	WTR predominant ATR with increasing age
Hong Kong	2020	5.5–10	4,058	≥ 0.5 D: 95.9% ≥ 1.0 D: 63.7% ≥ 2.0 D: 10.3%	Stable	No difference	WTR predominant > OBL > ATR \
Adults							
UK[206]	2011	30–91	746	≥ 1.0 D: 40.4%	N/A	N/A	N/A
Hong Kong[133]	2012	11–60	2,759	N/A	N/A	No difference	ATR shift with increasing age
Italy[207]	2013	33–96	380	≥ 1.0 D: 41.7%	N/A	No difference	N/A
Germany[136]	2017	35–74	13,558	≥ 1.0 D: 36.2%	N/A	N/A	ATR shift with increasing age
Hong Kong	2020	24–72	5,577	≥ 0.5 D: 75.3% ≥ 1.0 D: 45.3% ≥ 2.0 D: 7.1%	Stable	No difference	WTR predominant > ATR > OBL

Abbreviations: WTR, with-the-rule astigmatism; ATR, against-the-rule astigmatism; OBL, oblique astigmatism.

7.4.1 Prevalence of Hyperopia

Although hyperopia occurs in all people at the early stage of life, its prevalence varies by race, ethnicity, and geographic region.[145] In the Collaborative Longitudinal Evaluation of Ethnicity and Refractive Error (CLEERE) study of more than 2,500 children aged 5–17 years from four ethnic groups, white children had the highest prevalence of hyperopia (19.3%), while Asians had the lowest (6.3%).[147] In a recent multiethnic pooled analysis of four population-based studies of pediatric eye diseases, hyperopia was most prevalent in non-Hispanic white children (27.5%), followed by Hispanic white children (26.7%), 20.3% of black American children, and 11.6% of Asian children.[148] Girls tended to have a higher prevalence of low to moderate hyperopia than boys, but no sex difference was found among moderate to high hyperopes.[148]

Among children with hyperopia, more than two-thirds have hyperopia in both eyes. A significantly greater proportion of children with high hyperopia (≥+4.0 D) also had concurrent astigmatism compared to those who were emmetropic or had low to moderate hyperopia. Moreover, hyperopic children had significantly shorter axial lengths, flatter corneal curvatures, and hence lower corneal refractive power compared to emmetropic children.[145] Hyperopes also have difficulty converging incoming lights from nearby objects. They are thus associated with accommodation abnormalities. As accommodation brings about convergence, uncorrected hyperopia may lead to excessive convergence and accommodative esotropia.

7.4.2 Risk Factors for Hyperopia

Familial forms of extremely high hyperopia exist, although they are rare. Studies on twins demonstrated a high concordance of refractive errors between monozygotic twins, in particular a strong correlation in hyperopia, indicating genetic effect.[149] Maternal smoking during pregnancy was associated with a 28% higher risk of low to moderate hyperopia and a 64% higher risk of hyperopia of ≥+4.0 D in the pooled study. Such risks increased even when the consumption of cigarettes was modest and of a short duration. Furthermore, both longer smoking duration overall and smoking during the third trimester were linked to a greater risk of moderate to high hyperopia.[148]

7.5 PRESBYOPIA

Presbyopia is age-related loss of accommodation by the crystalline lens; the typical age of onset is around 45 years old. The reduction of accommodation amplitude progresses with time and increasing notice of difficulties in focusing on near objects in nearwork tasks such as reading fine print or using mobile phones. Age is the predominant factor for presbyopia.[150] Other associated conditions include habitual short reading distance, intensive use of small screens such as smartphone, persistent exposure to sunlight, comorbidity of glaucoma, or systemic diseases such as diabetes and hypertension, tobacco smoking, alcohol intake, and antipsychotic medications.[151] Women tend to develop presbyopia earlier, likely due to more near viewing tasks than physiological difference in accommodation between the two sexes.[152]

7.5.1 Prevalence of Presbyopia

A meta-analysis conducted in 2018[190] estimated that 800 million people had near visual impairment because of inadequate refractive correction among the 1.8 billion people suffering from presbyopia worldwide in 2015, an increase from an estimate of 1 billion in 2005[153] due to population aging globally (Table 7.5).[154-176] The prevalence of presbyopia increases with age in both urban and rural living environments. A cross-sectional study was conducted in different parts of the world – Shunyi (rural) and Guangzhou (urban) in China, Kaski (rural) in Nepal, Madurai (rural) in India, Dosso (rural) in Niger, Durban (semi-urban) in South Africa, and Los Angeles (urban) in the USA.[173] Compared to people aged younger than 40 years, presbyopia among people aged 40–49 years increased by at least 57% to almost eightfold.[173] Compared to those aged 50–59 years, the increase in prevalence slowed down by 1.36% to twofold. The prevalence reached up to 95% in people aged 60 or above; then the increase reached a plateau.[173] Other studies conducted in Andhra Pradesh in India,[174] Kaski in Nepal,[175] and Asa in Nigeria[161] demonstrated a similar pattern. The prevalences for Indian people aged 40–49, 50–59, 60–69, and 70 or above were 34%, 65%, 58%, and 50%;[174] for the Nepali aged 35–35, 40–49, 50–59, 60–69, and 70 or above they were 6%, 50%, 87%, 92%, and 55%;[175] and for the Nigerians aged under 75 and above 75 they were 54% and 83% respectively.[161]

7.5.2 Impact of Presbyopia

Presbyopia affects quality of life by imposing difficulties in near-vision tasks regardless of living environment, geographic location, or socioeconomic condition. In developed regions, there may be more intensive near work in reading and writing. A study conducted in the USA showed the association of presbyopia with substantial negative effects on health-related quality of life.[177] In developing areas reading and writing may be replaced by winnowing grain, sorting rice, weeding, and sewing.[170] A study in Tanzania

Table 7.5 Global prevalence of presbyopia

Location of study	Study year	Sample size	Presbyopia threshold	Prevalence
Pelotas and Rio Grande do Sul, Brazil (urban)[172]	2000	3007	N4 at 37 cm; unspecified	30–70y: 55%
Regional Tanzania (rural)[171]	2004	1562	N8 at 40 cm; 20/20	40–65y: 62%
Khyber Pakhtunkhwa, Pakistan (rural)[159]	2005	917	Unspecified; 20/20	≥ 30y: 58%
National Singapore (urban)[155]	2005, 2008, and 2010	7890	N8 at 40 cm; 20/30	40–85y: 70%
Nakuru, Kenya (urban and rural)[166]	2007–2008	3993	N8 at 40 cm; 20/40	≥ 50y: 92%
Shahroud, Iran (urban)[168]	2008	5019	N8 at 40 cm; unspecified	40–64y: 58%
Andhra Pradesh, India (urban and rural)[174]	2011	7378	N8 at 40 cm; 20/40	40–49y: 34%, 50–59y: 65%, ≥70y: 50%
Inner Mongolia, China (rural)[156]	2009	5158	N8 at 40 cm; 20/40	40–70y: 52%
Liaoning, China (rural)[169]	2009	1008	N8 at 40 cm; 20/60	40–70y: 67%
Viti Levu island, Fiji (urban and rural)[176]	2009	1381	N8 at 40 cm; 20/60	40–70y: 59%
Kaski, Nepal (rural)[175]	2010	2157	N6 at 40 cm; 20/40	35–39y: 6%, 50–59y: 87%, ≥70y: 55%
National Timor-Leste[167]	2010	2014	N8 at 40 cm; 20/60	40–70y: 52.5%
Durban, South Africa (semi-urban)[163]	2010	1939	N6 at 40 cm; 20/40	35–80y: 77%
Mbeere, Kenya (urban and rural)[164]	2012	3627	N8 at 40 cm; 20/40	35–75y: 25%
Zoba Ma'ekel, Eritrea (urban and rural)[165]	2012	3171	N6 at 40 cm; 20/40	35–50y: 33%
Zamfara, Nigeria (rural)[157]	2012	635	N8 at 40 cm; 20/60	40–70y: 30%
Asa, Nigeria[161]	2012	3899	N8 at 40 cm; 20/40	35–75y: 54%, ≥ 75y: 83%
Kahama, Tanzania (rural)[158]	2013	1663	N6 at 40 cm; 20/40	≥ 35y: 46.5%
Enugu, Nigeria (rural)[160]	2013	585	N8 at 40 cm; 20/20	35–65y: 63%
Oyo, Nigeria (suburban)[154]	2014	440	N8 at 40 cm; 20/60	40–60y: 75%
Shunyi, China (rural)[173]		3554	N6 at 40 cm; 20/40	35–39y: 2.6%, 40–49y: 28.4%, 50–59y: 85.9%, 60–69y: 95.3%, ≥70y: 98.9%
Kaski, Nepal (rural)[173]		1817	N6 at 40 cm; 20/40	35–39y: 15.3%, 40–49y: 41.6%, 50–59y: 76.7%, 60–69y: 83.9%, ≥70y: 93.6%
Madurai, India (rural)[173]		2156	N6 at 40 cm; 20/40	35–39y: 5.6%, 40–49y: 49.8%, 50–59y: 88.6%, 60–69y: 91.8%, ≥70y: 86.9%
Dosso, Niger (rural)[173]		2631	N6 at 40 cm; 20/40	35–39y: 51%, 40–49y: 88.4%, 50–59y: 89.6%, 60–69y: 91.1%, ≥70y: 94.9%
Durban, South Africa (semi-urban)[173]		1939	N6 at 40 cm; 20/40	35–39y: 53.3%, 40–49y: 83.6%, 50–59y: 94.8%, 60–69y: 98.5%, ≥70y: 96.3%

Table 7.5 (continued)

Location of study	Study year	Sample size	Presbyopia threshold	Prevalence
Guangzhou, China (urban)[173]		2045	N6 at 40 cm; 20/40	35–39y: 8.3%, 40–49y: 42.5%, 50–59y: 53.1%, 60–69y: 59%, ≥70y: 80.7%
Los Angeles, USA (urban)[173]		663	N6 at 40 cm; 20/40	35–39y: 7.1%, 40–49y: 49.2%, 50–59y: 86.7%, 60–69y: 85.9%, ≥70y: 89.5%
Guangzhou, China (urban)[208]	2008–2014	1817	N8 at 40 cm; 20/50	35–44y: 9.07%, 45–54y: 26.3%, 55–64y: 34.7%, ≥65y: 50.4%
Regional Bogotá, Colombia[209]	2015	2886	at 40 cm; 20/40	35–39y: 2.3%, 40–44y: 22.2%, 45–49y: 52.4%, 50–54y: 73%, 55–59y: 82.7%, 60–64y: 88.9%, 65–69y: 91.7%, 70–74y: 88.7%, 75–79y: 91.4%, ≥80y: 92.8%
Andhra Pradesh, India (urban and rural)[210]	2008	3095	N8 at customary distance; 20/40	35–49y: 63%
Andhra Pradesh, India (rural)[211]	2008	3203	N8 at customary distance; 20/40	35–49y: 64%
Andhra Pradesh, India (urban and rural)[212]	1997	5587	N8 at customary distance; 20/40	30–39y: 22.9%, 40–49y: 92.7%, 50–59y: 95.6%, 60–69y: 94.1%, ≥70y: 88.4%

showed that almost 80% of people were having difficulties in handling near-vision jobs and 71% of them were dissatisfied with their ability at work.[178] However, the global unmet need for presbyopia correction was estimated to be 45% in 2015, indicating a great need for improvement in awareness and treatment worldwide, particularly in the rural areas of low-resource regions.[190] While treatments for presbyopia, such as bifocal or progressive lenses, are easily accessible in affluent places, they are much less available in lower-income regions, where the rate of presbyopia correction can be as low as 10%.[179]

7.5.3 Correction of Presbyopia

Currently, correction of presbyopia is mainly by optical, surgical, and pharmaceutical methods. Optical correction of presbyopia can be achieved using spectacles, contact lenses, a refractive procedure, or intraocular lenses. Even though this approach is simple, direct, and relatively inexpensive, some people find it inconvenient in daily life and that it limits sport activities.[180] Keratorefractive procedures using laser ablation techniques to generate either monovision or a multifocal cornea, i.e., presbyLASIK, are among the surgical approaches. Since presbyLASIK can lead to irreversible compromise in distance vision, patient selection and pre-operative counseling are essential.[181] Another surgical approach is intracorneal or corneal inlays. An intracorneal inlay is reversible but it may create biological intolerance and affect optical performance. A corneal inlay is irreversible and provides monovision, but there are complications, including corneal haze, which requires the explantation of the inlay.[182] All the surgical approaches are invasive with risk for infection.

Pharmaceutical treatment is an alternative non-invasive approach appealing to people not wanting surgery. Conventional anti-presbyopia agents include miotics and non-steroidal anti-inflammatory drugs (NSAIDs). More recently, lipoic acid and oxymetazoline are also available. Earlier studies with miotics and NSAIDs failed to show objective improvement; recent clinical studies using EV06, a prodrug of lipoic acid, and oxymetazoline, an alpha-adrenoceptor agonist, demonstrated improvements in presbyopia.[183]

7.6 CONCLUSION

Refractive errors occur in most people but the epidemiology varies greatly around the world, due to ever-changing interactions between genetic and environmental factors as well as non-uniformity among diagnostic thresholds and criteria. These issues pose great difficulties when comparing data between regions and countries. Variations in the age ranges of study subjects and methodologies involved in epidemiological studies further complicated the interpretation of data generated from different parts of the world. Nonetheless, epidemiological studies, including ophthalmic, environmental, lifestyle, and genetic investigations, have greatly advanced the understanding of the complexity of refractive errors. Current knowledge has helped in designing preventive strategies by pharmacological, optical, or surgical means. The link to lifestyle factors, including near work and outdoor time in myopia, have led to the establishment of health policies targeting the younger generation, especially schoolchildren. Ultimately there should be a gradual change in human behaviors that leads to healthier vision.

ACKNOWLEDGMENTS

We would like to thank our colleagues Dr. Xiujuan Zhang, Dr. Fen Fen Li, Dr. Hei-Nga Chan, Dr. Arnold Chee, and Dr. Andre Ma for their contributions to this chapter. We would also like to thank Mr. John Tai for his service in the language editing for this work.

REFERENCES

1. Cho BJ, Shin JY, Yu HG. Complications of pathologic myopia. *Eye Contact Lens* 2016;42(1):9–15.

2. Bourne RR, Stevens GA, White RA, et al. Causes of vision loss worldwide, 1990–2010: a systematic analysis. *Lancet Glob Health* 2013;1(6):e339–49.

3. Haarman AEG, Enthoven CA, Tideman JWL, et al. The complications of myopia: a review and meta-analysis. *Invest Ophthalmol Vis Sci* 2020;61(4):49.

4. Morgan IG, Ohno-Matsui K, Saw S-M. Myopia. *Lancet* 2012;379(9827):1739–48.

5. Flitcroft DI. The complex interactions of retinal, optical and environmental factors in myopia aetiology. *Prog Retin Eye Res* 2012;31(6):622–60.

6. Fan DS, Lai C, Lau HH, et al. Change in vision disorders among Hong Kong preschoolers in 10 years. *Clin Exp Ophthalmol* 2011;39(5):398–403.

7. Dirani M, Chan YH, Gazzard G, et al. Prevalence of refractive error in Singaporean Chinese children: the strabismus, amblyopia, and refractive error in young Singaporean Children (STARS) study. *Invest Ophthalmol Vis Sci* 2010;51(3):1348–55.

8. Guo X, Fu M, Ding X, et al. Significant axial elongation with minimal change in refraction in 3- to 6-year-old chinese preschoolers: the Shenzhen Kindergarten Eye Study. *Ophthalmology* 2017;124(12):1826–38.

9. Ma Y, Qu X, Zhu X, et al. Age-specific prevalence of visual impairment and refractive error in children aged 3–10 years in Shanghai, China. *Invest Ophthalmol Vis Sci* 2016;57(14):6188–96.

10. Giordano L, Friedman DS, Repka MX, et al. Prevalence of refractive error among preschool children in an urban population: the Baltimore Pediatric Eye Disease Study. *Ophthalmology* 2009; 116(4):739–46, e1–4.

11. Wen G, Tarczy-Hornoch K, McKean-Cowdin R, et al. Prevalence of myopia, hyperopia, and astigmatism in non-Hispanic white and Asian children: multi-ethnic pediatric eye disease study. *Ophthalmology* 2013;120(10):2109–16.

12. Yam JC, Tang SM, Kam KW, et al. High prevalence of myopia in children and their parents in Hong Kong Chinese Population: the Hong Kong Children Eye Study. *Acta Ophthalmol* 2020; doi: 10.1111/aos.14350.

13. Saw SM, Carkeet A, Chia KS, et al. Component dependent risk factors for ocular parameters in Singapore Chinese children. *Ophthalmology* 2002;109(11):2065–71.

14. Hsu CC, Huang N, Lin PY, et al. Prevalence and risk factors for myopia in second-grade primary school children in Taipei: a population-based study. *J Chin Med Assoc* 2016;79(11):625–32.

15. He M, Zeng J, Liu Y, et al. Refractive error and visual impairment in urban children in southern China. *Invest Ophthalmol Vis Sci* 2004;45(3):793–9.

16. Li SM, Liu LR, Li SY, et al. Design, methodology and baseline data of a school-based cohort study in central China: the Anyang Childhood Eye Study. *Ophthalmic Epidemiol* 2013;20(6):348–59.

17. He M, Huang W, Zheng Y, et al. Refractive error and visual impairment in school children in rural southern China. *Ophthalmology* 2007;114(2):374–82.

18. Saxena R, Vashist P, Tandon R, et al. Prevalence of myopia and its risk factors in urban school children in Delhi: the North India Myopia Study (NIM Study). *PLoS One* 2015;10(2):e0117349.

19. Dandona R, Dandona L, Srinivas M, et al. Refractive error in children in a rural population in India. *Invest Ophthalmol Vis Sci* 2002;43(3):615–22.

20. Sheeladevi S, Seelam B, Nukella PB, et al. Prevalence of refractive errors in children in India: a systematic review. *Clin Exp Optom* 2018;101(4):495–503.

21. Goh PP, Abqariyah Y, Pokharel GP, Ellwein LB. Refractive error and visual impairment in school-age children in Gombak District, Malaysia. *Ophthalmology* 2005;112(4):678–85.

22. Ostadimoghaddam H, Fotouhi A, Hashemi H, et al. Prevalence of the refractive errors by age and gender: the Mashhad eye study of Iran. *Clin Exp Ophthalmol* 2011;39(8):743–51.

23. Pokharel GP, Negrel AD, Munoz SR, Ellwein LB. Refractive error study in children: results from Mechi Zone, Nepal. *Am J Ophthalmol* 2000; 129(4):436–44.

24. Naidoo KS, Raghunandan A, Mashige KP, et al. Refractive error and visual impairment in African children in South Africa. *Invest Ophthalmol Vis Sci* 2003;44(9):3764–70.

25. Maul E, Barroso S, Munoz SR, et al. Refractive error study in children: results from La Florida, Chile. *Am J Ophthalmol* 2000;129(4):445–54.

26. Wong TY, Foster PJ, Hee J, et al. Prevalence and risk factors for refractive errors in adult Chinese in Singapore. *Invest Ophthalmol Vis Sci* 2000;41(9):2486–94.

27. Cheng CY, Hsu WM, Liu JH, et al. Refractive errors in an elderly Chinese population in Taiwan: the Shihpai eye study. *Invest Ophthalmol Vis Sci* 2003;44(11):4630–8.

28. He M, Huang W, Li Y, et al. Refractive error and biometry in older Chinese adults: the Liwan eye study. *Invest Ophthalmol Vis Sci* 2009;50(11):5130–6.

29. Xu L, Li J, Cui T, et al. Refractive error in urban and rural adult Chinese in Beijing. *Ophthalmology* 2005;112(10):1676–83.

30. Liang YB, Wong TY, Sun LP, et al. Refractive errors in a rural Chinese adult population: the Handan eye study. *Ophthalmology* 2009;116(11):2119–27.

31. Saw SM, Chan YH, Wong WL, et al. Prevalence and risk factors for refractive errors in the Singapore Malay Eye Survey. *Ophthalmology* 2008;115(10):1713–19.

32. Pan CW, Ramamurthy D, Saw SM. Worldwide prevalence and risk factors for myopia. *Ophthalmic Physiol Opt* 2012;32(1):3–16.

33. Sawada A, Tomidokoro A, Araie M, et al. Refractive errors in an elderly Japanese population: the Tajimi study. *Ophthalmology* 2008;115(2):363–70 e3.

34. Raju P, Ramesh SV, Arvind H, et al. Prevalence of refractive errors in a rural South Indian population. *Invest Ophthalmol Vis Sci* 2004;45(12):4268–72.

35. Krishnaiah S, Srinivas M, Khanna RC, Rao GN. Prevalence and risk factors for refractive errors in the South Indian adult population: the Andhra Pradesh eye disease study. *Clin Ophthalmol* 2009;3:17–27.

36. Shah SP, Jadoon MZ, Dineen B, et al. Refractive errors in the adult Pakistani population: the national blindness and visual impairment survey. *Ophthalmic Epidemiol* 2008;15(3):183–90.

37. Saw SM, Gazzard G, Koh D, et al. Prevalence rates of refractive errors in Sumatra, Indonesia. *Invest Ophthalmol Vis Sci* 2002;43(10):3174–80.

38. Bourne RR, Dineen BP, Ali SM, et al. Prevalence of refractive error in Bangladeshi adults: results of the National Blindness and Low Vision Survey of Bangladesh. *Ophthalmology* 2004;111(6):1150–60.

39. Wickremasinghe S, Foster PJ, Uranchimeg D, et al. Ocular biometry and refraction in Mongolian adults. *Invest Ophthalmol Vis Sci* 2004;45(3):776–83.

40. Wang Q, Klein BE, Klein R, Moss SE. Refractive status in the Beaver Dam Eye Study. *Invest Ophthalmol Vis Sci* 1994;35(13):4344–7.

41. Katz J, Tielsch JM, Sommer A. Prevalence and risk factors for refractive errors in an adult inner city population. *Invest Ophthalmol Vis Sci* 1997;38(2):334–40.

42. Tarczy-Hornoch K, Ying-Lai M, Varma R, Los Angeles Latino Eye Study Group. Myopic refractive error in adult Latinos: the Los Angeles Latino Eye Study. *Invest Ophthalmol Vis Sci* 2006;47(5):1845–52.

43. Vitale S, Ellwein L, Cotch MF, et al. Prevalence of refractive error in the United States, 1999–2004. *Arch Ophthalmol* 2008;126(8):1111–19.

44. Varma R, Torres M, McKean-Cowdin R, et al. Prevalence and risk factors for refractive error in adult Chinese Americans: the Chinese American eye study. *Am J Ophthalmol* 2017;175:201–12.

45. Attebo K, Ivers RQ, Mitchell P. Refractive errors in an older population: the Blue Mountains Eye Study. *Ophthalmology* 1999;106(6):1066–72.

46. Wensor M, McCarty CA, Taylor HR. Prevalence and risk factors of myopia in Victoria, Australia. *Arch Ophthalmol* 1999;117(5):658–63.

47. Wu SY, Yoo YJ, Nemesure B, et al. Nine-year refractive changes in the Barbados Eye Studies. *Invest Ophthalmol Vis Sci* 2005;46(11):4032–9.

48. Midelfart A, Kinge B, Midelfart S, Lydersen S. Prevalence of refractive errors in young and middle-aged adults in Norway. *Acta Ophthalmol Scand* 2002;80(5):501–5.

49. Anton A, Andrada MT, Mayo A, et al. Epidemiology of refractive errors in an adult European population: the Segovia study. *Ophthalmic Epidemiol* 2009;16(4):231–7.

50. Rahi JS, Cumberland PM, Peckham CS. Myopia over the lifecourse: prevalence and early life influences in the 1958 British birth cohort. *Ophthalmology* 2011;118(5):797–804.

51. Matamoros E, Ingrand P, Pelen F, et al. Prevalence of myopia in France: a cross-sectional analysis. *Medicine (Baltimore)* 2015;94(45):e1976.

52. Sun J, Zhou J, Zhao P, et al. High prevalence of myopia and high myopia in 5060 Chinese university students in Shanghai. *Invest Ophthalmol Vis Sci* 2012;53(12):7504–9.

53. Chen M, Wu A, Zhang L, et al. The increasing prevalence of myopia and high myopia among high school students in Fenghua city, eastern China: a 15-year population-based survey. *BMC Ophthalmol* 2018;18(1):159.

54. Koh V, Yang A, Saw SM, et al. Differences in prevalence of refractive errors in young Asian males in Singapore between 1996–1997 and 2009–2010. *Ophthalmic Epidemiol* 2014;21(4):247–55.

55. Jung SK, Lee JH, Kakizaki H, Jee D. Prevalence of myopia and its association with body stature and educational level in 19-year-old male conscripts in Seoul, South Korea. *Invest Ophthalmol Vis Sci* 2012;53(9):5579–83.

56. Lee JH, Jee D, Kwon JW, Lee WK. Prevalence and risk factors for myopia in a rural Korean population. *Invest Ophthalmol Vis Sci* 2013;54(8):5466–71.

57. Bar Dayan Y, Levin A, Morad Y, et al. The changing prevalence of myopia in young adults: a 13-year series of population-based prevalence surveys. *Invest Ophthalmol Vis Sci* 2005;46(8):2760–5.

58. French AN, Morgan IG, Burlutsky G, et al. Prevalence and 5- to 6-year incidence and progression of myopia and hyperopia in Australian schoolchildren. *Ophthalmology* 2013;120(7):1482–91.

59. Jacobsen N, Jensen H, Goldschmidt E. Prevalence of myopia in Danish conscripts. *Acta Ophthalmol Scand* 2007;85(2):165–70.

60. Ohno-Matsui K, Kawasaki R, Jonas JB, et al. International photographic classification and grading system for myopic maculopathy. *Am J Ophthalmol* 2015;159(5):877–83 e7.

61. Ohno-Matsui K, Lai TY, Lai CC, Cheung CM. Updates of pathologic myopia. *Prog Retin Eye Res* 2016;52:156–87.

62. Liu HH, Xu L, Wang YX, et al. Prevalence and progression of myopic retinopathy in Chinese adults: the Beijing Eye Study. *Ophthalmology* 2010;117(9):1763–8.

63. Chen SJ, Cheng CY, Li AF, et al. Prevalence and associated risk factors of myopic maculopathy in elderly Chinese: the Shihpai eye study. *Invest Ophthalmol Vis Sci* 2012;53(8):4868–73.

64. Asakuma T, Yasuda M, Ninomiya T, et al. Prevalence and risk factors for myopic retinopathy in a Japanese population: the Hisayama study. *Ophthalmology* 2012;119(9):1760–5.

65. Jonas JB, Nangia V, Gupta R, et al. Prevalence of myopic retinopathy in rural central India. *Acta Ophthalmol* 2017;95(5):e399–e404.

66. Vongphanit J, Mitchell P, Wang JJ. Prevalence and progression of myopic retinopathy in an older population. *Ophthalmology* 2002;109(4):704–11.

67. Shi Y, Li Y, Zhang D, et al. Exome sequencing identifies ZNF644 mutations in high myopia. *PLoS Genet* 2011;7(6):e1002084.

68. Zhao F, Wu J, Xue A, et al. Exome sequencing reveals CCDC111 mutation associated with high myopia. *Hum Genet* 2013;132(8):913–21.

69. Wang B, Liu Y, Chen S, et al. A novel potentially causative variant of NDUFAF7 revealed by mutation screening in a Chinese family with pathologic myopia. *Invest Ophthalmol Vis Sci* 2017;58(10):4182–92.

70. Napolitano F, Di Iorio V, Testa F, et al. Autosomal-dominant myopia associated to a novel P4HA2 missense variant and defective collagen hydroxylation. *Clin Genet* 2018;93(5):982–91.

71. Guo H, Tong P, Liu Y, et al. Mutations of P4HA2 encoding prolyl 4-hydroxylase 2 are associated with nonsyndromic high myopia. *Genet Med* 2015;17(4):300–6.

72. Tran-Viet KN, Powell C, Barathi VA, et al. Mutations in SCO2 are associated with autosomal-dominant high-grade myopia. *Am J Hum Genet* 2013;92(5):820–6.

73. Feng L, Zhou D, Zhang Z, et al. Exome sequencing identifies a novel UNC5D mutation in a severe myopic anisometropia family: a case report. *Medicine (Baltimore)* 2017;96(24):e7138.

74. Jin ZB, Wu J, Huang XF, et al. Trio-based exome sequencing arrests de novo mutations in early-onset high myopia. *Proc Natl Acad Sci USA* 2017;114(16):4219–24.

75. Xiao X, Li S, Jia X, et al. X-linked heterozygous mutations in ARR3 cause female-limited early onset high myopia. *Mol Vis* 2016;22:1257–66.

76. Li J, Gao B, Xiao X, et al. Exome sequencing identified null mutations in LOXL3 associated with early-onset high myopia. *Mol Vis* 2016;22:161–7.

77. Guo H, Jin X, Zhu T, et al. SLC39A5 mutations interfering with the BMP/TGF-beta pathway in non-syndromic high myopia. *J Med Genet* 2014;51(8):518–25.

78. Aldahmesh MA, Khan AO, Alkuraya H, et al. Mutations in LRPAP1 are associated with severe myopia in humans. *Am J Hum Genet* 2013;93(2):313–20.

79. Ouyang J, Sun W, Xiao X, et al. CPSF1 mutations are associated with early-onset high myopia and involved in retinal ganglion cell axon projection. *Hum Mol Genet* 2019;28(12):1959–70.

80. Nakanishi H, Yamada R, Gotoh N, et al. A genome-wide association analysis identified a novel susceptible locus for pathological myopia at 11q24.1. *PLoS Genet* 2009;5(9):e1000660.

81. Shi Y, Qu J, Zhang D, et al. Genetic variants at 13q12.12 are associated with high myopia in the Han Chinese population. *Am J Hum Genet* 2011;88(6):805–13.

82. Lam CY, Tam PO, Fan DS, et al. A genome-wide scan maps a novel high myopia locus to 5p15. *Invest Ophthalmol Vis Sci* 2008;49(9):3768–78.

83. Meng W, Butterworth J, Bradley DT, et al. A genome-wide association study provides evidence for association of chromosome 8p23 (MYP10) and 10q21.1 (MYP15) with high myopia in the French population. *Invest Ophthalmol Vis Sci* 2012;53(13):7983–8.

84. Fan Q, Barathi VA, Cheng CY, et al. Genetic variants on chromosome 1q41 influence ocular axial length and high myopia. *PLoS Genet* 2012;8(6):e1002753.

85. Shi Y, Gong B, Chen L, et al. A genome-wide meta-analysis identifies two novel loci associated with high myopia in the Han Chinese population. *Hum Mol Genet* 2013;22(11):2325–33.

86. Khor CC, Miyake M, Chen LJ, et al. Genome-wide association study identifies ZFHX1B as a susceptibility locus for severe myopia. *Hum Mol Genet* 2013;22(25):5288–94.

87. Solouki AM, Verhoeven VJ, van Duijn CM, et al. A genome-wide association study identifies a susceptibility locus for refractive errors and myopia at 15q14. *Nat Genet* 2010;42(10):897–901.

88. Hysi PG, Young TL, Mackey DA, et al. A genome-wide association study for myopia and refractive error identifies a susceptibility locus at 15q25. *Nat Genet* 2010;42(10):902–5.

89. Meguro A, Yamane T, Takeuchi M, et al. Genome-wide association study in Asians identifies novel loci for high myopia and highlights a nervous system role in its pathogenesis. *Ophthalmology* 2020;127(12):1612–24.

90. Tedja MS, Wojciechowski R, Hysi PG, et al. Genome-wide association meta-analysis highlights light-induced signaling as a driver for refractive error. *Nat Genet* 2018;50(6):834–48.

91. Mirshahi A, Ponto KA, Hoehn R, et al. Myopia and level of education: results from the Gutenberg Health Study. *Ophthalmology* 2014;121(10):2047–52.

92. Mountjoy E, Davies NM, Plotnikov D, et al. Education and myopia: assessing the direction of causality by mendelian randomisation. *BMJ* 2018;361:k2022.

93. National Research Council Committee on Vision. *Myopia: Prevalence and Progression.* Washington, DC: National Academies Press (US), 1989.

94. Saw SM, Nieto FJ, Katz J, et al. Factors related to the progression of myopia in Singaporean children. *Optom Vis Sci* 2000;77(10):549–54.

95. Low W, Dirani M, Gazzard G, et al. Family history, near work, outdoor activity, and myopia in Singapore Chinese preschool children. *Br J Ophthalmol* 2010;94(8):1012–16.

96. French AN, Morgan IG, Mitchell P, Rose KA. Risk factors for incident myopia in Australian schoolchildren: the Sydney adolescent vascular and eye study. *Ophthalmology* 2013;120(10):2100–8.

97. Mutti DO, Mitchell GL, Moeschberger ML, et al. Parental myopia, near work, school achievement, and children's refractive error. *Invest Ophthalmol Vis Sci* 2002;43(12):3633–40.

98. Saw SM, Hong CY, Chia KS, et al. Nearwork and myopia in young children. *Lancet* 2001;357(9253):390.

99. Ip JM, Saw SM, Rose KA, et al. Role of near work in myopia: findings in a sample of Australian school children. *Invest Ophthalmol Vis Sci* 2008;49(7):2903–10.

100. Ku PW, Steptoe A, Lai YJ, et al. The associations between near visual activity and incident myopia in children: a nationwide 4-year follow-up study. *Ophthalmology* 2019;126(2):214–20.

101. Lu B, Congdon N, Liu X, et al. Associations between near work, outdoor activity, and myopia among adolescent students in rural China: the Xichang Pediatric Refractive Error Study report no. 2. *Arch Ophthalmol* 2009;127(6):769–75.

102. Huang HM, Chang DS, Wu PC. The association between near work activities and myopia in children – a systematic review and meta-analysis. *PLoS One* 2015;10(10):e0140419.

103. Wu PC, Tsai CL, Hu CH, Yang YH. Effects of outdoor activities on myopia among rural school children in Taiwan. *Ophthalmic Epidemiol* 2010;17(5):338–42.

104. Huang J, Wen D, Wang Q, et al. Efficacy comparison of 16 interventions for myopia control in children: a network meta-analysis. *Ophthalmology* 2016;123(4):697–708.

105. Norton TT, Siegwart JT, Jr. Light levels, refractive development, and myopia—a speculative review. *Exp Eye Res* 2013;114:48–57.

106. Sherwin JC, Reacher MH, Keogh RH, et al. The association between time spent outdoors and myopia in children and adolescents: a systematic review and meta-analysis. *Ophthalmology* 2012;119(10):2141–51.

107. Rose KA, Morgan IG, Ip J, et al. Outdoor activity reduces the prevalence of myopia in children. *Ophthalmology* 2008;115(8):1279–85.

108. Guggenheim JA, Northstone K, McMahon G, et al. Time outdoors and physical activity as predictors of incident myopia in childhood: a prospective cohort study. *Invest Ophthalmol Vis Sci* 2012;53(6):2856–65.

109. Tang SM, Kam KW, French AN, et al. Independent influence of parental myopia on childhood myopia in a dose-related manner in 2055 trios: the Hong Kong Children Eye Study. *Am J Ophthalmol* 2020;218:199–207.

110. Mutti DO, Zadnik K. The utility of three predictors of childhood myopia: a Bayesian analysis. *Vision Res* 1995;35(9):1345–52.

111. Wu PC, Chen CT, Lin KK, et al. Myopia prevention and outdoor light intensity in a school-based cluster randomized trial. *Ophthalmology* 2018;125(8):1239–50.

112. Wu PC, Tsai CL, Wu HL, et al. Outdoor activity during class recess reduces myopia onset and progression in school children. *Ophthalmology* 2013;120(5):1080–5.

113. He M, Xiang F, Zeng Y, et al. Effect of time spent outdoors at school on the development of myopia among children in China: a randomized clinical trial. *JAMA* 2015;314(11):1142–8.

114. Wu PC, Chen CT, Chang LC, et al. Increased time outdoors is followed by reversal of the long-term trend to reduced visual acuity in Taiwan primary school students. *Ophthalmology* 2020;127(11):1462–9.

115. Cho P, Cheung SW. Retardation of Myopia in Orthokeratology (ROMIO) study: a 2-year randomized clinical trial. *Invest Ophthalmol Vis Sci* 2012;53(11):7077–85.

116. Li SM, Kang MT, Wu SS, et al. Efficacy, safety and acceptability of orthokeratology on slowing axial elongation in myopic children by meta-analysis. *Curr Eye Res* 2016;41(5):600–8.

117. Lam CS, Tang WC, Tse DY, et al. Defocus Incorporated Soft Contact (DISC) lens slows myopia progression in Hong Kong Chinese schoolchildren: a 2-year randomised clinical trial. *Br J Ophthalmol* 2014;98(1):40–5.

118. Lam CSY, Tang WC, Tse DY, et al. Defocus Incorporated Multiple Segments (DIMS) spectacle lenses slow myopia progression: a 2-year randomised clinical trial. *Br J Ophthalmol* 2020;104(3):363–8.

119. Chua WH, Balakrishnan V, Chan YH, et al. Atropine for the treatment of childhood myopia. *Ophthalmology* 2006;113(12):2285–91.

120. Chia A, Chua WH, Cheung YB, et al. Atropine for the treatment of childhood myopia: safety and efficacy of 0.5%, 0.1%, and 0.01% doses (Atropine for the Treatment of Myopia 2). *Ophthalmology* 2012;119(2):347–54.

121. Yam JC, Jiang Y, Tang SM, et al. Low-concentration Atropine for Myopia Progression (LAMP) study: a randomized, double-blinded, placebo-controlled trial of 0.05%, 0.025%, and 0.01% atropine eye drops in myopia control. *Ophthalmology* 2019;126(1):113–24.

122. Yam JC, Li FF, Zhang X, et al. Two-year clinical trial of the Low-concentration Atropine for Myopia Progression (LAMP) study: phase 2 report. *Ophthalmology* 2020;127(7):910–19.

123. Li FF, Kam KW, Zhang Y, et al. Effects on ocular biometrics by 0.05%, 0.025%, and 0.01% atropine: Low-concentration Atropine for Myopia Progression (LAMP) study. *Ophthalmology* 2020;127(12):1603–11.

124. Schiefer U, Kraus C, Baumbach P, et al. Refractive errors. *Dtsch Arztebl Int* 2016;113(41):693–702.

125. Pascual M, Huang J, Maguire MG, et al. Risk factors for amblyopia in the vision in preschoolers study. *Ophthalmology* 2014;121(3):622–9 e1.

126. O'Leary CI, Evans BJ. Criteria for prescribing optometric interventions: literature review and practitioner survey. *Ophthalmic Physiol Opt* 2003;23(5):429–39.

127. Hashemi H, Fotouhi A, Yekta A, et al. Global and regional estimates of prevalence of refractive errors: systematic review and meta-analysis. *J Curr Ophthalmol* 2018;30(1):3–22.

128. Twelker JD, Mitchell GL, Messer DH, et al. Children's ocular components and age, gender, and ethnicity. *Optom Vis Sci* 2009;86(8):918–35.

129. Tong L, Saw SM, Carkeet A, et al. Prevalence rates and epidemiological risk factors for astigmatism in Singapore school children. *Optom Vis Sci* 2002;79(9):606–13.

130. Shih YF, Hsiao CK, Tung YL, et al. The prevalence of astigmatism in Taiwan schoolchildren. *Optom Vis Sci* 2004;81(2):94–8.

131. Xiao X, Liu WM, Ye YJ, et al. Prevalence of high astigmatism in children aged 3 to 6 years in Guangxi, China. *Optom Vis Sci* 2014;91(4):390–6.

132. Fan DS, Rao SK, Cheung EY, et al. Astigmatism in Chinese preschool children: prevalence, change, and effect on refractive development. *Br J Ophthalmol* 2004;88(7):938–41.

133. Leung TW, Lam AK, Deng L, Kee CS. Characteristics of astigmatism as a function of age in a Hong Kong clinical population. *Optom Vis Sci* 2012;89(7):984–92.

134. Huynh SC, Kifley A, Rose KA, et al. Astigmatism and its components in 6-year-old children. *Invest Ophthalmol Vis Sci* 2006;47(1):55–64.

135. Liu YC, Chou P, Wojciechowski R, et al. Power vector analysis of refractive, corneal, and internal astigmatism in an elderly Chinese population: the Shihpai Eye Study. *Invest Ophthalmol Vis Sci* 2011;52(13):9651–7.

136. Schuster AK, Pfeiffer N, Schulz A, et al. Refractive, corneal and ocular residual astigmatism: distribution in a German population and age-dependency – the Gutenberg health study. *Graefes Arch Clin Exp Ophthalmol* 2017;255(12):2493–501.

137. Fan Q, Zhou X, Khor CC, et al. Genome-wide meta-analysis of five Asian cohorts identifies PDGFRA as a susceptibility locus for corneal astigmatism. *PLoS Genet* 2011;7(12):e1002402.

138. Shah RL, Li Q, Zhao W, et al. A genome-wide association study of corneal astigmatism: the CREAM Consortium. *Mol Vis* 2018;24:127–42.

139. Shah RL, Guggenheim JA, UK Biobank Eye and Vision Consortium. Genome-wide association studies for corneal and refractive astigmatism in UK Biobank demonstrate a shared role for myopia susceptibility loci. *Hum Genet* 2018;137(11–12):881–96.

140. Twelker JD, Miller JM, Sherrill DL, Harvey EM. Astigmatism and myopia in Tohono O'odham Native American children. *Optom Vis Sci* 2013;90(11):1267–73.

141. Fulton AB, Hansen RM, Petersen RA. The relation of myopia and astigmatism in developing eyes. *Ophthalmology* 1982;89(4):298–302.

142. Yasuda A, Yamaguchi T. Steepening of corneal curvature with contraction of the ciliary muscle. *J Cataract Refract Surg* 2005;31(6):1177–81.

143. Buehren T, Collins MJ, Loughridge J, et al. Corneal topography and accommodation. *Cornea* 2003;22(4):311–16.

144. Ciner EB, Kulp MT, Maguire MG, et al. Visual function of moderately hyperopic 4- and 5-year-old children in the vision in preschoolers – hyperopia in preschoolers study. *Am J Ophthalmol* 2016;170:143–52.

145. Cotter SA, Varma R, Tarczy-Hornoch K, et al. Risk factors associated with childhood strabismus: the multi-ethnic pediatric eye disease and Baltimore pediatric eye disease studies. *Ophthalmology* 2011;118(11):2251–61.

146. Tarczy-Hornoch K. The epidemiology of early childhood hyperopia. *Optom Vis Sci* 2007;84(2):115–23.

147. Kleinstein RN, Jones LA, Hullett S, et al. Refractive error and ethnicity in children. *Arch Ophthalmol* 2003;121(8):1141–7.

148. Jiang X, Tarczy-Hornoch K, Stram D, et al. Prevalence, characteristics, and risk factors of moderate or high hyperopia among multiethnic children 6 to 72 months of age: a pooled analysis of individual participant data. *Ophthalmology* 2019;126(7):989–99.

149. Hammond CJ, Snieder H, Gilbert CE, Spector TD. Genes and environment in refractive error: the twin eye study. *Invest Ophthalmol Vis Sci* 2001;42(6):1232–6.

150. Ayoub SC, Ahmad M. Presbyopia: clinical update. *Insight* 2017;42(2):29–36.

151. Millodot M, Millodot S. Presbyopia correction and the accommodation in reserve. *Ophthalmic Physiol Opt* 1989;9(2):126–32.

152. Hickenbotham A, Roorda A, Steinmaus C, Glasser A. Meta-analysis of sex differences in presbyopia. *Invest Ophthalmol Vis Sci* 2012;53(6):3215–20.

153. Holden BA, Fricke TR, Ho SM, et al. Global vision impairment due to uncorrected presbyopia. *Arch Ophthalmol* 2008;126(12):1731–9.

154. Seidu MA, Bekibele CO, Ayorinde OO. Prevalence of presbyopia in a semi-urban population of south-west, Nigeria: a community-based survey. *Int Ophthalmol* 2016;36(6):767–73.

155. Kidd Man RE, Fenwick EK, Sabanayagam C, et al. Prevalence, correlates, and impact of uncorrected presbyopia in a multiethnic Asian population. *Am J Ophthalmol* 2016;168:191–200.

156. Cheng F, Shan L, Song W, et al. Distance- and near-visual impairment in rural Chinese adults in Kailu, Inner Mongolia. *Acta Ophthalmol* 2016;94(4):407–13.

157. Umar MM, Muhammad N, Alhassan MB. Prevalence of presbyopia and spectacle correction coverage in a rural population of North West Nigeria. *Clin Ophthalmol* 2015;9:1195–201.

158. Mashayo ER, Chan VF, Ramson P, et al. Prevalence of refractive error, presbyopia and spectacle coverage in Kahama District, Tanzania: a rapid assessment of refractive error. *Clin Exp Optom* 2015;98(1):58–64.

159. Abdullah AS, Jadoon MZ, Akram M, et al. Prevalence of uncorrected refractive errors in adults aged 30 years and above in a rural population in Pakistan. *J Ayub Med Coll Abbottabad* 2015;27(1):8–12.

160. Uche JN, Ezegwui IR, Uche E, et al. Prevalence of presbyopia in a rural African community. *Rural Remote Health* 2014;14(3):2731.

161. Senyonjo L, Lindfield R, Mahmoud A, et al. Ocular morbidity and health seeking behaviour in Kwara state, Nigeria: implications for delivery of eye care services. *PLoS One* 2014;9(8):e104128.

162. He M, Abdou A, Ellwein LB, et al. Age-related prevalence and met need for correctable and uncorrectable near vision impairment in a multi-country study. *Ophthalmology* 2014;121(1):417–22.

163. Naidoo KS, Jaggernath J, Martin C, et al. Prevalence of presbyopia and spectacle coverage in an African population in Durban, South Africa. *Optom Vis Sci* 2013;90(12):1424–9.

164. Kimani K, Lindfield R, Senyonjo L, et al. Prevalence and causes of ocular morbidity in Mbeere District, Kenya. Results of a population-based survey. *PLoS One* 2013;8(8):e70009.

165. Chan VF, Mebrahtu G, Ramson P, et al. Prevalence of refractive error and spectacle coverage in Zoba Ma'ekel Eritrea: a rapid assessment of refractive error. *Ophthalmic Epidemiol* 2013;20(3):131–7.

166. Bastawrous A, Mathenge W, Foster A, Kuper H. Prevalence and predictors of refractive error and spectacle coverage in Nakuru, Kenya: a cross-sectional, population-based study. *Int Ophthalmol* 2013;33(5):541–8.

167. Ramke J, Brian G, Naduvilath T. Refractive error and presbyopia in Timor-Leste: the impact of 5 years of a national spectacle program. *Invest Ophthalmol Vis Sci* 2012;53(1):434–9.

168. Hashemi H, Khabazkhoob M, Jafarzadehpur E, et al. Population-based study of presbyopia in Shahroud, Iran. *Clin Exp Ophthalmol* 2012;40(9):863–8.

169. Lu Q, He W, Murthy GV, et al. Presbyopia and near-vision impairment in rural northern China. *Invest Ophthalmol Vis Sci* 2011;52(5):2300–5.

170. Patel I, Munoz B, Burke AG, et al. Impact of presbyopia on quality of life in a rural African setting. *Ophthalmology* 2006;113(5):728–34.

171. Burke AG, Patel I, Munoz B, et al. Population-based study of presbyopia in rural Tanzania. *Ophthalmology* 2006;113(5):723–7.

172. Duarte WR, Barros AJ, Dias-da-Costa JS, Cattan JM. [Prevalence of near vision deficiency and related factors: a population-based study.] *Cad Saude Publica* 2003;19(2):551–9.

173. He M, Abdou A, Naidoo KS, et al. Prevalence and correction of near vision impairment at seven sites in China, India, Nepal, Niger, South Africa, and the United States. *Am J Ophthalmol* 2012;154(1): 107–16 e1.

174. Marmamula S, Khanna RC, Narsaiah S, et al. Prevalence of spectacles use in Andhra Pradesh, India: rapid assessment of visual impairment project. *Clin Exp Ophthalmol* 2014;42(3):227–34.

175. Sapkota YD, Dulal S, Pokharel GP, et al. Prevalence and correction of near vision impairment at Kaski, Nepal. *Nepal J Ophthalmol* 2012;4(1):17–22.

176. Brian G, Pearce MG, Ramke J. Refractive error and presbyopia among adults in Fiji. *Ophthalmic Epidemiol* 2011;18(2):75–82.

177. McDonnell PJ, Lee P, Spritzer K, et al. Associations of presbyopia with vision-targeted health-related quality of life. *Arch Ophthalmol* 2003;121(11):1577–81.

178. Patel I, West SK. Presbyopia: prevalence, impact, and interventions. *Community Eye Health* 2007;20(63):40–1.

179. Fricke TR, Tahhan N, Resnikoff S, et al. Global prevalence of presbyopia and vision impairment from uncorrected presbyopia: systematic review, meta-analysis, and modelling. *Ophthalmology* 2018;125(10):1492–9.

180. Balgos M, Vargas V, Alio JL. Correction of presbyopia: an integrated update for the practical surgeon. *Taiwan J Ophthalmol* 2018;8(3):121–40.

181. Luger MH, Ewering T, Arba-Mosquera S. One-year experience in presbyopia correction with biaspheric multifocal central presbyopia laser in situ keratomileusis. *Cornea* 2013;32(5):644–52.

182. Vargas V, Vejarano F, Alio JL. Near vision improvement with the use of a new topical compound for presbyopia correction: a prospective, consecutive interventional non-comparative clinical study. *Ophthalmol Ther* 2019;8(1):31–9.

183. Wolffsohn JS, Davies LN. Presbyopia: effectiveness of correction strategies. *Prog Retin Eye Res* 2019;68:124–43.

184. Fan DS, Lam DS, Lam RF, et al. Prevalence, incidence, and progression of myopia of school children in Hong Kong. *Invest Ophthalmol Vis Sci* 2004;45(4):1071–5.

185. Zhao J, Pan X, Sui R, et al. Refractive error study in children: results from Shunyi District, China. *Am J Ophthalmol* 2000;129(4):427–35.

186. Li Z, Xu K, Wu S, et al. Population-based survey of refractive error among school-aged children in rural northern China: the Heilongjiang eye study. *Clin Exp Ophthalmol* 2014;42(4):379–84.

187. Gao TY, Zhang P, Li L, et al. Rationale, design, and demographic characteristics of the Handan Offspring Myopia Study. *Ophthalmic Epidemiol* 2014;21(2):124–32.

188. Guo K, Yang DY, Wang Y, et al. Prevalence of myopia in schoolchildren in Ejina: the Gobi Desert Children Eye Study. *Invest Ophthalmol Vis Sci* 2015;56(3):1769–74.

189. Lin LL, Shih YF, Tsai CB, et al. Epidemiologic study of ocular refraction among schoolchildren in Taiwan in 1995. *Optom Vis Sci* 1999;76(5):275–81.

190. Fricke TR, Tahhan N, Resnikoff S, et al. Global prevalence of presbyopia and vision impairment from uncorrected presbyopia: Systematic review, meta-analysis, and modelling. *Ophthalmology* 2018;125(10):1492–9.

191. Murthy GV, Gupta SK, Ellwein LB, et al. Refractive error in children in an urban population in New Delhi. *Invest Ophthalmol Vis Sci* 2002;43(3):623–31.

192. Sapkota YD, Adhikari BN, Pokharel GP, et al. The prevalence of visual impairment in school children of upper-middle socioeconomic status in Kathmandu. *Ophthalmic Epidemiol* 2008;15(1):17–23.

193. Al Wadaani FA, Amin TT, Ali A, Khan AR. Prevalence and pattern of refractive errors among primary school children in Al Hassa, Saudi Arabia. *Glob J Health Sci* 2012;5(1):125–34.

194. Ip JM, Huynh SC, Robaei D, et al. Ethnic differences in refraction and ocular biometry in a population-based sample of 11–15-year-old Australian children. *Eye (Lond)* 2008;22(5):649–56.

195. Ojaimi E, Rose KA, Morgan IG, et al. Distribution of ocular biometric parameters and refraction in a population-based study of Australian children. *Invest Ophthalmol Vis Sci* 2005;46(8):2748–54.

196. Multi-Ethnic Pediatric Eye Disease Study Group. Prevalence of myopia and hyperopia in 6- to 72-month-old african american and Hispanic children: the multi-ethnic pediatric eye disease study. *Ophthalmology* 2010;117(1):140–7 e3.

197. Tideman JWL, Polling JR, Vingerling JR, et al. Axial length growth and the risk of developing myopia in European children. *Acta Ophthalmol* 2018;96(3):301–9.

198. Tan CS, Chan YH, Wong TY, et al. Prevalence and risk factors for refractive errors and ocular biometry parameters in an elderly Asian population: the Singapore Longitudinal Aging Study (SLAS). *Eye (Lond)* 2011;25(10):1294–301.

199. Pan CW, Zheng YF, Anuar AR, et al. Prevalence of refractive errors in a multiethnic Asian population:

the Singapore epidemiology of eye disease study. *Invest Ophthalmol Vis Sci* 2013;54(4):2590–8.

200. Shankar S, Bobier WR. Corneal and lenticular components of total astigmatism in a preschool sample. *Optom Vis Sci* 2004;81(7):536–42.

201. Pan CW, Wong TY, Lavanya R, et al. Prevalence and risk factors for refractive errors in Indians: the Singapore Indian Eye Study (SINDI). *Invest Ophthalmol Vis Sci* 2011;52(6):3166–73.

202. Pan CW, Klein BE, Cotch MF, et al. Racial variations in the prevalence of refractive errors in the United States: the multi-ethnic study of atherosclerosis. *Am J Ophthalmol* 2013;155(6):1129–38 e1.

203. Harvey EM, Twelker JD, Miller JM, et al. Visual motor and perceptual task performance in astigmatic students. *J Ophthalmol* 2017;2017:6460281.

204. Hashemi H, Rezvan F, Yekta AA, et al. The prevalence of astigmatism and its determinants in a rural population of Iran: the "Nooravaran Salamat" mobile eye clinic experience. *Middle East Afr J Ophthalmol* 2014;21(2):175–81.

205. Sanfilippo PG, Yazar S, Kearns L, et al. Distribution of astigmatism as a function of age in an Australian population. *Acta Ophthalmol* 2015;93(5):e377–85.

206. Khan MI, Muhtaseb M. Prevalence of corneal astigmatism in patients having routine cataract surgery at a teaching hospital in the United Kingdom. *J Cataract Refract Surg* 2011;37(10):1751–5.

207. De Bernardo M, Zeppa L, Cennamo M, et al. Prevalence of corneal astigmatism before cataract surgery in Caucasian patients. *Eur J Ophthalmol* 2014;24(4):494–500.

208. Han X, Lee PY, Keel S, He M. Prevalence and incidence of presbyopia in urban Southern China. *Br J Ophthalmol* 2018;102(11):1538–42.

209. Casas Luque L, Naidoo K, Chan VF, et al. Prevalence of refractive error, presbyopia, and spectacle coverage in Bogota, Colombia: a rapid assessment of refractive error. *Optom Vis Sci* 2019;96(8):579–86.

210. Marmamula S, Keeffe JE, Raman U, Rao GN. Population-based cross-sectional study of barriers to utilisation of refraction services in South India: Rapid Assessment of Refractive Errors (RARE) study. *BMJ Open* 2011;1(1):e000172.

211. Marmamula S, Keeffe JE, Rao GN. Uncorrected refractive errors, presbyopia and spectacle coverage: results from a rapid assessment of refractive error survey. *Ophthalmic Epidemiol* 2009;16(5):269–74.

212. Nirmalan PK, Krishnaiah S, Shamanna BR, et al. A population-based assessment of presbyopia in the state of Andhra Pradesh, south India: the Andhra Pradesh Eye Disease Study. *Invest Ophthalmol Vis Sci* 2006;47(6):2324–8.

8 Corneal Disorders

Darren S. J. Ting, Rashmi Deshmukh, Daniel S. W. Ting, and Marcus Ang

8.1 INTRODUCTION

The cornea is a vital transparent structure that forms "the front window of the eye," playing a key role in vision and ocular surface defense. Corneal damage from insults such as infection, inflammation, and trauma can lead to corneal opacity and resultant visual impairment. According to a recent World Health Organization (WHO) report, corneal opacity represents the fifth leading cause of blindness globally.[1] It is estimated that around 4.2 million people were suffering from moderate to severe visual impairment secondary to corneal diseases in 2019.[1] More importantly, avoidable corneal blindness has been shown to be significantly more prevalent (up to 90% of all blindness) in developing countries such as Africa (for example, Ethiopia), Myanmar, and many others, primarily attributed to poor sanitation, malnutrition, lower educational level, and limited access to healthcare facilities.[2–4]

Given the immensity of corneal blindness globally, there is a mismatch between the burden of corneal diseases and the healthcare resources required to alleviate the resultant visual impairment. As such, innovative measures in the field of research and healthcare delivery are urgently needed. In recent years, the considerable increase in the availability of electronic medical records (EMRs), diseases registries, biobanks, omics data, and information technology infrastructure has helped unlock the multi-faceted potential of big data research.[5–8] The wealth of information captured by these resources (e.g., corneal transplant registries, gene banks, etc.) not only helps improve the knowledge on the prevalence, causes, outcomes, and prognostic factors of many ocular diseases, but also enables more effective interventions and targeted public health resource planning,[8–11] which are particularly relevant for under-resourced countries where corneal blindness predominates.

With the ever-increasing pressure on healthcare services and prolonged patient waiting time, studies have shown that patients with ocular disease are at risk of suffering from significant and/or permanent visual impairment as a consequence of delayed ophthalmic review or treatment.[12] Digital innovations such as artificial intelligence (AI) and telemedicine have recently demonstrated their promise in increasing workflow efficiency whilst maintaining good diagnostic performance. For instance, Ting et al.[13] demonstrated that AI, based on a deep learning (DL) system, was able to evaluate >90,000 fundus photographs in approximately 1 month, compared to 2 years when performed by human assessors. In addition, telemedicine, using information and communication technologies, has greatly facilitated the delivery of healthcare services to inaccessible areas and rural populations in a more efficient and cost-effective manner.[14, 15] Currently, diabetic retinopathy and glaucoma are some of the fields that have already benefited from telemedicine in ophthalmology.[14, 16] Telemedicine also serves as a useful means of evaluating patients remotely during the recent COVID-19 pandemic to reduce the risk of disease transmission associated with face-to-face consultation.[17]

In view of the recent technological advancements, this chapter aims to provide an overview of the global burden of corneal blindness and the potential roles of big data and digital innovations in transforming the clinical approach to corneal diseases in the future.

8.2 EPIDEMIOLOGY OF CORNEAL BLINDNESS

The major causes of corneal blindness are trachoma, trauma, and infectious keratitis (IK), all of which are capable of causing corneal scarring and vascularization.[18, 19] Despite the reported decline in the incidence of corneal opacities (trachomatous and non-trachomatous) from WHO in 2010, ocular trauma and ulcerations remain a significant cause of unilateral blindness worldwide, causing 1.5–2 million new cases annually.[1, 18] These corneal diseases may also affect the younger population, potentially affecting education and economic productivity, translating to a greater socioeconomic burden that is reflected by the higher disability-adjusted life-years (DALYs) for corneal diseases compared to cataract or age-related macular degeneration.[2] A population-based study in south India showed that the average age of corneal blindness was 5 years, as compared to 69 years for cataract-related blindness.[20]

The epidemiology of corneal diseases also varies with age groups and socioeconomic status of the region. Childhood corneal blindness is due to xerophthalmia (vitamin A deficiency), neonatal conjunctivitis, and other ocular infections.[2, 19] Adults below the age of 30 years are more likely to suffer from corneal visual impairment

DOI: 10.1201/9781315146737-10

secondary to IK, keratoconus, corneal dystrophies, and corneal scars. On the other hand, diseases such as bullous keratopathy and corneal degenerations affect more elderly individuals.[2] Global regional estimates have also shown considerable variation of corneal causation of blindness, with India and Africa having a higher percentage of their visually impaired population suffering from corneal diseases. It is estimated that almost 98% of the global burden of corneal blindness comes from developing nations.[2] Poor hygiene, lack of sanitation facilities, and illiteracy are some of the factors responsible for an increased risk of infections in these regions.[2]

8.2.1 Trachoma

Trachoma is the most common cause of infectious blindness globally and is responsible for visual impairment in around 1.9 million people across 44 countries.[21] Nearly 90% of these individuals live in sub-Saharan Africa. According to a global report published in 2017, the number of people suffering from blindness due to trachoma was 0.4 million.[18] Trachoma is caused by *Chlamydia trachomatis*, which is a Gram-negative, obligate intracellular bacterium. The serotypes of *C. trachomatis* responsible for endemic trachoma include A, B, Ba, and C.[22] Recurrent episodes of infection and inflammation cause ocular surface complications, conjunctival scarring, and consequent lid abnormalities like entropion, trichiasis, and corneal scarring, eventually leading to blindness. A 4-year cohort study from Tanzania reported the progression of trachoma-related conjunctival scarring in 23% of affected children.[23] The scarring progression was strongly associated with papillary conjunctival inflammation. Another study from Ethiopia stressed the effects of trichiasis on the quality of life for adults suffering from trachomatous trichiasis.[24] This study concluded that scarring and trichiasis had a profound effect on vision-related as well as health-related quality of life, even in individuals having normal vision.[24]

The WHO has provided a grading system for the severity of trachoma, based on the presence or absence of clinical signs.[25] This simplified system was meant for health workers to reliably assess the affected population:

1. Trachomatous inflammation follicular (TF): Five or more follicles of >0.5 mm size on the upper tarsal conjunctiva

2. Trachomatous inflammation intense (TI): Inflammatory thickening obscuring more than half the normal deep tarsal vessels

3. Trachomatous conjunctival scarring (TS): Presence of easily visible scars in the tarsal conjunctiva

4. Trachomatous trichiasis (TT): At least one eyelash rubbing on the eyeball or evidence of recent removal of in-turned eyelashes

5. Corneal opacity (TO): Corneal opacity blurring part of the pupil margin

Chronic malnutrition, poor personal hygiene, and unsatisfactory sanitation facilities are known risk factors for endemic trachoma.[26] Several characteristics of trachoma indicate that eradication is possible. Humans are the only host of the organism, azithromycin is an effective antibiotic against chlamydia, and antibiotic resistance has not been reported yet.[27] The WHO came up with the SAFE (surgical treatment, antibiotics, face washing and environmental changes) strategy for prevention as well as treatment of the disease.[28] Surgical treatment includes surgeries for trichiasis and eyelid abnormalities. The WHO recommends bilamellar tarsal rotation and posterior lamellar tarsal rotation for treating trichiasis.[29] Antibiotic treatment includes single oral treatment with azithromycin 20 mg/kg up to 1 g or topical tetracycline for 6 weeks. When the prevalence is 5–10%, a targeted treatment for affected families is recommended. However, when prevalence exceeds 10%, mass treatment is preferred, which involves treating the entire village.[30] Facial cleanliness and environmental changes to prevent the spread of disease have been shown to be effective.[31] Implementation of the SAFE strategy has led to the successful elimination of trachoma from Cambodia, Ghana, Lao People's Democratic Republic, Mexico, Morocco, Nepal, Oman, and Iran.[21, 27]

8.2.2 Infectious Keratitis

IK is the most common cause of non-trachomatous corneal opacification, and as of 2015, is responsible for 3.5% of total blindness in the world.[18] The common causes of IK include bacteria, fungi, protozoa, and viruses.[22] Trachoma, onchocerciasis, and leprosy are other causes of IK that are designated as "neglected tropical diseases" (NTDs). These are associated with stigma, social isolation, and disfiguring complications. NTDs are preventable and treatable provided the actual epidemiological burden is recognized. Currently, the understanding of global epidemiology of IK is poorly understood owing to a lack of reporting.[32]

Similarly to trachoma, IK exhibits regional variations, with a higher incidence reported in the developing nations. Studies have estimated the incidence rates to be 2.5 per 100,000 in the USA[33] and 2.6–34.7 per 100,000 in the UK.[34, 35] In contrast to these numbers, studies from Asia have reported much higher incidence rates. A study from south India has reported the incidence to be 113 per 100,000.[36] Causative microorganisms of IK also demonstrate regional variation; for example, *Pseudomonas aeruginosa* is the most common pathogen in countries around Europe, the USA, and Australia,[37–39] attributed to the frequent use of contact lenses (CLs) in these regions. In tropical countries, however, fungi are a major cause of IK, with a prevalence of up to 49% of fungal culture-positive ulcers in south India.[40] Fungal IK is also prevalent in Ghana,[41] Tanzania,[42] and Bangladesh.[43]

CL wear and ocular trauma have been reported to be the two commonest risk factors for IK in many studies.[44–47] Other risk factors for IK include ocular surface diseases, exposure keratopathy, neurotrophic keratitis, chronic dacryocystitis, and iatrogenic causes such as post-corneal surgeries.[47–49] Since trauma is one of the most common risk factors for corneal ulcers, studies have been undertaken to examine the benefit of prophylactic antibiotic treatment to prevent IK following corneal trauma. The Bhaktapur Eye Study demonstrated that chloramphenicol 1% ointment started within 18 hours of injury prevented the development of IK following corneal abrasions.[49] The benefit of prophylactic topical antibiotic for preventing IK was similarly demonstrated by another study in India.[50]

8.2.3 Onchocerciasis

Onchocerciasis, also known as "river blindness," is caused by the filarial worm *Onchocerca volvulus*, which is transmitted by the bites of blackflies of *Simulum* spp. After trachoma, it is the second leading cause of corneal blindness in the world.[51] Approximately 37 million people are estimated to be infected worldwide, and 300,000 of them are permanently blind.[52]

Around 99% of the infected population lives in sub-Saharan African countries. It is also transmitted in Brazil, Yemen, and Venezuela.[52]

Onchocerciasis primarily affects the eyes and the skin with intense inflammatory response against the circulating microfilariae. There is no preventive medication or vaccine available. The major regional programs involved in controlling the disease include Onchocerciasis Control Programme (OCP), started in 1974, African Programme for Onchocerciasis Control (APOC), which began in 1995, and Onchocerciasis Elimination Program of the Americas (OEPA), which started in 1992.[52] The strategies used by these control programs are vector control to break the cycle of transmission, and widespread distribution of ivermectin. The OCP concentrated on vector control by spraying insecticides against blackflies using helicopters and planes, supplemented largely by distribution

of ivermectin since 1989. It helped relieve 40 million people from infection and prevented 600,000 individuals from turning blind. The APOC was launched in 1995 and closed in 2015. The strategy implemented was vector control along with community-directed treatment with ivermectin (CDTI). More than 119 million people were treated with ivermectin under the program and, as a result, several countries had reduced morbidity associated with onchocerciasis.[52]

The Expanded Special Project for the Elimination of Neglected Tropical Diseases in Africa (ESPEN) was set up with four objectives: (1) scale up treatments to achieve 100% geographical coverage; (2) scale down to stop treatment once control is achieved; (3) strengthen the control systems for evidence-based actions; and (4) enhance the supply chain management to use the distributed drugs effectively. The OEPA program concentrated on control of the disease in the Americas. It was launched in 1992 and, by 2006, all 13 foci in the region had achieved more than 85% coverage. Transmission was interrupted successfully in 11 of the 13 foci. Elimination has been achieved in Colombia, Ecuador, Mexico, and Guatemala and more than 500,000 people do not need ivermectin any more.[52]

8.2.4 Pseudophakic Bullous Keratopathy

Persistent corneal edema following cataract surgery (known as PBK) serves as one of the major indications for keratoplasty in developed countries. According to a report from Eye Bank Association of America (EBAA) in 2016, the commonest indication for corneal transplants in the USA was corneal edema secondary to PBK and/or Fuchs endothelial corneal dystrophy (FECD).[53] The Singapore national Corneal Transplant Study reported that, in Asian countries like Japan, Taiwan, Singapore, Philippines, and Hong Kong, PBK was the main indication for keratoplasties, ranging from 31 to 38% of all cases.[11] In India, a study found PBK to be the most frequent cause of bilateral corneal blindness post-cataract surgery.[54] Another study from the North Telangana region noted a rise in the prevalence of PBK in their population.[55] This rising trend could be attributed to the increase in the number of cataract surgeries.

8.2.5 Xerophthalmia

More than half the new cases of childhood blindness are caused by vitamin A deficiency and sometimes this is precipitated by measles, causing acute malnutrition.[56] Xerophthalmia refers to the spectrum of ocular conditions caused by deficiency of vitamin A. The earliest sign is night blindness which is sensitive and specific to the serum retinol levels.[57] According to the WHO estimate of 2009, around 5.2 million children in the preschool age group suffered from night blindness and around 290 million had low serum retinol concentration.[58] Night blindness is known to respond very well to vitamin A treatment and supplements given at this stage result in reversing the disease.[59] If left untreated, the condition progresses to conjunctival xerosis, where the conjunctiva appears dry and dull. The presence of whitish, opaque deposits with foamy appearance on the bulbar conjunctiva, called Bitot's spots, is the most characteristic appearance.[59] If vitamin A deficiency continues, progression to corneal xerosis and then keratomalacia is seen, which involves corneal melting and eventually corneal scarring.[60] The signs are classified as:

- Night blindness (XN)

- Conjunctival xerosis (X1A)

- Bitot's spots (X1B)

- Corneal xerosis (X2)

- Corneal ulceration/keratomalacia <1/3 corneal surface (X3A)

- Corneal ulceration/keratomalacia ≥1/3 corneal surface (X3B)

- Corneal scar (XS)

- Xerophthalmic fundus (XF)

Pregnancy and lactation are important causes of vitamin A deficiency as well. Vitamin A-deficient mothers can give birth to neonates at risk of xerophthalmia.[61] The 2009 WHO estimate revealed that 7.8% of pregnant women in at-risk areas suffer from night blindness.[58] In general, night blindness starts when serum retinol concentration falls below 1 μmol/L and severe xerophthalmia occurs at serum concentrations below 0.35 μmol/L.[62] Treatment strategies include dietary modification, vitamin A supplements, and fortification of food with vitamin A. Supplements include 100,000 IU of vitamin A to children aged 6–11 months and 200,000 IU in children aged 1–5 years.[63] Fortification of cereal-based products with up to 20–30% of vitamin A and cooking oil with up to 33 IU/g vitamin A has shown promising results.[64]

8.2.6 Ophthalmia Neonatorum

Conjunctivitis in a newborn is termed ophthalmia neonatorum (ON) or neonatal conjunctivitis. The incidence ranges from 2% to 12%.[65] Although ON is less common, it remains an important cause of childhood corneal blindness in developed countries, and even of mortality in developing regions of the world.[65,] [66] It is seen in babies of mothers affected by sexually transmitted diseases (STDs) caused by *C. trachomatis* (serotypes D–K) and *Neisseria gonorrhoeae*.[67] Chemical substances like erythromycin, tetracycline, or silver nitrate are also known to cause ON. Chemical conjunctivitis presents within 24 hours and is self-limiting. The bacterial causes of ON however need antibiotic treatment.[67] Affected babies present with congested, swollen eyes and sticky discharge usually within 2–14 days of birth. Chlamydial ON is more common than gonococcal ON. Most cases of chlamydial ON are mild to moderate in nature whereas gonococcal ON tends to be more severe.[66]

A swab should be taken to identify the causative organism. If access to microbiological investigation is not possible, the condition should be treated for both the organisms. The recommended treatment for gonococcal ON includes a single intramuscular injection of ceftriaxone in a dose of 50 mg/kg body weight. For chlamydial ON, the recommendation is erythromycin syrup 50 mg/kg in four divided doses for 2 weeks. Additional treatment includes frequent saline irrigation, cleaning the eyes, and erythromycin eye ointment.[66]

8.3 BIG DATA FOR CORNEAL DISEASES

Big data is commonly referred to mean data that display the characteristics of "3Vs" – high variety, high volume, and high velocity.[9] Compared to traditional epidemiological studies, the wealth of information provided by these big data resources (which may sometimes capture millions of patients and data) greatly facilitates the conduct of large-scale or nationwide epidemiological studies for many diseases, providing a comprehensive examination of incidence/prevalence, demographic factors, risk factors, outcomes, and impact of the diseases.[9] Results gleaned from these large-scale epidemiological studies could also help inform and guide public health policies in terms of modulation of risk factors, introduction of interventions for better disease control and prevention, and provision of research funding targeting more prevalent diseases.[10] Furthermore, with the increased availability of digital technologies such as AI, these rich datasets can be utilized to train and validate AI algorithms to screen and diagnose a wide range of conditions and discover new patterns or associations of the diseases that were previously unknown.[68]

Within the field of the cornea, there is an increasing pool of large corneal registries and epidemiological studies through which big data can be accessed. These include corneal transplant registries, IK studies, corneal genetic studies, large ophthalmology-related registries, and EMR-based big data resources.[8, 69, 70] These cornea-related big data enable a better grasp of the prevalence, risk factors, outcomes, and impact of corneal diseases, which in turn allows for more effective and targeted therapeutic and preventive strategies in reducing the burden of corneal blindness. In this section, we summarize the main cornea-related registries and studies in various countries and the impact of these databases.

8.3.1 Infectious Keratitis Studies and Registries

IK is the leading cause of corneal blindness in the world, particularly in developing countries. It is therefore not surprising to observe a vast amount of literature on IK, including the epidemiology, risk factors, clinical characteristics, causative organisms, management, and outcomes of the disease.[35, 40, 47, 71–78] A tabulated summary of the main IK studies in each continent is provided in Table 8.1.

Many of the IK studies have included thousands of patients with clinical and/or laboratory datasets, allowing the clinicians and researchers to gain a better understanding of the causes and impact of the disease, and more importantly to focus on the most-needed areas to reduce the risk and improve the outcome of this clinical entity. In the recent Asia Cornea Society Infectious Keratitis Study (ACSIKS), Khor et al.[47] included over 6,000 patients with IK from 13 study centers in Asia and observed that

bacterial and fungal infections were most commonly observed in developed and developing countries, respectively. More than half of the eyes developed moderate visual impairment (defined as less than 6/18). In addition, approximately 50% of the performed therapeutic keratoplasty failed by 6-month follow-up, highlighting the severity of the clinical entity and the need for further improvement in management. These large-scale studies could also help identify any interesting patterns concerning IK. In the UK, several studies[35, 74, 79] have observed an increasing trend of *Moraxella* keratitis – a type of keratitis that is often associated with chronic infection and longer healing time[80] – over the past decade, suggesting a potential endemic issue within the UK.

As outcomes of IK are often dictated by the initial presenting severity of the disease, identification of important risk factors to reduce and prevent the occurrence of IK remains the cornerstone in tackling IK. CL-related IK has been shown to be a major public health problem, which could pose significant visual impairment. By studying over 2,000 patients, Sauer et al.[81] identified important risk factors of CL-related IK, including the use of expired CL and overnight CL wear. They also devised a risk equation tool to educate the public and patients in reducing the risk of CL-related IK.

Several large-scale IK studies have also helped identify the emerging issue of antimicrobial resistance (AMR) against the common antimicrobial agents used for IK.[82, 83] Broad-spectrum

Table 8.1 Summary of large-scale infectious keratitis studies (>1000 cases) in the world, in descending order of chronology

Authors	Year of publication	Study period	Region	No. of scrapes	Culture positivity (%)	Bacteria (%)	Fungi (%)	Acanthamoeba (%)
Ting et al.[35]	2020	2007–2019	UK	1,333	37.7	92.8	3.0	4.2
Green et al.[72a]	2019	2005–2015	Australia	3,182	100.0	93.1	6.3	0.5
Kowalski et al.[73a, b]	2019	1993–2018	USA	1,387	100.0	72.1	6.7	5.2
Khor et al.[47]	2018	2012–2014	Asia	6,563	43.1	38	32.7	2.26
Tan et al.[74]	2017	2004–2015	UK	4,229	32.6	90.6	7.1	2.3
Lin et al.[75]	2017	2009–2013	China	2,973	46.1	41.9	44.6	13.6
Lalitha et al.[76]	2015	2002–2012	India	23,897	61.7	24.7	34.3	–
Hernandez-Camarena et al.[77]	2015	2002–2011	Mexico	1,638	37.6	88.3	11.7	–
Cariello et al.[78]	2011	1975–2007	Brazil	6804	48.6	78.9	11	7.4
Bharathi et al.[40]	2007	1999–2002	India	3183	70.6	46.4	48.7	1.5

Note: [a] These studies only included culture-proven infectious keratitis cases. [b] This study also included viral keratitis cases.

topical antimicrobial therapy serves as the current gold standard for treating IK, and AMR has been shown to negatively affect the outcome and healing time of IK.[84] In the Antibiotic Resistance Among Ocular Microorganisms (ARMOR) trial with data from 6091 ocular isolates, Asbell et al.[82] observed that 35% and 49% of the *Staphylococcus aureus* and coagulase-negative staphylococci were methicillin-resistant. Moreover, these microorganisms were often associated with multidrug resistance. In contrast, the Nottingham Infectious Keratitis Study, UK, demonstrated a low rate (<5%) of AMR against the commonly employed antibiotic regimens used for IK, namely fluoroquinolone monotherapy and cephalosporin–aminoglycoside dual therapy.[35] These findings highlight the geographical variations in AMR for IK and the importance of up-to-date examination in each region.

8.3.2 Corneal Transplant Registries

Since the first successful penetrating keratoplasty performed more than 100 years ago, corneal transplantation remains the main method for restoring corneal clarity and vision in patients with visually debilitating corneal diseases.[85] It is the most common transplantation performed worldwide, with >40,000 cases/year and ~3,500 cases/year performed in the USA and the UK, respectively.[85] However, shortage of donor corneas remains a persistent global issue, with around one cornea available for 70 needed.[69] This has led to a range of innovative measures being considered and implemented to improve the eye donation rate and utilization of donor corneas.[86–89]

In view of the limited pool of donor corneas, national corneal graft registries and eye banks have been established in many countries, including Singapore, India, the USA, the UK, Europe, Australia, and others,[11, 69, 90] to enable nationwide standardization of the corneal donation-to-transplantation pathway and control of usage and distribution of donor corneas (Table 8.2). In addition, the database could also provide a plethora of clinical and research information that is valuable to clinicians, researchers, policymakers, and relevant stakeholders.

First, the database can facilitate the examination of the availability and utilization of donor corneas, as well as the trends in the types and indications of corneal transplantation.[91, 92] Understanding the reasons for unutilized donor corneas (i.e., retrieved but not transplanted) allows introduction of effective changes to improve the utilization rate of donor corneas.[87, 93, 94] For instance, Ting et al.[87] demonstrated a significant improvement in the utilization rate of donor corneas by 14% in the North East of

England, UK, following refinement of the serological testing methods adopted by the UK eye bank system. In terms of the types of keratoplasty, regional/national studies have shown a paradigm shift from penetrating (full-thickness) keratoplasty to lamellar (partial-thickness) keratoplasty over the past decades in many countries, with FECD, keratoconus, and PBK being the main indications.[91, 92, 95–97]

Second, data collected through corneal transplant registries enable researchers to examine for important risk factors and prognostic factors of corneal transplantation, ultimately improving anatomical and visual outcomes.[98–101] Ang et al.[102] observed that patients who underwent Descemet membrane endothelial keratoplasty (DMEK) for FECD and bullous keratopathy achieved a better long-term graft survival when compared to Descemet stripping automated endothelial keratoplasty (DSAEK) and penetrating keratoplasty. National corneal transplant registries have also facilitated the identification of important prognostic factors for graft survival rate, including the indication for graft, number of previous grafts, corneal neovascularization, history of ocular inflammation or glaucoma, and postoperative events such as graft rejection or infection.[103–107] Studies have shown that corneal transplantation performed for the most common causes of blindness mentioned above, such as IK and PBK, generally fare worse than those performed for "low-risk" conditions such as keratoconus and FECD,[85] highlighting the need for improvement in management for the former indications and risk factors for graft failure.[108] In addition, the registries enable examination and monitoring for any significant postoperative adverse events such as infection and endophthalmitis. Based on a UK nationwide study of 11,320 patients, Chen et al.[109] demonstrated that the incidence of endophthalmitis after penetrating keratoplasty was only 0.7% in the UK. More importantly, they observed that the increased risk of endophthalmitis was associated with the cause of death, indications for graft, high-risk cases, and presumed transmission of infection from the donor corneas.

8.3.3 Corneal Genetic Studies

The surge in large-scale genetic studies, such as genome-wide linkage studies (GWLS) and genome-wide association studies (GWAS), has greatly improved our understanding of many diseases, including corneal diseases (Table 8.3).[110–122] GWLS is a valuable methodology used to genotype a particular disease by examining families with affected and unaffected individuals, whereas GWAS is a useful tool

Table 8.2 Summary of main corneal transplant registries and institutions in the world, categorized by continents

Countries	Corneal transplant registries (and institutions)
Global	Global Alliance of Eye Bank Associations (GAEBA)
Asia	
China	Beijing Tongren Eye Centre Shandong Eye Institute
Hong Kong	Lions Eye Bank of Hong Kong
Japan	Cornea Centre and Eye Bank, Tokyo Dental College Kyoto Prefectural University of Medicine
India	Eye Bank Association of India (EBAI)
Philippines	Santa Lucia International Eye Bank of Manila
Russia	S. N. Fyodorov Eye Microsurgery State Institution
Saudi Arabia	King Khaled Eye Specialist Hospital
Singapore	Singapore Corneal Transplant Study, Singapore Eye Bank
South Korea	Korean Network for Organ Sharing (KONOS) Seoul St. Mary's Eye Hospital
Taiwan	National Taiwan University Hospital
North and South America	
Brazil	Brazilian Association of Organ Transplantation (ABTO)
USA	Eye Bank Association of America (EBAA) Pan American Association of Eye Banks
UK and Europe	
Europe	European Cornea and Cell Transplantation Registry
France	Centre François Xavier Michelet, CHU de Bordeaux, Site Pellegrin
Germany	German Ophthalmological Society (GOS)
Italy	Società Italiana Trapianto di Cornea (SITRAC) Veneto Eye Bank Foundation
Netherlands	Netherlands Institute for Innovative Ocular Surgery
Sweden	Swedish Registry for Corneal Transplant
UK	UK National Health Service (NHS) Blood and Transplant
Australasia	
Australia	Australian Cornea Graft Registry (ACGR)
New Zealand	New Zealand National Eye Centre
Africa	
Ethiopia	Addis Ababa University
South Africa	Pretoria Eye Institute

Source: Adapted from the thesis published by Tan et al.[11]

designed to genotype common genetic variations across the genome, particularly single-nucleotide polymorphisms (SNPs), by analyzing the genotype–phenotype associations of a disease in case–control cohorts with a large number of individuals.[123, 124]

Amongst all, keratoconus and FECD are two of the most commonly investigated corneal diseases. This is primarily attributed to the high disease prevalence and the need for corneal transplantation for the severe form of these diseases, which places substantial burden on the

Table 8.3 Summary of the main genetic mutations of two main corneal dystrophies, namely keratoconus and Fuchs endothelial corneal dystrophy, identified through genome-wide linkage studies and genome-wide association studies

Corneal conditions	Gene	Genetic loci (variants)	References
Keratoconus	COL5A1	Chr 9 (rs1536482, rs7044529)	110, 111
	DOCK9	Chr 13 (c.2262A>C)	112
	FOXO1	Chr 13 (rs2721051)	111
	HGF	Chr 7 (rs3735520, rs1014091)	113, 114
	PNPLA2	Chr 11 (rs61876744)	115
	LOX	Chr 5 (rs10519694)	113, 116
	ZNF469	Chr 16 (rs9938149)	111
FECD	AGBL1	Chr 15 (c.3082C>T)	118
	ATP1B1	Chr 1 (rs1200114)	119
	FCD1	Chr 13 (D13S1236-D13S1304)	120
	FCD3	Chr 5 (D5S209-D5S425)	120
	FCD4	Chr 9 (D9S168-D9S1869)	121
	KANK4	Chr 1 (rs79742895)	119
	LAMC1	Chr 1 (rs3768617)	119
	TCF4	Chr 18 (rs613872)	122

limited pool of donor corneas.[95] Over the years, GWLS have successfully identified a number of genetic mutations implicated in keratoconus, including COL8A1, CAST, LOX, TCEB1, and TGFBI genes, amongst others.[124] GWAS has increasingly been used to identify genetic susceptibility regions in keratoconus and FECD.[124, 125] For instance, McComish et al.[115] recently identified a novel genetic locus in PNPLA2 at chromosome 11 for keratoconus based on over 6 million genetic variants. Several novel genetic loci for FECD, including TCF4, KANK4 rs79742895, LAMC1 rs3768617, and LINC00970/ ATP1B1 rs1200114, have also been discovered through GWAS.[119] Next-generation sequencing (NGS), which represents the most comprehensive tool in identifying genomic variants,[126] has recently been utilized to unravel novel mutations associated with other types of corneal dystrophy.[127]

In addition to the large-scale genomic studies conducted by independent research groups, genetic banks or databases containing comprehensive genetic information of most, if not all, human diseases are also made available through different web-based resources, including www. omim.org/, www.ncbi.nlm.nih.gov/gtr/, and www.gene2function.org/, amongst others.

8.3.4 Other Large-Scale and Electronic Health Record-Based Registries

With the increasing shift from traditional paper-based medical records to EHRs in healthcare systems, millions of valuable data can now be captured, synthesized, and utilized by clinicians and researchers.[128, 129] The Intelligent Research in Sight (IRIS) registry, a US-based ophthalmic EHR registry established by the American Academy of Ophthalmology, represents one of the most notable examples in the field of ophthalmology.[8, 130] In 2006, the IRIS registry had captured data from >17 million eye patients, including over a million of patients with dry-eye disease (DED), and >35 million visits, offering a wealth of information on prevalence, demographic factors, risk factors, management, and outcome of a range of ocular diseases. Donthineni et al.[70] similarly demonstrated the significant value of utilizing EHR-derived big data to estimate the incidence of DED in India as well as predisposing factors such as age, gender, socioeconomic status, and profession.

Beyond the world of ophthalmology, there are nationwide databases such as the UK Biobank which may also contain pertinent information related to the eye (and cornea).[131] Corneal hysteresis, an important biomechanical aspect of cornea, has been shown to play a role in the measurement of intraocular pressure, risk of developing glaucoma, and glaucoma management.[132] Based on the data of 93,345 participants derived from the UK Biobank, Zhang et al.[127] were able to demonstrate a significant association between corneal hysteresis and various demographic factors, such as age, sex, and ethnicity. In addition, GWAS based on the UK Biobank data successfully identified four novel genetic loci, including ZC3H11B, NPLOC4, LINC00340, and HERC2 genes, for corneal astigmatism.[133]

8.4 FUTURE TECHNOLOGIES FOR CORNEAL DISEASES

8.4.1 Role of Artificial Intelligence

Ophthalmology is a heavily imaging-centric specialty that utilizes advanced imaging technologies to assist the diagnosis and management of a wide range of ocular diseases. The widespread availability of ophthalmic images has made ophthalmology one of the best specialties for harnessing the power of AI, particularly those that employ DL-based algorithms. While the majority of ophthalmology-related AI research previously focused on the screening and diagnosis of posterior-segment diseases (e.g., diabetic retinopathy, age-related macular degeneration, and glaucoma), AI research is now starting to gain traction in the realm of corneal diseases, particularly for keratoconus, refractive surgery, and IK.[134]

8.4.1.1 Keratoconus

Keratoconus is the most common corneal ectatic disorder, with an estimated prevalence of 13.3–265 per 100,000 population.[135] Traditionally, depending on the severity of the disease, keratoconus is managed with glasses, CL, intracorneal ring segments (ICRS), and corneal transplantation, if all measures fail.[136] However, the innovation of corneal collagen cross-linking (CXL) in 2003 has revolutionized the management of keratoconus as it could halt the disease progression.[137] That said, treatment success relies on early detection of the disease as CXL does not reverse the progression of keratoconus.[138]

Currently, Placido disc-based, scanning-slit, and Scheimpflug imaging represent the commonly used imaging techniques to diagnose and monitor the progression of keratoconus.[139] To improve the detection rate of keratoconus, several AI algorithms, such as support vector machine learning, conventional neural network, and feedforward neural network, have been incorporated with these imaging systems.[134, 140–144] Studies have shown that the diagnostic accuracy for distinguishing between normal eyes and keratoconic eyes was as high as 92–97%.[134] In addition, AI algorithms could also help differentiate between normal eyes and preclinical keratoconus or forme fruste keratoconus,[142] which remains a challenging area in clinical practice. Moreover, AI such as artificial neural network has been utilized to guide the ICRS implantation for treating keratoconus.[145]

8.4.1.2 Refractive Surgery

Refractive surgery is one of the most common ophthalmic surgeries performed in the world. It has been shown to improve spectacle independence, cosmesis, and, more importantly, the quality of life of many people.[146] However, meticulous preoperative assessment is critical to optimize the visual and refractive outcomes, patient satisfaction, and safety, as well as to minimize postoperative complications such as corneal ectasia following corneal refractive surgery.[146] AI has demonstrated its clinical potential in detecting patients who are at higher risk of developing post-laser in situ keratomileusis (LASIK) ectasia.[147, 148] For instance, Xie et al.[148] developed a DL-based AI classification, using Pentacam InceptionResNetV2 Screening System (PIRSS), to screen candidates for corneal refractive surgery. Based on 1,385 patients and 6,465 corneal tomographic images, the AI algorithm was able to achieve an overall detection accuracy of 95%, which was comparable to senior refractive surgeons. Another study similarly demonstrated a detection accuracy of 93% in predicting suitability for corneal refractive surgery.[149]

8.4.1.3 Infectious Keratitis

IK is one of the commonest ocular emergencies that requires immediate medical attention and intervention to preserve vision and the eye. It is primarily diagnosed on clinical grounds with supplementation from microbiological investigations, most commonly in the form of corneal scraping. However, the diagnosis is challenged by the low yield of culture, slow turnaround time for positive microbiological results, and polymicrobial infection.[35, 74, 150] Several studies have demonstrated the potential value of AI in diagnosing and differentiating types of IK.[151–153] Liu et al.[153] demonstrated that a novel AI algorithm, based on convolutional neural network, could improve the diagnostic accuracy of in vivo confocal microscopy (IVCM) for fungal keratitis. Another DL-based AI algorithm similarly demonstrated a superior accuracy of 94% in automatically detecting fungal keratitis based on IVCM images.[152]

8.4.2 Role of Telemedicine

The convergence of 4G/5G technologies, enhanced imaging systems, and digital technologies has greatly facilitated the implementation of telemedicine in clinical practice. Its clinical deployment has also been emphasized and expedited by the recent COVID-19 pandemic lockdown where conventional face-to-face consultation is avoided whenever possible.[17]

Telemedicine is not a new concept in the field of ophthalmology. One of the best ophthalmic examples relates to the use of telemedicine in screening and diagnosing diabetic retinopathy and maculopathy in the community using fundus photography and a store-and-forward method for tele-consultation. Such services have been implemented in many countries, including the UK, USA, Singapore, and many others, to help cope with the oppressive volume of patients requiring diabetic eye checks.[14, 154] In addition, incorporation of AI with telemedicine could provide a synergistic effect in terms of enhancing the workflow efficiency of service provision.[134]

So far, telemedicine is not routinely used for assessing or diagnosing corneal diseases. However, within the research setting of cornea, telemedicine has been trialed in several areas, including the assessment and diagnosis of corneal diseases,[155, 156] monitoring of DED,[157] and evaluation of the suitability of donor corneal tissue for transplantation.[158]

Maamari et al.[155] developed a novel telemedicine platform using smartphones, combined with a +25-D lens and white/blue light sources, to detect and diagnose corneal abrasions and ulcers in Thailand. Based on photographic assessment only, the diagnostic performance of detecting IK by off-site ophthalmologists was very good (83–89% sensitivity and 91–97% specificity).[155] On the other hand, another pilot study evaluated the use of portable cameras in assessing and detecting a range of corneal diseases, including corneal abrasions, IK, pterygia, and corneal scarring.[156] Although the detection specificity was high (82–98%), the sensitivity was reported to be moderate (54–75%), suggesting that the quality of the anterior-segment images obtained was not sufficiently adequate for tele-cornea applications, highlighting further need for refinement before clinical deployment can be considered.[156]

8.5 CONCLUSION

Corneal diseases represent an important cause of blindness in the world, with IK (trachomatous and non-trachomatous) and PBK being the main causes of adult corneal blindness, and xerophthalmia and ON being the commonest causes of childhood corneal blindness. Through the successful implementation of various initiatives and programs, including the SAFE strategy, OEPA, and ESPEN, amongst others, the number of people being affected by trachoma and onchocerciasis is likely to continue to reduce significantly over the next decade. On the other hand, IK remains a persistent problem in both developed and developing countries, warranting further improvement in the diagnostic and therapeutic approaches for this clinical entity.

The establishment of data platforms such as corneal transplant registries, gene banks, and EHRs has so far provided a vast amount of valuable clinical and research information on a wide range of corneal diseases, including those that are sight-threatening (e.g., IK, PBK, etc.) and non-sight-threatening but functionally debilitating (e.g., DED). However, it is noteworthy to mention that the establishment and maintenance of these large-scale platforms and registries often require substantial financial resources and workforce, which explains why they normally exist in developed countries but not in under-resourced countries. Such mismatch and deficit highlight the need for increased effort and work to be invested in the under-resourced countries where the problem of corneal blindness predominates.[11, 159]

With the continued maturation of big data research and digital technologies, it is anticipated that telemedicine and AI-assisted platforms will become the "new normal" in medicine, including ophthalmology. Currently, telemedicine such as virtual clinics has already been deployed in several clinical areas of ophthalmology, including screening and monitoring of diabetic retinopathy and glaucoma, albeit primarily taking place in developed countries. Tele-consultation for corneal diseases has been explored but the performance and robustness of current imaging technologies need to be further enhanced before clinical implementation is possible. On the other hand, AI has demonstrated its clinical potential in several cornea-related territories, including screening and diagnosis of keratoconus, preoperative planning for refractive surgery, and diagnosis of IK.

As the digital technologies become fully developed for clinical use in the coming decade, increased effort, resources, and training need to be invested in under-resourced countries where corneal diseases are most prevalent so that these under-served populations can be assessed and managed more efficiently and effectively, ultimately ameliorating the global burden of corneal blindness.

REFERENCES

1. World Health Organization. *Blindness and Vision Impairment.* www.who.int/news-room/fact-sheets/detail/blindness-and-visual-impairment [accessed on 5 May 2020].

2. Oliva MS, Schottman T, Gulati M. Turning the tide of corneal blindness. *Indian J Ophthalmol* 2012;60(5):423–7.

3. Robaei D, Watson S. Corneal blindness: a global problem. *Clin Exp Ophthalmol* 2014;42(3):213–14.

4. Porth JM, Deiotte E, Dunn M, Bashshur R. A review of the literature on the global epidemiology of corneal blindness. *Cornea* 2019;38(12):1602–9.

5. Seyed Tabib NS, Madgwick M, Sudhakar P, et al. Big data in IBD: big progress for clinical practice. *Gut* 2020; gutjnl-2019-320065.

6. Kortüm KU, Müller M, Kern C, et al. Using electronic health records to build an ophthalmologic data warehouse and visualize patients' data. *Am J Ophthalmol* 2017;178:84–93.

7. Johnston RL, Taylor H, Smith R, Sparrow JM. The Cataract National Dataset electronic multi-centre audit of 55,567 operations: variation in posterior capsule rupture rates between surgeons. *Eye (Lond)* 2010;24(5):888–93.

8. Chiang MF, Sommer A, Rich WL, et al. The 2016 American Academy of Ophthalmology IRIS(®) Registry (Intelligent Research in Sight) database: characteristics and methods. *Ophthalmology* 2018;125(8):1143–8.

9. Mooney SJ, Westreich DJ, El-Sayed AM. Commentary: Epidemiology in the era of big data. *Epidemiology* 2015;26(3):390–4.

10. Roski J, Bo-Linn GW, Andrews TA. Creating value in health care through big data: opportunities and policy implications. *Health Aff (Millwood)* 2014;33(7):1115–22.

11. Tan D, Ang M, Arundhati A, Khor WB. Development of selective lamellar keratoplasty within an Asian corneal transplant program: the Singapore Corneal Transplant Study (an American Ophthalmological Society thesis). *Trans Am Ophthalmol Soc* 2015;113:T10.

12. Foot B, MacEwen C. Surveillance of sight loss due to delay in ophthalmic treatment or review: frequency, cause and outcome. *Eye (Lond)* 2017;31(5):771–5.

13. Ting DSW, Cheung CY, Nguyen Q, et al. Deep learning in estimating prevalence and systemic risk factors for diabetic retinopathy: a multi-ethnic study. *NPJ Digit Med* 2019;2:24.

14. Sim DA, Mitry D, Alexander P, et al. The evolution of teleophthalmology programs in the United Kingdom: beyond diabetic retinopathy screening. *J Diabetes Sci Technol* 2016;10(2):308–17.

15. Ting DSJ, Ang M, Mehta JS, Ting DSW. Artificial intelligence-assisted telemedicine platform for cataract screening and management: a potential model of care for global eye health. *Br J Ophthalmol* 2019;103(11):1537–8.

16. Gan K, Liu Y, Stagg B, et al. Telemedicine for glaucoma: guidelines and recommendations. *Telemed J E Health* 2020;26(4):551–5.

17. Ting DSW, Carin L, Dzau V, Wong TY. Digital technology and COVID-19. *Nat Med* 2020;26(4):459–61.

18. Flaxman SR, Bourne RRA, Resnikoff S, et al. Global causes of blindness and distance vision impairment 1990–2020: a systematic review and meta-analysis. *Lancet Glob Health* 2017;5(12):e1221–34.

19. Ting DSJ, Ho CS, Deshmukh R, et al. Infectious keratitis: an update on epidemiology, causative organisms, risk factors, and antimicrobial resistance. *Eye (Lond)* 2021;35(4):1084–101.

20. Dandona L, Dandona R, Naduvilath TJ, et al. Is current eye-care-policy focus almost exclusively on cataract adequate to deal with blindness in India? *Lancet* 1998;351(9112):1312–16.

21. World Health Organization. *Trachoma*. www.who.int/news-room/fact-sheets/detail/trachoma [accessed on 10 May 2020].

22. Mariotti SP, Pascolini D, Rose-Nussbaumer J. Trachoma: global magnitude of a preventable cause of blindness. *Br J Ophthalmol* 2009;93(5):563–8.

23. Ramadhani AM, Derrick T, Macleod D, et al. Progression of scarring trachoma in Tanzanian children: a four-year cohort study. *PLoS Negl Trop Dis* 2019;13(8):e0007638.

24. Habtamu E, Wondie T, Aweke S, et al. The impact of trachomatous trichiasis on quality of life: a case control study. *PLoS Negl Trop Dis* 2015;9(11):e0004254.

25. Thylefors B, Dawson CR, Jones BR, et al. A simple system for the assessment of trachoma and its complications. *Bull World Health Organ* 1987;65(4):477–83.

26. Taylor HR, Rapoza PA, West S, et al. The epidemiology of infection in trachoma. *Invest Ophthalmol Vis Sci* 1989;30(8):1823–33.

27. Lietman TM, Oldenburg CE, Keenan JD. Trachoma: time to talk eradication. *Ophthalmology* 2020;127(1):11–13.

28. Lavett DK, Lansingh VC, Carter MJ, et al. Will the SAFE strategy be sufficient to eliminate trachoma by 2020? Puzzlements and possible solutions. *Sci World J* 2013;2013:648106.

29. Burton M, Habtamu E, Ho D, Gower EW. Interventions for trachoma trichiasis. *Cochrane Database Syst Rev 2015*;2015(11):Cd004008.

30. Frick KD, Lietman TM, Holm SO, et al. Cost-effectiveness of trachoma control measures: comparing targeted household treatment and mass treatment of children. *Bull World Health Organ* 2001;79(3):201–7.

31. Ngondi J, Onsarigo A, Matthews F, et al. Effect of 3 years of SAFE (surgery, antibiotics, facial cleanliness, and environmental change) strategy for trachoma control in southern Sudan: a cross-sectional study. *Lancet* 2006;368(9535):589–95.

32. Ung L, Acharya NR, Agarwal T, et al. Infectious corneal ulceration: a proposal for neglected tropical disease status. *Bull World Health Organ* 2019;97(12):854–6.

33. Erie JC, Nevitt MP, Hodge DO, Ballard DJ. Incidence of ulcerative keratitis in a defined population from 1950 through 1988. *Arch Ophthalmol* 1993; 111(12):1665–71.

34. Seal DV, Kirkness CM, Bennett HG, Peterson M. Population-based cohort study of microbial keratitis in Scotland: incidence and features. *Cont Lens Anterior Eye* 1999;22(2):49–57.

35. Ting DSJ, Ho CS, Cairns J, et al. A 12-year analysis of incidence, microbiological profiles, and in vitro antimicrobial susceptibility of infectious keratitis: the Nottingham infectious keratitis study. *Br J Ophthalmol* 2021;105(3):328–33.

36. Gonzales CA, Srinivasan M, Whitcher JP, Smolin G. Incidence of corneal ulceration in Madurai district, South India. *Ophthalmic Epidemiol* 1996;3(3):159–66.

37. Schein OD, Ormerod LD, Barraquer E, et al. Microbiology of contact lens-related keratitis. *Cornea* 1989;8(4):281–5.

38. Green M, Apel A, Stapleton F. Risk factors and causative organisms in microbial keratitis. *Cornea* 2008;27(1):22–7.

39. Dart JK, Radford CF, Minassian D, et al. Risk factors for microbial keratitis with contemporary contact lenses: a case-control study. *Ophthalmology* 2008;115(10):1647–54, 54.e1-3.

40. Bharathi MJ, Ramakrishnan R, Meenakshi R, et al. Microbial keratitis in South India: influence of risk factors, climate, and geographical variation. *Ophthalmic Epidemiol* 2007;14(2):61–9.

41. Hagan M, Wright E, Newman M, et al. Causes of suppurative keratitis in Ghana. *Br J Ophthalmol* 1995;79(11):1024–8.

42. Poole TR, Hunter DL, Maliwa EM, Ramsay AR. Aetiology of microbial keratitis in northern Tanzania. *Br J Ophthalmol* 2002;86(8):941–2.

43. Dunlop AA, Wright ED, Howlader SA, et al. Suppurative corneal ulceration in Bangladesh. A study of 142 cases examining the microbiological diagnosis, clinical and epidemiological features of bacterial and fungal keratitis. *Aust N Z J Ophthalmol* 1994;22(2):105–10.

44. Xie L, Zhong W, Shi W, Sun S. Spectrum of fungal keratitis in north China. *Ophthalmology* 2006;113(11):1943–8.

45. Ormerod LD, Hertzmark E, Gomez DS, et al. Epidemiology of microbial keratitis in southern California. A multivariate analysis. *Ophthalmology* 1987;94(10):1322–33.

46. Stehr-Green JK, Bailey TM, Visvesvara GS. The epidemiology of *Acanthamoeba* keratitis in the United States. *Am J Ophthalmol* 1989;107(4):331–6.

47. Khor WB, Prajna VN, Garg P, et al. The Asia Cornea Society Infectious Keratitis Study: a prospective multicenter study of infectious keratitis in Asia. *Am J Ophthalmol* 2018;195:161–70.

48. Dart JK, Stapleton F, Minassian D. Contact lenses and other risk factors in microbial keratitis. *Lancet* 1991;338(8768):650–3.

49. Upadhyay MP, Karmacharya PC, Koirala S, et al. The Bhaktapur eye study: ocular trauma and antibiotic prophylaxis for the prevention of corneal ulceration in Nepal. *Br J Ophthalmol* 2001;85(4):388–92.

50. Srinivasan M, Upadhyay MP, Priyadarsini B, et al. Corneal ulceration in south-east Asia III: prevention of fungal keratitis at the village level in south India using topical antibiotics. *Br J Ophthalmol* 2006;90(12):1472–5.

51. Brattig NW, Cheke RA, Garms R. Onchocerciasis (river blindness): more than a century of research and control. *Acta Trop* 2021;218:105677.

52. World Health Organization. *Onchocerciasis.* www.who.int/news-room/fact-sheets/detail/onchocerciasis. [accessed on 13 May 2020]

53. Eye Bank Association of America. http://restoresight.org/wp-content/uploads/2017/04/2016_Statistical_Report-Final-040717.pdf [accessed on 13 May 2020].

54. Gupta N, Vashist P, Tandon R, et al. Prevalence of corneal diseases in the rural Indian population: the Corneal Opacity Rural Epidemiological (CORE) study. *Br J Ophthalmol* 2015;99(2):147–52.

55. Veladanda R, Ch SS, Pallapolu L, et al. A hospital based clinical study on corneal blindness in a tertiary eye care centre in North Telangana. *JKIMSU* 2016;5:12–17.

56. World Health Organization. Xerophthalmia and night blindness for the assessment of clinical vitamin A deficiency in individuals and populations. www.who.int/publications/i/item/WHO-NMH-NHD-EPG-14.4 [accessed on 13 December 2020].

57. Sommer A, Hussaini G, Muhilal, et al. History of nightblindness: a simple tool for xerophthalmia screening. *Am J Clin Nutr* 1980;33(4):887–91.

58. World Health Organization. *Global Prevalence of Vitamin A Deficiency in Populations at Risk. 1995–2005 WHO Global Database on Vitamin A Deficiency* 2009. Available at: https://apps.who.int/iris/bitstream/handle/10665/44110/9789241598019_eng.pdf?sequence=1.

59. Spence JC. A clinical study of nutritional xerophthalmia and night-blindness. *Arch Dis Child* 1931;6(31):17–26.

60. McLaren DS, Kraemer K. Xerophthalmia. *World Rev Nutr Diet* 2012;103:65–75.

61. Katz J, Khatry SK, West KP, et al. Night blindness is prevalent during pregnancy and lactation in rural Nepal. *J Nutr* 1995;125(8):2122–7.

62. Natadisastra G, Wittpenn JR, West KP, Jr., et al. Impression cytology for detection of vitamin A deficiency. *Arch Ophthalmol* 1987;105(9):1224–8.

63. Villamor E, Fawzi WW. Vitamin A supplementation: implications for morbidity and mortality in children. *J Infect Dis* 2000;182 Suppl 1:S122–33.

64. Kielmann AA, Ajello CA, Kielmann NS. Nutrition intervention: an evaluation of six studies. *Stud Fam Plann* 1982;13(8–9):246–57.

65. Zloto O, Gharaibeh A, Mezer E, et al. Ophthalmia neonatorum treatment and prophylaxis: IPOSC global study. *Graefes Arch Clin Exp Ophthalmol* 2016;254(3):577–82.

66. Whitcher JP, Srinivasan M, Upadhyay MP. Corneal blindness: a global perspective. *Bull World Health Organ* 2001;79(3):214–21.

67. Chandler JW, Rapoza PA. Ophthalmia neonatorum. *Int Ophthalmol Clin* 1990;30(1):36–8.

68. Ting DSW, Pasquale LR, Peng L, et al. Artificial intelligence and deep learning in ophthalmology. *Br J Ophthalmol* 2019;103(2):167–75.

69. Gain P, Jullienne R, He Z, et al. Global survey of corneal transplantation and eye banking. *JAMA Ophthalmol* 2016;134(2):167–73.

70. Donthineni PR, Kammari P, Shanbhag SS, et al. Incidence, demographics, types and risk factors of dry eye disease in India: electronic medical records driven big data analytics report I. *Ocul Surf* 2019;17(2):250–6.

71. Ung L, Bispo PJM, Shanbhag SS, et al. The persistent dilemma of microbial keratitis: global burden, diagnosis, and antimicrobial resistance. *Surv Ophthalmol* 2019;64(3):255–71.

72. Green M, Carnt N, Apel A, Stapleton F. Queensland Microbial Keratitis Database: 2005–2015. *Br J Ophthalmol* 2019;103(10):1481–6.

73. Kowalski RP, Nayyar SV, Romanowski EG, et al. The prevalence of bacteria, fungi, viruses, and *Acanthamoeba* from 3,004 cases of keratitis, endophthalmitis, and conjunctivitis. *Eye Contact Lens* 2020;46(5):265–8.

74. Tan SZ, Walkden A, Au L, et al. Twelve-year analysis of microbial keratitis trends at a UK tertiary hospital. *Eye (Lond)* 2017;31(8):1229–36.

75. Lin L, Lan W, Lou B, et al. Genus distribution of bacteria and fungi associated with keratitis in a large eye center located in southern China. *Ophthalmic Epidemiol* 2017;24(2):90–6.

76. Lalitha P, Prajna NV, Manoharan G, et al. Trends in bacterial and fungal keratitis in South India, 2002–2012. *Br J Ophthalmol* 2015;99(2):192–4.

77. Hernandez-Camarena JC, Graue-Hernandez EO, Ortiz-Casas M, et al. Trends in microbiological and antibiotic sensitivity patterns in infectious keratitis: 10-year experience in Mexico City. *Cornea* 2015;34(7):778–85.

78. Cariello AJ, Passos RM, Yu MC, Hofling-Lima AL. Microbial keratitis at a referral center in Brazil. *Int Ophthalmol* 2011;31(3):197–204.

79. Ting DSJ, Settle C, Morgan SJ, et al. A 10-year analysis of microbiological profiles of microbial keratitis: the North East England Study. *Eye (Lond)* 2018;32(8):1416–17.

80. Das S, Constantinou M, Daniell M, Taylor HR. *Moraxella* keratitis: predisposing factors and clinical review of 95 cases. *Br J Ophthalmol* 2006;90(10):1236–8.

81. Sauer A, Greth M, Letsch J, et al. Contact lenses and infectious keratitis: from a case-control study to a computation of the risk for wearers. *Cornea* 2020;39(6):769–74.

82. Asbell PA, Sanfilippo CM, Sahm DF, DeCory HH. Trends in antibiotic resistance among ocular microorganisms in the United States from 2009 to 2018. *JAMA Ophthalmol* 2020;138(5):1–12.

83. Lalitha P, Manoharan G, Karpagam R, et al. Trends in antibiotic resistance in bacterial keratitis isolates from South India. *Br J Ophthalmol* 2017;101(2):108–13.

84. Kaye S, Tuft S, Neal T, et al. Bacterial susceptibility to topical antimicrobials and clinical outcome in bacterial keratitis. *Invest Ophthalmol Vis Sci* 2010;51(1):362–8.

85. Tan DT, Dart JK, Holland EJ, Kinoshita S. Corneal transplantation. *Lancet* 2012;379(9827):1749–61.

86. Ting DS, Potts J, Jones M, et al. Impact of telephone consent and potential for eye donation in the UK: the Newcastle Eye Centre study. *Eye (Lond)* 2016;30(3):342–8.

87. Ting DS, Potts J, Jones M, et al. Changing trend in the utilisation rate of donated corneas for keratoplasty in the UK: the North East England Study. *Eye (Lond)* 2016;30(11):1475–80.

88. Gupta N, Vashist P, Ganger A, et al. Eye donation and eye banking in India. *Natl Med J India* 2018;31(5):283–6.

89. Singh R, Gupta N, Vanathi M, Tandon R. Corneal transplantation in the modern era. *Indian J Med Res* 2019;150(1):7–22.

90. Tan JCK, Ferdi AC, Gillies MC, Watson SL. Clinical registries in ophthalmology. *Ophthalmology* 2019;126(5):655–62.

91. Keenan TD, Jones MN, Rushton S, Carley FM. Trends in the indications for corneal graft surgery in the United Kingdom: 1999 through 2009. *Arch Ophthalmol* 2012;130(5):621–8.

92. Park CY, Lee JK, Gore PK, et al. Keratoplasty in the United States: a 10-year review from 2005 through 2014. *Ophthalmology* 2015;122(12):2432–42.

93. Sharma N, Arora T, Singhal D, et al. Procurement, storage and utilization trends of eye banks in India. *Indian J Ophthalmol* 2019;67(7):1056–9.

94. Gogia V, Gupta S, Agarwal T, et al. Changing pattern of utilization of human donor cornea in India. *Indian J Ophthalmol* 2015;63(8):654–8.

95. Ting DS, Sau CY, Srinivasan S, et al. Changing trends in keratoplasty in the west of Scotland: a 10-year review. *Br J Ophthalmol* 2012;96(3):405–8.

96. Fuest M, Ang M, Htoon HM, et al. Long-term visual outcomes comparing Descemet stripping automated endothelial keratoplasty and penetrating keratoplasty. *Am J Ophthalmol* 2017;182:62–71.

97. Ang M, Wilkins MR, Mehta JS, Tan D. Descemet membrane endothelial keratoplasty. *Br J Ophthalmol* 2016;100(1):15–21.

98. Ang M, Htoon HM, Cajucom-Uy HY, et al. Donor and surgical risk factors for primary graft failure following Descemet's stripping automated endothelial keratoplasty in Asian eyes. *Clin Ophthalmol* 2011;5:1503–8.

99. Ang M, Mehta JS, Lim F, et al. Endothelial cell loss and graft survival after Descemet's stripping automated endothelial keratoplasty and penetrating keratoplasty. *Ophthalmology* 2012;119(11):2239–44.

100. Bose S, Ang M, Mehta JS, et al. Cost-effectiveness of Descemet's stripping endothelial keratoplasty versus penetrating keratoplasty. *Ophthalmology* 2013;120(3):464–70.

101. Ang M, Lim F, Htoon HM, et al. Visual acuity and contrast sensitivity following Descemet stripping automated endothelial keratoplasty. *Br J Ophthalmol* 2016;100(3):307–11.

102. Ang M, Soh Y, Htoon HM, et al. Five-year graft survival comparing Descemet stripping automated endothelial keratoplasty and penetrating keratoplasty. *Ophthalmology* 2016;123(8):1646–52.

103. Sibley D, Hopkinson CL, Tuft SJ, et al. Differential effects of primary disease and corneal vascularisation on corneal transplant rejection and survival. *Br J Ophthalmol* 2020;104(5):729–34.

104. Williams KA, Lowe M, Bartlett C, et al. Risk factors for human corneal graft failure within the Australian corneal graft registry. *Transplantation* 2008;86(12):1720–4.

105. Ang M, Mehta JS, Sng CC, et al. Indications, outcomes, and risk factors for failure in tectonic keratoplasty. *Ophthalmology* 2012;119(7):1311–19.

106. Ang M, Li L, Chua D, et al. Descemet's stripping automated endothelial keratoplasty with anterior chamber intraocular lenses: complications and 3-year outcomes. *Br J Ophthalmol* 2014;98(8):1028–32.

107. Ang M, Ting DSJ, Kumar A, et al. Descemet membrane endothelial keratoplasty in Asian eyes: intraoperative and postoperative complications. *Cornea* 2020;39(8):940–5.

108. Ang M, Sng CCA. Descemet membrane endothelial keratoplasty and glaucoma. *Curr Opin Ophthalmol* 2018;29(2):178–84.

109. Chen JY, Jones MN, Srinivasan S, et al. Endophthalmitis after penetrating keratoplasty. *Ophthalmology* 2015;122(1):25–30.

110. Li X, Bykhovskaya Y, Canedo AL, et al. Genetic association of COL5A1 variants in keratoconus patients suggests a complex connection between corneal thinning and keratoconus. *Invest Ophthalmol Vis Sci* 2013;54(4):2696–704.

111. Lu Y, Vitart V, Burdon KP, et al. Genome-wide association analyses identify multiple loci associated with central corneal thickness and keratoconus. *Nat Genet* 2013;45(2):155–63.

125

112. Czugala M, Karolak JA, Nowak DM, et al. Novel mutation and three other sequence variants segregating with phenotype at keratoconus 13q32 susceptibility locus. *Eur J Hum Genet* 2012;20(4):389–97.

113. Dudakova L, Palos M, Jirsova K, et al. Validation of rs2956540:G>C and rs3735520:G>A association with keratoconus in a population of European descent. *Eur J Hum Genet* 2015;23(11):1581–3.

114. Burdon KP, Macgregor S, Bykhovskaya Y, et al. Association of polymorphisms in the hepatocyte growth factor gene promoter with keratoconus. *Invest Ophthalmol Vis Sci* 2011;52(11):8514–19.

115. McComish BJ, Sahebjada S, Bykhovskaya Y, et al. Association of genetic variation with keratoconus. *JAMA Ophthalmol* 2019;138(2):174–81.

116. Bykhovskaya Y, Li X, Epifantseva I, et al. Variation in the lysyl oxidase (LOX) gene is associated with keratoconus in family-based and case-control studies. *Invest Ophthalmol Vis Sci* 2012;53(7):4152–7.

117. Sahebjada S, Schache M, Richardson AJ, et al. Evaluating the association between keratoconus and the corneal thickness genes in an independent Australian population. *Invest Ophthalmol Vis Sci* 2013;54(13):8224–8.

118. Riazuddin SA, Vasanth S, Katsanis N, Gottsch JD. Mutations in AGBL1 cause dominant late-onset Fuchs corneal dystrophy and alter protein–protein interaction with TCF4. *Am J Hum Genet* 2013;93(4):758–64.

119. Afshari NA, Igo RP, Jr., Morris NJ, et al. Genome-wide association study identifies three novel loci in Fuchs endothelial corneal dystrophy. *Nat Commun* 2017;8:14898.

120. Riazuddin SA, Eghrari AO, Al-Saif A, et al. Linkage of a mild late-onset phenotype of Fuchs corneal dystrophy to a novel locus at 5q33.1-q35.2. *Invest Ophthalmol Vis Sci* 2009;50(12):5667–71.

121. Riazuddin SA, Zaghloul NA, Al-Saif A, et al. Missense mutations in TCF8 cause late-onset Fuchs corneal dystrophy and interact with FCD4 on chromosome 9p. *Am J Hum Genet* 2010;86(1):45–53.

122. Baratz KH, Tosakulwong N, Ryu E, et al. E2-2 protein and Fuchs's corneal dystrophy. *N Engl J Med* 2010;363(11):1016–24.

123. Tam V, Patel N, Turcotte M, et al. Benefits and limitations of genome-wide association studies. *Nat Rev Genet* 2019;20(8):467–84.

124. Karolak JA, Gajecka M. Genomic strategies to understand causes of keratoconus. *Mol Genet Genomics* 2017;292(2):251–69.

125. Iliff BW, Riazuddin SA, Gottsch JD. The genetics of Fuchs' corneal dystrophy. *Expert Rev Ophthalmol* 2012;7(4):363–75.

126. Londin E, Yadav P, Surrey S, et al. Use of linkage analysis, genome-wide association studies, and next-generation sequencing in the identification of disease-causing mutations. *Methods Mol Biol* 2013;1015:127–46.

127. Zhang B, Shweikh Y, Khawaja AP, et al. Associations with corneal hysteresis in a population cohort: results from 96 010 UK Biobank participants. *Ophthalmology* 2019;126(11):1500–10.

128. Evans RS. Electronic health records: then, now, and in the future. *Yearb Med Inform* 2016;Suppl 1:S48–61.

129. Day AC, Donachie PH, Sparrow JM, Johnston RL. The Royal College of Ophthalmologists' National Ophthalmology Database study of cataract surgery: report 1, visual outcomes and complications. *Eye (Lond)* 2015;29(4):552–60.

130. Parke Ii DW, Lum F, Rich WL. The IRIS® Registry: purpose and perspectives. *Ophthalmologe* 2017;114(Suppl 1):1–6.

131. Chua SYL, Thomas D, Allen N, et al. Cohort profile: design and methods in the eye and vision consortium of UK Biobank. *BMJ Open* 2019;9(2):e025077.

132. Deol M, Taylor DA, Radcliffe NM. Corneal hysteresis and its relevance to glaucoma. *Curr Opin Ophthalmol* 2015;26(2):96–102.

133. Shah RL, Guggenheim JA. Genome-wide association studies for corneal and refractive astigmatism in UK Biobank demonstrate a shared role for myopia susceptibility loci. *Hum Genet* 2018;137(11–12):881–96.

134. Ting DSJ, Foo VH, Yang LWY, et al. Artificial intelligence for anterior segment diseases: emerging applications in ophthalmology. *Br J Ophthalmol* 2021;105(2):158–68.

135. Godefrooij DA, de Wit GA, Uiterwaal CS, et al. Age-specific incidence and prevalence of keratoconus: a nationwide registration study. *Am J Ophthalmol* 2017;175:169–72.

136. Rabinowitz YS. Keratoconus. *Surv Ophthalmol* 1998;42(4):297–319.

137. Wollensak G, Spoerl E, Seiler T. Riboflavin/ultraviolet-A-induced collagen crosslinking for the treatment of keratoconus. *Am J Ophthalmol* 2003;135(5):620–7.

138. Ting DSJ, Rana-Rahman R, Chen Y, et al. Effectiveness and safety of accelerated (9 mW/cm 2) corneal collagen cross-linking for progressive keratoconus: a 24-month follow-up. *Eye (Lond)* 2019;33(5):812–18.

139. Masiwa LE, Moodley V. A review of corneal imaging methods for the early diagnosis of pre-clinical keratoconus. *J Optom* 2020;S1888–4296(19)30104-9.

140. Lavric A, Valentin P. KeratoDetect: keratoconus detection algorithm using convolutional neural networks. *Comput Intell Neurosci* 2019;2019:8162567.

141. Arbelaez MC, Versaci F, Vestri G, et al. Use of a support vector machine for keratoconus and subclinical keratoconus detection by topographic and tomographic data. *Ophthalmology* 2012;119(11):2231–8.

142. Smadja D, Touboul D, Cohen A, et al. Detection of subclinical keratoconus using an automated decision tree classification. *Am J Ophthalmol* 2013;156(2):237–46 e1.

143. Issarti I, Consejo A, Jiménez-García M, et al. Computer aided diagnosis for suspect keratoconus detection. *Comput Biol Med* 2019;109:33–42.

144. Ruiz Hidalgo I, Rodriguez P, Rozema JJ, et al. Evaluation of a machine-learning classifier for keratoconus detection based on Scheimpflug tomography. *Cornea* 2016;35(6):827–32.

145. Fariselli C, Vega-Estrada A, Arnalich-Montiel F, Alio JL. Artificial neural network to guide intracorneal ring segments implantation for keratoconus treatment: a pilot study. *Eye Vis (Lond)* 2020;7:20.

146. Kim TI, Alió Del Barrio JL, Wilkins M, et al. Refractive surgery. *Lancet* 2019;393(10185):2085–98.

147. Lopes BT, Ramos IC, Salomão MQ, et al. Enhanced tomographic assessment to detect corneal ectasia based on artificial intelligence. *Am J Ophthalmol* 2018;195:223–32.

148. Xie Y, Zhao L, Yang X, et al. Screening candidates for refractive surgery with corneal tomographic-based deep learning. *JAMA Ophthalmol* 2020;e200507.

149. Yoo TK, Ryu IH, Lee G, et al. Adopting machine learning to automatically identify candidate patients for corneal refractive surgery. *NPJ Digit Med* 2019;2:59.

150. Ting DSJ, Bignardi G, Koerner R, et al. Polymicrobial keratitis with *Cryptococcus curvatus*, *Candida parapsilosis*, and *Stenotrophomonas maltophilia* after penetrating keratoplasty: a rare case report with literature review. *Eye Contact Lens* 2019;45(2):e5–10.

151. Saini JS, Jain AK, Kumar S, et al. Neural network approach to classify infective keratitis. *Curr Eye Res* 2003;27(2):111-6.

152. Lv J, Zhang K, Chen Q, et al. Deep learning-based automated diagnosis of fungal keratitis with in vivo confocal microscopy images. *Ann Transl Med* 2020;8(11):706.

153. Liu Z, Cao Y, Li Y, et al. Automatic diagnosis of fungal keratitis using data augmentation and image fusion with deep convolutional neural network. *Comput Methods Programs Biomed* 2020;187:105019.

154. Horton MB, Brady CJ, Cavallerano J, et al. practice guidelines for ocular telehealth-diabetic retinopathy, third edition. *Telemed J E Health* 2020;26(4):495–543.

155. Maamari RN, Ausayakhun S, Margolis TP, et al. Novel telemedicine device for diagnosis of corneal abrasions and ulcers in resource-poor settings. *JAMA Ophthalmol* 2014;132(7):894–5.

156. Woodward MA, Musch DC, Hood CT, et al. Teleophthalmic approach for detection of corneal diseases: accuracy and reliability. *Cornea* 2017;36(10):1159–65.

157. Amparo F, Dana R. Web-based longitudinal remote assessment of dry eye symptoms. *Ocul Surf* 2018;16(2):249–53.

158. Alabi RO, Ansin A, Clover J, et al. Novel use of telemedicine for corneal tissue evaluation in eye banking: establishing a standardized approach for the remote evaluation of donor corneas for transplantation. *Cornea* 2019;38(4):509–14.

159. Pineda R. Corneal transplantation in the developing world: lessons learned and meeting the challenge. *Cornea* 2015;34 Suppl 10:S35–40.

9 Dry-Eye Disease

Fiona Stapleton and Revathy Mani

9.1 INTRODUCTION

Dry-eye disease (DED) is a chronic, multifactorial disease of the ocular surface, where the pathophysiology is underpinned by tear film instability, hyperosmolarity, ocular surface inflammation, and neurosensory abnormalities (Bron et al., 2017; Craig et al., 2017). The disease is associated with significant morbidity and societal impact where affected individuals report ocular discomfort or pain, and reduced visual function and quality of life. The major societal burden of disease is related to indirect costs due to reduced productivity at work. The public health impact of the disease is anticipated to increase with population aging, and there is considerable interest in characterizing and potentially modifying risk factors associated with the disease as a means of prevention. This chapter will focus on evidence for risk factors and burden of disease and will particularly focus on publications in the last 10 years.

9.2 BURDEN, COST, AND IMPACT OF DRY-EYE DISEASE

9.2.1 Burden of Dry-Eye Disease

Prevalence estimates for DED vary significantly based on disease definition (Stapleton et al., 2017), severity, and demographic characteristics of the population. Several large population-based studies using the Women's Health Study (WHS) criteria, arguably capturing more severe disease (severe symptoms of dryness or irritation constantly or often, and/or a prior diagnosis of DED by a clinician) have reported age-adjusted prevalence rates of 4.3 (males only)–9.1% in Caucasian populations (Schaumberg et al., 2009; Vehof et al., 2021) and 16–23.7% in Asian populations (Ahn et al., 2014; Um et al., 2014). The prevalence of DED characterized by both signs and symptoms has been reported at 8.7–11.0% in Caucasians (Viso et al., 2009; Hashemi et al., 2014; Vehof et al., 2014) and 30.1% (Tian et al., 2009) in Asian populations. Female sex and older age are consistently identified as risk factors in prevalence studies using symptoms-based criteria or a prior diagnosis of dry eye made by a clinician.

The majority of published studies, using symptoms or a prior diagnosis of dry eye, however, have explored rates of disease in the over-40s population. The Lifelines cohort study in the Netherlands (Vehof et al., 2021) established an overall prevalence of dry eye using the WHS criteria of 9.1%, also that prevalence increased with age above 50 years, women had twice the rate of disease compared with men but individuals aged 20–30 years had a similar rate of disease to those aged 40–50 years. Similarly, the National Health and Wellness Survey in the USA examined rates of diagnosed dry eye and undiagnosed but symptomatic disease (combined prevalence of 9.3%) and showed broadly similar findings to the Lifelines study with respect to the younger age groups (Farrand et al., 2017). While this has not been confirmed, the unexpectedly high rates of disease in younger age groups are speculated to be a consequence of greater exposure to contact lens wear or digital device use.

The prevalence of DED characterized by both signs and symptoms has been reported at 8.7–11.0% in Caucasians (Viso et al., 2009; Hashemi et al., 2014; Malet et al., 2014; Vehof et al., 2014), 16.7–33.4% (Tian et al., 2009; Ahn et al., 2014; Gong et al., 2017; Arita et al., 2019; Viet Vu et al., 2019) in South-East Asian populations, and 26.2% in India (Tandon et al., 2020). In an older Caucasian population (over 65), the prevalence was 21.4% (Ferrero et al., 2018). Limited studies have been carried out in Africa and one small community study ($n = 363$) has estimated signs and symptoms of dry eye to be present in 32.5% of residents (Olaniyan et al., 2016).

Signs of meibomian gland dysfunction (MGD) are present in 30–35% of Caucasian individuals (Viso et al., 2009, 2012, 2014; Hashemi et al., 2014) and in 33–50% of Asian individuals (Tian et al., 2009; Han et al., 2011; Siak et al., 2012; Arita et al., 2019), rising to 51.8–60.8% in the over-65 age group (Lin et al., 2003; Han et al., 2011; Siak et al., 2012). In an Iranian population-based study, the prevalence of MGD was 26.3% in an adult population (Hashemi et al., 2017), rising to 71.2% in the over-60s age group (Hashemi et al., 2021). It is recognized, however, that up to two-thirds of the disease may be asymptomatic (Viso et al., 2012) and that age-related lid and gland changes underpin high rates of asymptomatic disease in older adults. A systematic review of interethnic disparities in the natural history of DED suggested that meibomian gland changes were apparent earlier in life in South-East Asian compared with Caucasian eyes (Wang and Craig, 2019). In comparison with studies exploring signs and symptoms of dry eye, several studies have suggested a higher prevalence of MGD in males (up to 2.5×) compared with females (Arita et al., 2019; Hashemi et al., 2021).

DOI: 10.1201/9781315146737-11

In conclusion, as a conservative estimate, 10–20% of the population over 40 report severe symptoms and/or seek treatment for DED. Irrespective of the definition of disease, the prevalence consistently varies with age and race, although the impact of sex on MGD is equivocal. Importantly, from a public health perspective, there is some evidence from an audit of health records for the disease prevalence having increased in a US population over time (Dana et al., 2019).

A recent systematic review investigated the relationship between economic status of countries and the prevalence of DED (Yu et al., 2021). Using the gross domestic product (GDP) per capita and gross national income (GNI) per capita as an indicator of economic status, the prevalence of DED progressively declined in countries from lower-middle-income, upper middle-income, to high-income. This finding is perhaps confounded by access to services, education, lifestyle, and societal factors.

9.2.2 Cost and Impact of Dry-Eye Disease

The economic cost of DED can be measured in terms of direct medical expenses, resource utilization, impact on work productivity and quality of life, causing societal and mental health burden. It is recognized that most approaches to capture the costs are incomplete and depend on healthcare systems, access to healthcare, societal factors, and reimbursement for diagnostic and treatment costs. Historically, studies have focused on severe DED, particularly keratoconjunctivitis sicca and Sjögren's syndrome.

The following key words were used to search the literature using PubMed, Embase Ovid, and Google Scholar to retrieve potential articles: (dry eye disease OR dry eye) AND (economic burden OR economic cost OR work productivity OR productivity loss OR quality of life). Articles were included if they were observational studies conducted in humans published after 2015 and had reported economic burden in terms of work productivity cost and/or loss, medical expenses, and had evaluated quality-of-life assessment (ocular, visual, physical, mental, and pyschosocial and general health) using a questionnaire or qualitative research. Studies were excluded if they were reviews or editorials.

In Canada, the annual cost of DED, based on a practitioner diagnosis, was $24,331 per patient (Chan et al., 2020). The annual cost was determined from the annual salary of the patients and included direct costs from resource utilization and out-of-pocket expenses and indirect costs from work-related productivity impairment. The mean direct and indirect costs

were $2,324 and $21,052 per year respectively. Dry eye was stratified into mild, moderate, and severe on the basis of symptoms measured using a visual analog scale. Direct out-of-pocket costs for severe disease were $2,766, followed by moderate and mild disease costing $1,303 and $958 per year respectively. Similarly, indirect costs were highest for severe ($25,485), followed by moderate and mild disease, costing $16,525 and $5,961 respectively (see below).

Several studies have explored costs through insurance claims. While hospitalization is rare in DED, related hospitalization costs from an insurance claims database derived from a private and public healthcare center in Spain increased over time between 1999 and 2015 (Darbà and Ascanio, 2021), where *International Classification of Diseases*, ninth revision (ICD-9) codes were used to identify DED. The annual cost for hospitalization increased nearly six times from €4.9 (USD 5.8) million in 1999 to €30.3 million (USD 35.95) in 2015. These costs included hospitalization charges, inpatient emergency admissions, readmissions, discharge to home, and/or transfer to another hospital. The total annual cost to the patient also doubled from €4,301 (US$5,102) to €9,801 (US$11,627) over the same period. The annual cost by dry-eye subtype was €4,570 for non-Sjögren keratoconjunctivitis sicca, followed by Sjögren's syndrome keratoconjunctivitis sicca (€4,243), dry-eye syndrome (€4,238), xerophthalmia due to vitamin A deficiency (€4,015), and vitamin A deficiency with xerophthalmia scars (€3,036).

A study in China assessed the treatment expenditure on medications for 64 patients with DED (Yao and Le, 2018) diagnosed using the Ocular Surface Disease Index (OSDI) questionnaire and a panel of ocular surface assessments. The annual medication out-of-pocket costs for dry eye in Sjögren's syndrome was CNY7,637.2 (US$1,173.8) and for non-Sjögren disease was CNY1,179 (US$183).

9.2.3 Quality of Life

DED consistently impacts all aspects of vision-related quality of life, including physical, psychological, and emotional wellbeing, social functioning, daily living activities, and independence. The impact of symptoms associated with dry eye, including soreness, discomfort, eye irritation, itching, grittiness, watering, redness, eye strain, fatigue, heavy eyelids, blurred vision and/or fluctuating vision, higher-order aberrations, glare, and sensitivity to light and wind, and their chronicity underpin those adverse findings.

Social and physical functioning, including independence, is impacted due to poor participation in outdoor/recreational activities such as sports and games and daily life activities such as watching television, reading, using computers and digital devices, and driving during day and night. Aspects of general and mental health, social functioning, physical, emotional states, bodily pain, and vitality are significantly poorer in patients with symptomatic DED compared with those without disease after controlling for several confounding factors, including contact lens wear, autoimmune disease, nutritional deficiencies, and psychiatric conditions (Morthen et al., 2021). Similarly, in a recent European study, when controlling for chronic pain syndromes, poor sleep quality, depression, stress, and anxiety, the adverse impact of DED on vision-related quality of life persists (Vehof et al., 2021).

These adverse vision-related quality-of-life findings are consistent over time, geographic regions, and variations in ethnicity (Tong et al., 2010; Li et al., 2012). Importantly, and perhaps less widely appreciated, the vision-related population burden of DED is higher than other common age-related ocular diseases, including glaucoma and macular degeneration (Vehof et al., 2021).

Questionnaires for dry-eye assessment have been previously reviewed (Stapleton et al., 2017); however there is no single valid tool that provides a holistic measure of quality of life in dry eye or ocular surface disease. The current questionnaires were designed to be specific to either frequency of ocular symptoms (OSDI) or severity (Dry Eye Questionnaire 5: DEQ-5) and generally do not include symptoms specific to psychological, social, and treatment effect, although the Impact of Dry Eye on Everyday Life (IDEEL) instrument is fairly comprehensive. Frequently ocular symptomatology instruments are administered with a more generalized quality-of-life tool, such as the Visual Function Questionnaire (VFQ). Recent evidence would suggest the relevance of capturing vision-related quality of life in patients with dry eye to better understand disease impact.

9.2.4 Work Productivity

Work productivity has been assessed through absenteeism, presenteeism, and productivity impairment and non-work-related productivity using the Work Productivity and Activity Impairment (WPAI) (Reilly et al., 1993) and Valuation of Lost Productivity (VOLP) questionnaires (McCormick et al., 2019). Perhaps unexpectedly, multiple studies suggest that the impact of dry eye on reduced productivity during work time is significantly higher than the cost due to work time missed.

The mean indirect costs of presenteeism and absenteeism for a cohort of 151 patients with dry eyes in Canada were $19,304 and $2,702 per year, respectively (Chan et al., 2020). This study is one of the few to stratify by disease severity and has determined that indirect costs are more than four times higher in severe ($25,485) compared with mild ($5,961) disease.

In a study of 158 patients with DED in the USA, the impact on non-work-related performance (30%) was similar to the work-related loss (29%) caused by dry eye (Nichols et al., 2016). Non-work-related performance includes impairment of daily activities. Work productivity loss was calculated based on the number of hours missed due to absenteeism (working hours missed), presenteeism (impairment of work performance), and productivity impairment (both absenteeism and presenteeism) over a period of 7 days. Work-related productivity loss (28.6%) was considerably more than the total work time missed due to absenteeism (0.36%).

In Saudi Arabia, 463 patients with DED were stratified by disease severity on the basis of their OSDI score (Binyousef et al., 2021). As anticipated, there was greater impairment in work productivity amongst those with more severe disease, compared with mild to moderate DED. Although most patients (>90%) did not report missing work, dry eye affected performance during working hours in 37%, which was five times more common in the severe group. Amongst those with severe dry eyes, almost 40% lost 1–2 hours of working hours performance, 59% had difficulty focusing, 79% had to take a break during work, and 76% avoided air-conditioning or modified their environment at work.

9.3 RISK FACTORS FOR DRY-EYE DISEASE

Risk factors for DED have been extensively reviewed in the literature (see Stapleton et al., 2017, for a review). A literature search was conducted to review recent studies of DED both to determine new risk factors and to establish whether there was supportive evidence for stronger links between known risk factors and dry eye. The following key words were used for the search: (dry eye OR dry eye disease) AND (risk factors OR correlation OR association) AND (diabetes OR rosacea OR viral infection OR psychiatric conditions OR thyroid disease OR pterygium OR refractive surgery OR allergic conjuncitivtis OR hispanic ethnicity OR menopause OR acne OR sarcoidosis OR smoking OR alcohol OR pregnancy OR demodex OR botulinum toxin OR pain OR digital device OR smart phone OR sleep quality). Table 9.1 shows an updated summary of risk factors based on consistent, probable, and possible associations with

Table 9.1 Risk factors categorized by the level of available evidence

	Consistent[a]	Probable[b]	Inconclusive[c]
Non-modifiable	Aging Female sex Asian race Meibomian gland dysfunction Connective tissue diseases Autoimmune disease Sjögren's syndrome Diabetes Psychiatric conditions	Rosacea Viral infection Thyroid disease Pterygium	Hispanic ethnicity Menopause Acne Sarcoidoisis

Modifiable	Computer use
	Contact lens wear
	Androgen deficiency
	Hormone replacement therapy
	Certain medications, including
	  antidepressants
	Environment
	Hematopoietic stem cell
	  transplantation
		Refractive surgery
		Allergic conjunctivitis
		Smoking
		Sleep quality
			Pregnancy, *Demodex*,
			  multivitamins
			Contraceptive pill use
			Botulinum
			Digital device use
			Chronic pain syndromes

Note: [a] Consistent evidence implies the existence of at least one adequately powered, and otherwise well-conducted, study published in a peer-reviewed journal, along with the existence of a plausible biological rationale and corroborating basic research or clinical data. [b] Suggestive evidence implies the existence of either inconclusive information from peer-reviewed publications or inconclusive or limited information to support the association, but either not published or published somewhere other than in a peer-reviewed journal. [c] Inconclusive evidence implies either directly conflicting information in peer-reviewed publications, or inconclusive information but with some basis for a biological rationale.

dry eye according to the quality of the evidence available.

New risk factors, including systemic pain syndromes (Vehof et al., 2016), digital device and smartphone use (Moon et al., 2016; Baabdullah et al., 2019; Chaterjee et al., 2021), and sleep quality (Hanyuda et al., 2020; Kawashima et al., 2016; Magno et al., 2021), were identified as either probable or inconclusive risk factors. Diabetes (Shaikh and Ameen, 2015; Rathnakumar et al., 2017; Shujaat et al., 2017; Ma et al., 2018; Masmali et al., 2018) and psychiatric conditions (Um et al., 2018; Hyon et al., 2019; Inomata et al., 2020; Liang et al., 2020) were characterized as consistent risk factors. Smoking was characterized as a probable risk factor (Graue-Hernández et al., 2019; Sherry et al., 2020; Chatterjee et al., 2021; Vehof et al., 2021). There were no other major changes to other risk factors identified in the 2017 report. Adequately powered studies are lacking specifically for digital device and smartphone use.

9.4 CONCLUSION

As a conservative estimate, 10–20% of the population over 40 report and/or seek treatment for DED, which would arguably represent the prevalence of more severe disease. Age and South-East Asian race are consistently associated

with a higher risk of DED, irrespective of the disease definition. While most studies of dry eye identify women as having twice the risk of men in studies evaluating dry-eye symptoms, signs and symptoms of dry eye or a prior diagnosis of dry eye, recent evidence suggests that the effect of sex on MGD is equivocal, with two well-conducted studies showing a higher risk in males. Recent studies have identified new risk factors, including a strong association between DED and sleep quality and chronic pain syndromes. The focus of most studies has been on individuals over the age of 40; however, there are high rates of symptom reporting in younger Asian and Caucasian adults. The impact of younger age and the importance of specific risk factors in youth remain unclear and prevalence data in future studies should be disaggregated by age and sex to better explore these associations.

Studies of vision-related quality of life confirm the significant public health burden of DED and that the adverse impact on vision-related quality of life persists when controlling for co-morbidities. Future epidemiological studies should include measures of vision-related quality of life disaggregated by disease severity to better understand the impact of disease and allocation of health resources.

REFERENCES

Ahn, J. M., Lee, S. H., Rim, T. H. T., Park, R. J., Yang, H. S., Im Kim, T., Yoon, K. C., Seo, K. Y., Epidemiologic Survey Committee of the Korean Ophthalmological Society. 2014. Prevalence of and Risk Factors Associated with Dry Eye: The Korea National Health and Nutrition Examination Survey 2010–2011. *American Journal of Ophthalmology*, 158, 1205–1214. E7.

Arita, R., Mizochuchi, T., Kawashima, M., Fukuoka, S., Koh, S., Shirakawa, R., Suzuki, T. & Morishige, N. 2019. Meibomian Gland Dysfunction and Dry Eye Are Similar but Different Based on a Population-Based Study: The Hirado-Takushima Study in Japan. *American Journal of Ophthalmology*, 207, 410–418.

Baabdullah, A. M., Abumohssin, A. G., Alqahtani, Y. A., Nemri, I. A., Sabbahi, D. A. & Alhibshi, N. M. 2019. The Association between Smartphone Addiction and Dry Eye Disease: A Cross-Sectional Study. *Journal of Nature and Science of Medicine*, 2, 81–85.

Binyousef, F. H., Alruwaili, S. A., Alatmmami, A. F., Alharbi, A. A., Alrakaf, F. A. & Almazrou, A. A. 2021. Impact of Dry Eye Disease on Work Productivity among Saudi Workers in Saudi Arabia. *Clinics in Ophthalmology*, 15, 2675–2681.

Bron, A. J., De Paiva, C. S., Chauhan, S. K., Bonini, S., Gabison, E. E., Jain, S., Knop, E., Markoulli, M., Ogawa, Y., Perez, V., Uchino, Y., Yokoi, N., Zoukhri, D. & Sullivan, D. A. 2017. TFOS Dews II Pathophysiology Report. *Ocular Surface*, 15, 438–510.

Chan, C. C., Ziai, S., Myageri, V., Burns, J. G. & Prokopich, C. L. 2020. Dry Eye Disease: A Canadian Quality of Life and Productivity Loss Survey. *medRxiv*, 2020.10.07.20207225.

Chatterjee, S., Agrawal, D., Sanowar, G. & Kandoi, R. 2021. Prevalence of Symptoms of Dry Eye Disease in an Urban Indian Population. *Indian Journal of Ophthalmology*, 69, 1061–1066.

Craig, J. P., Nelson, J. D., Azar, D. T., Belmonte, C., Bron, A. J., Chauhan, S. K., De Paiva, C. S., Gomes, J. A. P., Hammitt, K. M., Jones, L., Nichols, J. J., Nichols, K. K., Novack, G. D., Stapleton, F. J., Willcox, M. D. P., Wolffsohn, J. S. & Sullivan, D. A. 2017. TFOS DEWS II Report Executive Summary. *Ocular Surface*, 15, 802–812.

Dana, R., Bradley, J. L., Guerin, A., Pivneva, I., Stillman, I., Evans, A. M. & Schaumberg, D. A. 2019. Estimated Prevalence and Incidence of Dry Eye Disease Based on Coding Analysis of a Large, All-Age United States Health Care System. *American Journal of Ophthalmology*, 202, 47–54.

Darbà, J. & Ascanio, M. 2021. Economic Impact of Dry Eye Disease in Spain: A Multicentre Retrospective Insurance Claims Database Analysis. *European Journal of Ophthalmology*, 31, 328–333.

Farrand, K. F., Fridman, M., Stillman, I. Ö. & Schaumberg, D. A. 2017. Prevalence of Diagnosed Dry Eye Disease in the United States Among Adults Aged 18 Years and Older. *American Journal of Ophthalmology*, 182, 90–98.

Ferrero, A., Alassane, S., Binquet, C., Bretillon, L., Acar, N., Arnould, L., Museelier-Mathieu, A., Delcourt, C., Bron, A. M. & Creuzot-Garcher, C. 2018. Dry Eye Disease in the Elderly in a French Population-Based Study (the Montrachet Study: Maculopathy, Optic Nerve, eurovasc, eurovascular and HearT Diseases): Prevalence and Associated Factors. *Ocular Surface*, 16, 112–119.

Gong, Y. Y., Zhang, F., Zhou, J., Li, J., Zhang, G. H., Wang, J. L. & Gu, Z. S. 2017. Prevalence of Dry Eye in Uyghur and Han Ethnic Groups in Western China. *Ophthalmic Epidemiology*, 24, 181–187.

Graue-Hernández, E. O., Serna-Ojeda, J. C., Estrada-Reyes, C., Navas, A., Arrieta-Camacho, J. & Jiménez-Corona, A. 2019. Dry Eye Symptoms and Associated Risk Factors among Adults Aged 50 or More Years in Central Mexico. *Salud Pública de México*, 60, 520–527.

Han, S. B., Hyon, J. Y., Woo, S. J., Lee, J. J., Kim, T. H. & Kim, K. W. 2011. Prevalence of Dry Eye Disease in an Elderly Korean Population. *Archives of Ophthalmology*, 129, 633–638.

Hanyuda, A., Sawada, N., Uchino, M., Kawashima, M., Yuki, K., Tsubota, K., Yamagushi, K., Iso, H., Yasuda, N., Saito, I., Kato, T., Abe, Y., Arima, K., Tanno, K., Sakata, K., Shimazu, T., Yamaji, T., Goto, A., Inoue, M., Iwasaki, M. & Tsugane, S. 2020. Relationship Between Unhealthy Sleep Status and Dry Eye Symptoms in a Japanese Population: The Jphc-Next Study. *Ocular Surface*, 18, 56–63.

Hashemi, H., Asharlous, A., Aghamirsalim, M., Yekta, A., Pourmatin, R., Sajjadi, M., Pakbin, M., Asadollahi, M. & Khabazkhoob, M. 2021. Meibomian Gland Dysfunction in Geriatric Population: Tehran Geriatric Eye Study. *International Ophthalmology*, 41, 2539–2546.

Hashemi, H., Khabazkhoob, M., Kheirkhah, A., Emamian, M. H., Mehravaran, S., Shariati, M. & Fotouhi, A. 2014. Prevalence of Dry Eye Syndrome in an Adult Population. *Clinical Experiments in Ophthalmology*, 42, 242–248.

Hashemi, H., Rastad, H., Emamian, M. H. & Fotouhi, A. 2017. Meibomian Gland Dysfunction and its Determinants in Iranian Adults: A Population-Based Study. *Contact Lens and Anterior Eye*, 40, 213–216.

Hyon, J. Y., Yang, H. K. & Han, S. B. 2019. Association Between Dry Eye Disease and Psychological Stress Among Paramedical Workers in Korea. *Scientific Reports*, 9, 1–6.

Inomata, T., Iwagami, M., Nkamura, M., Shiang, T., Yoshimura, Y., Fujimoto, K., Okumura, Y., Eguchi, A., Iwata, N. & Miura, M. 2020a. Characteristics and Risk Factors Associated with Diagnosed and Undiagnosed Symptomatic Dry Eye Using a Smartphone Application. *JAMA Ophthalmology*, 138, 58–68.

Kawashima, M., Uchino, M., Yokoi, N., Uchino, Y., Dogru, M., Komuro, A., Sonomura, Y., Kato, H., Kinoshita, S. & Tsubota, K. 2016. The Association of Sleep Quality with Dry Eye Disease: The Osaka Study. *Clinics in Ophthalmology*, 10, 1015–1021.

Li, M., Gong, L., Chapin, W. J. & Zhu, M. 2012. Assessment of Vision-Related Quality of Life in Dry Eye Patients. *Investigative Ophthalmology & Visual Science*, 53, 5722–5727.

Liang, C.-Y., Cheang, W.-M., Wang, C.-Y., Lin, K.-H., Wei, L.-C., Chen, Y.-Y. & Shen, Y.-C. 2020. The Association of Dry Eye Syndrome and Psychiatric Disorders: A Nationwide Population-Based Cohort Study. *BMC Ophthalmology*, 20, 1–6.

Lin, P. Y., Tsai, S. Y., Cheng, C. Y., Liu, J. H., Chou, P. & Hsu, W. M. 2003. Prevalence of Dry Eye Among an Elderly Chinese Population in Taiwan: The Shihpai Eye Study. *Ophthalmology*, 110, 1096–1101.

Ma, A., Mak, M. S. Y., Shih, K. C., Tsui, C. K. Y., Cheung, R. K. Y., Lee, S. H., Leung, H., Leung, J. N. S., Leung, J. T. H., Van-Boswell, M. Z., Wong, M. T. L., Ng, A. L. K., Lee, C. H., Jhanji, V. & Tong, L. 2018. Association of Long-Term Glycaemic Control on Tear Break-up Times and Dry Eye Symptoms in Chinese Patients with Type 2 Diabetes. *Clinical and Experimental Ophthalmology*, 46, 608–615.

Magno, M. S., Utheim, T. P., Snieder, H., Hammond, C. J. & Vehof, J. 2021. The Relationship Between Dry Eye and Sleep Quality. *Ocular Surface*, 20, 13–19.

Malet, F., Le Goff, M., Colin, J., Schweitzer, C., Delyfer, M. N., Korobelnik, J. F., Rougier, M. B., Radeau, T., Dartigues, J. F. & Delcourt, C. 2014. Dry Eye Disease in French Elderly Subjects: The Alienor Study. *Acta Ophthalmologica,* 92, e429–e436.

Masmali, A. M., Maeni, Y. A., El-Hiti, G. A., Murphy, P. J. & Almubrad, T. 2018. Investigation of Ocular Tear Ferning in Controlled and Uncontrolled Diabetic Subjects. *Eye & Contact Lens,* 44, S70–S75.

McCormick, N., Marra, C. A., Sadatsafavi, M., Kopec, J. A. & Aviña-Zubieta, J. A. 2019. Excess Productivity Costs of Systemic Lupus Erythematosus, Systemic Sclerosis, and Sjögren's Syndrome: A General Population-Based Study. *Arthritis Care & Research,* 71, 142–154.

Moon, J. H., Kim, K. W. & Moon, N. J. 2016. Smartphone Use Is a Risk Factor for Pediatric Dry Eye Disease According to Region and Age: A Case Control Study. *BMC Ophthalmology,* 16, 1–7.

Morthen, M. K., Magno, M. S., Utheim, T. P., Snieder, H., Hammond, C. J. & Vehof, J. 2021. The Physical and Mental Burden of Dry Eye Disease: A Large Population-Based Study Investigating the Relationship with Health-Related Quality of Life and its Determinants. *Ocular Surface,* 21, 107–117.

Nichols, K. K., Bacharach, J., Holland, E., Kislan, T., Shettle, L., Lunacsek, O., Lennert, B., Burk, C. & Patel, V. 2016. Impact of Dry Eye Disease on Work Productivity, and Patients' Satisfaction with over-the-Counter Dry Eye Treatments. *Investigative Ophthalmology & Visual Science,* 57, 2975–2982.

Olaniyan, S. I., Fasina, O., Bekibele, C. O. & Ogundipe, A. O. 2016. Dry Eye Disease in an Adult Population in South-West Nigeria. *Contact Lens and Anterior Eye,* 39, 359–364.

Rathnakumar, K., Ramachandran, K., Ramesh, V., Anebaracy, V., Vidhya, R., Vinothkumar, R. & Geetha, R. 2017. Prevalence of Dry Eye Disease in Type 2 Diabetic Patients and its Association with Retinopathy. *International Journal of Pharmaceutics and Scientific Research,* 8, 4298–4304.

Reilly, M. C., Zbrozek, A. S. & Dukes, E. M. 1993. The Validity and Reproducibility of a Work Productivity and Activity Impairment Instrument. *Pharmacoeconomics,* 4, 353–365.

Schaumberg, D. A., Dana, R., Buring, J. E. & Sullivan, D. A. 2009. Prevalence of Dry Eye Disease Among US Men: Estimates from the Physicians' Health Studies. *Archives of Ophthalmology,* 127, 763–768.

Shaikh, R. & Ameen, J. 2015. Prevalence of Dry Eye Disease in Type 2 Diabetic Patients and Its Co-Relation with the Duration, Glycemic Control and Retinopathy. *Al Ameen Journal of Medical Science,* 8, 225–229.

Sherry, A., Aridi, M. & Ghach, W. 2020. Prevalence and Risk Factors of Symptomatic Dry Eye Disease in Lebanon. *Contact Lens and Anterior Eye,* 43, 355–358.

Shujat, S., Jawed, M., Memon, S. & Talpur, K. I. 2017. Determination of Risk Factors and Treatment of Dry Eye Disease in Type 1 Diabetes before Corneal Complications at Sindh Institute of Ophthalmology and Visual Sciences. *The Open Ophthalmology Journal,* 11, 355.

Siak, J. J., Tong, L., Wong, W. L., Cajucom-Uy, H., Rosman, M., Saw, S. M. & Wong, T. Y. 2012. Prevalence and Risk Factors of Meibomian Gland Dysfunction: The Singapore Malay Eye Study. *Cornea,* 31, 1223–1228.

Stapleton, F., Alves, M., Bunya, V. Y., Jalbert, I., Lekhanont, K., Malet, F., Na, K. S., Schaumberg, D., Uchino, M., Vehof, J., Viso, E., Vitale, S. & Jones, L. 2017. TFOS DEWS II Epidemiology Report. *Ocular Surface,* 15, 334–365.

Tandon, R., Vashist, P., Gupta, N., Gupta, V., Sahay, P., Deka, D., Singh, S., Vishwanath, K. & Murthy, G. V. S. 2020. Association of Dry Eye Disease and Sun Exposure in Geographically Diverse Adult (≥40 Years) Populations of India: The SEED (Sun Exposure, Environment and Dry Eye Disease) Study – Second Report of the ICMR-EYE SEE Study Group. *Ocular Surface,* 18, 718–730.

Tian, Y. J., Liu, Y., Zou, H. D., Jiang, Y. J., Liang, X. Q., Sheng, M. J., Li, B. & Xu, X. 2009. [Epidemiologic Study of Dry Eye in Populations Equal or Over 20 years Old in Jiangning District of Shanghai.] *Zhonghua Yan Ke Za Zhi,* 45, 486–91.

Tong, L., Waduthantri, S., Wong, T., Saw, S., Wang, J., Rosman, M. & Lamoureux, E. 2010. Impact of Symptomatic Dry Eye on Vision-Related Daily Activities: The Singapore Malay Eye Study. *Eye,* 24, 1486–1491.

Um, S. B., Kim, N. H., Lee, H. K., Song, J. S. & Kim, H. C. 2014. Spatial Epidemiology of Dry Eye Disease: Findings from South Korea. *International Journal of Health Geography,* 13, 31.

Um, S.-B., Yeom, H., Kim, N. H., Kim, H. C., Lee, H. K. & Suh, I. 2018. Association Between Dry Eye Symptoms and Suicidal Ideation in a Korean Adult Population. *PloS One,* 13, e0199131.

Vehof, J., Kozareva, D., Hysi, P. G. & Hammond, C. J. 2014. Prevalence and Risk Factors of Dry Eye Disease in a British Female Cohort. *British Journal of Ophthalmology,* 98, 1712–1717.

Vehof, J., Smitt-Kamminga, N. S., Kozareva, D., Nibourg, S. A. & Hammond, C. J. 2016. Clinical Characteristics of Dry Eye Patients With Chronic Pain Syndrome. *American Journal of Ophthalmology,* 162, 59–65.

Vehof, J., Snieder, H., Jansonius, N. & Hammond, C. J. 2021. Prevalence and Risk Factors of Dry Eye in 79,866 Participants of the Population-Based Lifelines Cohort Study in the Netherlands. *Ocular Surface,* 19, 83–93.

Viet Vu, C. H., Uchino, M., Kawashima, M., Yuki, K., Tsubota, K., Nishi, A., German, C. A., Sakata, K., Tanno, K., Iso, H., Yamagishi, K., Yasuda, N., Saito, I., Kato, T., Arima, K., Tomita, Y., Shimazu, T., Yamaji, T., Goto, A., Inoue, M., Iwasaki, M., Sawad, N. & Tsugane, S. 2019. Lack of Social Support and Social Trust as Potential Risk Factors for Dry Eye Disease: JPHC-NEXT Study. *Ocular Surface,* 17, 278–284.

Viso, E., Rodríguez-Ares, M. T., Abelenda, D., Oubina, B. & Gude, F. 2012. Prevalence of Asymptomatic and Symptomatic Meibomian Gland Dysfunction in the General Population of Spain. *Investigative Ophthalmology & Visual Science,* 53, 2601–2606.

Viso, E., Rodríguez-Ares, M. T., Bóveda, F. J., Touriño, R. & Gude, F. 2014. Prevalence of Conjunctival Shrinkage and its Association with Dry Eye Disease: Results from a Population-Based Study in Spain. *Cornea,* 33, 442–447.

Viso, E., Rodríguez-Ares, M. T. & Gude, F. 2009. Prevalence of and Associated Factors for Dry Eye in a Spanish Adult Population (the Salnes Eye Study). *Ophthalmic Epidemiology,* 16, 15–21.

Wang, M. T. M. & Craig, J. P. 2019. Natural History of Dry Eye Disease: Perspectives from Inter-Ethnic Comparison Studies. *Ocular Surface,* 17, 424–433.

Yao, W. & Le, Q. 2018. Social-Economic Analysis of Patients with Sjögren's Syndrome Dry Eye in East China: A Cross-Sectional Study. *BMC Ophthalmology,* 18, 1–9.

Yu, W., Mingzhou, Z. & Xuemin, L. 2021. The Global Prevalence of Dry Eye Disease and its Association with Economy: A Systematic Review. *Research Square,* unpublished.

10 Cataract and Cataract Surgical Coverage

Olusola Olawoye, Priya Adhisesha Reddy, Ving Fai Chan,
Prabhath Piyasena, and Nathan Congdon

10.1 INTRODUCTION

The human lens is an optically clear structure that lies between the iris and the vitreous body of the eye. It is transparent, biconvex, composed of lens fibers, and surrounded by capsule. The lens is supported by zonules on either side. The nucleus of the lens is made up of older lens fibers, while newer fibers are located in the cortex at the outer layers of the lens. The clear lens focuses light rays on the retina, while providing accommodation and maintaining its own clarity. Cataract occurs when the lens loses its optical clarity for any reason and becomes opacified. Specifically, cataracts are defined as lens opacities associated with some degree of visual impairment.[1] Lens opacity is a direct result of oxidative stress.[2] There are different causes of cataract, but by far the most common is aging. Other causes include congenital and developmental factors, trauma, various ocular and metabolic diseases, radiation of different kinds, allergic dermatitis, and medications.

10.2 AGE-RELATED CATARACTS

10.2.1 Classification and Aetiology of Age-Related Cataracts

There are three main types of age-related cataracts based on the anatomic location of the opacification: nuclear, posterior sub-capsular, and cortical. These can occur alone or in combination. Nuclear cataract is the most common.[3] It begins with gradual yellowing, sclerosis, and hardening of the nucleus. This is a normal aging process which may affect vision or cause a change in refraction of light with a myopic shift.[3] Cortical cataracts may develop within the anterior or posterior cortex of the lens, and often do not cause visual symptoms unless the visual axis is affected. Posterior sub-capsular cataracts occur mainly in the central posterior aspect of the posterior cortex of the lens and can develop rapidly. They are often associated with glare and reduced near and distance vision, even early in their development.

10.2.1.1 Secondary Cataracts

Cataracts can be secondary to ocular or systemic diseases, such as diabetes, which causes a two- to five-fold increased risk of developing lens opacity.[4] Other systemic causes of cataracts include allergic dermatitis, myotonic dystrophy, hypoparathyroidism, and neurofibromatosis.

Cataracts can also occur secondary to ocular diseases such as uveitis, or from steroid medications used to treat uveitis. Other ocular diseases which may cause cataracts are acute angle closure glaucoma ("Glaukomflecken"), and hereditary conditions such as retinitis pigmentosa and Stickler's syndrome. Cataracts can result from both blunt and penetrating trauma, electric shock, and irradiation. This will be discussed in more detail under disease-related risk factors.

10.2.2 Epidemiology and Prevalence

According to the World Health Organization (WHO), there were 95 million people with visual impairment due to cataracts in 2014.[5] The prevalence of cataract increases with age, growing from <5% between ages 55 and 64 years to >90% at 80 years and older.[6–8] Cataract is still the leading cause of blindness and visual impairment globally, especially in low- and middle-income countries (LMIC),[9, 10] where cataracts account for 50% of blindness.[5] As at 2010, there were 32.4 million people blind and 191 million visually impaired worldwide,[11] among whom 10.8 million of the blind and 35.1 million of those visually impaired were due to cataract.[12]

The number of cataract blind persons globally fell from 12.3 million in 1990 to 10.8 million in 2010, representing an 11.4% reduction.[9, 10] Moderate and severe visual impairment (MSVI) due to cataract also fell from 44.0 million to 35.2 million people over the same period, a reduction of 20.2%.[12] The prevalence of cataracts has been on a downward trend over the past two decades because of increasing rates of cataract surgery, improved techniques, and various surgical outreach and capacity-building initiatives. In 1990, cataract was responsible for 47.8–51% of all global blindness but by 2010 this proportion had fallen to 33.4%.[12]

The age-standardized prevalence of blindness in adults older than 50 years remains highest in sub-Saharan Africa (SSA), with a rate of 6.0% in West Africa and 5.7% in East Africa,[13] and cataract is still the most common cause of blindness in most of SSA.[13, 14]

10.2.3 Risk Factors for Age-Related Cataract

The aetiology of age-related cataracts is multifactorial.[1] Older age is associated with increasing prevalence of nuclear and cortical cataracts. Other risk factors include personal

DOI: 10.1201/9781315146737-12

and individual issues, lifestyle, genetics, diet, systemic and ocular factors.[1]

10.2.3.1 Personal and Individual Factors

Several population-based, cross-sectional studies have reported increased age-adjusted risk of cataract in women,[15, 16] particularly for cortical opacities. The Lens Opacities case–control study reported that women had higher odds (1.51) of more cortical opacities compared to men in the same age group.[17] The risk of cortical opacities was less in women who were older at the age of menopause, suggesting the female hormonal milieu might resist cataractogenesis and that excess risk among women observed in some settings might be due to other factors, such as reduced access to care.[18]

Another individual factor associated with a higher prevalence of cataract is low education. In the Framingham Eye Study, Kahn et al. reported higher cataract rates among persons with seventh-grade education or less.[19] Other studies have also reported higher prevalence rates of cataracts among persons with no formal education. Rates remained significantly higher even after adjusting for personal, dietary, and environmental factors.[20] Studies in Italy and Boston also reported higher prevalence of cataracts in persons with low education after adjusting for gender, sunlight exposure, anti-oxidative enzyme levels, personal, environmental, medical, nutritional, and occupational factors.[17, 21] It is likely that this association between lower education and greater risk of cataract is mediated through diminished access to healthcare services, as has been seen with numerous other diseases.

10.2.3.2 Lifestyle Factors

The main lifestyle risk factor for cataract is cigarette smoking. Several studies, including the Beaver Dam study,[22, 23] and other case–control studies such as the Lens Opacities Case Control Studies,[17] have reported an association between cigarette smoking and age-related cataracts. Other prospective cohort studies, such as the Physician's Health Study,[24] the Nurses' Health Study,[25] and the City Eye study,[26] have also reported a positive association between cigarette smoking and cataracts. West et al., in their study[23] where cigarette smoking was the main exposure, reported a dose–response relationship between cigarette smoking and cataracts. Cigarette smoking plays an important role in the development of nuclear sclerosis and may also increase the risk of posterior sub-capsular opacities.[3]

Heavy alcohol consumption is also associated with an increase in the risk of cataract. Studies have shown a J-shaped effect of alcohol on risk of cataract. This means a higher risk among both total abstainers and heavy drinkers compared to occasional drinkers.[27, 28] Heavy drinkers are more at risk of developing posterior sub-capsular cataracts, nuclear, and cortical cataracts.[29] The mechanism of action by which alcohol leads to cataract is not yet well understood. Harding and van Heyningen[30] have suggested that it may be related to the conversion of alcohol to acetaldehyde, which can react with lens proteins.

10.2.3.3 Environmental Factors

The effect of ultraviolet B radiation on cataract has been reported in ecologic prevalence and case–control studies.[31] Some studies have found a dose–response relationship between ultraviolet radiation and cortical cataracts.[32, 33] Use of sunglasses and hats may be a practical strategy to reduce cataract associated with sunlight.

10.2.3.4 Disease-Related Risk Factors

Diabetes mellitus is a strong risk factor for cortical and posterior sub-capsular cataracts, increasing risk of opacity by two- to five-fold.[32, 34] Abnormalities in the levels of electrolyte, gluthathione, glucose, or galactose may be responsible for this. When aldose reductase reacts with glucose and glutathione, it forms sugar alcohols which lead to hyperosmotic effects, resulting in lens fiber swelling, vacuole formation, and opacification. Corticosteroid treatment (oral[17] and systemic) is also a risk factor predisposing to posterior sub-capsular cataracts.[21] Several population surveys, case–control studies, and a matched retrospective investigation have all confirmed the enhanced risk of posterior sub-capsular cataract with the use of steroids.[32, 35]

10.3 CONGENITAL CATARACT

10.3.1 Incidence and Risk Factors

Congenital cataract is the leading cause of life-long visual loss in children globally, especially in LMICs.[36–38] Congenital cataract occurs in about 1–6 cases per 10,000 live births in high-income countries (HICs)[39, 40] and 5–15 per 10,000 in the poorest regions of the world.[41]

Congenital cataracts refer to a lens opacity that appears at birth whereas an infantile cataract develops during the first year of life. Each year, 20,000–40,000 new cases of bilateral congenital cataract are diagnosed globally.[40, 42] About a third of all pediatric cataracts are inherited, a third are associated with ocular abnormalities or systemic syndromes, and a third have undetermined causes. Specific causes of congenital cataracts include intrauterine infections such as rubella, ocular toxoplasmosis, congenital syphilis, meta-bolic disorders such as galactosemia, chromo-somal abnormalities, systemic syndromes such as Down's, Wilson's syndrome, and myotonic dystrophy. The etiology of many cases of con-genital/infantile cataracts remains unknown.

Bilateral congenital cataracts are inherited in 8–25% of cases,[42] 27% among bilateral cataracts, and 2% of unilateral cataracts.[43] The majority of inherited non-syndromic cataracts have an autosomal-dominant inheritance with high penetrance in non-consanguineous populations. However, autosomal-recessive and X-linked inheritance has also been reported.[44]

Other risk factors for idiopathic congenital/infantile cataracts are low birth weight and older maternal age. In studies conducted in blind schools in West Africa, Chile, and South India, it has been reported that lens abnormalities accounted for 15.5%, 9.2%, and 7.4% of blindness in these countries respectively.[45] More reliable region-specific data on prevalence and incidence are needed for policy makers to make evidence-based decisions on resource allocation.

10.3.2 Genetic Mutations in Cataractogenesis

More than 25 loci and genes on different chromosomes have been identified in congenital cataracts.[46] Distinct gene mutations which encode the cytoplasmic proteins of human lens are associated with cataracts of different morpholo-gies. These include genes coding for crystallins (*CRYA*, *CRYB*, and *CRYG*),[47] connexins (Cx43, Cx46, and Cx50),[48] major intrinsic proteins,[49] cyto-skeletal structural proteins,[50] and heat shock tran-scription factor 4 (HSF4).[51]

10.4 CATARACT-GRADING METHODS

A grading scale is a tool that is used to quan-tify the severity of a condition with reference to a standard set of descriptions or illustrations.[52] Standardized grading systems are used to quan-tify the severity of cataracts rather than the use of qualitative terminologies such as mild, mod-erate, or severe cataracts. This standardized description enables future comparisons of the cataract to determine either progression or stability.

Cataract-grading systems are useful both clin-ically and for the purposes of research. Clinically ophthalmologists are able to monitor cataract progression over a period of time. In addition, it provides a standardized way to share patients' reports and data with other physicians. Cataract-grading systems also help ophthalmologists give information about the diagnosis, progression, and importance of treatments to patients.

10.4.1 Oxford Clinical Grading System

The Oxford clinical grading system was the first grading system to score several characteristics of cataract, but it has largely been replaced by the Lens Opacification Classification System III (LOCS III), which is simpler for clinicians to use compared with the Oxford grading system. The Oxford cataract-grading system is complex. It involves the analysis of a large variety of cataract characteristics, including different morphologies of cataracts, like focal dots, nuclear brunescence, vacuoles, retro dots, and white nuclear scatter.[53] Its complexity makes it difficult to apply it clinically.

10.4.2 WHO Simplified Cataract-Grading System

The WHO simplified cataract-grading system is a WHO initiative. This grading system was developed to unify and simplify lens classifications. The cortex of the lens is divided into two zones: anterior and posterior cortex, with each of the zones having four sections: C1–C4. C1 is the outer clear shell and an inner shell of increased light scattering. Zones 3 and 4 of the cortex are close to the nucleus. The cataract features which are graded are anterior and pos-terior sub-capsular opacities and cortical spoke opacities: vacuoles, waterclefts, focal dots. retro dots, and anterior clear zone thickness, nuclear brunescence, and white nuclear scatter (nuclear features). Each feature is graded on a scale from 1 to 5. It is important that patients are fully dilated before cataract grading. Figure 10.1 shows the Oxford cataract-grading recording sheet. In addition, image degradation is done using reso-lution target projection. This is performed using a modified ophthalmoscope to assess the effect of cataract on retinal image formation.

10.4.3 Lens Opacities Classification System

The Lens Opacities Classification System (LOCS I) provides a reproducible and reliable grading system. It uses the slit lamp or retro-illuminated photographs to classify cataracts. LOCS I[54] grades cataract severity using only the morph-ology of the cataracts rather than visual acuity, as in the Oxford grading system. LOCS II[55] is an improved version of LOCS I, and differentiates the degrees of cortical, sub-capsular, and nuclear opacification in addition to using standardized colored photographs for comparison. In the LOCS II visual acuity was not included in the grading system since there are other path-ologies that could affect visual acuity apart from an abnormal lens. There was good intra-observer agreement at the slit lamp and also in the photographic readings. The slit lamp had

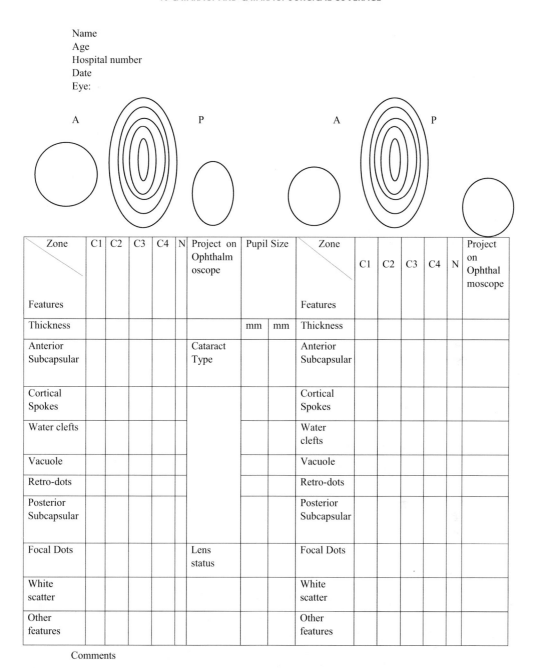

Figure 10.1 Recording chart for the Oxford cataract clinical classification and grading system.

better sensitivity at detecting opacification due to the photographic technology available at that time. LOCS III removed some of the limitations of LOCS II, with improvement in capturing early stages of cataract formation. It examines posterior sub-capsular cataracts and cortical cataracts on a scale of 1–5 using slit-lamp retro-illumination images and examines nuclear opalescence (NO) and nuclear color (NC) on a scale of 1–6. Currently the LOCS III system of classification[56] is still widely used in clinical practice. Figure 10.2 shows the LOCS III photos against which the cataract should be graded.

It is important to characterize cataract type and determine its severity to better understand the treatment needed. Vision-specific functioning decreases for different types and grades of cataract in the LOCS III grading system. As the grades of the different morphologies increase, vision-specific function reduces. However, each cataract type produces symptoms at different cataract grades depending on the cataract type. For instance, posterior sub-capsular cataract affects vision-specific functions at all grades and affects vision more than other types of cataract. The LOCS III grading system is also an important preoperative tool in determining a surgical plan and approach for nuclear cataracts. The grading system can be used preoperatively to determine case complexity and postoperative outcome. It can be used to counsel patients on the risks and possible outcomes of surgery. Figure 10.2 shows photographic evaluations of the cataract using the LOCS III classification.

10.4.4 Other Cataract-Grading Methods

Other methods have been developed that grade nuclear sclerotic cataracts using slit-lamp photographs to focus on the visual axis. The BCN 10 is an example of a clinical and surgical guidance grading system that focuses primarily on the nucleus of the lens. This grading system mainly uses the nucleus, since it is the most important determinant of the most appropriate surgical technique based on the hardness of the nucleus. This grading system places more emphasis on advanced stages of cataract. Other grading methods include the automatic diagnostic system for nuclear cataracts, where the system is trained to locate the lens and extract lens features such as color, intensity, and entropy inside the nucleus and the lens.

10.4.5 Newer Technologies to Grade Cataract

The slit lamp has been used both for examination and photographs for several years to grade cataracts, but other methods for cataract assessment have been proposed. These methods can be useful when time and resources are limited since they vary in their accuracy compared to standard slit-lamp photographs. Some authors have used retinal images.[57, 58] They quantified the optical degradation in retinal images using an automated method to detect cataract and this had good correlation with LOCS III. The disadvantage of this method is that the vitreous cavity could not be evaluated separately from the cataract and also there was no automated grading of the cataract. The anterior-segment optical coherence tomogram (ASOCT) has also been used to compare nucleus density measurement with LOCS III grading of color and opalescence of the nucleus with significant correlation. Opalescence has a higher association compared

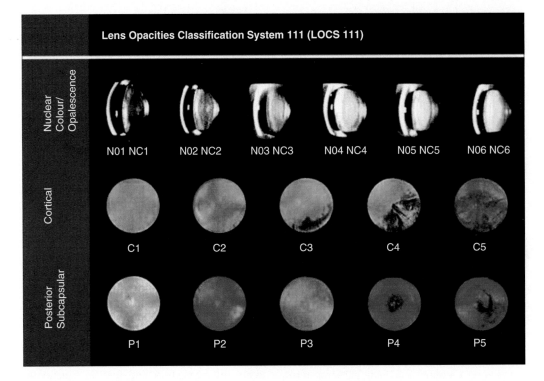

Figure 10.2 Standard photos for grading cataracts. Nuclear opalescence (NO) and nuclear color (NC) are graded from 1 to 6 while cortical and posterior sub-capsular opacities are graded from 1 to 5 (C1–C5 and P1–P5), respectively.

to nuclear color.[59] The use of ASOCT to grade lens density can be objective, fast, and reliable and requires less training compared to the LOCS III grading system.

Deep learning and artificial intelligence can also be used to grade cataract. Systems can be trained to learn the features of the lens used for grading, and filtered and fed into a cataract-grading system. Gao et al.[60] in their study demonstrated that deep learning could be a powerful and effective tool to grade cataracts.

10.5 CATARACT SURGICAL COVERAGE AND ITS MEASUREMENT

Cataract surgical coverage (CSC) is an indicator used to measure the impact of cataract intervention programs. It is a community-based parameter comparing the proportion of persons who have received surgery with the total who still need or have had surgery in a defined area or cohort.[61] This output measure indicates the extent to which local cataract services have covered existing needs, and as such is crucial to the monitoring of progress in reducing avoidable blindness.[61] Importantly, CSC does not measure quality of cataract surgical outcomes, but it does give important information about the uptake of cataract surgical services.[62] According to the Global Action Plan (GAP) 2014–2019,[63] CSC is defined as the "The proportion of people with bilateral cataract eligible for cataract surgery who have received cataract surgery in one or both eyes (at 3/60 and 6/18 level)." While CSC can be calculated for persons or for eyes, in the GAP it is computed by person.

Because CSC does not take into account quality of cataract services, limiting its usefulness to monitor progress towards universal eye health,[64] therefore, "effective cataract surgical coverage (eCSC)" has been promoted as an alternative which does reflect quality of outcomes. eCSC is the proportion of a population who need cataract surgeries, used available cataract surgical services, and obtained the desired results.[64–66] Postoperative visual acuity is a useful measure in the context of universal health coverage (UHC),[67–69] as an indicator of the effectiveness of cataract surgery in restoring vision.

Cataract remains the leading cause of avoidable blindness worldwide despite the wealth of evidence showing the cost-effectiveness, the socioeconomic benefits, and relative simplicity of carrying out cataract surgery, not to mention the impact that the treatment of cataract is shown to have on the lives of beneficiaries and their families.[70] Cataract surgery is one of the most widely undertaken surgical procedures globally. It has recently been recognized by the World Bank as an "essential surgery,"[71] and is one of a group of 44 surgical procedures deemed essential on the basis that they address substantial needs, are cost-effective, and can be feasibly implemented.

10.5.1 Brief Review of Cataract Surgical Rate by Regions

Another useful term is cataract surgical rate (CSR), which is defined as the number of surgeries performed annually per million population. The CSR can be as high as 10,000 in some developed market economies, and less than 1,000 in some countries with a young population and/or inadequate eye care services.[72]

In HICs (such as the USA, Europe, Australia, and Japan), the general CSR ranges from 4,000 to 10,000, and cataract blindness in the community is very rare. Comparatively, across LMICs in Latin America (such as Peru, Mexico, and Paraguay) and Asia (such as China and Vietnam), the CSR typically ranges from 500 to 2,000. In many African countries, such as Ethiopia and Kenya, the CSR has been <500 as recently as the last 10 years.[73–75] Over this time period, CSRs have increased with the implementation of Vision 2020 and socioeconomic development.[76, 77] Although the CSR appears to be closely associated with the economic development of countries, this is not always true, as evidenced in the cases of India (CSR > 6,000) and China (CSR = 2,000–2,500).[75, 78–80] It has been recognized that there are three main determinants of CSR: the age structure of the community, visual acuity cut-off for cataract surgery, and the CSC rate.[81]

One in three of the world's 32.4 million blind people (<3/60 presenting visual acuity in the better-seeing eye) are blind due to cataract, and this proportion is closer to one-half in SSA.[9, 10] In addition, there are many millions more who have significant visual impairment from cataract. This is despite an effective, low-cost cure for cataract having been known for decades.[82]

The availability of cataract surgical services in SSA is by no means universal, but even where services are available, uptake has mostly been below the level required for elimination of cataract blindness.[83] CSR of around 500 operations/million population/annum are frequently reported, well below the target of 2,000 suggested by the WHO.[84, 85] A commonly cited barrier to acceptance of surgery is concern about poor outcomes amongst potential beneficiaries.[70, 86–88]

Factors influencing uptake of cataract surgical services differ in different regions. Important socioeconomic barriers exist to the acceptance of surgery in many areas.[89] These include: both direct and indirect costs of surgery, lack of awareness, fear of surgery, transport difficulties, lack of an escort, family responsibilities, ageism, fatalism, and an attitude of being able to cope with existing poor vision.[90-94]

10.5.2 Gender and Access to Cataract Surgery

Existing data suggest that women do not receive cataract surgery at the same rate as men, and that closing the gender gap could decrease the global prevalence of cataract blindness by >10%.[95] Evidence however is limited, in that the data are mostly from a few regions of Asia, with only two African countries and no Latin American countries represented.[94, 96]

There are probably many reasons for the gender gap. In general, differences in surgical coverage rates could be attributed to gender-defined social roles, which could be confounded by socioeconomic factors, such as literacy, socioeconomic status, and marital status. Documented reasons for low use of services vary by location, and include the following:

- *The cost of cataract surgery may be prohibitive*: Costs include transportation to the hospital; loss of work for the patient or the guardian accompanying the patient; and living expenses for the guardian while the patient is in hospital. Also, poor rural women often have less disposable income, or control of finances, than men.[97]

- *Cataract surgery requires transport to a hospital*: This reduces the use of cataract services by women because they are less likely than men to travel outside their village for services.[98]

- *Family factors*: The perceived "value" of cataract surgery is often gender-dependent.[90] Research in Malawi showed that widowed women were more likely to have cataract surgery than married ones, while the opposite was true for men.[99] After divorce or widowhood, the probability that a woman would have surgery increased when there was a grown child or sibling to assist her in seeking surgery.

- *Community-based education about cataract has not been undertaken in most areas*: When it is, the demand for surgery will increase, and women who meet other women who have had successful surgery are more likely to accept surgery themselves.[99] Currently, however, educational programs are usually not gender-specific. Cataract programs in which women have lower coverage rates than men should investigate other local barriers that might exist.

- *Other factors*: Gender-specific access to surgery can also vary by age group. In Nepal, men aged 65–74 years received 40% more surgery than women, while above the age of 75 years the gap was 70%.[100] Cataract programs should not assume that women have equal access to cataract surgery compared to men, just because women receive 50% of the surgery performed. Due to the higher prevalence of cataract in women (due to increased risk, as well as longer life expectancy), women will comprise approximately 60–70% of all cataract surgeries when coverage rates are equal.[101] Although cataract surgical coverage rates have rarely been calculated for industrialized countries, data from the USA, Canada, the UK, and Sweden indicate that women receive 60–70% of the cataract operations there.[102-108] For most of the ten Latin American countries with existing data CSC is at parity or tends to favor women, whilst in all but one of 16 African, Asian, and Eastern Mediterranean countries with data, men generally have greater access.[62]

10.5.3 Alternative Measures of Coverage

It has also been proposed that the "sight restoration rate" be used to measure cataract surgical access. This is defined as the proportion of cataract operations that restore eyesight in people bilaterally blind from cataract.[109] In contrast, CSC does not take into account the outcome of the surgery, and the proportion of persons or eyes operated that were initially blind.

10.6 COMMUNITY INTERVENTION PROGRAMS TO INCREASE CATARACT SURGICAL COVERAGE

10.6.1 Examples from India

In the rural areas of India where healthcare facilities are primitive or non-existent, blindness is more common (1.62%) than in urban areas (1.03%). In order to develop and maintain a high-quality, large-volume, sustainable cataract surgery program, it is essential to be proactive about attracting patients instead of simply waiting for them to arrive spontaneously. In other words, it is necessary to generate demand for service through community outreach. A study of factors associated with 3-year increase in CSR among several dozen rural Chinese hospitals concluded that the single most important among these was the existence of high-volume community outreach.[110]

Outreach programs for eye care should aim at reaching the unreached. Many healthcare institutions organize outreach activities to create awareness in the community, to educate the community on health, and to provide possible medical intervention. There is a need to extend health care facilities to rural masses in order to cover the vast majority of the population.

10.6.1.1 Involving the Community

Poverty, ignorance, superstition, and socio-economic factors play key roles in keeping poor blind people from accessing the eye care services of urban areas. Active community involvement and health education contribute to the success of any outreach program. Urban hospitals should identify influential people in rural villages and convince them of the need to extend eye care services. They must also explain the benefits the community will reap. It is the responsibility of hospitals to ensure effective coordination and harmonious working relationships with these leaders in order to provide eye care services to their communities.

A key to a successful outreach program is active community involvement leading to community participation. This increases patient attendance, promotes credibility of the program, and reduces the cost considerably since the community members volunteer their services and quite often provide "in-kind" support (donations other than financial, for example, time, furniture, supplies). Community involvement also ensures that a good balance is maintained between altruism and self-interest.

10.6.1.2 Eye Health Education

This may be deemed to include the following:[111] (1) a process of bringing about a social change, which in this instance relates to changing attitudes towards eye health and eye health behavior patterns; (2) a process of generating awareness of and demand for healthcare services in the community by those who need health intervention but are not seeking it; and (3) a process that enables families and communities to improve their health and, in this case, their eyesight by improving or increasing their knowledge, attitudes, and skills. This is one of the fundamental principles of primary healthcare as spelled out by the WHO.

10.6.1.3 Eye Camps

An eye camp is an activity in which a medical team from a base hospital visits a community and carries out vision exams to detect problems. Those with eye problems are offered necessary treatment, either at the camp itself or at the base hospital, depending on the nature of the problem. Free eye camps are a major step in the campaign against avoidable blindness in LMICs. There are two types of eye camp:

1. *Diagnostic camps*: The medical team examines patients for eye problems and treats minor problems on the spot with medication. People who need surgery or specialty care are advised to come to the base hospital. No surgery is performed at the screening camp.

2. *Mobile surgery camps*: Patients are examined for eye problems and the necessary surgery is then performed at the camp itself. These camps are difficult as well as highly expensive to conduct in rural and underserved areas due to the lack of proper facilities. However, in some situations, they are the only way to reach the needlessly blind in remote areas.

10.6.1.4 Key Informants or Volunteers to Strengthen Referral Systems

In India, over two-thirds of the population live in small villages, where there are no voluntary organizations to organize eye camps. Hence it is neither cost-effective nor feasible to cover all villages. In addition, people in rural areas have their own socioeconomic problems, due to illiteracy and ignorance, that keep them from accessing facilities and services in eye hospitals. Many LMICs face similar challenging problems. As an alternative strategy, methods can be adopted to train healthcare volunteers in communities to screen people for operable cataract and to motivate them to accept surgery.

10.7 CONCLUSION

In conclusion, the prevalence of cataracts will continue to rise because of the rapid increase in aging populations worldwide. Therefore, it is important to continue to improve and develop new strategies to increase CSC. It is important that these strategies are practical and region-specific.

REFERENCES

1. West SK, Valmadrid CT. Epidemiology of risk factors for age-related cataract. *Surv Ophthalmol*. 1995;39(4): 323–334. Doi:10.1016/s0039-6257(05)80110-9

2. Vinson JA. Oxidative stress in cataracts. *Pathophysiol Off J Int Soc Pathophysiol*. 2006;13(3):151–162. Doi:10.1016/j.pathophys.2006.05.006

3. Hodge WG, Whitcher JP, Satariano W. Risk factors for age-related cataracts. *Epidemiol Rev*. 1995;17(2):336–346. Doi:10.1093/oxfordjournals.epirev.a036197

4. Klein BE, Klein R, Wang Q, Moss SE. Older-onset diabetes and lens opacities. The Beaver Dam Eye Study. *Ophthalmic Epidemiol*. 1995;2(1):49–55. Doi:10.3109/09286589509071451

5. WHO. *WHO Visual Impairment and Blindness*. 2014. Www.Who.Int/ Mediacentre/ Factsheets/ Fs282/ En/

6. Mitchell P, Cumming RG, Attebo K, Panchapakesan J. Prevalence of cataract in Australia: the Blue Mountains

Eye Study. *Ophthalmology*. 1997;104(4):581–588. Doi:https://doi.org/10.1016/S0161-6420(97)30266-8

7. Varma R, Torres M, Los Angeles Latino Eye Study Group. Prevalence of lens opacities in Latinos: the Los Angeles Latino Eye Study. *Ophthalmology*. 2004;111(8):1449–1456. Doi:10.1016/j.ophtha.2004.01.024

8. Chua J, Koh JY, Tan AG, et al. Ancestry, socio-economic status, and age-related cataract in Asians: the Singapore Epidemiology of Eye Diseases study. *Ophthalmology*. 2015;122(11):2169–2178. Doi:10.1016/j.ophtha.2015.06.052

9. Bourne RRA, Stevens GA, White RA, et al. Causes of vision loss worldwide, 1990–2010: a systematic analysis. *Lancet Glob Heal*. 2013;1(6):e339–e349. Doi:10.1016/S2214-109X(13)70113-X

10. Pascolini D, Mariotti SP. Global estimates of visual impairment: 2010. *Br J Ophthalmol*. 2012;96(5):614–618. Doi:10.1136/bjophthalmol-2011-300539

11. Stevens GA, White RA, Flaxman SR, et al. Global prevalence of vision impairment and blindness: magnitude and temporal trends, 1990–2010. *Ophthalmology*. 2013;120(12):2377–2384. Doi:10.1016/j.ophtha.2013.05.025

12. Khairallah M, Kahloun R, Bourne R, et al. Number of people blind or visually impaired by cataract worldwide and in world regions, 1990 to 2010. *Invest Ophthalmol Vis Sci*. 2015;56(11):6762–6769. Doi:10.1167/iovs.15-17201

13. Bastawrous A, Dean WH, Sherwin JC. Blindness and visual impairment due to age-related cataract in sub-Saharan Africa: a systematic review of recent population-based studies. *Br J Ophthalmol*. 2013;97(10):1237–1243. Doi:10.1136/bjophthalmol-2013-303135

14. Bourne R, Jonas J, Flaxman S, et al. Prevalence and causes of vision loss in high-income countries and in Eastern and Central Europe: 1990–2010. *Br J Ophthalmol*. 2014;98. Doi:10.1136/bjophthalmol-2013-304033

15. Chatterjee A, Milton RC, Thyle S. Prevalence and aetiology of cataract in Punjab. *Br J Ophthalmol*. 1982;66(1):35–42. Doi:10.1136/bjo.66.1.35

16. Hiller R, Sperduto RD, Ederer F. Epidemiologic associations with cataract in the 1971–1972 National Health and Nutrition Examination Survey. *Am J Epidemiol*. 1983;118(2):239–249. Doi:10.1093/oxfordjournals.aje.a113631

17. Leske MC, Chylack LTJ, Wu SY. The Lens Opacities Case-Control Study. Risk factors for cataract. *Arch Ophthalmol (Chicago, Ill 1960)*. 1991;109(2):244–251. Doi:10.1001/archopht.1991.01080020090051

18. Klein BE, Klein R, Ritter LL. Is there evidence of an estrogen effect on age-related lens opacities? The Beaver Dam Eye Study. *Arch Ophthalmol (Chicago, Ill 1960)*. 1994;112(1):85–91. Doi:10.1001/archopht.1994.01090130095025

19. Kahn HA, Leibowitz HM, Ganley JP, et al. The Framingham Eye Study. II. Association of ophthalmic pathology with single variables previously measured in the Framingham Heart Study. *Am J Epidemiol*. 1977;106(1):33–41. Doi:10.1093/oxfordjournals.aje.a112429

20. Mohan M, Sperduto RD, Angra SK, et al. India-US case-control study of age-related cataracts. India-US Case-Control Study Group. *Arch Ophthalmol (Chicago, Ill 1960)*. 1989;107(5):670–676. Doi:10.1001/archopht.1989.01070010688028

21. The Italian-American Cataract Study Group. Risk factors for age-related cortical, nuclear, and posterior subcapsular cataracts. *Am J Epidemiol*. 1991;133(6):541–553.

22. Klein BE, Klein R, Linton KL, Franke T. Cigarette smoking and lens opacities: the Beaver Dam Eye Study. *Am J Prev Med*. 1993;9(1):27–30.

23. West S, Munoz B, Emmett EA, Taylor HR. Cigarette smoking and risk of nuclear cataracts. *Arch Ophthalmol (Chicago, Ill 1960)*. 1989;107(8):1166–1169. Doi:10.1001/archopht.1989.01070020232031

24. Christen WG, Manson JE, Seddon JM, et al. A prospective study of cigarette smoking and risk of cataract in men. *JAMA*. 1992;268(8):989–993.

25. Hankinson SE, Willett WC, Colditz GA, et al. A prospective study of cigarette smoking and risk of cataract surgery in women. *JAMA*. 1992;268(8):994–998. Doi:10.1001/jama.1992.03490080068026

26. Flaye DE, Sullivan KN, Cullinan TR, Silver JH, Whitelocke RA. Cataracts and cigarette smoking. The City Eye Study. *Eye (Lond)*. 1989;3 (Pt 4):379–384. Doi:10.1038/eye.1989.56

27. Clayton RM, Cuthbert J, Duffy J, et al. Some risk factors associated with cataract in S.E. Scotland: a pilot study. *Trans Ophthalmol Soc UK*. 1982;102 Pt 3:331–336.

28. Clayton RM, Cuthbert J, Seth J, Phillips CI, Bartholomew RS, Reid JM. Epidemiological and other studies in the assessment of factors contributing to cataractogenesis. *Ciba Found Symp*. 1984;106:25–47. Doi:10.1002/9780470720875.ch3

29. Ritter LL, Klein BE, Klein R, Mares-Perlman JA. Alcohol use and lens opacities in the Beaver Dam Eye Study. *Arch Ophthalmol (Chicago, Ill 1960)*. 1993;111(1):113–117. Doi:10.1001/archopht.1993.01090010117037

30. Harding JJ, van Heyningen R. Beer, cigarettes and military work as risk factors for cataract. *Dev Ophthalmol*. 1989;17:13–16. Doi:10.1159/000416990

31. Brilliant LB, Grasset NC, Pokhrel RP, et al. Associations among cataract prevalence, sunlight hours, and altitude in the Himalayas. *Am J Epidemiol*. 1983;118(2):250–264. Doi:10.1093/oxfordjournals.aje.a113632

32. Bochow TW, West SK, Azar A, Munoz B, Sommer A, Taylor HR. Ultraviolet light exposure and risk of posterior subcapsular cataracts. *Arch Ophthalmol*. 1989;107(3):369–372. Doi:10.1001/archopht.1989.01070010379027

33. Taylor HR. Ultraviolet radiation and the eye: an epidemiologic study. *Trans Am Ophthalmol Soc*. 1989;87:802–853.

34. Hiller R, Sperduto RD, Ederer F. Epidemiologic associations with nuclear, cortical, and posterior subcapsular cataracts. *Am J Epidemiol*. 1986;124(6):916–925. Doi:10.1093/oxfordjournals.aje.a114481

35. Harding JJ, van Heyningen R. Drugs, including alcohol, that act as risk factors for cataract, and possible protection against cataract by aspirin-like analgesics and cyclopenthiazide. *Br J Ophthalmol*. 1988;72(11):809–814. Doi:10.1136/bjo.72.11.809

36. Ezegwui IR, Umeh RE, Ezepue UF. Causes of childhood blindness: results from schools for the

blind in south eastern Nigeria. *Br J Ophthalmol.* 2003;87(1):20–23. Doi:10.1136/bjo.87.1.20

37. Waddell KM. Childhood blindness and low vision in Uganda. *Eye (Lond).* 1998;12 (Pt 2):184–192. Doi:10.1038/eye.1998.45

38. Eckstein MB, Foster A, Gilbert CE. Causes of childhood blindness in Sri Lanka: results from children attending six schools for the blind. *Br J Ophthalmol.* 1995;79(7):633–636. Doi:10.1136/bjo.79.7.633

39. Rahi JS, Sripathi S, Gilbert CE, Foster A. Childhood blindness in India: causes in 1318 blind school students in nine states. *Eye (Lond).* 1995;9 (Pt 5):545–550. Doi:10.1038/eye.1995.137

40. Gilbert C, Foster A. Childhood blindness in the context of VISION 2020—the right to sight. *Bull World Health Organ.* 2001;79(3):227–232.

41. Apple DJ, Ram J, Foster A, Peng Q. Elimination of cataract blindness: a global perspective entering the new millenium. *Surv Ophthalmol.* 2000;45 Suppl 1:S1–196.

42. Messina-Baas OM, Gonzalez-Huerta LM, Cuevas-Covarrubias SA. Two affected siblings with nuclear cataract associated with a novel missense mutation in the CRYGD gene. *Mol Vis.* 2006;12:995–1000.

43. Rahi JS, Dezateux C. National cross sectional study of detection of congenital and infantile cataract in the United Kingdom: role of childhood screening and surveillance. The British Congenital Cataract Interest Group. *BMJ.* 1999;318(7180):362–365. Doi:10.1136/bmj.318.7180.362

44. Deng H, Yuan L. Molecular genetics of congenital nuclear cataract. *Eur J Med Genet.* 2014;57(2-3):113–122. Doi:10.1016/j.ejmg.2013.12.006

45. Gilbert C, Awan H. Blindness in children. *BMJ.* 2003;327(7418):760–761. Doi:10.1136/bmj.327.7418.760

46. Guleria K, Sperling K, Singh D, Varon R, Singh JR, Vanita V. A novel mutation in the connexin 46 (GJA3) gene associated with autosomal dominant congenital cataract in an Indian family. *Mol Vis.* 2007;13:1657–1665.

47. Bhat SP. Crystallins, genes and cataract. *Prog Drug Res Fortschritte der Arzneimittelforschung Prog des Rech Pharm.* 2003;60:205–262. Doi:10.1007/978-3-0348-8012-1_7

48. Hansen L, Yao W, Eiberg H, et al. Genetic heterogeneity in microcornea-cataract: five novel mutations in CRYAA, CRYGD, and GJA8. *Invest Ophthalmol Vis Sci.* 2007;48(9):3937–3944. Doi:10.1167/iovs.07-0013

49. Berry V, Francis P, Kaushal S, Moore A, Bhattacharya S. Missense mutations in MIP underlie autosomal dominant 'polymorphic' and lamellar cataracts linked to 12q. *Nat Genet.* 2000;25(1):15–17. Doi:10.1038/75538

50. Jakobs PM, Hess JF, FitzGerald PG, Kramer P, Weleber RG, Litt M. Autosomal-dominant congenital cataract associated with a deletion mutation in the human beaded filament protein gene BFSP2. *Am J Hum Genet.* 2000;66(4):1432–1436. Doi:10.1086/302872

51. Forshew T, Johnson CA, Khaliq S, et al. Locus heterogeneity in autosomal recessive congenital cataracts: linkage to 9q and germline HSF4 mutations. *Hum Genet.* 2005;117(5):452–459. Doi:10.1007/s00439-005-1309-9

52. Efron N, Morgan PB, Katsara SS. Validation of grading scales for contact lens complications.

53. Sparrow JM, Bron AJ, Brown NA, Ayliffe W, Hill AR. The Oxford clinical cataract classification and grading system. *Int Ophthalmol.* 1986;9(4):207–225. Doi:10.1007/BF00137534

54. Chylack LTJ, Leske MC, Sperduto R, Khu P, McCarthy D. Lens opacities classification system. *Arch Ophthalmol (Chicago, Ill 1960).* 1988;106(3):330–334. Doi:10.1001/archopht.1988.01060130356020

55. Chylack LTJ, Leske MC, McCarthy D, Khu P, Kashiwagi T, Sperduto R. Lens opacities classification system II (LOCS II). *Arch Ophthalmol (Chicago, Ill 1960).* 1989;107(7):991–997. Doi:10.1001/archopht.1989.01070020053028

56. Chylack LTJ, Wolfe JK, Singer DM, et al. The lens opacities classification system III. The longitudinal study of cataract study group. *Arch Ophthalmol (Chicago, Ill 1960).* 1993;111(6):831–836. Doi:10.1001/archopht.1993.01090060119035

57. Xiong L, Li H, Xu L. An approach to evaluate blurriness in retinal images with vitreous opacity for cataract diagnosis. *J Healthc Eng.* 2017;2017:5645498. Doi:10.1155/2017/5645498

58. Abdul-Rahman AM, Molteno T, Molteno ACB. Fourier analysis of digital retinal images in estimation of cataract severity. *Clin Experiment Ophthalmol.* 2008;36(7):637–645. Doi:10.1111/j.1442-9071.2008.01819.x

59. Wong AL, Leung CK-S, Weinreb RN, et al. Quantitative assessment of lens opacities with anterior segment optical coherence tomography. *Br J Ophthalmol.* 2009;93(1):61–65. Doi:10.1136/bjo.2008.137653

60. Gao X, Lin S, Wong TY. Automatic feature learning to grade nuclear cataracts based on deep learning. *IEEE Trans Biomed Eng.* 2015;62(11):2693–2701. Doi:10.1109/TBME.2015.2444389

61. Limburg H, Foster A. Cataract surgical coverage: an indicator to measure the impact of cataract intervention programmes. *Community Eye Heal.* 1998;11(25):3–6.

62. Gray Z, Ackland P. *Cataract Surgical Coverage. An Important Indicator for Eye Health and for Monitoring Progress Towards Universal Health Coverage.* London: International Agency for the Prevention of Blindness, 2015.

63. World Health Organization. WHA Res. 66.4. *Universal Eye Health: A Global Action Plan 2014–2019.* www.who.int/blindness/actionplan/en/.

64. Ramke J, Gilbert CE, Lee AC, Ackland P, Limburg H, Foster A. Effective cataract surgical coverage: an indicator for measuring quality-of-care in the context of universal health coverage. *PloS One.* 2017;12(3):e0172342. Doi:10.1371/journal.pone.0172342

65. World Health Organization. Background paper for the technical consultation on effective coverage health systems. Geneva: World Health Organization; 2001.

66. Hogan D, Hosseinpoor AR, Boerma T. *Developing an Index for the Coverage of Essential Health Services. Technical Note for World Health Statistics 2016.* Geneva: World Health Organization; 2016.

67. Boerma T, AbouZahr C, Evans D, Evans T. Monitoring intervention coverage in the context of universal health coverage. *PloS Med.* 2014;11(9):e1001728. Doi:10.1371/journal.pmed.1001728

Ophthalmic Physiol Opt J Br Coll Ophthalmic Opt. 2001;21(1):17–29.

68. Ng M, Fullman N, Dieleman J, Flaxman A, Murray C, Lim S. Effective coverage: a metric for monitoring universal health coverage. *PloS Med.* 2014;11:e1001730. Doi:10.1371/journal.pmed.1001730

69. Eballe AO, Owono D, Bella AL, Ebana C, Long D, Aboutou R. [Clinical and epidemiological characteristics of chronic open angle glaucoma at a Yaounde Hospital.] *Sante.* 2008;18(1):19–23. Doi:10.1684/san.2008.0095

70. Syed A, Polack S, Eusebio C, et al. Predictors of attendance and barriers to cataract surgery in Kenya, Bangladesh and the Philippines. *Disabil Rehabil.* 2013;35(19):1660–1667. Doi:10.3109/09638288.2012.748843

71. Debas HT, Donkor P, Gawande A, et al., eds. *Essential Surgery: Disease Control Priorities,* third edition (Volume 1). Washington, DC: The International Bank for Reconstruction and Development.

72. Wang W, Yan W, Fotis K, et al. Cataract surgical rate and socioeconomics: a global study. *Invest Ophthalmol Vis Sci.* 2016;57(14):5872–5881. Doi:10.1167/iovs.16-19894

73. Rao GN, Khanna R, Payal A. The global burden of cataract. *Curr Opin Ophthalmol.* 2011;22(1):4–9. Doi:10.1097/ICU.0b013e3283414fc8

74. Lansingh VC, Resnikoff S, Tingley-Kelley K, et al. Cataract surgery rates in Latin America: a four-year longitudinal study of 19 countries. *Ophthalmic Epidemiol.* 2010;17(2):75–81. Doi:10.3109/09286581003624962

75. Murthy G, John N, Shamanna B, Pant H. Elimination of avoidable blindness due to cataract: where do we prioritize and how should we monitor this decade? *Indian J Ophthalmol.* 2012;60(5):438–445. Doi:10.4103/0301-4738.100545

76. Foster A, Resnikoff S. The impact of Vision 2020 on global blindness. *Eye (Lond).* 2005;19(10):1133–1135. Doi:10.1038/sj.eye.6701973

77. Pararajasegaram R. Vision 2020 – the right to sight: from strategies to action. *Am J Ophthalmol.* 1999;128(3):359–360. Doi:10.1016/s0002-9394(99)00251-2

78. Habtamu E, Eshete Z, Burton MJ. Cataract surgery in Southern Ethiopia: distribution, rates and determinants of service provision. *BMC Health Serv Res.* 2013;13:480. Doi:10.1186/1472-6963-13-480

79. Hashemi H, Rezvan F, Fotouhi A, et al. Distribution of cataract surgical rate and its economic inequality in Iran. *Optom Vis Sci Off Publ Am Acad Optom.* 2015;92(6):707–713. Doi:10.1097/OPX.0000000000000590

80. Zhu M, Zhu J, Lu L, He X, Zhao R, Zou H. Four-year analysis of cataract surgery rates in Shanghai, China: a retrospective cross-sectional study. *BMC Ophthalmol.* 2014;14:3. Doi:10.1186/1471-2415-14-3

81. Tin KY, Tsoi PK, Lee YH, et al. Hong Kong domestic health spending: financial years 1989/90 to 2011/12. = Xianggang yi xue za zhi. *Hong Kong Med J.* 21(3 Suppl 3):1.24.

82. Buchan JC, Dean WH, Foster A, Burton MJ. What are the priorities for improving cataract surgical outcomes in Africa? Results of a Delphi exercise. *Int Ophthalmol.* 2018;38(4):1409–1414. Doi:10.1007/s10792-017-0599-y

83. Lewallen S, Schmidt E, Jolley E, et al. Factors affecting cataract surgical coverage and outcomes: a retrospective cross-sectional study of eye health systems in sub-Saharan Africa. *BMC Ophthalmol.* 2015;15:67. Doi:10.1186/s12886-015-0063-6

84. Lecuona K, Cook C. South Africa's cataract surgery rates: why are we not meeting our targets? *S Afr Med J.* 2011;101(8):510–512.

85. Lewallen S, Williams TD, Dray A, et al. Estimating incidence of vision-reducing cataract in Africa: a new model with implications for program targets. *Arch Ophthalmol (Chicago, Ill 1960).* 2010;128(12):1584–1589. Doi:10.1001/archophthalmol.2010.307

86. Rotchford AP, Rotchford KM, Mthethwa LP, Johnson GJ. Reasons for poor cataract surgery uptake – a qualitative study in rural South Africa. *Trop Med Int Health.* 2002;7(3):288–292. Doi:10.1046/j.1365-3156.2002.00850.x

87. Adepoju FG, Adekoya BJ, Ayanniyi AA, Olatunji V. Poor cataract surgical output: eye care workers perspective in north central Nigeria. *Niger J Clin Pract.* 2012;15(4):408–414. Doi:10.4103/1119-3077.104513

88. Briesen S, Geneau R, Roberts H, Opiyo J, Courtright P. Understanding why patients with cataract refuse free surgery: the influence of rumours in Kenya. *Trop Med Int Health.* 2010;15(5):534–539. Doi:10.1111/j.1365-3156.2010.02486.x

89. Tiwari A, Verma N, Bhawnami D, Srivastava N. Assessment of the cataract surgical coverage among people aged 50 years and above residing in urban slums of Raipur city, Chhattisgarh. *Int J Res Heal Sci.* 2014;2(2):621–628.

90. Fletcher AE, Donoghue M, Devavaram J, et al. Low uptake of eye services in rural India: a challenge for programs of blindness prevention. *Arch Ophthalmol (Chicago, Ill 1960).* 1999;117(10):1393–1399. Doi:10.1001/archopht.117.10.1393

91. Johnson JG, Goode Sen V, Faal H. Barriers to the uptake of cataract surgery. *Trop Doct.* 1998;28(4):218–220. Doi:10.1177/004947559802800410

92. Shen W, Yang Y, Yu M, Li J, Wei T, Li X et al. Prevalence and outcomes of cataract surgery in adult rural Chinese populations of the Bai nationality in Dali: the Yunnan minority eye study. *PloS One.* 2013;8:e60236.

93. Athanasiov PA, Edussuriya K, Senaratne T, Sennanayake S, Selva D, Casson RJ. Cataract in central Sri Lanka: cataract surgical coverage and self-reported barriers to cataract surgery. *Clin Experiment Ophthalmol.* 2009;37(8):780–784. Doi:10.1111/j.1442-9071.2009.02152.x

94. Lewallen S, Courtright P. Gender and use of cataract surgical services in developing countries. *Bull World Health Organ.* 2002;80(4):300–303.

95. Courtright P. Gender and blindness: taking a global and a local perspective. *Oman J Ophthalmol.* 2009;2(2):55–56. Doi:10.4103/0974-620X.53032

96. Ramke J, Kyari F, Mwangi N, Piyasena M, Murthy G, Gilbert CE. Cataract services are leaving widows behind: examples from national cross-sectional surveys in Nigeria and Sri Lanka. *Int J Environ Res Public Health.* 2019;16(20):3854.

97. Brilliant GE, Brilliant LB. Using social epidemiology to understand who stays blind and who gets operated for cataract in a rural setting. *Soc Sci Med.* 1985;21(5):553–558. Doi:10.1016/0277-9536(85)90040-1

98. Gupta SK, Murthy GV. Distances travelled to reach surgical eye camps. *World Health Forum.* 1995;16(2):180–181.

99. Courtright P, Kanjaloti S, Lewallen S. Barriers to acceptance of cataract surgery among patients presenting to district hospitals in rural Malawi. *Trop Geogr Med*. 1995;47(1):15–18.

100. Marseille E, Brand R. The distribution of cataract surgery services in a public health eye care program in Nepal. *Health Policy*. 1997;42(2):117–133. Doi:10.1016/s0168-8510(97)00063-8

101. Abou-Gareeb I, Lewallen S, Bassett K, Courtright P. Gender and blindness: a meta-analysis of population-based prevalence surveys. *Ophthalmic Epidemiol*. 2001;8(1):39–56. Doi:10.1076/opep.8.1.39.1540

102. Klein BE, Klein R, Moss SE. Incident cataract surgery: the Beaver Dam eye study. *Ophthalmology*. 1997;104(4):573–580. Doi:10.1016/s0161-6420(97)30267-x

103. Javitt JC, Kendix M, Tielsch JM, et al. Geographic variation in utilization of cataract surgery. *Med Care*. 1995;33(1):90–105. Doi:10.1097/00005650-199501000-00008

104. Meddings DR, McGrail KM, Barer ML, et al. The eyes have it: cataract surgery and changing patterns of outpatient surgery. *Med Care Res Rev*. 1997;54(3):285–286. Doi:10.1177/107755879705400303

105. Baratz KH, Gray DT, Hodge DO, Butterfield LC, Ilstrup DM. Cataract extraction rates in Olmsted County, Minnesota, 1980 through 1994. *Arch Ophthalmol (Chicago, Ill 1960)*. 1997;115(11):1441–1446. Doi:10.1001/archopht.1997.01100160611015

106. Mönestam E, Wachtmeister L. Cataract surgery from a gender perspective—a population based study in Sweden. *Acta Ophthalmol Scand*. 1998;76(6):711–716. Doi:10.1034/j.1600-0420.1998.760617.x

107. Williams ES, Seward HC. Cataract surgery in South West Thames region: an analysis of age-adjusted surgery rates and length of stay by district. *Public Health*. 1993;107(6):441–449. Doi:10.1016/s0033-3506(05)80170-2

108. Desai P, Reidy A, Minassian DC. Profile of patients presenting for cataract surgery in the UK: national data collection. *Br J Ophthalmol*. 1999;83(8):893–896. Doi:10.1136/bjo.83.8.893

109. Limburg H, Kumar R, Bachani D. Monitoring and evaluating cataract intervention in India. *Br J Ophthalmol*. 1996;80(11):951–955. Doi:10.1136/bjo.80.11.951

110. Liu T, Ong EL, Yan X, et al. Factors influencing the success of rural cataract surgery programs in China: the Study of Hospital Administration and Relative Productivity (SHARP). *Invest Ophthalmol Vis Sci*. 2013;54(1):266–273. Doi:10.1167/iovs.12-10906

111. Sundaram M. Community outreach initiatives. In: *Community Outreach Initiatives*. Aravind Eye Hospital and Postgraduate Institute of Ophthalmology; 2001:1–33.

11 Glaucoma

Zhi Da Soh, Victor Koh, and Ching-Yu Cheng

11.1 INTRODUCTION

Glaucoma is a significant global health concern, despite the availability of medical and surgical interventions.[1] Although the ill effects of glaucoma can be mitigated with early treatment, it remains the leading cause of irreversible vision loss globally.[2] Thus, it is of foremost importance to understand the magnitude of disease burden associated with glaucoma worldwide, and the risk and impact associated with it. To achieve this, establishing the epidemiology of glaucoma is mandatory.

Epidemiology is the study of the distribution and determinants of health-related events in specific populations, and the application of these data to prevent diseases, control disease co-morbidities, and to promote healthy living.[3] Thus, it provides the foundation needed for researchers and clinicians to better understand disease risk factors and to evaluate new therapies, as well as a rational basis for policy makers to plan and prioritize public health policies.

Glaucoma is an optic neuropathy that is characterized by progressive degeneration of the retinal ganglion cells, resulting in the thinning of retinal nerve fiber layer (RNFL) and optic disc excavation (cupping).[1] This leads to the eventual development of a distinctive pattern of visual field defect.[1] Intra-ocular pressure (IOP) is no longer regarded as a defining criterion for glaucoma, although it remains the most important and modifiable risk factor.[2]

11.2 GLAUCOMA CLASSIFICATION
11.2.1 Clinic Classification

In clinic, glaucoma is classified according to the configuration of the anterior-chamber angle, and the presence of an identifiable cause (Figure 11.1).[4] Glaucoma is classified as *open angle* in cases where the anterior-chamber angle space is unobstructed, and aqueous humor can flow freely into the trabecular meshwork. In contrast, *angle closure* is diagnosed when there is a physical impediment to aqueous outflow (e.g., irido-trabecular contact). In open-angle glaucoma, raised IOP is commonly attributed to outflow resistance from within the trabecular meshwork itself. *Primary* glaucoma is used to describe cases with no discernible cause, and vice versa for *secondary*. Secondary glaucoma often results as a sequela to neovascularization, uveitis, trauma, or lens-related complications.[4] Angle closure is further classified into primary

angle closure suspect (PACS), primary angle closure (PAC), and primary angle closure glaucoma (PACG) (Table 11.1).

11.2.2 Epidemiological Classification

In epidemiologic studies, glaucoma is often classified according to the International Society of Geographical and Epidemiological Ophthalmology (ISGEO) classification after its inception in 2002 (Table 11.2).[5] This scheme comprises three levels of evidence, and emphasizes diagnosis based on structural and functional damage that is pathognomonic of glaucoma (level 1). However, provisions are made for cases where functional assessment is impeded by severe vision loss (level 2), and for cases where structural and functional assessment is hindered by severe media opacities (level 3).

Structural assessment focuses on vertical cup-to-disc ratio (VCDR) elongation, which is a pathognomonic sign of glaucoma that can be easily assessed. The 97.5th percentile value of VCDR observed among healthy individuals in a population denotes the upper limit of normality, and it is used arbitrarily to distinguish cases from normal. When functional assessment is not possible, the 99.5th percentile value is used instead to indicate advanced structural damage. The distribution of VCDR varies between different populations, but modal values of 0.70 (97.5th) and 0.80 (99.5th) are often utilized in epidemiology studies (Figure 11.2). Functional assessment relies on visual field results obtained from the threshold test strategy with 24-2 test pattern.

The ISGEO classification is a conceptually simple-to-use scheme that allows classification to be made without the need for sophisticated imaging tools such as optical coherence tomography (OCT). This standardizes the definition of glaucoma, and allows for prevalence data to be compared across studies and over time.

11.3 GLOBAL PREVALENCE OF GLAUCOMA
11.3.1 Prevalence of Primary Glaucoma

In 2013, the global prevalence of primary glaucoma among adults aged 40–80 years old was 3.54% (95% credible interval [CrI] 2.09, 5.82), affecting 64.3 million individuals (Figure 11.3).[6] Primary open-angle glaucoma (POAG) affected 3.05% (95% CrI 1.69, 5.27) adults globally, which was sixfold higher than the global PACG prevalence of 0.5% (95% CrI 0.11, 1.36).[6]

 DOI: 10.1201/9781315146737-13

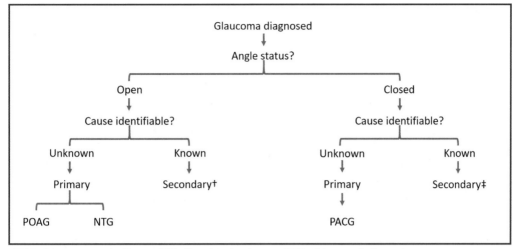

POAG – Primary open angle glaucoma, NTG – Normal tension glaucoma, PACG – Primary angle closure glaucoma
† e.g. Pigmentary, exfoliative, steroid-induced, angle recession, aphakic glaucoma
‡ e.g. neovascular, irido-corneal endothelial syndrome, phacomorphic cataract, aqueous misdirection

Figure 11.1 Clinical classification of glaucoma.

Table 11.1 Angle closure classification

Angle closure	ITC[a]	Elevated IOP	PAS	ONH damage
PACS	>=180°	–	–	–
PAC	>=180°	±	+	–
PACG	>=180°	±	+	+

Abbreviations: ITC, irido-trabecular contact; IOP, intra-ocular pressure; PAS, posterior anterior synechiae; ONH, optic nerve head; PACS, primary angle closure suspect; PAC, primary angle closure; PACG, primary angle closure glaucoma.

Note: [a] 180° or more of posterior trabecular meshwork not seen on gonioscopy at primary gaze without indentation.

Table 11.2 International Society of Geographical and Epidemiological Ophthalmology classification of ophthalmic epidemiology studies

Level 1 (presence of structural and functional evidence)
■ Vertical cup-to-disc ratio (VCDR) or VCDR asymmetry ≥97.5th percentile for the normal population, or
■ Neural retinal rim (NRR) ≤0.1 VCDR between 11 and 1 o'clock and 5 and 7 o'clock
■ Definite glaucomatous visual field defect

Level 2 (advanced structural evidence, absence of functional evidence)
■ VCDR or VCDR asymmetry ≥99.5th percentile for the normal population

Level 3 (absence of structural and functional evidence)
■ Visual acuity <3/60 and intra-ocular pressure >99.5th percentile for normal population, or
■ Visual acuity <3/60 and evidence of glaucoma-filtering surgery or medical records confirm glaucomatous visual morbidity

Africa has the highest prevalence of primary glaucoma (4.79%, 95% CrI 2.63, 8.03) and POAG (4.20%, 95% CrI 2.08, 7.35), whereas Asia is affected disproportionately by PACG (1.09%, 95% 0.43, 2.32). Nonetheless, Asia accounts for 60% of all glaucoma cases globally, or 1 in 2 POAG and 3 in 4 PACG, due to its sheer population size.[6] Within Asia, East Asia has the highest

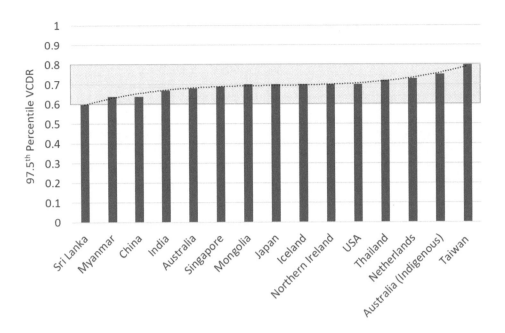

Figure 11.2 The average 97.5th percentile value of vertical cup-to-disc ratio (VCDR) reported in population-based studies from different countries.

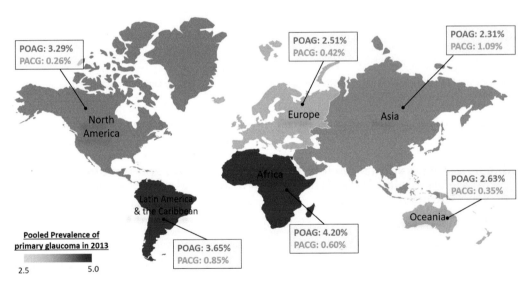

Figure 11.3 Global prevalence of primary glaucoma in 2013. POAG, primary open-angle glaucoma; PACG, primary angle closure glaucoma.

prevalence of PACG (1.07%, 95% CrI 0.28, 2.74) whereas the prevalence of POAG was similarly distributed.[7]

In addition, Asia consists of the largest number of POAG with "statistically normal" IOP (Figure 11.4). This variant of glaucoma was first described by Von Graefe in 1957,[8] and has been referred to as *normal-tension* (NTG) or *low-tension glaucoma* (LTG). However, controversies remain with regard to its classification as a separate disease entity or as a variant form of POAG.[9] NTG makes up 47–92% of POAG cases in Asia,[10–28] which is much higher than the 33–57% observed in Africa,[29–31] and 11–43% in Europe.[32–39] In the United States, NTG accounts for 17% and 82% of POAG among Hispanics

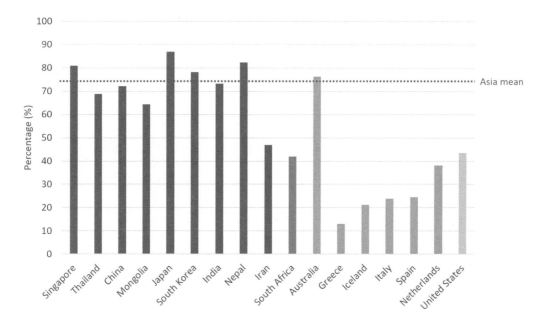

Figure 11.4 Average proportion of primary open-angle glaucoma (POAG) with "statistically normal" intra-ocular pressure (IOP) across countries. Bar graphs are color-coded according to geographical region: blue: Asia; orange: Africa; gray: Oceania; green: Europe; yellow: America. "Asia mean" represents the average proportion of open-angle glaucoma with statistically normal IOP derived from Asian countries in the figure.

and Latinos respectively.[40, 41] Among Asians, NTG is particularly prevalent among Japanese, accounting for 9 in 10 POAG cases.[15] However, it is noteworthy that cross-sectional estimates on NTG are limited by a single measurement of IOP, which varies diurnally.[42]

11.3.2 Prevalence of Secondary Glaucoma

In Asia, the overall prevalence of secondary glaucoma was 0.47% (95% CrI 0.09, 1.48) in 2013, making up 11.9% of all glaucoma cases and affecting 6.13 million individuals.[7] Among Caucasian populations, the prevalence of secondary glaucoma ranges from 0.20% in Australia and Brazil to 0.29% in Italy.

The major causes of secondary glaucoma in Asia included pseudo-exfoliation, pigment dispersion, neovascularization, trauma, and steroid-induced.[7] There are limited population-based data on the prevalence of pseudo-exfoliation glaucoma (PXG) and available prevalence figures vary widely from 0.1% (95% confidence interval [CI] 0.0, 0.2) in Japan to 2.2% (95% CI 1.7, 2.7) in Australia (Table 11.3). In addition, the National Blindness and Visual Impairment survey in Nigeria reported that couching, an ancient non-medical method of manipulating the crystalline lens, remains the most prevalent cause

of secondary glaucoma, accounting for 38% of cases.[43]

11.3.3 Projected Number of People with Glaucoma

Primary glaucoma is projected to affect 76 million individuals globally in 2020, and 111.8 million by 2040 (Figure 11.5).[6] This represents an 18.3% and 74% increase from the global estimates in 2013. POAG is projected to affect 52.7 million adults in 2020 and 74.8 million by 2040, while PACG is projected to affect 23.4 million in 2020 and 32 million by 2040.[6]

The surge in global prevalence of glaucoma will be driven largely by Africa and Asia.[6] In Africa, the prevalence of glaucoma is projected to increase by 130.8% or 10.9 million from 2013 to 2040. Nonetheless, Asia will still contain the highest absolute numbers of primary glaucoma in 2040, with 18.8 million POAG and 9 million PACG cases.

Within Asia, South Central Asia is projected to record the steepest increase in prevalence of primary glaucoma, increasing from 17.1 million in 2013 to 32.9 million by 2040.[7] In 2040, South Central Asia is poised to overtake East Asia as the Asia sub-region with the highest number of primary glaucoma and POAG cases, although

Table 11.3 Prevalence of pseudo-exfoliation glaucoma in population-based studies

Study, year	Country	Prevalence (95% confidence interval)
Blue Mountains Eye Study, 1996[44]	Australia	2.20 (1.70, 2.70)
Reykjavik Eye Study, 2003[38]	Finland	1.90 (–)
Thessaloniki Eye Study, 2007[39]	Greece	1.70 (–)
Hlabisa study, 2002[29]	South Africa	1.10 (–)
Aravind Comprehensive Eye Survey, 2003[19]	India	0.40 (0.30, 0.43)
Tehran Study, 2008[45]	Iran	0.23 (0.03, 0.43)
Yazd Eye Study, 2013[18]	Iran	0.40 (0.10, 0.70)
Tajimi Study, 2005[46]	Japan	0.20 (0.0, 0.30)
Kumejima Study, 2020[47]	Japan	0.10 (0.0, 0.20)
Singapore Malay Eye Study, 2008[21]	Singapore	0.18 (–)
Singapore Indian Eye Study, 2013[17]	Singapore	0.06 (–)

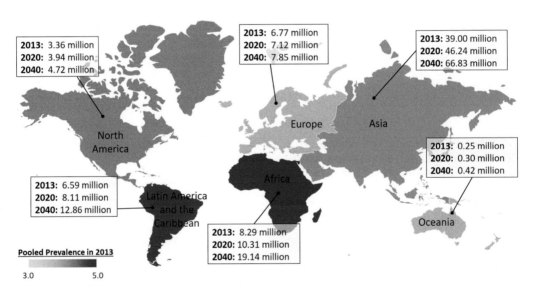

Figure 11.5 Global projection of number of people with primary glaucoma from 2013 to 2040.

East Asia will remain as the sub-region with the highest number of PACG cases.[7]

11.4 INCIDENCE OF PRIMARY GLAUCOMA

Incidence data indicate the number of new cases in a specific population over a specific period of time, and are important in identifying disease risk factors.[3] However, incidence data are more challenging to collect, and are less common as a result. Nonetheless, available data show that incident POAG varies widely between different populations (Table 11.4).

The incidence of PACS ranged from 16.9% (95% CI 14.1, 20.1) over 10 years in China,[56]

to 20.4% (95% CI 14.8, 25.7) over 6 years in Mongolia.[57] The incidence of PAC from the general population was 2.4% (95% CI 1.4, 4.0) over 10 years[56] or 7.97 per 1,000 eye-years (95% CI 5.75, 11.0) in China,[58] and 1.1% (95% CI 0.7, 1.5) over 6 years in India.[59] Furthermore, 22% (95% CI 9.8, 34.2) of PACS progressed to PAC and 28.5% (95% CI 12.0, 45.0) PAC cases developed PACG over 5 years.[60, 61] The incidence of PACG was 0.5% (95% CI 0.1, 1.8) over 12 years in Italy,[54] 0.3% (95% CI 0.1, 0.4) over 6 years in India,[59] and 1.1% (95% CI 0.5, 2.3) over 10 years in China.[56] In addition, the incidence of acute angle closure (AAC) was 2 per 100,000 persons annually in

Table 11.4 Incidence of primary open-angle glaucoma from population-based ophthalmic studies

Country	Baseline age	Follow-up, years	Follow-up rates, %	Cumulative incidence, % (95% confidence interval)
The Visual Impairment Project[48]	≥40	5	85.0	1.1 (0.8, 1.4)
The Yunnan Minority Eye Study[49]	≥50	5	80.6	1.3 (0.7, 1.9)
Chennai Eye Disease Incidence Study[50]	≥40	6	81.3	2.9 (2.4, 3.4)
Tema Eye Study[51]	≥40	8	80.3	4.6 (3.5, 6.0)
The Barbados Eye Studies[52]	≥40	9	81.0	4.4 (3.7, 5.2)
The Rotterdam Study[53]	≥55	5	78.0	1.2 (–)
Ponza Eye Study[54]	≥40	12	70.6	3.8 (2.3, 6.2)
The Los Angeles Latino Eye Study[55]	≥40	4	77.0	2.3 (1.8, 2.8)

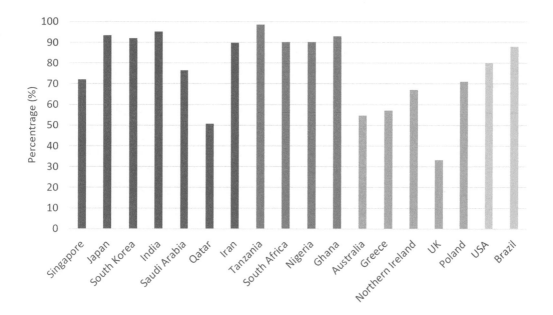

Figure 11.6 Average proportion of undiagnosed primary glaucoma across countries. See Figure 11.4 for key to color coding.

Scotland.[62] In contrast, incident AAC was 1.11 per 1,000 eye-years in China,[58] and 49.54 per 100,000 persons in Taiwan.[63] The highest incidence of AAC in Taiwan occurred among adults aged 60–69 years, accounting for approximately 1 in 3 cases.[64]

11.5 UNDETECTED GLAUCOMA

Glaucoma is the leading cause of irreversible vision impairment globally despite the availability of advanced medical treatments, and the good prognosis that is attainable with early treatment. However, a large proportion of glaucoma cases are undetected across communities worldwide, which impedes timely interventions and increases the risk of visual impairment.

11.5.1 Magnitude of Undiagnosed Glaucoma

The proportion of previously undetected glaucoma ranges from 33.3% in the United Kingdom (UK),[36] 72.1% in Singapore,[65] 80% of POAG in the United States,[41, 66] to over 90% in parts of Africa[29, 43, 67, 68] and India (Figure 11.6).[69] This proportion further varies by ethnicity and geographical area.

In the United States, approximately 2.4 million Americans suffer from glaucoma that is either undetected or untreated, with ethnic minorities affected disproportionately.[66] Black Americans were 4.4 times (95% CI 2.9, 6.7), and Hispanics 2.3 times (95% CI 1.5, 4.3) more likely to suffer from undetected glaucoma than non-Hispanic whites, after adjusting for age differences.[66] Hispanics are the largest minority in the United States, and are projected to account for half of all POAG cases by 2030.[70] In addition, glaucoma was 3.65-fold more likely to be undetected among Malay than Chinese adults in Singapore,[65] whereas 72.0–80.8% of indigenous Australians had undetected glaucoma compared to 46.6–63.0% of non-indigenous Australians.[71, 72] Furthermore, 71% of Australians in rural areas were undetected for glaucoma as compared to 58% in urban settings.[71]

11.5.2 Reasons for Undetected Glaucoma

11.5.2.1 Lack of Disease Knowledge

Glaucoma is often referred to as the "silent thief of sight" due to its asymptomatic nature in the early stages, and the reduced sensitivity of humans towards peripheral visual field defects.[2] Thus, knowledge on the debilitating effects of glaucoma may not be readily appreciated by the general public,[73] and glaucoma screening may not be prioritized. Consequently, individuals may only seek medical attention in the later stages when vision loss is more pronounced.

In Singapore, the higher prevalence of undetected glaucoma among Malays, despite having similar access to the same healthcare system and government subsidies as the rest of the population, is postulated to be related to their poorer health-seeking behavior.[65] For example, Malay adults may prefer to seek traditional healers for illnesses first, thereby delaying a formal assessment and diagnosis.

11.5.2.2 Lack of Service Utilization

Glaucoma is at least sixfold more likely to be diagnosed in individuals who consult both an optometrist and ophthalmologist within a 12-month period.[74] However, inadequate utilization of eye care services is among the most consistent factors associated with undetected glaucoma.[66, 75, 76]

In Australia, approximately 50% of undetected glaucoma cases did not have an eye check by an optometrist or ophthalmologist in the past year.[71] Factors deterrent to utilization of eye care services include lack of medical insurance, inability to speak English, and rural residence.[66] In the United States, immigrants were threefold less likely to utilize optometry services due to language barriers and lack of financial resources and health insurance.[77] In Singapore, the odds of undiagnosed glaucoma were 9.29-fold (95% CI 3.43, 25.21) higher in individuals with no annual assessment for spectacle prescription.[65]

11.5.2.3 Lack of Access to Services

While lack of utilization refers to the presence of services that are under-used, lack of access refers to the absence of services or restrictions that impedes access. Lack of access to essential eye care services is often associated with low socioeconomic status (SES), and affects ethnic minorities disproportionately.[78, 79]

SES is significantly associated with health outcomes, and eye health is no exception. For example, people with low SES may be diagnosed with advanced glaucoma by the time they seek medical attention.[80, 81] Individuals with poverty–income ratio <1.5 (poverty indicated for ratio <1) had much lower access to eye care services as compared to those with ratio ≥5.[82] Globally, many rural towns are not equipped with an ophthalmology clinic.[76] In India, 3 in 4 adults in rural regions require eye care services but only 1 in 3 have had an eye examination in their lifetime.[83]

In addition, ethnic minorities such as Hispanic Americans and indigenous Australians may have less access to healthcare services, which may explain the higher rates of undetected glaucoma.[70, 71] The cost of care and distance between service providers and area of residence were cited as barriers that inhibit access to eye care services in Africa, India, and among Hispanics in the United States.[70, 78, 79]

11.5.2.4 Lack of Accurate Diagnosis

The problem of undetected glaucoma goes beyond the barriers posed by inadequate disease knowledge, utilization, or access to essential eye care services. In India, glaucoma is as likely to be undetected in urban (94.1%) as compared to rural areas (98.4%), despite the increase in availability of eye care services in urban areas.[69] Furthermore, 50% of newly detected glaucoma from the Aravind Comprehensive Eye Survey had previously consulted an ophthalmologist, but less than 20% of them were diagnosed.[19] Based on the natural progression of glaucoma, it is likely that individuals with undetected glaucoma have had the disease for several years prior to detection.[84] Similarly, 49% of undetected glaucoma in the Visual Impairment Project had visited an eye care practitioner in the preceding 12 months.[74]

11.5.2.5 Lack of Adequate Resources

In Africa, glaucoma assessment is hindered by poor healthcare infrastructure, lack of appropriate equipment, limited treatment options, and inadequate number of ophthalmologists and support staff for surgical treatment such as trabeculectomy.[85, 86]

In addition, the diagnostic ability of practitioners may differ between geographical localities, which further explains the higher prevalence of undetected glaucoma in rural regions.[66] Also, poor examination techniques, over-reliance on IOP measurements, and poor clinical training have been attributed to the lack of diagnosis rather than inadequate equipment.[78, 87] The majority of glaucomatous cases may present with IOP <21 mmHg, which highlights the importance of optic disc assessment.[71, 79]

11.5.2.6 Lack of Participatory Effort

Optometrists are primary providers of eye care services and, thus, represent a valuable avenue for disease detection. Importantly, optometrists with adequate training are capable of making appropriate diagnostic and management decisions.[88, 89] However, optometrists' participation in glaucoma detection varies widely between countries, depending on the maturity and training of the profession, among other factors.[90, 91] In Australia, individuals who consulted an optometrist were 1.87-fold (95% CI 1.50, 2.30) more likely to be diagnosed with age-related macular degeneration, cataract, and glaucoma.[76] However, many optical practices across the world do not offer additional examination beyond refraction and prescription of optical aids.[79] Furthermore, the top-down approach in medical care often renders patients in a passive role, which may affect compliance with eye care advice.

11.5.2.7 Lack of Effective Screening Tools

A major factor that hinders glaucoma detection is the lack of a screening tool that is accurate in distinguishing disease from normal cases, applicable for mass screening, and practical in terms of resource requirements. For example, objective structural assessment with OCT is more accurate than VCDR assessment. However, the logistic feasibility, cost, and need for technical expertise often limit its applicability in community screening. A summary of the performances reported from simple and commonly administered screening tools is presented in Table 11.5. Nonetheless, the current stymie in glaucoma screening is increasingly addressed by the potentials shown in tele-medicine and artificial intelligence (AI)-assisted case detection.

11.6 IMPACT OF GLAUCOMA

A thorough knowledge of the burden of glaucoma aids in our understanding of its impact on finances, social well-being, and quality of life.[101] The chief concern for undetected glaucoma is the risk of irreversible vision loss,[66] which is a major contributor to the ill effects of glaucoma.[102, 103]

11.6.1 Visual Impairment

According to the Global Burden of Disease (GBD) study, glaucoma is the leading cause of irreversible vision loss.[104] In 2010, 2.1 million or 1 in every 15 individuals with glaucoma were blind (presenting visual acuity worse than 3/60 Snellen in the better eye). This represented 6.6% of global blindness in 2010, and a 62% increase from two decades ago.[104] A further 4.2 million or 1 in every 45 individuals with glaucoma suffered from moderate to severe vision impairment (MSVI, presenting visual acuity worse than 6/18 and no worse than 3/60 Snellen). This represented 2.2% of global vision impairment, and an 83% increase from two decades ago.[104] In addition, glaucoma-related visual morbidities were 2–3 times higher in low-income countries as compared to high-income countries.[105]

Although the prevalence of PACG is less than half of POAG, it is associated with a 2–3

Table 11.5 Sensitivity and specificity of common parameters for glaucoma screening

Screening test	Sensitivity (%)	Specificity (%)
IOP ≥21 mmHg[36,79]	25.1–47.1	86.9–95.3
VCDR ≥0.70[92–94]	45.3–53.6	95.4–98.9
Frequency-doubling technique[79, 95]	56.0–94.0	55.0–96.0
Van Herick[96, 97]	62.0–80.0	89.0–92.3
Shadow test[98, 99]	80.0–86.0	69.0–70.0
Combination 1. VCDR ≥0.70 or IOP asymmetry ≥4 mmHg[100] 2. VCDR ≥0.70 or VCDR asymmetry ≥0.30 or NRR ≤0.15[35]	68.8 76.0	94.2 73.0

Abbreviations: IOP, intra-ocular pressure; VCDR, vertical cup-to-disc ratio; NRR, neural retinal rim.

times higher risk of vision impairment and blindness.[106] In China, PACG accounts for 91% of vision impairment attributed to glaucoma.[107] In Singapore, 30.5% of Chinese with PACG were visually impaired as compared to 17.5% of Chinese with POAG.[10] In India, 2.9–16.6% of PACG cases were bilaterally blind as compared to 1.5–11.1% of POAG.[28, 69] In addition, glaucoma affects Africans and African Americans earlier in life and tends to follow a more aggressive clinical cause, resulting in visual impairment at an earlier age.[78, 108]

11.6.2 Quality of Life and Burden of Disease

Glaucomatous individuals with vision loss suffer from reduced quality of life, increased difficulties in performing activities of daily living, and increased risk of falls.[102, 109, 110] Individuals with moderate and severe glaucoma were 2.81- and 3.72-fold more at risk of falls respectively.[111] In addition, blindness could lead to increased social isolation, even in developed countries.[112]

Furthermore, glaucoma-related blindness or MSVI accounted for 5.99 million years lived with disability in 2017,[113] while age-standardized disability-adjusted life-years (DALY: 1 DALY = 1 year of healthy life lost) increased by 15% globally from 1990 to 2015.[102] In addition, glaucomatous individuals who received laser treatment had an increase of 2.5 quality-adjusted life-years (QALY: 1 QALY = 1 year of healthy life lived), and those on medical therapy had an increase of 5 QALYs as compared to untreated individuals.[114]

11.6.3 Socio-Economic Impact

Low SES is both a cause and consequence of glaucoma. As mentioned in the previous section, lower SES results in lower utilization and higher barriers to access essential eye care services, thus increasing the risk of late diagnosis and vision impairment from glaucoma.[81] This in turn worsens SES through increased cost of treatment, loss of personal income from reduced work productivity, and loss of family income from increased dependence on care givers.[112, 115, 116]

In Nigeria, the cost of treatment for glaucoma may take up 50% of monthly income for the middle class, and almost the entire monthly income for low-income earners.[115] This leads to poor compliance or the inability to pay for continued treatment. In India, glaucoma treatment is out of reach for low-income earners, requiring 23–37% more than their monthly income.[116] Furthermore, 92% of Indians with glaucoma are not covered by insurance or government subsidies, thus affecting access to treatment.[116]

In addition, the cost of glaucoma treatment is high and increasing. In the United States, the cost of glaucoma care incurred by Medicare beneficiaries was US$748 million in 2009, with POAG accounting for 61% of resources disbursed.[117] In Australia, the cost of POAG treatment is projected to increase from A$1.9 billion in 2005 to A$4.3 million by 2025.[111]

11.7 RISK FACTORS OF PRIMARY GLAUCOMA

11.7.1 Primary Open-Angle Glaucoma

11.7.1.1 Demographic Factors

11.7.1.1.1 Age

Age is a significant risk factor for the development and progression of glaucoma, after adjusting for the association between older age and increased IOP.[4] Globally, the odds of POAG increase by 73% (odds ratio [OR] 1.73, 95% CI 1.63, 1.82) per decade increase in age.[6]

11.7.1.1.2 Ethnicity

The risk of POAG is 2.8-fold (95% CI 1.83, 4.06) higher among Africans as compared to people of European ancestry.[6] Similarly, Africans were 2.05 times (95% CI 1.11, 3.43) more likely to develop POAG as compared to Asians.[6]

Gender

The association between gender and glaucoma is less consistent.[2] However, men were 1.36 times (95% CI 1.23, 1.51) more likely to develop POAG in a global meta-analysis on POAG.[6]

11.7.1.2 Ocular Factors

11.7.1.2.1 IOP

The general consensus is that there is no single IOP threshold that denotes normality.[1, 2] This is evident from the considerable overlap in IOP distribution between glaucomatous and normal individuals (Figure 11.7).[118] Nonetheless, IOP remains an important risk factor and the only one that is modifiable.[1] The risk of glaucoma increases greatly with higher IOP even if it remains below IOP <21 mmHg.[1]

The relative risk of glaucoma with IOP ≥22 mmHg ranged from 1.5 (95% CI 1.2, 1.9) in the Tema Eye Survey[51] to 8.1 (95% CI 2.7, 24.5) in the Ponza Eye Study.[54] In addition, the risk of glaucoma increased by 20% (relative risk [RR] 1.2, 95% CI 1.08, 1.16) for every 1 mmHg increase in IOP,[52] or by twofold (OR 2.0, 95% CI 1.5, 2.6) for every 10 mmHg increase.[50]

11.7.1.2.2 Myopia

Myopic eyes are more susceptible to glaucomatous damage.[119] The odds of glaucoma were 1.92 (95% CI 1.54, 2.38) for any myopia, 1.65

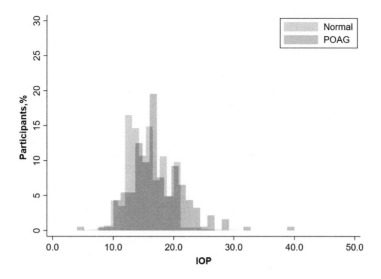

Figure 11.7 Intra-ocular pressure (IOP) distribution from the Singapore Epidemiology Eye Diseases Study showing extensive overlap between individuals with and without primary open-angle glaucoma (POAG). (Unpublished results from the Singapore Epidemiology of Eye Diseases Study.)

(95% CI 1.26, 2.17) for myopia less than –3 D, and 2.46 (95% 1.93, 3.15) for myopia –3 D or more.[119] In addition, the risk of glaucoma (RR 7.2, 95% CI 1.3, 39.9) is significantly higher in high myopia (<–6D),[54] and the odds of glaucoma (OR 1.5, 95% CI 1.0, 2.2) increased with every millimeter increase in axial elongation.[50]

11.7.1.2.3 Central Corneal Thickness
Thinner central corneal thickness (CCT) may increase the risk of glaucoma partly due to under-estimation of IOP measurements.[4] In addition, it may act as a biomarker for disease susceptibility, with thinner CCT being observed more in blacks as compared to whites.[4]

The odds of glaucoma for every 40 μm thinner in CCT ranged from 1.20 (95% CI 1.03, 1.50) in the Tema Eye Survey[51] to 1.41 (95% CI 1.01, 1.96) in the Barbados Eye Study.[52] In addition, POAG was more likely to develop in thin corneas with higher IOP.[50]

11.7.1.2.4 Ocular Perfusion Pressure
Ocular perfusion pressure (OPP = diastolic blood pressure [BP] + 1/3 systolic BP – IOP) is a proxy of ocular blood flow, and it is measured to ascertain the effect of inadequate or unstable ocular blood flow in causing ischemic glaucomatous damage.[4] In the Singapore Malay Eye Study, the odds of glaucoma (OR 1.73, 95% CI 1.05, 3.15) among Malay adults in the lowest quartile of mean OPP (≤46 mmHg) were significantly higher than those in the highest quartile

(>58 mmHg).[120] However, the Rotterdam study reported that the effect of OPP may have been driven by IOP (lower OPP results from high IOP).[121] The association between every mmHg increase in OPP and incident POAG was not significant (hazard ratio [HR] 0.995, 95% CI 0.971, 1.019) when adjusted for IOP.[121]

11.7.1.3 Family History and Genetic Factors
The development of POAG appears to consist of a familial or genetic component, either through a multi-factorial or polygenic transmission.[122] The Barbados Eye Study reported an increase in risk of POAG (RR 2.40, 95% CI 1.30, 4.60) with positive family history,[52] as did the Ponza Eye Study (RR 3.80, 95% CI 1.20, 11.70).[54]

In addition, genome-wide association studies (GWAS) have identified several single-nucleotide polymorphisms (SNPs) at different loci that are either associated directly with POAG itself, or through its quantitative traits (e.g., IOP, VCDR, CCT).[123, 124] These loci include, are not limited to, *CAV1/CAV2*,[125, 126] *TMC01*,[127] *CDKN2BAS*,[127, 128] *SIX6*,[128, 129] *AFAP1*,[130] *GMDS*,[130] *ABCA1*,[130, 131] *PMM2*,[131] *TGFBR3*,[132] *FNDC3B*,[132] *ARHGEF12*,[133] *TXNRD2*,[134] *ATXN2*,[134] *FOXC1*,[134] and *GAS7*.[134]

11.7.1.4 Systemic Factors
Chronic systemic conditions, such as hypertension and diabetes, are hypothesized to be associated with glaucoma through elevated IOP and/or reduced vascular supply to the optic

disc.[135] However, these associations remain inconclusive from current literatures, which are mainly cross-sectional studies that are limited by lack of temporality and reverse causation bias.

Hypertension was reported to be a significant risk factor in epidemiological studies such as the Blue Mountains Eye Study (OR 1.56, 95% CI 1.01, 2.40)[136] and Harbin study (OR 2.40, 95% CI 1.17, 5.16),[137] but not in others such as the Barbados Eye Study (OR 0.80, 95% CI 0.50, 1.20)[52] and Beijing Eye Study (OR 1.35, 95% CI 0.86, 2.14).[138] Among Hispanics, the odds of glaucoma were significantly higher (OR 2.0, 95% CI 1.1, 4.0) for systolic BP (SBP) above 161 mmHg as compared to SBP between 111 and 120 mmHg.[139] However, the Rotterdam Study reported an insignificant increase in odds of glaucoma with increased SBP (OR 1.20 per 23 mmHg increase, 95% CI 0.97, 1.48).[140]

Diabetes was reported to be a significant risk factor for glaucoma among Hispanics (OR 1.40, 95% CI 1.03, 1.80),[141] but not among Malay in Singapore (OR 1.02, 95% CI 0.58, 1.79),[142] the Rotterdam Study (OR 0.65, 95% CI 0.25, 1.64),[143] and the Barbados Eye Study (OR 1.20, 95% CI 0.70, 1.80).[52]

Likewise, the association between body mass index (BMI) and glaucoma development is inconclusive. Lower BMI was a significant risk factor for POAG in central India (OR 1.11, 95% CI 1.03, 1.19)[144] and in the Rotterdam Study (HR 1.06 per unit lower in BMI, 95% CI 1.01, 1.12),[145] but not in studies such as the Kumejima Study (OR 0.99, 95% CI 0.94, 1.04).[146] Furthermore, lower BMI was also associated with lower IOP, which is counter-intuitive to its association with POAG.[135]

In addition, NTG is further associated with systemic vascular dysregulation.[147, 148] Systemic conditions, such as vasospastic disorders (e.g., migraine, Raynaud phenomenon), systemic hypotension, sleep apnea syndrome, autoimmune and ischemic vascular diseases, are observed more frequently among NTG cases than POAG, albeit inconsistently.[4, 9, 147, 148]

11.7.2 Primary Angle Closure Glaucoma

11.7.2.1 Demographic Factors

11.7.2.1.1 Age

Age may increase the risk of PACG through a combination of increasing lens thickness, forward budging of the lens, and pupil miosis, thereby increasing the risk of pupillary block.[149] In Asia, the odds of PACG increase by 121% (95% CrI 92.0, 157.0) per decade increase in age.[7]

11.7.2.1.2 Ethnicity

Asians are consistently associated with higher risk of PACG.[6, 149] The prevalence of PACG among Asians was 1.82-fold higher than in Africans, and 1.28–4.19-fold higher than in Caucasians.[6] Within Asia, the odds of PACG were 5.5 times (95% CrI 1.52, 14.73) higher among East Asians as compared to South East Asians.[7] The prevalence of PACG is higher among the Chinese and Mongolian populations in Asia,[150, 151] as well as the Inuit population in the west.[152]

11.7.2.1.3 Gender

Women are consistently associated with higher risk of PACG.[4, 7] The association between women and PACG may be attributed to a shallower anterior chamber.[4] In a meta-analysis of PACG in Asia, the odds of men developing PACG were almost half (OR 0.54, 95% CI 0.41, 0.71) those of women.[7] In India, women were 2.07 times (95% CI 1.09, 3.93) more likely to develop PACG.[153] In Korea, the incidence rate of PACG among women was 85.85 (95% CI 84.03, 87.66) per 1 million person-years, which was 2.56-fold higher than the incidence rate of 33.48 (95% CI 32.33, 34.62) per 1 million person-years among men.[154]

11.7.2.2 Ocular Factors

Our understanding of angle closure has improved considerably with the advent of anterior-segment OCT (ASOCT). ASOCT has identified several new anatomical parameters that are associated with angle closure in addition to conventional risk factors such as shallow anterior-chamber depth, short axial length, and a large lens.[149, 155] These ASOCT parameters, such as anterior-chamber width,[156] lens vault,[157] iris thickness,[158] and iris area[159] or volume,[160] are found to be independently associated with angle closure in various studies, albeit inconsistently. Nonetheless, a combination of six ASOCT parameters was found to be able to identify 95% of narrow angles determined from gonioscopy.[161] However, anatomical features remain insufficient in explaining why angle closure affects Asians disproportionately.[162]

Physiological factors, such as iris fluid conductivity, are increasingly regarded as integral to the development of angle closure.[163] In eyes with open angle, the iris loses approximately 4% of its volume per millimeter of pupil dilation.[164] In contrast, a retention or gain in iris volume has been observed in eyes with angle closure, which narrows the anterior-chamber space by two- to three-fold, bringing the iris and trabecular meshwork closer into apposition.[160, 164] However, our understanding of iris fluid conductivity remains inadequate, although iris surface features such as iris crypts and furrows have been found to be predictive of iris fluid conductivity.[165, 166] Furthermore, the odds of acute angle closure glaucoma were lower in Asian eyes with more crypts.[167]

11.7.2.3 Family History and Genetic Factors

Familial association observed in cases of PAC suggests some extent of hereditary influence.[149] The odds of PAC were 4.82 (95% CI 2.08, 11.19) and 1.65 (95% CI 1.16, 2.34) for PACG in people with a family history of PAC and PACG respectively.[168] Furthermore, similarities in quantitative traits of PACG (i.e., iris and angle parameters) have been observed among first-degree relatives of people with PACG.[169–171] For example, hereditary or genetic effect accounted for 90.1% (95% CI 88.2, 91.7) of variation in anterior-chamber depth, even after accounting for axial myopia, in the Guangzhou Twin Eye Study.[169]

In addition, GWAS have identified several SNPs at different loci that are either associated directly with PACG itself, or through ocular features involved in its pathogenesis (e.g., anterior-chamber depth, trabecular meshwork, iris).[124, 172] These loci include, but are not limited to, *PLEKHA7, COL11A1, PCMTD1, EPDR1, CHAT, GLIS3, FERMT2*, and *DRM2-FAM102*.[172, 173] Taken together, these loci explain less than 2% of genetic variation in PACG,[124] and exhibit little overlap between the genetic etiology of POAG and PACG.[172]

11.8 GLAUCOMA SCREENING

Glaucoma screening is necessary to distinguish between people in the population with the disease from those who do not have it, so as to unravel its true burden and mitigate against its ill effects. Although screening is difficult in the absence of symptoms in the early stages, it is not a Sisyphean task with the advent of imaging and information technologies. Furthermore, heightened motivation can be garnered from the good prognosis that is attainable with early treatment.[1]

The US Preventive Services Task Force (USPSTF) presented evidence that glaucoma screening results in early detection of POAG, which may lead to earlier treatment that mitigates against the development or progression of functional defects.[174] However, USPSTF released a statement of neutrality with regard to glaucoma screening, citing insufficient evidence to determine the impact that screening had on vision-related function and quality of life, as well as concerns regarding side effects from early treatment.[174, 175] The World Glaucoma Association further cited cost-effectiveness as the main roadblock for glaucoma screening.[176] However, almost a decade has passed since the release of these statements, and major developments, such as the internet of things (IoT) and AI, have ushered in a new era of data-driven healthcare.

AI provides the computational prowess to develop machines that expertly learn, think, and act like humans in real time.[177] This enables the development of predictive algorithms through deep learning that accurately distinguish between health statuses, including glaucoma.[178, 179] Overall, these algorithms are able to distinguish glaucoma cases of varying definitions with an accuracy of 87.2–98.6% and sensitivity/specificity of >80% (Table 11.6).[179]

Table 11.6 Summary of artificial intelligence algorithms in detecting glaucoma

Authors	Image type	Disease definition	AUC	Sensitivity	Specificity
Ting et al.[182]	CFP	Possible glaucoma	0.942	0.964	0.872
Li et al.[183]	HVF	UKGTS guideline	0.876	0.826	0.932
Asaoka et al.[184]	OCT	Early glaucoma	0.937	0.833	0.866
Li et al.[185]	CFP	Referable glaucoma	0.986	0.956	0.920
Shibata et al.[186]	CFP	JGS guideline	0.965	–	–
Masumoto et al.[187]	SLO	Any glaucoma	0.872	0.813	0.802
		Early glaucoma	0.830	0.838	0.753
		Moderate glaucoma	0.864	0.775	0.902
		Severe glaucoma	0.934	0.909	0.958
Medeiros et al.[180]	CFP + OCT	Glaucomatous neural loss	0.944	–	–
Thompson et al.[188]	CFP + OCT	Glaucomatous NRR loss	0.945	–	–
Hamelings et al.[181]	CFP	ICD standards	0.995	0.980	0.910

Abbreviations: AUC, area under curve; CFP, color fundus photograph; HVF, Humphrey visual fields; UKGTS, United Kingdom Glaucoma Treatment Study; OCT, optical coherence tomography; JGS, Japanese Glaucoma Society; SLO, scanning laser ophthalmoscope; NRR, neural retinal rim; ICD, *International Classification of Disease.*

Further developments have resulted in an algorithm that predicts RNFL thickness based on fundus photographs without the need for OCT imaging,[180] and an algorithm that utilizes less input to achieve similar performances.[181]

In addition, IoT has given rise to tele-medicine through its ability to harness enormous data from inter-connected mobiles, wireless, and digital devices.[189] Telemedicine extends the reach of medical care by mitigating barriers to care posed by lack of financial resources, medical staff, and healthcare facilities in remote localities. In a recent meta-analysis, 83.3% of glaucoma cases (sensitivity 0.83, 95% CI 0.77, 0.88) and 79% of normal cases (specificity 0.79, 95% CI 0.67, 0.88) were correctly identified through tele-consultation.[190] Glaucoma detection through tele-consultation was more specific but less sensitive as compared to in-patient examination, and cost less (US$922.77 vs. US$1,098.67) for each detected case.[190]

In recent years, cost-effective glaucoma screenings have been reported in India and China.[191–193] In urban China, a combined POAG and PACG screening was considered cost-effective by World Health Organization (WHO) standards, when incurred cost of detection was compared to gains in QALY and years of blindness avoided.[193] Over a 30-year period, every 100,000 rural and urban Chinese residents screened would result in an estimated total of 246 and 1,325 years of blindness avoided respectively.[193] Glaucoma screening is likely to be more cost-effective in Asia due to the high prevalence of PACG in the region, the high absolute number of primary glaucoma cases, and the lower cost of staffing.[193, 194] Furthermore, screening may be required more in some countries in Asia and in developing countries due to the poorer access to eye care services.[194] Nonetheless, screening is redundant in the absence of universal coverage and continuity of care. Thus, it is imperative that screening initiatives are accessible to all, and arrangements for follow-up consultation are acceptable, affordable, and tailored to the local context.

11.9 FUTURE DIRECTIONS

The dawn of humanity's fourth industrial revolution is upon us, and with this comes a time of reflection and reaction. Also known as the era of big data and AI, this revolution promises to transform the way ophthalmology is practiced.

For decades, the hazards of glaucoma have persisted despite improvements in disease interventions. Over the years, epidemiology studies have provided us with much-needed information on the disease burden that glaucoma

brings to communities worldwide. Yet, it remains one thing to get an updated perspective on the problem, and quite another to act on it. For this, inter-disciplinary collaboration to find solutions, along with masterful communication of scientific discoveries, must be endeavored moving forward. In fact, both aspects are needed more than ever as we navigate the complexity of big data to harness its full potential.

Moving forward, the adoption of AI will be more of an implantation challenge rather than a proof of concept. AI will have an important role in disease detection and could potentially provide a cost-effective tool for mass screening. In addition, big data will provide the foundation for developing new models of care for glaucoma, and initial results on the viability of virtual glaucoma clinics[195] and monitoring of IOP with "smart" contact lenses are encouraging.[196, 197]

More significantly, the time has perhaps arrived to relook into the definition of glaucoma in both clinic and research settings. The ISGEO classification scheme was conceptualized almost two decades ago when OCT technology was in its infancy stage. However, OCT has not only developed rapidly from time domain to swept-source capabilities with enhanced image resolution and angiography measurements; it is now commonly available and routinely utilized in glaucoma diagnosis and monitoring. The use of OCT provides further insights on disease mechanism, and reduces over-reliance on subjective measures such as VCDR and gonioscopy assessment. This, in turn, may lead to more accurate and objective diagnosis and further aid in standardizing the definition of glaucoma. Moreover, accurate diagnoses and classification of glaucoma will become more important clinically as surgical interventions, such as minimally invasive glaucoma surgeries (MIGS) and selective laser trabeculoplasty (SLT), are targeted for mild and early cases of glaucoma.

11.10 CONCLUSION

The problem of glaucoma is not new, and its global impact will exacerbate in the coming decades. Africans are affected disproportionately by POAG, while PACG is the predominant form of glaucoma among Asians. This is a cause for concern as access to eye care is generally poorer in both regions, and PACG is visually more debilitating. Furthermore, a large proportion of glaucoma cases are undetected globally, fueling concerns regarding the effectiveness of current case detection strategies. The chief concern for glaucoma is visual impairment, which drastically affects quality of life and the financial and social well-being of those affected.

Therefore, screening should be endeavored and the adoption of AI should be explored further. Importantly, screening initiatives must be accessible, affordable, and acceptable to all, and continuity of care is germane.

REFERENCES

1. Weinreb RN, Khaw PT. Primary open-angle glaucoma. *The Lancet*. 2004;363(9422):1711–1720.

2. Jonas JB, Aung T, Bourne RR, Bron AM, Ritch R, Panda-Jonas S. Glaucoma. *The Lancet*. 2017;390(10108): 2183–2193.

3. Gordis L. *Epidemiology*. Fifth ed. Philadelphia, PA: Elsevier/Saunders; 2013.

4. Girkin CA, Crowston JG, Giaconi JA, Medeiros FA, Sit AJ, Tanna AP. *Basic and Clinical Science Course 2019–2020: Glaucoma*. San Francisco, CA: American Acadey of Ophthalmology, 2016.

5. Foster PJ, Buhrmann R, Quigley HA, Johnson GJ. The definition and classification of glaucoma in prevalence surveys. *British Journal of Ophthalmology*. 2002;86(2):238–242.

6. Tham Y-C, Li X, Wong TY, Quigley HA, Aung T, Cheng C-Y. Global prevalence of glaucoma and projections of glaucoma burden through 2040: a systematic review and meta-analysis. *Ophthalmology*. 2014;121(11):2081–2090.

7. Chan EWe, Li X, Tham Y-C, et al. Glaucoma in Asia: regional prevalence variations and future projections. *British Journal of Ophthalmology*. 2016;100(1):78–85.

8. Zhao J, Solano MM, Oldenburg CE, et al. Prevalence of normal-tension glaucoma in the Chinese population: a systematic review and meta-analysis. *American Journal of Ophthalmology*. 2019;199:101–110.

9. Fan N, Tan J, Liu X. Is "normal tension glaucoma" glaucoma? *Medical Hypotheses*. 2019;133:109405.

10. Baskaran M, Foo RC, Cheng C-Y, et al. The prevalence and types of glaucoma in an urban Chinese population: the Singapore Chinese Eye Study. *JAMA Ophthalmology*. 2015;133(8):874–880.

11. Bourne RRA, Sukudom P, Foster PJ, et al. Prevalence of glaucoma in Thailand: a population based survey in Rom Klao District, Bangkok. *British Journal of Ophthalmology*. 2003;87(9):1069–1074.

12. He J, Zou H, Lee RK, et al. Prevalence and risk factors of primary open-angle glaucoma in a city of Eastern China: a population-based study in Pudong New District, Shanghai. *BMC Ophthalmology*. 2015;15(1):134.

13. He M, Foster PJ, Ge J, et al. Prevalence and clinical characteristics of glaucoma in adult Chinese: a population-based study in Liwan District, Guangzhou. *Investigative Ophthalmology & Visual Science*. 2006;47(7):2782.

14. Li H, Zhang Y-Y, Liu S-C, He X-g, Li C-j, Li C-h, Li G, Wu Y-f, Song S-f. Prevalence of open-angle glaucoma in Southwestern China : the Yongchuan Glaucoma Study. *Journal of Huazhong University Science and Technology Medical Science*. 2014;34(1):137–141.

15. Iwase A, Suzuki Y, Araie M, et al. The prevalence of primary open-angle glaucoma in Japanese: the Tajimi Study. *Ophthalmology*. 2004;111(9):1641–1648.

16. Liang YB, Friedman DS, Zhou Q, et al. Prevalence of primary open angle glaucoma in a rural adult Chinese population: the Handan eye study. *Investigative Ophthalmology & Visual Science*. 2011;52(11):8250.

17. Narayanaswamy A, Baskaran M, Zheng Y, et al. The prevalence and types of glaucoma in an urban Indian population: the Singapore Indian Eye Study. *Investigative Ophthalmology & Visual Science*. 2013;54(7):4621.

18. Pakravan M, Yazdani S, Javadi M-A, et al. A population-based survey of the prevalence and types of glaucoma in central Iran: the Yazd eye study. *Ophthalmology*. 2013;120(10):1977–1984.

19. Ramakrishnan R, Nirmalan PK, Krishnadas R, et al. Glaucoma in a rural population of southern India: the Aravind comprehensive eye survey. *Ophthalmology*. 2003;110(8):1484–1490.

20. Raychaudhuri A, Lahiri S, Bandyopadhyay M, Foster P, Reeves B, Johnson G. A population based survey of the prevalence and types of glaucoma in rural West Bengal: the West Bengal Glaucoma Study. *British Journal of Ophthalmology*. 2005;89(12):1559–1564.

21. Shen SY, Wong TY, Foster PJ, et al. The prevalence and types of glaucoma in Malay people: the Singapore Malay Eye Study. *Investigative Ophthalmology & Visual Science*. 2008;49(9):3846.

22. Song W, Shan L, Cheng F, et al. Prevalence of glaucoma in a rural northern china adult population: a population-based survey in Kailu county, Inner Mongolia. *Ophthalmology*. 2011;118(10):1982–1988.

23. Sun J, Zhou X, Kang Y, et al. Prevalence and risk factors for primary open-angle glaucoma in a rural northeast China population: a population-based survey in Bin County, Harbin. *Eye (London, England)*. 2012;26(2):283–291.

24. Thapa SS, Paudyal I, Khanal S, et al. A population-based survey of the prevalence and types of glaucoma in Nepal: the Bhaktapur Glaucoma Study. *Ophthalmology*. 2012;119(4):759–764.

25. Vijaya L, George R, Paul PG, et al. Prevalence of open-angle glaucoma in a rural south Indian population. *Investigative Ophthalmology & Visual Science*. 2005;46(12):4461–4467.

26. Yamamoto S, Sawaguchi S, Iwase A, et al. Primary open-angle glaucoma in a population associated with high prevalence of primary angle-closure glaucoma: the Kumejima Study. *Ophthalmology*. 2014;121(8):1558–1565.

27. Zhong H, Li J, Li C, et al. The prevalence of glaucoma in adult rural Chinese populations of the Bai nationality in Dali: the Yunnan Minority Eye Study. *Investigative Ophthalmology & Visual Science*. 2012;53(6):3221.

28. Garudadri C, Senthil S, Khanna RC, Sannapaneni K, Rao HBL. Prevalence and risk factors for primary glaucomas in adult urban and rural populations in the Andhra Pradesh Eye Disease Study. *Ophthalmology*. 2010;117(7):1352–1359.

29. Rotchford AP, Johnson GJ. Glaucoma in Zulus: a population-based cross-sectional survey in a rural district in South Africa. *Archives of Ophthalmology*. 2002;120(4):471–478.

30. Rotchford AP, Kirwan JF, Muller MA, Johnson GJ, Roux P. Temba glaucoma study: a population-based cross-sectional survey in urban South Africa. *Ophthalmology*. 2003;110(2):376–382.

31. Salmon JF, Mermoud A, Ivey A, Swanevelder SA, Hoffman M. The prevalence of primary angle closure glaucoma and open angle glaucoma in Mamre, western Cape, South Africa. *Archives of Ophthalmology.* 1993;111(9):1263–1269.

32. Antón A, Andrada MT, Mujica V, Calle MA, Portela J, Mayo A. Prevalence of primary open-angle glaucoma in a Spanish population: the Segovia study. *Journal of Glaucoma.* 2004;13(5):371–376.

33. Bonomi L, Marchini G, Marraffa M, et al. Prevalence of glaucoma and intraocular pressure distribution in a defined population: the Egna-Neumarkt Study. *Ophthalmology.* 1998;105(2):209–215.

34. Cedrone C, Culasso F, Cesareo M, Zapelloni A, Cedrone P, Cerulli L. Prevalence of glaucoma in Ponza, Italy: a comparison with other studies. *Ophthalmic Epidemiology.* 1997;4(2):59–72.

35. Dielemans I, Vingerling JR, Wolfs RC, Hofman A, Grobbee DE, de Jong PT. The prevalence of primary open-angle glaucoma in a population-based study in the Netherlands: the Rotterdam Study. *Ophthalmology.* 1994;101(11):1851–1855.

36. Foster PJ, Broadway DC, Garway-Heath DF, et al. Intraocular pressure and corneal biomechanics in an adult British population: the EPIC-Norfolk eye study. *Investigative Ophthalmology & Visual Science.* 2011;52(11):8179–8185.

37. Jóhannesson G, Guðmundsdóttir GJ, Lindén C. Can the prevalence of open-angle glaucoma be estimated from a retrospective clinical material? A study on the west coast of Iceland. *Acta Ophthalmologica Scandinavica.* 2005;83(5):549–553.

38. Jonasson F, Damji K, Arnarsson A, et al. Prevalence of open-angle glaucoma in Iceland: Reykjavik Eye Study. *Eye.* 2003;17(6):747–753.

39. Topouzis F, Wilson MR, Harris A, et al. Prevalence of open-angle glaucoma in Greece: the Thessaloniki Eye Study. *American Journal of Ophthalmology.* 2007;144(4):511–519. e511.

40. Quigley HA, West SK, Rodriguez J, Munoz B, Klein R, Snyder R. The prevalence of glaucoma in a population-based study of Hispanic subjects: Proyecto VER. *Archives of Ophthalmology.* 2001;119(12):1819–1826.

41. Varma R, Ying-Lai M, Francis BA, et al. Prevalence of open-angle glaucoma and ocular hypertension in Latinos: the Los Angeles Latino Eye Study. *Ophthalmology.* 2004;111(8):1439–1448.

42. Liu JH, Zhang X, Kripke DF, Weinreb RN. Twenty-four-hour intraocular pressure pattern associated with early glaucomatous changes. *Investigative Ophthalmology & Visual Science.* 2003;44(4):1586–1590.

43. Kyari F, Entekume G, Rabiu M, et al. A population-based survey of the prevalence and types of glaucoma in Nigeria: results from the Nigeria National Blindness and Visual Impairment Survey. *BMC Ophthalmology.* 2015;15(1):176.

44. Mitchell P, Smith W, Attebo K, Healey PR. Prevalence of open-angle glaucoma in Australia. The Blue Mountains Eye Study. *Ophthalmology.* 1996;103(10):1661.

45. Amini H, Javadi M-A, Yazdani S, et al. The prevalence of glaucoma in Tehran, Iran. *Journal of Ophthalmic & Vision Research.* 2008;2(2):93–100.

46. Yamamoto T, Iwase A, Araie M, et al. The Tajimi Study report 2: prevalence of primary angle closure and secondary glaucoma in a Japanese population. *Ophthalmology.* 2005;112(10):1661–1669.

47. Arakaki Y, Sawaguchi S, Iwase A, Tomidokoro A, Araie M. Pseudoexfoliation syndrome and relating factors in a rural Japanese population: the Kumejima Study. *Acta Ophthalmologica.* 2020;98(7):e888–e894.

48. Mukesh BN, McCarty CA, Rait JL, Taylor HR. Five-year incidence of open-angle glaucoma: The visual impairment project. *Ophthalmology.* 2002;109(6):1047–1051.

49. Pan C-W, Yang W-Y, Hu D-N, et al. Longitudinal cohort study on the incidence of primary open-angle glaucoma in Bai Chinese. *American Journal of Epidemiology.* 2017;176:127–133.

50. Vijaya L, Rashima A, Panday M, et al. Predictors for incidence of primary open-angle glaucoma in a South Indian population: the Chennai eye disease incidence study. *Ophthalmology.* 2014;121(7):1370–1376.

51. Mwanza J-C, Tulenko SE, Barton K, et al. Eight-year incidence of open-angle glaucoma in the Tema eye survey. *Ophthalmology* 2019;126(3):372–380.

52. Leske MC, Wu S-Y, Hennis A, Honkanen R, Nemesure B, BES Study Group. Risk factors for incident open-angle glaucoma: the Barbados Eye Studies. *Ophthalmology.* 2008;115(1):85–93.

53. de Voogd S, Ikram MK, Wolfs RCW, Jansonius NM, Hofman A, de Jong PTVM. Incidence of open-angle glaucoma in a general elderly population: the Rotterdam Study. *Ophthalmology.* 2005;112:1487–1493.

54. Cedrone C, Mancino R, Ricci F, Cerulli A, Culasso F, Nucci C. The 12-year incidence of glaucoma and glaucoma-related visual field loss in Italy: the Ponza Eye Study. *Journal of Glaucoma* 2012;21(1):1–6.

55. Varma R, Wang D, Wu C, et al. Four-year incidence of open-angle glaucoma and ocular hypertension: the Los Angeles Latino Eye Study. *American Journal of Ophthalmology.* 2012;154:315–325.e311.

56. Wang L, Huang W, Huang S, et al. Ten-year incidence of primary angle closure in elderly Chinese: the Liwan Eye Study. *British Journal of Ophthalmology.* 2019;103:355–360.

57. Yip JLY, Foster PJ, Gilbert CE, et al. Incidence of occludable angles in a high-risk Mongolian population. *British Journal of Ophthalmology.* 2008;92:30–33.

58. He M, Jiang Y, Huang S, et al. Laser peripheral iridotomy for the prevention of angle closure: a single-centre, randomised controlled trial. *The Lancet.* 2019;393(10181):1609–1618.

59. Vijaya L, Asokan R, Panday M, et al. Six-year incidence of angle-closure disease in a South Indian population: the Chennai Eye Disease Incidence Study. *American Journal of Ophthalmology.* 2013;156(6):1308–1315. e1302.

60. Thomas R, George R, Parikh R, Muliyil J, Jacob A. Five year risk of progression of primary angle closure suspects to primary angle closure: a population based study. *Acta Ophthalmologica Scandinavica.* 2003;87:450–454.

61. Thomas R, Parikh R, Muliyil J, Kumar RS. Five-year risk of progression of primary angle closure to primary angle closure glaucoma: a population-based study. *Acta Ophthalmologica Scandinavica.* 2003;81:480–485.

62. Chua PY, Day AC, Lai KL, et al. The incidence of acute angle closure in Scotland: a prospective surveillance study. *British Journal of Ophthalmology.* 2018;102:539.

63. Chiu S-L, Chu C-L, Muo C-H, Chen C-L, Lan S-J. The prevalence and the incidence of diagnosed open-angle glaucoma and diagnosed angle-closure glaucoma: changes from 2001 to 2010. *Journal of Glaucoma.* 2016;25:e514–e519.

64. Zhu J, Xu Y, Wang H, Liu D, Zhu J, Wu H. The seasonality of acute attack of primary angle-closure glaucoma in Beijing, China. *Scientific Report.* 2018;8:4036–4037.

65. Chua J, Baskaran M, Ong PG, et al. Prevalence, risk factors, and visual features of undiagnosed glaucoma: the Singapore Epidemiology of Eye Diseases Study. *JAMA Ophthalmology.* 2015;133(8):938–946.

66. Shaikh Y, Yu F, Coleman AL. Burden of undetected and untreated glaucoma in the United States. *American Journal of Ophthalmology.* 2014;158(6):1121–1129. e1121.

67. Buhrmann RR, Quigley HA, Barron Y, West SK, Oliva MS, Mmbaga BB. Prevalence of glaucoma in a rural East African population. *Investigative Ophthalmology & Visual Science.* 2000;41(1):40–48.

68. Ntim-Amponsah C, Amoaku W, Ofosu-Amaah S, et al. Prevalence of glaucoma in an African population. *Eye.* 2004;18(5):491–497.

69. Vijaya L, George R, Baskaran M, et al. Prevalence of primary open-angle glaucoma in an urban south Indian population and comparison with a rural population: the Chennai Glaucoma Study. *Ophthalmology.* 2008;115(4):648–654. e641.

70. Nathan N, Joos KM. Glaucoma disparities in the Hispanic population. Paper presented at: Seminars in Ophthalmology 2016.

71. Keel S, Xie J, Foreman J, et al. Prevalence of glaucoma in the Australian National Eye Health Survey. *British Journal of Ophthalmology.* 2019;103(2):191–195.

72. Chua BE, Xie J, Arnold A-L, Koukouras I, Keeffe JE, Taylor HR. Glaucoma prevalence in Indigenous Australians. *British Journal of Ophthalmology.* 2011;95(7):926–930.

73. Sathyamangalam RV, Paul PG, George R, et al. Determinants of glaucoma awareness and knowledge in urban Chennai. *Indian Journal of Ophthalmology.* 2009;57(5):355–360.

74. Wong EYH, Keeffe JE, Rait JL, et al. Detection of undiagnosed glaucoma by eye health professionals. *Ophthalmology.* 2004;111(8):1508–1514.

75. Weih LM, Nanjan M, McCarty CA, Taylor HR. Prevalence and predictors of open-angle glaucoma: results from the visual impairment project. *Ophthalmology.* 2001;108(11):1966–1972.

76. Keeffe JE, Weih LM, McCarty CA, Taylor HR. Utilisation of eye care services by urban and rural Australians. *British Journal of Ophthalmology.* 2002;86(1):24–27.

77. Wilson FA, Wang Y, Stimpson JP. Do immigrants underutilize optometry services? *Optometry and Vision Science.* 2015;92(11):1113–1119.

78. Kyari F, Abdull M, Bastawrous A, Gilbert C, Faal H. Epidemiology of glaucoma in sub-Saharan Africa: prevalence, incidence and risk factors. *Middle East African Journal of Ophthalmology.* 2013;20(2):111–125.

79. Ronnie G, Ve RS, Velumuri L, Asokan R, Vijaya L. Importance of population-based studies in clinical practice. *Indian Journal of Ophthalmology.* 2011;59(Suppl 1):S11.

80. Ng WS, Agarwal PK, Sidiki S, McKay L, Townend J, Azuara-Blanco A. The effect of socio-economic deprivation on severity of glaucoma at presentation. *British Journal of Ophthalmology.* 2010;94(1):85–87.

81. Fraser S, Bunce C, Wormald R, Brunner E. Deprivation and late presentation of glaucoma: case-control study. *BMJ.* 2001;322(7287):639–643.

82. Zhang X, Beckles GL, Chou C-F, et al. socioeconomic disparity in use of eye care services among US adults with age-related eye diseases: National Health Interview Survey, 2002 and 2008. *JAMA Ophthalmology.* 2013;131(9):1198–1206.

83. Robin AL, Nirmalan PK, Krishnadas R, et al. The utilization of eye care services by persons with glaucoma in rural south India. *Transactions of the American Ophthalmological Society.* 2004;102:47–56.

84. Heijl A, Bengtsson B, Oskarsdottir SE. Prevalence and severity of undetected manifest glaucoma: results from the early manifest glaucoma trial screening. *Ophthalmology.* 2013;120(8):1541.

85. Patel D, Mercer E, Mason I. Ophthalmic equipment survey 2010: preliminary results. *Community Eye Health.* 2010;23(73):22–25.

86. Resnikoff S, Felch W, Gauthier T-M, Spivey B. The number of ophthalmologists in practice and training worldwide: a growing gap despite more than 200 000 practitioners. *British Journal of Ophthalmology.* 2012;96(6):783–787.

87. Thomas R, Dogra M. An evaluation of medical college departments of ophthalmology in India and change following provision of modern instrumentation and training. *Indian Journal of Ophthalmology.* 2008;56(1):9–16.

88. Baker H, Ratnarajan G, Harper RA, Edgar DF, Lawrenson JG. Effectiveness of UK optometric enhanced eye care services: a realist review of the literature. *Ophthalmic and Physiological Optics.* 2016;36(5):545–557.

89. Keenan J, Shahid H, Bourne RR, White AJ, Martin KR. Cambridge community optometry glaucoma scheme. *Clinical & Experimental Ophthalmology.* 2015;43(3):221–227.

90. Dandona R. Optometry and eye care in India. *Indian Journal of Ophthalmology.* 1998;46(3):175–175.

91. Barrett C, O'Brien C, Butler JS, Loughman J. Barriers to glaucoma case finding as perceived by optometrists in Ireland. *Clinical and Experimental Optometry.* 2018;101(1):90–99.

92. Garway-Heath DF, Ruben ST, Viswanathan A, Hitchings RA. Vertical cup/disc ratio in relation to optic disc size: its value in the assessment of the glaucoma suspect. *The British Journal of Ophthalmology.* 1998;82(10):1118–1124.

93. Buhrmann RR, Quigley HA, Barron Y, West SK, Oliva MS, Mmbaga BBO. Prevalence of glaucoma in a rural East African population. *Investigative Ophthalmology & Visual Science.* 2000;41(1):40.

94. Robin TA, Müller A, Rait J, Keeffe JE, Taylor HR, Mukesh BN. Performance of community-based glaucoma screening using frequency doubling technology and Heidelberg retinal tomography. *Ophthalmic Epidemiology.* 2005;12(3):167–178.

95. Iwasaki A, Sugita M, for The Glaucoma Screening Project Study Group. Performance of glaucoma mass screening with only a visual field test using

frequency-doubling technology perimetry. *American Journal of Ophthalmology.* 2002;134(4):529–537.

96. Devereux JG, Foster PJ, Baasanhu J, et al. Anterior chamber depth measurement as a screening tool for primary angle-closure glaucoma in an East Asian population. *Archives of Ophthalmology.* 2000;118(2):257–263.

97. Foster PJ, Devereux JG, Alsbirk PH, et al. Detection of gonioscopically occludable angles and primary angle closure glaucoma by estimation of limbal chamber depth in Asians: modified grading scheme. *British Journal of Ophthalmology.* 2000;84(2):186–192.

98. Congdon NG, Quigley HA, Hung PT, Wang TH, Ho TC. Screening techniques for angle-closure glaucoma in rural Taiwan. *Acta Ophthalmologica Scandinavica.* 1996;74(2):113–119.

99. Thomas R, George T, Braganza A, Muliyil J. The flashlight test and van Herick's test are poor predictors for occludable angles. *Australian and New Zealand Journal of Ophthalmology.* 1996;24(3):251–256.

100. Unpublished results from the Singapore Epidemiology of Eye Diseases (SEED) Study.

101. Wang Y, Alnwisi S, Ke M. The impact of mild, moderate, and severe visual field loss in glaucoma on patients' quality of life measured via the Glaucoma Quality of Life-15 Questionnaire: a meta-analysis. *Medicine.* 2017;96(48):e8019.

102. Wang W, He M, Li Z, Huang W. Epidemiological variations and trends in health burden of glaucoma worldwide. *Acta Ophthalmologica.* 2019;97(3):e349–e355.

103. Quaranta L, Riva I, Gerardi C, Oddone F, Floriano I, Konstas AGP. Quality of life in glaucoma: a review of the literature. *Advances in Therapy.* 2016;33(6):959–981.

104. Bourne RRA, Taylor HR, Flaxman SR, et al. Number of people blind or visually impaired by glaucoma worldwide and in world regions 1990–2010: a meta-analysis. *PloS One.* 2016;11(10):e0162229.

105. Freeman EE, Roy-Gagnon M-H, Samson E, et al. The global burden of visual difficulty in low, middle, and high income countries. *PloS One.* 2013;8(5):e63315.

106. Friedman DS, Foster PJ, Aung T, He M. Angle closure and angle-closure glaucoma: what we are doing now and what we will be doing in the future. *Clinical & Experimental Ophthalmology.* 2012;40(4):381–387.

107. Foster PJ, Johnson GJ. Glaucoma in China: how big is the problem? *British Journal of Ophthalmology.* 2001;85(11):1277–1282.

108. Sommer A, Tielsch JM, Katz J, et al. Racial differences in the cause-specific prevalence of blindness in east Baltimore. *The New England Journal of Medicine.* 1991;325(20):1412–1417.

109. Ramulu PYMDP, van Landingham SWBS, Massof RWP, Chan ESMS, Ferrucci LMDP, Friedman DSMDP. Fear of falling and visual field loss from glaucoma. *Ophthalmology.* 2012;119(7):1352–1358.

110. Adachi S, Yuki K, Awano-Tanabe S, et al. Factors associated with developing a fear of falling in subjects with primary open-angle glaucoma. *BMC Ophthalmology.* 2018;18(1):39–37.

111. Dirani M, Crowston JG, Taylor PS, et al. Economic impact of primary open-angle glaucoma in Australia. *Clinical & Experimental Ophthalmology.* 2011;39(7):623–632.

112. Gilbert CE, Shah SP, Jadoon MZ, et al. Poverty and blindness in Pakistan: results from the Pakistan national blindness and visual impairment survey. *BMJ.* 2008;336(7634):29–32.

113. James SL, Abate D, Abate KH, et al. Global, regional, and national incidence, prevalence, and years lived with disability for 354 diseases and injuries for 195 countries and territories, 1990–2017: a systematic analysis for the Global Burden of Disease Study 2017. *Lancet.* 2018;392:1789–1858.

114. Guedes RAP, Guedes VMP, Gomes CEdM, Chaoubah A. Maximizing cost-effectiveness by adjusting treatment strategy according to glaucoma severity. *Medicine.* 2016;95(52):e5745.

115. Adio AO, Onua AA. Economic burden of glaucoma in Rivers State, Nigeria. *Clinical Ophthalmology (Auckland, NZ).* 2012;6:2023–2031.

116. Nayak B, Gupta S, Kumar G, Dada T, Gupta V, Sihota R. Socioeconomics of long-term glaucoma therapy in India. *Indian Journal of Ophthalmology.* 2015;63(1):20–24.

117. Quigley HAMD, Cassard SDS, Gower EWP, Ramulu PYMDP, Jampel HDMDMHS, Friedman DSMDP. The cost of glaucoma care provided to medicare beneficiaries from 2002 to 2009. *Ophthalmology.* 2013;120(11):2249–2257.

118. Cho H-k, Kee C. Population-based glaucoma prevalence studies in Asians. *Survey of Ophthalmology.* 2014;59(4):434–447.

119. Marcus MWM, de Vries MMMD, Montolio FGJMD, Jansonius NMMDP. Myopia as a risk factor for open-angle glaucoma: a systematic review and meta-analysis. *Ophthalmology.* 2011;118:1989–1994. e1982.

120. Zheng Y, Wong TY, Mitchell P, Friedman DS, He M, Aung T. Distribution of ocular perfusion pressure and its relationship with open-angle glaucoma: the Singapore Malay Eye Study. *Investigative Ophthalmology and Visual Science.* 2010;51:3399.

121. Ramdas WD, Wolfs RCW, Hofman A, de Jong PTVM, Vingerling JR, Jansonius NM. Ocular perfusion pressure and the incidence of glaucoma: real effect or artifact? The Rotterdam Study. *Investigative Ophthalmology and Visual Science.* 2011;52:6875–6881.

122. Abu-Amero K, Kondkar AA, Chalam KV. An updated review on the genetics of primary open angle glaucoma. *International Journal of Molecular Science.* 2015;16:28886–28911.

123. Abu-Amero K, Kondkar AA, Chalam KV. An updated review on the genetics of primary open angle glaucoma. *International Journal of Molecular Sciences.* 2015;16(12):28886–28911.

124. Wiggs JL, Pasquale LR. Genetics of glaucoma. *Human Molecular Genetics.* 2017;26(R1):R21–R27.

125. Thorleifsson G, Walters GB, Hewitt AW, et al. Common variants near CAV1 and CAV2 are associated with primary open-angle glaucoma. *Nature Genetics.* 2010;42(10):906–909.

126. Wiggs JL, Hee Kang J, Yaspan BL, et al. Common variants near CAV1 and CAV2 are associated with primary open-angle glaucoma in Caucasians

from the USA. *Human Molecular Genetics.* 2011;20(23):4707–4713.

127. Burdon KP, Macgregor S, Hewitt AW, et al. Genome-wide association study identifies susceptibility loci for open angle glaucoma at TMCO1 and CDKN2B-AS1. *Nature Genetics.* 2011;43(6):574.

128. Osman W, Low S-K, Takahashi A, Kubo M, Nakamura Y. A genome-wide association study in the Japanese population confirms 9p21 and 14q23 as susceptibility loci for primary open angle glaucoma. *Human Molecular Genetics.* 2012;21(12):2836–2842.

129. Wiggs JL, Yaspan BL, Hauser MA, et al. Common variants at 9p21 and 8q22 are associated with increased susceptibility to optic nerve degeneration in glaucoma. *PLoS Genetics.* 2012;8(4).

130. Gharahkhani P, Burdon KP, Fogarty R, et al. Common variants near ABCA1, AFAP1 and GMDS confer risk of primary open-angle glaucoma. *Nature Genetics.* 2014;46(10):1120.

131. Chen Y, Lin Y, Vithana EN, et al. Common variants near ABCA1 and in PMM2 are associated with primary open-angle glaucoma. *Nature Genetics.* 2014;46(10):1115.

132. Li Z, Allingham RR, Nakano M, et al. A common variant near TGFBR3 is associated with primary open angle glaucoma. *Human Molecular Genetics.* 2015;24(13):3880–3892.

133. Springelkamp H, Iglesias AI, Cuellar-Partida G, et al. ARHGEF12 influences the risk of glaucoma by increasing intraocular pressure. *Human Molecular Genetics.* 2015;24(9):2689–2699.

134. Bailey JNC, Loomis SJ, Kang JH, et al. Genome-wide association analysis identifies TXNRD2, ATXN2 and FOXC1 as susceptibility loci for primary open-angle glaucoma. *Nature Genetics.* 2016;48(2):189.

135. Tham YC, Cheng CY. Associations between chronic systemic diseases and primary open angle glaucoma: an epidemiological perspective. *Clinical Experiments in Ophthalmology.* 2017;45:24–32.

136. Mitchell P, Lee AJ, Rochtchina E, Wang JJ. Open-angle glaucoma and systemic hypertension: the Blue Mountains Eye Study. *Journal of Glaucoma.* 2004;13:319–326.

137. Sun J, Zhou X, Kang Y, et al. Prevalence and risk factors for primary open-angle glaucoma in a rural northeast China population: a population-based survey in Bin County, Harbin. *Eye (London).* 2012;26:283–291.

138. Wang S, Xu L, Jonas JB, et al. Major eye diseases and risk factors associated with systemic hypertension in an adult Chinese population: the Beijing Eye Study. *Ophthalmology.* 2009;116:2373.

139. Memarzadeh F, Ying-Lai M, Chung J, Azen SP, Varma R, Los Angeles Latino Eye Study Group. Blood pressure, perfusion pressure, and open-angle glaucoma: the Los Angeles Latino Eye Study. *Investigative Ophthalmology and Visual Science.* 2010;51:2872–2877.

140. Hulsman CAA, Vingerling JR, Hofman A, Witteman JCM, de Jong PTVM. Blood pressure, arterial stiffness, and open-angle glaucoma: the Rotterdam Study. *Archives of Ophthalmology.* 2007;125:805–812.

141. Chopra V, Varma R, Francis BA, et al. Type 2 diabetes mellitus and the risk of open-angle glaucoma: the Los Angeles Latino Eye Study. *Ophthalmology.* 2008;115:227–232.e221.

142. Tan GS, Wong TY, Fong C-W, Aung T. Diabetes, metabolic abnormalities, and glaucoma: the Singapore Malay eye study. *Archives of Ophthalmology.* 2009;127:1354–1361.

143. de Voogd S, Ikram MK, Wolfs RCW, et al. Is diabetes mellitus a risk factor for open-angle glaucoma? The Rotterdam Study. *Ophthalmology.* 2006;113:1827–1831.

144. Nangia V, Jonas JB, Matin A, et al. Prevalence and associated factors of glaucoma in rural central India. The Central India Eye and Medical Study. *Plos One.* 2013;8:e76434.

145. Ramdas WD, Wolfs RCW, Hofman A, de Jong PTVM, Vingerling JR, Jansonius NM. Lifestyle and risk of developing open-angle glaucoma: the Rotterdam study. *Archives of Ophthalmology.* 2011;129:767–772.

146. Nakamura M, Kanamori A, Negi A. Diabetes mellitus as a risk factor for glaucomatous optic neuropathy. *Ophthalmologica.* 2005;219:1–10.

147. Fan N, Wang P, Tang L, Liu X. Ocular blood flow and normal tension glaucoma. *Biomedical Research International.* 2015;2015:308505–308507.

148. Trivli A, Koliarakis I, Terzidou C, et al. Normal-tension glaucoma: pathogenesis and genetics. *Experimental and Therapeutic Medicine.* 2019;17:563–574.

149. Sun X, Dai Y, Chen Y, et al. Primary angle closure glaucoma: what we know and what we don't know. *Progress in Retinal Eye Research.* 2017;57:26.

150. Wright C, Tawfik MA, Waisbourd M, Katz LJ. Primary angle-closure glaucoma: an update. *Acta Ophthalmologica.* 2016;94(3):217–225.

151. Foster PJ, Baasanhu J, Alsbirk PH, Munkhbayar D, Uranchimeg D, Johnson GJ. Glaucoma in Mongolia: a population-based survey in Hövsgöl Province, Northern Mongolia. *Archives of Ophthalmology.* 1996;114(10):1235–1241.

152. Arkell SM, Lightman DA, Sommer A, Taylor HR, Korshin OM, Tielsch JM. The prevalence of glaucoma among Eskimos of Northwest Alaska. *Archives of Ophthalmology.* 1987;105(4):482–485.

153. Senthil SF, Garudadri CF, Khanna RCMD, Sannapaneni KMPS. Angle closure in the Andhra Pradesh Eye Disease Study. *Ophthalmology.* 2010;117:1729–1735.

154. Park SJ, Park KH, Kim TW, Park BJ. Nationwide incidence of acute angle closure glaucoma in Korea from 2011 to 2015. *Journal of Korean Medical Science.* 2019;34:e306–308.

155. Porporato N, Baskaran M, Aung T. Role of anterior segment optical coherence tomography in angle-closure disease: a review. *Clinical Experiments in Ophthalmology.* 2018;46:147–157.

156. Nongpiur MEMD, Sakata LMMDP, Friedman DSMDP, et al. Novel association of smaller anterior chamber width with angle closure in Singaporeans. *Ophthalmology.* 2010;117:1967–1973.

157. Guzman CP, Gong T, Nongpiur ME, et al. Anterior segment optical coherence tomography parameters in subtypes of primary angle closure. *Investigative Ophthalmology and Visual Science.* 2013;54:5281.

158. Wang BMD, Sakata LMMDP, Friedman DSMD, et al. Quantitative iris parameters and association with narrow angles. *Ophthalmology*. 2010;117:11–17.

159. Moghimi S, Torkashvand A, Mohammadi M, et al. Classification of primary angle closure spectrum with hierarchical cluster analysis. *Plos One*. 2018;13:e0199157.

160. Aptel FMDM, Denis PMDP. Optical coherence tomography quantitative analysis of iris volume changes after pharmacologic mydriasis. *Ophthalmology*. 2010;117:3–10.

161. Nongpiur MEMD, Haaland BAP, Friedman DSMDP, et al. Classification algorithms based on anterior segment optical coherence tomography measurements for detection of angle closure. *Ophthalmology*. 2013;120:48–54.

162. Congdon NG, Youlin Q, Quigley H, et al. Biometry and primary angle-closure glaucoma among Chinese, white, and black populations. *Ophthalmology*. 1997;104:1489–1495.

163. Quigley HA. Angle-closure glaucoma – simpler answers to complex mechanisms: LXVI Edward Jackson memorial lecture. *American Journal of Ophthalmology*. 2009;148:657–669.e651.

164. Quigley HA, Silver DM, Friedman DS, et al. Iris cross-sectional area decreases with pupil dilation and its dynamic behavior is a risk factor in angle closure. *Journal of Glaucoma*. 2009;18:173–179.

165. Chua JP, Thakku SGB, Tun TAMD, et al. Iris crypts influence dynamic changes of iris volume. *Ophthalmology*. 2016;123:2077–2084.

166. Chua J, Thakku SG, Pham TH, et al. Automated detection of iris furrows and their influence on dynamic iris volume change. *Scientific Report*. 2017;7:17894–17898.

167. Koh V, Chua J, Shi Y, et al. Association of iris crypts with acute primary angle closure. *British Journal of Ophthalmology*. 2017;101:1318–1322.

168. Kong X, Chen Y, Chen X, Sun X. Influence of family history as a risk factor on primary angle closure and primary open angle glaucoma in a Chinese population. *Ophthalmic Epidemiology*. 2011;18:226–232.

169. He M, Wang D, Zheng Y, et al. Heritability of anterior chamber depth as an intermediate phenotype of angle-closure in Chinese: the Guangzhou Twin Eye Study. *Investigative Ophthalmology & Visual Science*. 2008;49:81.

170. He M, Ge J, Wang D, et al. Heritability of the iridotrabecular angle width measured by optical coherence tomography in Chinese children: the Guangzhou Twin Eye Study. *Investigative Ophthalmology & Visual Science*. 2008;49(4):1356.

171. He M, Wang D, Console JW, Zhang J, Zheng Y, Huang W. Distribution and heritability of iris thickness and pupil size in Chinese: the Guangzhou Twin Eye Study. *Investigative Ophthalmology & Visual Science*. 2009;50(4):1593.

172. Khor CC, Do T, Jia H, et al. Genome-wide association study identifies five new susceptibility loci for primary angle closure glaucoma. *Nature Genetics*. 2016;48(5):556–562.

173. Vithana EN, Khor C-C, Qiao C, et al. Genome-wide association analyses identify three new susceptibility loci for primary angle closure glaucoma. *Nature Genetics*. 2012;44(10):1142–1146.

174. Calonge N, Force USPST. Screening for glaucoma: recommendation statement. *Annals of Family Medicine*. 2005;3:171–172.

175. Moyer VA, US Preventive Services Task Force. Screening for glaucoma: U.S. Preventive Services Task Force recommendation statement. *Annals of Internal Medicine*. 2013;159:484.

176. Weinreb RN, Healey PR, Topouzis F, World Glaucoma Association. *Glaucoma Screening: The 5th Consensus Report of the World Glaucoma Association*. Amsterdam: Kugler Publications; 2008.

177. Joshi AV. *Machine Learning and Artificial Intelligence*. Cham: Springer International Publishing; 2020.

178. Panesar A. *Machine Learning and AI for Healthcare*: *Big Data for Improved Health Outcomes*. Berkeley, CA: Apress; 2019.

179. Mayro EL, Wang M, Elze T, Pasquale LR. The impact of artificial intelligence in the diagnosis and management of glaucoma. *Eye (London)*. 2020;34:1–11.

180. Medeiros FA, Jammal AA, Thompson AC. From machine to machine: an OCT-trained deep learning algorithm for objective quantification of glaucomatous damage in fundus photographs. *Ophthalmology*. 2019;126:513–521.

181. Hemelings R, Elen B, Barbosa-Breda J, et al. Accurate prediction of glaucoma from colour fundus images with a convolutional neural network that relies on active and transfer learning. *Acta Ophthalmologica*. 2020;98:e94–e100.

182. Ting DSW, Cheung CY-L, Lim G, et al. Development and validation of a deep learning system for diabetic retinopathy and related eye diseases using retinal images from multiethnic populations with diabetes. *JAMA*. 2017;318(22):2211–2223.

183. Li F, Wang Z, Qu G, et al. Automatic differentiation of glaucoma visual field from non-glaucoma visual filed using deep convolutional neural network. *BMC Medical Imaging*. 2018;18:35–37.

184. Asaoka R, Murata H, Hirasawa K, et al. Using deep learning and transfer learning to accurately diagnose early-onset glaucoma from macular optical coherence tomography images. *American Journal of Ophthalmology*. 2019;198:136–145.

185. Li Z, He Y, Keel S, Meng W, Chang RT, He M. Efficacy of a deep learning system for detecting glaucomatous optic neuropathy based on color fundus photographs. *Ophthalmology*. 2018;125:1199–1206.

186. Shibata N, Tanito M, Mitsuhashi K, et al. Development of a deep residual learning algorithm to screen for glaucoma from fundus photography. *Scientific Reports*. 2018;8(1):1–9.

187. Masumoto H, Tabuchi H, Nakakura S, Ishitobi N, Miki M, Enno H. Deep-learning classifier with an ultrawide-field scanning laser ophthalmoscope detects glaucoma visual field severity. *Journal of Glaucoma*. 2018;27:647–652.

188. Thompson AC, Jammal AA, Medeiros FA. A deep learning algorithm to quantify neuroretinal rim loss from optic disc photographs. *American Journal of Ophthalmology*. 2019;201:9–18.

189. Dimitrov DV. Medical internet of things and big data in healthcare. *Korea (South)*: *Korean Society of Medical Informatics*; 2016;22:156–163.

190. Thomas S-M, Jeyaraman MM, Jeyaraman M, et al. The effectiveness of teleglaucoma versus in-patient

examination for glaucoma screening: a systematic review and meta-analysis. *Plos One.* 2014;9:e113779.

191. John D, Parikh R. Cost-effectiveness and cost utility of community screening for glaucoma in urban India. *Public Health.* 2017;148:37–48.

192. John D, Parikh R. Cost-effectiveness of community screening for glaucoma in rural India: a decision analytical model. *Public Health.* 2018;155:142–151.

193. Tang J, Liang Y, O'Neill C, Kee F, Jiang J, Congdon N. Cost-effectiveness and cost-utility of population-based glaucoma screening in China: a decision-analytic Markov model. *Lancet Global Health.* 2019;7:e968–e978.

194. Tan NYQ, Friedman DS, Stalmans I, Ahmed IIK, Sng CCA. Glaucoma screening: where are we and where do we need to go? *Current Opinion in Ophthalmology.* 2020;31:91–100.

195. Jones L, Bryan SR, Miranda MA, Crabb DP, Kotecha A. Example of monitoring measurements in a virtual eye clinic using 'big data'. *British Journal of Ophthalmology.* 2018;102:911–915.

196. Lindell J. Contact lens-based 24-hour continuous IOP monitoring is well tolerated. *Contact Lens and Anterior Eye.* 2012;35:e44–e45.

197. Mansouri K, Weinreb RN, Liu JHK. Efficacy of a contact lens sensor for monitoring 24-h intraocular pressure related patterns. *Plos One.* 2015;10:e0125530.

12 Age-Related Macular Degeneration

Jost B. Jonas and Songhomitra Panda-Jonas

12.1 INTRODUCTION

Due to a marked increase in the life expectancy and general aging of populations, age-related ocular diseases, namely glaucoma and age-related macular degeneration (AMD), have markedly increased in importance as causes of irreversible vision impairment and blindness within the last two decades.[1–60] As a progressive chronic disease of the central retina, AMD leads to vision loss mostly in its medium advanced and late stages.

As a disorder affecting probably first the retinal pigment epithelium (RPE), AMD is characterized in its early and medium advanced stage by structural and pigmentary irregularities of the RPE, including the formation of drusen as deposits beneath the RPE and above Bruch's membrane.[61] In addition, a detachment of the RPE may develop and subretinal drusenoid deposits may form. In the late stage of AMD, the RPE can get lost in the case of geographic atrophy and/or a fibrovascular scar with proliferation of the RPE can develop as a sequel of a choroidal neovascularization in the foveal region. These changes result in a central relative or absolute scotoma while the peripheral visual field is usually not affected. Since landmark clinical trials demonstrated in 2006 the therapeutic benefit of intravitreally applied antibodies against vascular endothelial growth factor (VEGF), repeated intravitreal injections of ranibizumab, bevacizumab, aflibercept, and conbercept significantly improved vision in treated patients compared to untreated patients in control groups.[62–64] Correspondingly, recent population-based data have suggested that legal AMD-related blindness has been reduced by 50% in some countries since the introduction of VEGF antagonists.[65, 66]

12.2 PREVALENCE OF AMD

Population-based investigations have revealed that AMD as the most common form of the maculopathies is a major cause of vision loss in elderly people and that it shows a steep increase in prevalence beyond an age of 75 years.[3, 8, 13, 23, 25, 42] Wong and colleagues estimated in their landmark study as the most recent meta-analysis of preceding population-based investigations the number of individuals affected by AMD.[42] It revealed that, within an age range of 45–85 years, early and late-stage AMD together had a prevalence of 8.69% (95% credible interval

[CrI]: 4.26–17.40) with a prevalence of early-stage AMD of 8.01% (95% CrI: 3.95–15.49) and a prevalence of late-stage AMD of 0.37% (0.18–0.77). The early stage of AMD occurred more frequently in individuals of European ancestry (11.2%) than in Asian individuals (6.8%), and correspondingly, any AMD was more common in populations of European ancestry (12.3%) than of Asian ancestry (7.4%). In agreement with these findings, the prevalence of any AMD and of early, intermediate, and late AMD was lower in the ethnically mixed study population of the recent Russian Ural Eye and Medical Study than in previous investigations on study populations of European descent, and it was slightly higher in the population of the Russian study than in study populations from East Asia.[67] Early AMD, late AMD, or any AMD were markedly less common in populations of African ancestry than in populations of European ancestry.[42] In a similar manner, if the late stage of AMD was stratified into geographic atrophy and neovascular AMD, geographic atrophy was more common among Europeans (1.11%; 95% CrI: 0.53–2.08) than among Africans (0.14%; 95% CrI: 0.04–0.45), among Asians (0.21%; 95%CrI: 0.04–0.87), and among Hispanics (0.16%; 95%CrI: 0.05–0.46), while neovascular AMD did not differ between various ethnic groups.[42] Correspondingly, the prevalence of geographic atrophy in the Ural Eye and Medical Study was 0.4% (95% confidence interval [CI]: 0.2, 0.6), a value between the value for Europeans and the values for Asians or Africans.[67]

The association of a higher prevalence of AMD with older age was not linear but showed a more pronounced increase beyond the age of 75 years in all ethnicities examined. It held true in particular for the late stage of AMD, especially in individuals of European descent. It suggested a non-linear relationship of the prevalence of AMD with age.

12.3 VISUAL IMPAIRMENT AND BLINDNESS CAUSED BY AMD

The number of persons being blind or visually impaired due to AMD was assessed in the meta-analysis performed by the Vision Loss Expert Group for 2015.[35, 36, 68–77] Macular diseases, i.e., AMD, was the cause of blindness (defined as presenting visual acuity worse than 3/60) for 2.0 million (80% uncertainty interval [UI]: 0.2, 7.3) individuals out of 36.0 million individuals blind worldwide, and AMD was the cause for

DOI: 10.1201/9781315146737-14

moderate to severe vision impairment (MSVI) (defined as presenting visual acuity worse than 6/18 to 3/60 inclusive) in 8.4 million (80% UI: 0.9–29.5) persons out of 216.6 million people with MSVI.[75, 77] By 2020, among the global population who are blind (38.5 million), the number of people affected by AMD is anticipated to remain mostly unchanged, with a figure of 2.0 million (80% UI: 0.2–7.6 million), and among the global population with MSVI (237.1 million), the number of people affected by AMD is anticipated to rise in 2020 to 8.8 million (80% UI: 0.8–32.1 million). In the meta-analysis conducted by Wong and colleagues, the projected number of individuals with AMD was 196 million (95% CrI: 140–261) in 2020, and 288 million (95% CrI: 205–399) in 2040. Per geographical region, the number of patients afflicted by AMD in 2040 was expected to be highest in Asia (113 million; 95% CrI: 60–203), followed by Europe (69 million; 95% CrI: 40–109), Africa (39 million; 95% CrI: 12–93), Latin America and the Caribbean (39 million; 95% CrI: 15–82), North America (25 million; 95% CrI: 15–38), and finally Oceania (2 million; 95% CrI: 1–5).

Interestingly, the number of persons being blind due to AMD decreased slightly from 1990 (2.2 million; 80% UI: 0.2–8.3 million) to 2015 (2.0 million; 80% UI: 0.2–7.3 million), and the number of persons with AMD-related MSVI also decreased slightly from 1990 (8.5 million; 80% UI: 1.0–29.4 million) to 2015 (8.4 million; 80% UI: 0.9–29.5 million).[77] Since during the same period global population increased by >30%, the decrease in the number of individuals affected by AMD-related blindness and MSVI corresponded to a decrease in the age-adjusted prevalence of AMD-related blindness and AMD-related MSVI. The slight reduction in the total number of individuals affected by AMD-related blindness or AMD-related MSVI is even more remarkable if one takes into account the worldwide demographic transition with a substantial increase in the average age in most regions and falling death rates.[78] Since the drop in the age-standardized prevalence of macular degeneration-related blindness took place mostly in high-income regions, one may infer that it was due to the clinical introduction of intravitreally applied anti-VEGF drugs.[50–53] The reduction in the age-standardized prevalence of macular degeneration-related blindness was markedly less profound than the global decrease in the age-standardized prevalence of blindness due to cataract, under-corrected refractive error, and trachoma.[35, 76, 77]

In 2015, macular diseases, namely AMD, were the cause of blindness in 5.9% of all blind individuals and the cause of MSVI in 4.4% of all visually impaired persons.[76, 77] The proportion of blindness caused by macular diseases, including AMD, showed geographic variation. It was lowest in South Asia (2.4%) and highest in Eastern Europe (19.5%), followed by high-income Asia Pacific (16.7%), Australasia (16.6%), Central Europe (15.9%), high-income North America (15.9%), Western Europe (15.4%), and Southern Latin America (14.3%).[77] In a parallel manner, Eastern Europe (13.4%) showed the highest proportion of MSVI caused by macular diseases, followed by high-income Asia Pacific (11.6%), Central Europe (10.9%), high-income North America (10.9%), Western Europe (10.7%), and Southern Latin America (10.1%). The percentage of MSVI caused by macular diseases was the lowest in South Asia (1.3%) and South-East Asia (1.6%). This ranking followed the tendency that world regions with older populations, such as the high-income regions and Southern Latin America, as compared to world regions with younger populations showed a higher percentage of blindness and MSVI caused by macular diseases, namely AMD.[76, 77] Overall, AMD was in 2015 the fourth most common cause of blindness globally after cataract, under-correction of refractive errors, and glaucoma. In the ranking list of causes of MSVI, AMD ranked third after under-corrected refractive error and cataract, and it was followed by glaucoma.[77] The estimated figures for 2020 suggested a similar ranking.

In 2015 as compared with 1990, the global percentage of blindness and of MSVI related to macular diseases, namely AMD, as compared to all causes of blindness and MSVI decreased globally from 7.9% to 5.9%, and from 6.0% to 4.4%, respectively. This decline was observed in all world regions.[77]

The increasing number of patients with late AMD, in particular of neovascular AMD, will markedly increase the necessity of sufficient financial funds to treat this stage of the disease as it is currently performed by intravitreal application of anti-VEGF. Future developments will show whether a more common use of non-expensive bevacizumab in an off-label fashion and/or the expiration of patent rights for ranibizumab and other approved drugs in 2020 onwards will have an effect on the general availability of this hitherto only proven treatment of neovascular AMD. In that context, it may also be of interest that the steepest rise in the number of patients with late AMD will be in Asia due to the foreseeable demographical development. The future increase in the prevalence of AMD may be most marked in regions which have a relatively young population and where aging of the population has just started, in contrast to regions which already have a relatively old population. One may also consider that the impact of anti-VEGF therapy in areas in Asia where polypoidal choroidal vasculopathy is a predominant subtype is less certain.

From 1990 onwards, the percentage of individuals blind or visually impaired due to AMD in comparison to the total number of blind or visually impaired people has continuously increased, reflecting the success in reducing the amount of blindness and vision impairment due to cataract and refractive error. The findings obtained by the Vision Loss Expert Group revealed that in 2015 AMD was globally the fourth most common cause of blindness and the third most common cause of MSVI. It shows the future importance of AMD for public health. If one anticipates that treatment modalities may also become available for non-exudative forms of AMD, for which currently no treatment modalities exist, the treatment costs for AMD may increase in future. Several therapies directed against geographic atrophy as one form of late AMD are currently under development, and their potential impact on the incidence of blindness due to geographic atrophy of the macula will need to be evaluated in future studies.

12.4 RISK FACTORS OF AMD

12.4.1 Gender

Gender was not markedly associated with the prevalence of AMD or with the frequency of AMD as the cause of vision impairment or blindness, nor did men and women differ significantly in the prevalence of any type of AMD.[40] While in some studies, female gender was considered a weak risk factor for late AMD, other investigations on individuals of European ancestry did not show a significant gender difference in the prevalence of neovascular AMD or geographic atrophy.[79–81] This is in agreement with other studies on Asians.[14, 21, 22]

12.4.2 Ocular Factors

In several investigations, a higher prevalence of AMD was associated with shorter axial length.[82–85] The reasons for the association between shorter axial length and an increased AMD prevalence have remained elusive so far. Studies have suggested that a potentially lower concentration of VEGF in myopic eyes and differences in the properties of the vitreous body in association with a potentially faster turn-over of VEGF in the vitreous body of myopic eyes as compared to hyperopic eyes could be etiologically important.[85] If longer axial length is a protective factor against AMD, the worldwide shift towards myopia in the young generation,

observed in particular in East Asia, may predict a decrease in the age-standardized prevalence rates of AMD in the future.[86,87]

Significant correlations between AMD prevalence and prior cataract surgery have been reported in some previous studies, while other studies did not report on such an association.[88, 89]

12.4.3 Systemic Factors

In the recent Ural Eye and Medical Study, the AMD prevalence was not significantly correlated with the systemic parameters of body mass index, physical activity score, prevalence of alcohol consumption, history of cardiovascular or cerebrovascular disorders, serum concentration of hepatic enzymes, blood lipids and creatinine, stage of chronic kidney disease, parameters of systemic inflammation (erythrocyte sedimentation rate, rheumatoid factor, C-reactive protein), blood pressure and arterial hypertension, and manual dynamometry.[55] These observations suggest that the presence and severity of AMD were mostly independent of the general health of patients in terms of cardiovascular and cerebrovascular disorders and internal medical diseases. It corresponded to the results of previous investigations, which mostly showed that the prevalence of AMD was independent of extraocular conditions.[89] By the same token, AMD prevalence was not correlated with systemic parameters of inflammation, such as erythrocyte sedimentation rate and serum concentrations of rheumatoid factor and C-reactive protein. A similar result was recently reported by Cipriani and colleagues.[90] It points against a systemic inflammation playing a major role in the etiology of AMD.

AMD prevalence was not associated with serum concentration of creatinine and the presence and stage of a chronic kidney disease in the Ural Eye and Medical Study, while in contrast, Leisy and associates reported on an association between reticular macular drusen as part of AMD and renal dysfunction.[55, 91] A reason for the discrepancy between the studies may be that the subgroup analysis focused on reticular drusen in the study by Leisy and colleagues. Future studies may further explore the topic. There are conflicting reports of an association of arterial hypertension and AMD in the literature as well as about a relationship between diet and prevalence of AMD.[55, 92, 93]

12.4.4 Diet

In a study conducted by Chiu and colleagues, a higher prevalence of AMD was associated more with Western food than with Oriental food.[94] In a study by Chong and associates, a diet low in trans-unsaturated fat and rich in omega-3 fatty acids and olive oil was associated with a reduced risk of AMD.[95]

12.4.5 Smoking

An association between AMD and smoking may not have completely been explored yet, with most studies agreeing that smoking is a risk factor for neovascular AMD.[96, 97] There was no consistent association with early and inter-mediate AMD stage and smoking.[55, 96, 97] Care may be taken to include axial length into the multivariate analysis for exploring the relation-ship between AMD and smoking, since AMD is associated with shorter axial length, which is associated with a lower socioeconomic back-ground and a higher prevalence of smoking.

12.4.6 Others

In the Ural Eye and Medical Study, AMD prevalence was not significantly correlated with hearing loss or with the prevalence of pseudoexfoliation of the lens.[55] It was in contrast to the study by Kozobolis and colleagues.[98]

12.5 LIMITATIONS OF CURRENT POPULATION-BASED STUDIES AND FUTURE WORKS

Many population-based studies on the preva-lence of AMD have limitations which should be discussed and which may be improved in future investigations. First, most primary studies did not reliably differentiate between polypoidal choroidal vasculopathy and exudative AMD which can have a similar appearance on ophthal-moscopy. It may have led to an overestimation of the prevalence of late (neovascular) AMD in the Asian subgroup in the present study, since polypoidal choroidal vasculopathy is more common in Asians than in Europeans.[44, 45, 99] Second, some studies did not clearly differen-tiate between AMD and myopic maculopathy as a cause of blindness or vision impairment.[68–77] It may again have led to an overestimation of AMD as a cause of blindness or vision impair-ment. Third, a meta-analysis is only as strong as its underlying primary studies are weak. Due to the relatively low number of studies exam-ining the prevalence of AMD, many country-years as assessed in the meta-analyses remained without data, or only sub-national data were available for a relatively large number of coun-tries. Only a few national studies reported vision impairment for all ages and all causes, including AMD. Fourth, the number of patients with late AMD was relatively small in the pri-mary studies, so that the statistical power of

the statistical analyses was limited. Fifth, some population-based studies reported only the major cause of blindness or vision impairment so that in an individual with cataract and AMD, only cataract might have been noted as the cause of vision impairment. Also in eyes with dense cataract, the lens opacification might have prevented a clear examination of the fundus and the detection of a concomitant AMD. It resulted in an underestimation of the prevalence of AMD. Sixth, in most population-based studies, AMD was usually diagnosed based on fundus photographs, supported in some investigations by available optical coherence tomography (OCT) images. For clinical studies a consensus group has recently recommended a multimodal imaging approach, so that fundus abnormalities might have been missed or misinterpreted in the population-based studies.[100] Seventh, AMD could be diagnosed on the fundus photographs if the clarity of the optic media allowed the visibility of the fundus. It may have led to an underdiagnosis of AMD in eyes with advanced cataract.

12.6 CONCLUSIONS

The global prevalence of any AMD, early AMD, and late AMD in the age group of 45–85 years has been estimated to be 8.7%, 8.0%, and 0.4%, respectively, with higher prevalence figures for Europeans than for Asians and the lowest figures for sub-Saharan Africans. The global number of individuals with AMD was estimated to be 196 million in 2020, and 288 million in 2040. The worldwide number of persons blind or with MSVI due to AMD in 2010 was 2.1 million indi-viduals out of 32.4 million individuals blind, and 6.0 million persons out of 191 million people with MSVI. Age-standardized prevalence of macular diseases, namely AMD, as cause of blindness in adults aged 50+ years worldwide decreased from 0.2% in 1990 to 0.1% in 2010, and as the cause of MSVI, it remained mostly unchanged (1990: 0.4%; 2010: 0.4%), with no sig-nificant gender difference. In 2015, AMD was the fourth most common cause of blindness (and second most common cause of irrevers-ible blindness) globally, making up 5.93% of all causes of blindness, and it was the third most common cause of MSVI, making out 4.38% of all causes with MSVI.

REFERENCES

1. Gibson JM, Rosenthal AR, Lavery J. A study of the prevalence of eye disease in the elderly in an English community. *Trans Ophthalmol Soc UK.* 1985;104:196–203.

2. Rouhiainen H, Terasvirta M. Kuopio eye survey (KEYS). *Acta Ophthalmol (Copenh).* 1990;68:554–8.

3. Klein R, Klein BE, Linton KL. Prevalence of age-related maculopathy. The Beaver Dam Eye Study. *Ophthalmology*. 1992;99:933–43.

4. Das BN, Thompson JR, Patel R, et al. The prevalence of eye disease in Leicester: a comparison of adults of Asian and European descent. *J R Soc Med*. 1994;87:219–22.

5. Vinding T. Age-related macular degeneration. An epidemiological study of 1000 elderly individuals. With reference to prevalence, funduscopic findings, visual impairment and risk factors. *Acta Ophthalmol Scand Suppl*. 1995;217:1–32.

6. Vingerling JR, Dielemans I, Hofman A, et al. The prevalence of age-related maculopathy in the Rotterdam Study. *Ophthalmology*. 1995;102:205–10.

7. Ramrattan RS, Wolfs RC, Panda-Jonas S, et al. Prevalence and causes of visual field loss in the elderly and associations with impairment in daily functioning: the Rotterdam Study. *Arch Ophthalmol*. 2001;119:1788–94.

8. Mitchell P, Smith W, Attebo K, et al. Prevalence of age-related maculopathy in Australia. The Blue Mountains Eye Study. *Ophthalmology*. 1995;102:1450–60.

9. Mitchell P, Hayes P, Wang JJ. Visual impairment in nursing home residents: the Blue Mountains Eye Study. *Med J Aust*. 1997;166:73–6.

10. Klein R, Klein BE, Cruickshanks KJ. The prevalence of age-related maculopathy by geographic region and ethnicity. *Prog Retin Eye Res*. 1999;18:371–89.

11. Friedman DS, Katz J, Bressler NM, et al. Racial differences in the prevalence of age-related macular degeneration: the Baltimore Eye Survey. *Ophthalmology*. 1999;106(6):1049–55.

12. Van der Pols JC, Bates CJ, McGraw PV, et al. Visual acuity measurements in a national sample of British elderly people. *Br J Ophthalmol*. 2000 84:165–70.

13. Klaver CC, Assink JJ, van Leeuwen R, et al. Incidence and progression rates of age-related maculopathy: the Rotterdam Study. *Invest Ophthalmol Vis Sci*. 2001;42:2237–41.

14. Oshima Y, Ishibashi T, Murata T, et al. Prevalence of age related maculopathy in a representative Japanese population: the Hisayama study. *Br J Ophthalmol*. 2001;85:1153–7.

15. Bressler NM. Age-related macular degeneration is the leading cause of blindness. *JAMA*. 2004 291:1900–1.

16. Klein R, Klein BE, Knudtson MD, et al. Prevalence of age-related macular degeneration in 4 racial/ethnic groups in the multi-ethnic study of atherosclerosis. *Ophthalmology*. 2006;113:373–80.

17. Augood CA, Vingerling JR, de Jong PT, et al. Prevalence of age-related maculopathy in older Europeans: the European Eye Study (EUREYE). *Arch Ophthalmol*. 2006;124:529–35.

18. Iwase A, Araie M, Tomidokoro A, et al. Prevalence and causes of low vision and blindness in a Japanese adult population: the Tajimi Study. *Ophthalmology*. 2006;113:1354–62.

19. Xu L, Wang Y, Li Y, et al. Causes of blindness and visual impairment in an urban and rural area in Beijing: the Beijing Eye Study. *Ophthalmology*. 2006 113:1141.e1–3.

20. Maruko I, Iida T, Saito M, et al. Clinical characteristics of exudative age-related macular degeneration in Japanese patients. *Am J Ophthalmol*. 2007;144:15–22.

21. Kawasaki R, Wang JJ, Aung T, et al. Prevalence of age-related macular degeneration in a Malay population: the Singapore Malay Eye Study. *Ophthalmology*. 2008;115:1735–41.

22. Chen SJ, Cheng CY, Peng KL, et al. Prevalence and associated risk factors of age-related macular degeneration in an elderly Chinese population in Taiwan: the Shihpai Eye Study. *Invest Ophthalmol Vis Sci*. 2008 49:3126–33.

23. Wong TY, Chakravarthy U, Klein R, et al. The natural history and prognosis of neovascular age-related macular degeneration: a systematic review of the literature and meta-analysis. *Ophthalmology*. 2008;115:116–26.

24. Klein BE, Klein R. Forecasting age-related macular degeneration through 2050. *JAMA*. 2009;301:2152–3.

25. Kawasaki R, Yasuda M, Song SJ, et al. The prevalence of age-related macular degeneration in Asians: a systematic review and meta-analysis. *Ophthalmology*. 2010;117:921–7.

26. Klein R, Chou CF, Klein BE, et al. Prevalence of age-related macular degeneration in the US population. *Arch Ophthalmol*. 2011;129:75–80.

27. Jenchitr W, Ruamviboonsuk P, Sanmee A, et al. Prevalence of age-related macular degeneration in Thailand. *Ophthalmic Epidemiol*. 2011;18:48–52.

28. Yang K, Liang YB, Gao LQ, et al. Prevalence of age-related macular degeneration in a rural Chinese population: the Handan Eye Study. *Ophthalmology*. 2011;118:1395–401.

29. Nangia V, Jonas JB, Kulkarni M, et al. Prevalence of age-related macular degeneration in rural central India: the Central India Eye and Medical Study. *Retina*. 2011;31:1179–85.

30. Wu L, Sun X, Zhou X, et al. Causes and 3-year-incidence of blindness in Jing-An District, Shanghai, China 2001–2009. *BMC Ophthalmol*. 2011;11:10.

31. Rudnicka AR, Jarrar Z, Wormald R, et al. Age and gender variations in age-related macular degeneration prevalence in populations of European ancestry: a meta-analysis. *Ophthalmology*. 2012;119:571–580.

32. He M, Abdou A, Naidoo KS, et al. Prevalence and correction of near vision impairment at seven sites in China, India, Nepal, Niger, South Africa, and the United States. *Am J Ophthalmol*. 2012;154:107–116 e1.

33. Cheung CM, Tai ES, Kawasaki R, et al. Prevalence of and risk factors for age-related macular degeneration in a multiethnic Asian cohort. *Arch Ophthalmol*. 2012;130:480–486.

34. Lim LS, Mitchell P, Seddon JM, et al. Age-related macular degeneration. *Lancet*. 2012;379:1728–38.

35. Bourne R, Stevens GA, White RA, et al. Causes of vision loss worldwide: 1990–2010: a systematic analysis. *Lancet Global Health*. 2013;1:339–49.

36. Stevens G, White R, Flaxman SR, et al. Global prevalence of visual impairment and blindness: magnitude and temporal trends, 1990–2010. *Ophthalmology*. 2013;120:2377–84.

37. Gemmy Cheung CM, Li X, Cheng C-Y, et al. Prevalence and risk factors for age-related macular degeneration in Indians: a comparative study in Singapore and India. *Am J Ophthalmol*. 2013;155:764–73.e3.

38. Klein R, Klein BE. The prevalence of age-related eye diseases and visual impairment in aging:

current estimates. *Invest Ophthalmol Vis Sci*. 2013;54:ORSF5-ORSF13.

39. Cheung CM, Li X, Cheng CY, et al. Prevalence, racial variations, and risk factors of age-related macular degeneration in Singaporean Chinese, Indians, and Malays. *Ophthalmology*. 2014;121:1598–603.

40. Wong WL, Su X, Li X, et al. Global prevalence of age-related macular degeneration and disease burden projection for 2020 and 2040: a systematic review and meta-analysis. *Lancet Glob Health*. 2014;2:e106–16.

41. Klein R, Myers CE, Buitendijk GH, et al. Lipids, lipid genes, and incident age-related macular degeneration: the three continent age-related macular degeneration consortium. *Am J Ophthalmol*. 2014;158:513–24.e3.

42. Wong WL, Su X, Li X, et al. Global prevalence and burden of age-related macular degeneration: A meta-analysis and disease burden projection for 2020 and 2040. *Lancet Glob Health*. 2014;2:e106–116.

43. Rudnicka AR, Kapetanakis VV, Jarrar Z, et al. Incidence of late-stage age-related macular degeneration in American Whites: systematic review and meta-analysis. *Am J Ophthalmol*. 2015;160:85–93.e3.

44. Wong CW, Wong TY, Cheung CM. Polypoidal choroidal vasculopathy in Asians. *J Clin Med*. 2015;4:782–821.

45. Wong CW, Yanagi Y, Lee WK, et al. Age-related macular degeneration and polypoidal choroidal vasculopathy in Asians. *Prog Retin Eye Res*. 2016;53:107–39.

46. Taylor HR. The global issue of vision loss and what we can do about it: José Rizal Medal 2015. *Asia Pac J Ophthalmol (Phila)*. 2016;5:95–6.

47. Mitchell P, Liew G, Gopinath B, Wong TY. Age-related macular degeneration. *Lancet*. 2018 Sep 29;392 (10153):1147–59.

48. RAAB Repository. Available at: www.raabdata.info. Accessed 10th October, 2019.

49. Rudnicka AR, Kapetanakis VV, Jarrar Z, et al. Incidence of late-stage age-related macular degeneration in American Whites: systematic review and meta-analysis. *Am J Ophthalmol*. 2015;160(1):85–93.

50. Park SJ, Kwon KE, Choi NK, et al. Prevalence and incidence of exudative age-related macular degeneration in South Korea: a nationwide population-based study. *Ophthalmology*. 2015;122(10):2063–70.

51. Joachim N, Mitchell P, Burlutsky G, et al. The incidence and progression of age-related macular degeneration over 15 years: the Blue Mountains Eye Study. *Ophthalmology*. 2015;122(12):2482–9.

52. Reibaldi M, Longo A, Pulvirenti A, et al. Geo-epidemiology of age-related macular degeneration: new clues into the pathogenesis. *Am J Ophthalmol*. 2016;161:78–93.

53. Raman R, Pal SS, Ganesan S, et al. The prevalence and risk factors for age-related macular degeneration in rural-urban India, Sankara Nethralaya Rural-Urban Age-related Macular degeneration study, report no. 1. *Eye (Lond)*. 2016;30(5):688–97.

54. Song P, Du Y, Chan KY, et al. The national and subnational prevalence and burden of age-related macular degeneration in China. *J Glob Health*. 2017;7(2):020703.

55. Colijn JM, Buitendijk GHS, Prokofyeva E, et al. Prevalence of age-related macular degeneration in Europe: the past and the future. *Ophthalmology*. 2017;124(12):1753–63.

56. Keel S, Xie J, Foreman J, et al. Prevalence of age-related macular degeneration in Australia: the Australian National Eye Health Survey. *JAMA Ophthalmol*. 2017;135(11):1242–9.

57. Cheung CMG, Ong PG, Neelam K, et al. Six-year incidence of age-related macular degeneration in Asian Malays: the Singapore Malay Eye Study. *Ophthalmology*. 2017;124(9):1305–13.

58. Cruickshanks KJ, Nondahl DM, Johnson LJ, et al. Generational differences in the 5-year incidence of age-related macular degeneration. *JAMA Ophthalmol*. 2017;135(12):1417–23.

59. Obata R, Yanagi Y, Inoue T, et al. Prevalence and factors associated with age-related macular degeneration in a southwestern island population of Japan: the Kumejima Study. *Br J Ophthalmol*. 2018;102(8):1047–53.

60. Jin G, Zou M, Chen A, et al. Prevalence of age-related macular degeneration in Chinese populations worldwide: a systematic review and meta-analysis. *Clin Exp Ophthalmol*. 2019 Jul 3. doi: 10.1111/ceo.13580. [Epub ahead of print.]

61. Wong EN, Chew AL, Morgan WH, et al. The use of microperimetry to detect functional progression in non-neovascular age-related macular degeneration: a systematic review. *Asia Pac J Ophthalmol (Phila)*. 2017;6:70–9.

62. Rosenfeld PJ, Brown DM, Heier JS, et al. Ranibizumab for neovascular age-related macular degeneration. *N Engl J Med*. 2006;355:1419–31.

63. Rush RB, Rush SW. Ranibizumab versus bevacizumab for neovascular age-related macular degeneration with an incomplete posterior vitreous detachment. *Asia Pac J Ophthalmol (Phila)*. 2016;5:171–5.

64. Koh A, Lanzetta P, Lee WK, et al. Recommended guidelines for use of intravitreal aflibercept with a treat-and-extend regimen for the management of neovascular age-related macular degeneration in the Asia-Pacific Region: Report from a consensus panel. *Asia Pac J Ophthalmol (Phila)*. 2017;6:296–302.

65. Bressler NM, Doan QV, Varma R, et al. Estimated cases of legal blindness and visual impairment avoided using ranibizumab for choroidal neovascularization: non-Hispanic white population in the United States with age-related macular degeneration. *Arch Ophthalmol*. 2011;129:709–17.

66. Bloch SB, Larsen M, Munch IC. Incidence of legal blindness from age-related macular degeneration in Denmark: year 2000 to 2010. *Am J Ophthalmol*. 2012;153:209–13.

67. Bikbov MM, Zainullin RM, Gilmanshin TR, Kazakbaeva GM, Rakhimova EM, Rusakova YA, Bolshakova NI, Safiullina KR, Yakupova DF, Uzianbayeva YV, Khalimov TA, Salavatova VF, Panda-Jonas S, Arslangareeva II, Nuriev IF, Bikbova GM, Zaynetdinov AF, Zinatullin AA, Jonas JB. Prevalence and associated factors of age-related macular degeneration in a Russian population. The Ural Eye and Medical Study. *Am J Ophthalmol* 2020;210:146–57.

68. Wong TY, Zheng Y, Jonas JB, et al. Prevalence and causes of vision loss in East Asia: 1990–2010. *Br J Ophthalmol*. 2014;98:599–604.

69. Naidoo K, Gichuhi S, Basáñez MG, et al. Prevalence and causes of vision loss in Sub-Saharan Africa: 1990–2010. *Br J Ophthalmol*. 2014;98:612–18.

70. Jonas JB, George R, Asokan R, et al. Prevalence and causes of vision loss in Central and South Asia: 1990–2010. *Br J Ophthalmol*. 2014;98:592–8.

71. Leasher JL, Lansingh V, Flaxman SR, et al. Prevalence and causes of vision loss in Latin America and the Caribbean: 1990–2010. *Br J Ophthalmol*. 2014;98:619–28.

72. Khairallah M, Kahloun R, Flaxman SR, et al. Prevalence and causes of vision loss in North Africa and the Middle East: 1990–2010. *Br J Ophthalmol*. 2014;98:605–11.

73. Bourne RR, Jonas JB, Flaxman SR, et al. Prevalence and causes of vision loss in high-income countries and in Eastern and Central Europe: 1990–2010. *Br J Ophthalmol*. 2014;98:629–38.

74. Keeffe J, Taylor HR, Pesudovs K, et al. Prevalence and causes of vision loss in Southeast Asia and Oceania: 1990–2010. *Br J Ophthalmol*. 2014;98:586–91.

75. Jonas JB, Bourne RR, White RA, et al. Visual impairment and blindness due to macular diseases globally: a systematic review and meta-analysis. *Am J Ophthalmol*. 2014;158:808–15.

76. Bourne RRA, Flaxman SR, Braithwaite T, Cicinelli MV, Das A, Jonas JB, Keeffe J, Kempen JH, Leasher J, Limburg H, Naidoo K, Pesudovs K, Resnikoff S, Silvester A, Stevens GA, Tahhan N, Wong TY, Taylor HR; Vision Loss Expert Group. Magnitude, temporal trends, and projections of the global prevalence of blindness and distance and near vision impairment: a systematic review and meta-analysis. *Lancet Glob Health*. 2017;5(9):e888–e97.

77. Flaxman SR, Bourne RRA, Resnikoff S, Ackland P, Braithwaite T, Cicinelli MV, Das A, Jonas JB, Keeffe J, Kempen JH, Leasher J, Limburg H, Naidoo K, Pesudovs K, Silvester A, Stevens GA, Tahhan N, Wong TY, Taylor HR; Vision Loss Expert Group of the Global Burden of Disease Study. Global causes of blindness and distance vision impairment 1990–2020: a systematic review and meta-analysis. *Lancet Glob Health*. 2017;5(12):e1221–e34.

78. GBD 2017 Population and Fertility Collaborators. Population and fertility by age and sex for 195 countries and territories, 1950–2017: a systematic analysis for the Global Burden of Disease Study 2017. *Lancet*. 2018;392(10159):1995–2051.

79. Chakravarthy U, Wong TY, Fletcher A, et al. Clinical risk factors for age-related macular degeneration: a systematic review and meta-analysis. *BMC Ophthalmol*. 2010;10:31.

80. Evans JR. Risk factors for age-related macular degeneration. *Prog Retin Eye Res*. 2001;20:227–53.

81. Smith W, Assink J, Klein R, et al. Risk factors for age-related macular degeneration: pooled findings from three continents. *Ophthalmology*. 2001;108:697–704.

82. Ikram MK, van Leeuwen R, Vingerling JR, Hofman A, de Jong PT. Relationship between refraction and prevalent as well as incident age-related maculopathy: the Rotterdam Study. *Invest Ophthalmol Vis Sci*. 2003;44(9):3778–82.

83. Xu L, Li Y, Zheng Y, Jonas JB. Associated factors for age related maculopathy in the adult population in China: the Beijing eye study. *Br J Ophthalmol*. 2006;90(9):1087–90.

84. Cheung CM, Tai ES, Kawasaki R, et al. Prevalence of and risk factors for age-related macular degeneration in a multiethnic Asian cohort. *Arch Ophthalmol*. 2012;130(4):480–6.

85. Jonas JB, Nangia V, Kulkarni M, Gupta R, Khare A. Factors associated with early age-related macular degeneration in Central India. The Central India Eye and Medical Study. *Acta Ophthalmol*. 2012;90(3):e185–91.

86. Jonas JB, Tao Y, Neumaier M, Findeisen P. VEGF and refractive error. *Ophthalmology*. 2010;117(11):2234 e1.

87. Morgan IG, Ohno-Matsui K, Saw SM. Myopia. *Lancet*. 2012;379(9827):1739–48.

88. Klein R, Klein BE, Wong TY, et al. The association of cataract and cataract surgery with the long-term incidence of age-related maculopathy: the Beaver Dam Eye Study. *Arch Ophthalmol*. 2002;120(11):1551–8.

89. Krishnaiah S, Das T, Nirmalan PK, et al. Risk factors for age-related macular degeneration: findings from the Andhra Pradesh Eye Disease Study in South India. *Invest Ophthalmol Vis Sci*. 2005;46(12):4442–9.

90. Cipriani V, Hogg RE, Sofat R, et al. Association of C-reactive protein genetic polymorphisms with late age-related macular degeneration. *JAMA Ophthalmol*. 2017;135(9):909–16.

91. Leisy HB, Ahmad M, Marmor M, Smith RT. Association between decreased renal function and reticular macular disease in age-related macular degeneration. *Ophthalmol Retina*. 2017;1(1):42–8.

92. Smith W, Assink J, Klein R, et al. Risk factors for age-related macular degeneration: pooled findings from three continents. *Ophthalmology*. 2001;108(4):697–704.

93. La TY, Cho E, Kim EC, Kang S, Jee D. Prevalence and risk factors for age-related macular degeneration: Korean National Health and Nutrition Examination Survey 2008–2011. *Curr Eye Res*. 2014;39(12):1232–9.

94. Chiu CJ, Chang ML, Zhang FF, et al. The relationship of major American dietary patterns to age-related macular degeneration. *Am J Ophthalmol*. 2014;158(1):118–27.e1.

95. Chong EW, Robman LD, Simpson JA, et al. Fat consumption and its association with age-related macular degeneration. *Arch Ophthalmol*. 2009;127(5):674–80.

96. Chakravarthy U, Augood C, Bentham GC, et al. Cigarette smoking and age-related macular degeneration in the EUREYE study. *Ophthalmology*. 2007;114(6):1157–63.

97. Complications of Age-related Macular Degeneration Prevention Trial (CAPT) Research Group. Risk factors for choroidal neovascularization and geographic atrophy in the complications of age-related macular degeneration prevention trial. *Ophthalmology*. 2008;115(9):1474–9.

98. Kozobolis VP, Detorakis ET, Tsilimbaris MK, et al. Correlation between age-related macular degeneration and pseudoexfoliation syndrome in the population of Crete (Greece). *Arch Ophthalmol*. 1999;117(5):664–9.

99. Maruko I, Iida T, Saito M, et al. Clinical characteristics of exudative age-related macular degeneration in Japanese patients. *Am J Ophthalmol*. 2007;144:15–22.

100. Holz FG, Sadda SR, Staurenghi G, et al. Imaging protocols in clinical studies in advanced age-related macular degeneration: recommendations from classification of atrophy consensus meetings. *Ophthalmology*. 2017;124(4):464–7.

13 Polypoidal Choroidal Vasculopathy

Shinji Ono and Yasuo Yanagi

13.1 INTRODUCTION

Polypoidal choroidal vasculopathy (PCV) was first described by Yannuzzi in 1982, as "idiopathic polypoidal choroidal vasculopathy."[1] PCV shares similarities with neovascular age-related macular degeneration (nAMD), i.e., PCV typically evokes recurrent exudative changes and subretinal or sub-retinal pigment epithelial (RPE) bleeding in the macula, resulting in subretinal fibrosis if left untreated. It sometimes causes massive subretinal hemorrhage or vitreous hemorrhage, which may result in severe loss of vision.

The most characteristic feature of PCV is polypoidal (or aneurysmal) dilatation of the vessels at the terminal of "branching vascular networks (BNN) (or branching neovascular networks)." There has been a long debate as to whether PCV is a form of choroidal neovascularization (CNV) or abnormal remodeling of the choroidal vessels. Recent evidence suggests that BNN grows between Bruch's membrane and RPE, and morphologically shares similarities with macular neovascularization (MNV) due to nAMD. Therefore, PCV can be classified as a subtype of nAMD.

However, PCV also has distinct clinical characteristics from typical nAMD; it typically lacks drusen, and is more prevalent in Asian populations compared to Caucasian populations. Most importantly, natural history and treatment responses of PCV are different from those of typical nAMD in Caucasians.[2] The disease concepts of PCV have been changing,[3] and pachychoroid plays an important role in the pathogenesis of PCV. This chapter summarizes the current understanding of the definition, pathogenesis, and epidemiology of PCV.

13.2 DEFINITION OF PCV

Clinically, PCV is characterized by recurrent exudative and hemorrhagic maculopathy and the presence of characteristic red-orange nodules typically in the macula. Initially, PCV was reported as a peculiar type of nAMD found in black women,[4] and subsequently, many reports followed from Asian countries. However, it is now generally accepted that PCV can be found in all races despite some ethnic differences in prevalence. Diagnosis of PCV is based on multimodal imaging (Figure 13.1). Commonly used diagnostic criteria for PCV are either the Japanese Study Group of PCV or the EVEREST Study, both of which were developed when the dye angiographies and fundus photographs were the only commonly available tools for the diagnostics of the retina. The Japanese Study Group of PCV proposed a set of diagnostic criteria for PCV. Definite PCV cases were diagnosed when one or both of the following criteria were met: protruding orange-red elevated lesions on fundus examination, and characteristic polypoidal lesions seen on ICGA. Criteria for probable PCV cases included the following findings: only an abnormal vascular network seen on ICGA, or recurrent hemorrhagic and/or serous PED. Later in 2012, the EVEREST Study Group proposed their criteria for a multicenter randomized controlled clinical trial evaluating treatments for PCV. In their proposal, the diagnosis of PCV was based on the presence of focal subretinal hyperfluorescence on confocal ICGA within the first 6 minutes, *plus* one of the following criteria: nodular appearance of polyp(s) on stereoscopic examination, hypofluorescent halo around nodule(s), presence of a branching vascular network, pulsation of polyp(s) on dynamic ICGA, orange subretinal nodules on color fundus photography, or massive submacular hemorrhage (Table 13.1). Although the validity of these criteria has not been tested thoroughly, either of these diagnostic criteria is used for the diagnosis of PCV. In many Asian countries where the prevalence of PCV is high among nAMD patients, ICGA is routinely performed to diagnose PCV when patients present with exudative or hemorrhagic maculopathy.

In both criteria, ICGA is an indispensable tool to diagnose PCV. Single or multiple polyps can be clearly seen in the early phase of ICGA, but polyps may be obscured due to fluorescent blocking by dense bleeding or PED in some cases. Additionally, ICGA gives clinically useful information other than diagnosis. For example, a pulsatile polyp and cluster of grape-like polypoidal dilations of the vessels confer a high risk for massive bleeding. ICGA is also useful because it is the only imaging modality that can detect choroidal vascular hyperpermeability (CVH). CVH was first reported in eyes with central serous chorioretinopathy (CSC), but subsequent studies showed CVH is also observed in PCV. It has been reported that photodynamic therapy (PDT) is more effective in PCV with CVH compared to those without.[5] Therefore, detecting CVH by ICGA is important in deciding treatment. Regarding diagnostics, there is a

DOI: 10.1201/9781315146737-15

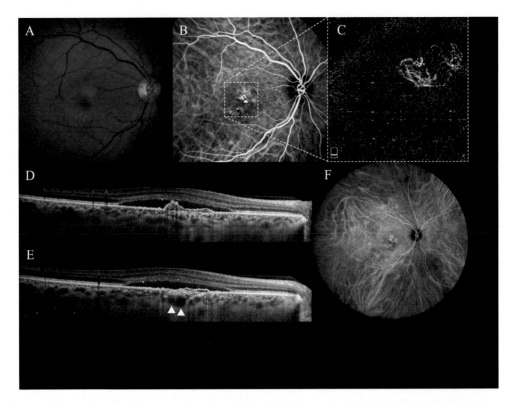

Figure 13.1 A 67-year-old man with polypoidal choroidal vasculopathy. Color photograph showed grayish-white lesions in the fovea, but red-orange nodule is not clear (A). Early phase of ICGA image evidenced polypoidal lesions and BNN (B). OCTA outer retina slab clearly exhibited BNN, but the OCTA image alone cannot distinguish between polypoidal lesions and BNN (C). Cross-sectional OCT showed steep RPE elevation and double-layer sign, which mean polypoidal lesions and BNN respectively (D). Pachyvessels (arrow heads) were found below BNN, accompanied by thinning of the choroid inner layer (E). Wide-angle image of late phase of ICGA showed CVH spreading to the posterior pole (F). BNN, branching neovascular networks; CVH, choroidal vascular hyperpermeability; ICGA, indocyanine green angiography; OCT, optical coherence tomography; OCTA, OCT angiography; RPE, retinal pigment epithelium.

Table 13.1 Polypoidal choroidal vasculopathy diagnostic criteria

Japanese Study Group Guidelines	EVEREST criteria
Definite	Focal hyperfluorescent lesions appearing within the first 5 minutes of ICG dye injection and at least one of the following diagnostic criteria:
Elevated orange-red nodules on fundus examination, and/or polypoidal lesions on ICGA	■ Nodular appearance of the polyp on stereoscopic viewing ■ Hypofluorescent halo around the nodule ■ Abnormal vascular channel(s) supplying the polyps ■ Pulsatile filling of polyps
Probable	■ Orange subretinal nodules corresponding to the hyperfluorescent area on ICGA
Only abnormal BVN seen on ICGA and/or recurrent hemorrhagic or serous PED	■ Massive submacular hemorrhage

Abbreviations: ICGA, indocyanine green angiography; BNN, branching vascular network; PED, pigment epithelial detachment.

debate as to whether we still need to use ICGA to diagnose PCV or other imaging modalities, such as optical coherence tomography (OCT) and OCT angiography (OCTA), can replace ICGA, as discussed in the last section of this chapter.

13.3 PATHOGENESIS OF PCV

There is controversy as to whether PCV is a peculiar type of CNV or abnormal inner choroidal vessels.[6] Initially, it was assumed that PCV originates in the abnormality of inner choroidal vessels.[7] Reportedly, PCV could be classified into two types according to ICGA findings.[8] The first type was "PCV in the narrow sense" or "typical PCV," which was caused by inner choroidal vessel abnormalities, and not by CNV. The characteristics of this type of PCV were the paucity of network vessels; there were neither feeder nor draining vessels to the lesion. Besides, this type had small lesions with polyps, typically a pigment epithelial detachment (PED) containing the polyps in the margin. The second type was the "polypoidal CNV," which had numerous polyps with BNN (as a feeder vessel), and it tended to repeat bleeding under RPE, resulting in large scar lesions and a poor prognosis. In recent studies, however, PCV is generally considered a variant of type 1 MNV, and the polyps are thought to originate from the vascular network, instead of directly from choroidal vessels. The polyps can be aneurysmal dilation of the vessel walls of the vascular network, and therefore, a new nomenclature "aneurysmal type 1 CNV" has been proposed instead of PCV.

Recently, a concept called "pachychoroid" has been proposed, which integrates the functional and anatomical abnormalities of the choroid, and it is proposed that pachychoroid may be involved in the pathogenesis of PCV.[3] Pachychoroid refers to the functional and structural abnormalities of the choroid, and is associated with retinal diseases, including those without exudative changes such as pachychoroid pigment epitheliopathy (PPE),[9] those with exudative changes such as CSC, and those with neovascularization such as pachychoroid neovasculopathy (PNV),[3] which are now collectively called pachychoroid diseases.[10] Although the prefix "pachy-" means thick, pachychoroid does not simply refer to the thickened choroid, but it also manifests other abnormalities such as CVH observed by ICGA, dilation of choroidal vessels in the Haller's layer called pachyvessels, and thinning of the inner layer of the choroid at the site corresponding to the pachyvessels. The recent expansion of our understanding of pachychoroid has raised fundamental questions as to whether PCV differs from PNV and that these two conditions are not distinct diseases but simply represent different stages of the same spectrum disorder. It was proposed that polypoidal lesions are formed at the terminal of PNV (i.e., BNN) and finally cause PCV.[3] Specifically, PNV is sometimes found at an indolent stage without exudation. Although such quiescent PNV may develop flank exudation without polypoidal lesions, over a long term, aneurysmal dilatations may arise at the outer border of the BNN to form the characteristic polypoidal lesions.[11] These aberrant BNN and polypoidal lesions can cause exudation, breaching the RPE, and may rupture, causing hemorrhage. Additionally, even when the BNN and polypoidal lesions are "inactive," pachychoroid can contribute to outer blood–retinal barrier breakdown and exudative changes through a similar mechanism as with CSC. Although it is controversial whether all cases of PCV belong to pachychoroid spectrum diseases[12, 13] (note that the choroid thickness of PCV is bimodal[14]), experts regard 40–60% of cases of PCV as pachychoroid spectrum diseases. BNN or the type 1 MNV in PCV likely arises as a consequence of local ischemia or inflammatory responses. Angiogenic factors such as vascular endothelial growth factor (VEGF) have been implicated in the development of PCV since VEGF has been found to be higher in eyes with PCV,[15] albeit less higher than typical nAMD.[16,17]

13.4 EPIDEMIOLOGY OF PCV

13.4.1 Population-Based Studies

There is growing evidence that the prevalence of AMD is increasing worldwide. In Asian population-based studies, the prevalence of late AMD is reported to be 5.16 per 1,000 persons (95% confidence interval [CI], 3.93–6.38).[18] With the presumption that PCV is a subtype of nAMD, epidemiological data of PCV have largely been derived from studies on AMD so far; it is, however, difficult to estimate the prevalence of PCV due to the difficulties in diagnosing PCV based on fundus photographs alone as performed in traditional epidemiological studies. As such, there are few studies that have investigated the prevalence of PCV in Asian countries, and there is a total lack of data regarding its prevalence in Caucasian populations. Nonetheless, PCV appears to have different epidemiological profiles among various racial groups and seems to have a predilection for Asian populations and other pigmented races.

To date, only two studies have attempted to estimate the prevalence rate of PCV in the general East Asian population. The Beijing Eye Study, which was conducted in northern China involving 3,468 participants, reported the prevalence of PCV based on color fundus photographs and OCT.[19] PCV was diagnosed by an elevated orange-red lesion on fundus photographs characterized by a double-layer sign and a high dome-shaped pigment epithelial detachment on OCT. As a result, PCV was found in 18 eyes of 17 subjects and the prevalence of PCV was 0.3%. However, the accuracy of this study of PCV is limited because ICGA was not performed. Another study is from Hisayama; this was conducted in southern Japan and evaluated the prevalence rate of PCV using fundus photographs and ICGA among 2,663 participants.[20] Participants were first screened with fundus photographs, and 43 subjects were suspected of having characteristic features of late AMD. These 43 subjects then underwent dye angiographies using both fluorescein angiography and ICGA. Consequently, 10 were diagnosed as PCV and 22 as nAMD without PCV. As a result, the estimated prevalence rate of PCV was 0.4%, which accounted for 30.3% among the study subjects with late AMD. Although ICGA is required for the diagnosis of PCV, it is an invasive test and it is not practical to obtain ICGA images from all participants in epidemiological studies. Future advancements in non-invasive assessment tools, together with the establishment of multimodal imaging diagnostic criteria, will clarify the precise prevalence of PCV in the general population.

13.4.2 Hospital-Based Studies

Despite the paucity of the data in population-based studies, many hospital- and clinic-based studies reported the proportion of PCV among patients presenting with presumed nAMD based on ICGA findings. The prevalence of PCV among the nAMD cases has been reported to range from 22.3% to 61.6% in Asian patients; 22.3–24.5% in Chinese,[21, 22] 24.6% in Korean,[23] 49.0% in Taiwanese,[24] 55.4% in Singaporeans,[25] and 23.4–54.7% in Japanese,[26–29] whereas it is 4–13.9% in Caucasians,[29–33] with a recent meta-analysis showing that the pooled prevalence of PCV with exudative AMD was 8.7% (95% CI: 7.2–10.3%).[34] As such, the prevalence of PCV seems to be higher in Asians than in whites. Moreover, when compared with typical nAMD patients, there is a lower prevalence of bilateral disease and younger disease onset in PCV patients. However, it should also be noted that, among Asians, unilateral typical nAMD is also common and the frequency of bilateral involvement was not different between PCV and typical nAMD.[28]

13.4.3 Incidence

The incidence of PCV remains unclear in the general population. However, several hospital- and clinic-based studies reported the incidence of PCV in the fellow eyes of patients presenting with unilateral PCV. Initially PCV was reported to affect both eyes, but later studies from Asian populations found that PCV is typically a unilateral condition at presentation. Not only PCV, but also MNV (without polypoidal lesions) may develop in the fellow eyes of unilateral PCV. With a follow-up period of approximately 3 years, the incidence of fellow eye involvement ranges from 9 to 19.1%. In a retrospective observational consecutive case series including 91 patients with typical AMD and 125 patients with PCV, the cumulative incidence of involvement in fellow eyes with overall exudative AMD, including both PCV and typical nAMD, was 3.4% in 1 year, 9.3% in 3 years, and 11.3% in 5 years. It was 3.6%, 7.3%, and 11.2% in typical nAMD, and 3.2%, 11.1%, and 11.1% in PCV in 1, 3, and 5 years, respectively, with an average follow-up period of 25.1 and 33.6 months for PCV and typical nAMD patients. Another study reported that the development of active PCV was noted in 19.1% with a mean follow-up period of 30.3 ± 12.2 months.[35] In a retrospective observational consecutive case series, 10.9% of 129 eyes developed exudative changes in the fellow eye with a median follow-up of 3.2 years.[36] In a study enrolling 263 patients with unilateral PCV, 9% (20/233) of eyes had MNV (12 PCV and 8 type 1 MNV) during a 27.6-month mean follow-up period.[37] Recently, another study from Korea reported that PCV or MNV developed in 17% of fellow eyes in 5 years.[38]

13.4.4 Risk Factors

A number of hospital- and clinic-based studies have identified shared, as well as distinct, risk factors between PCV and typical nAMD. Regarding gender, iPCV was thought to be more prevalent in females in white and black patients initially. However, subsequent reports from Asian populations have demonstrated a male preponderance.[39] A population-based Hisayama Study confirmed that male sex is a significant risk factor for PCV.[20] Several other studies have confirmed that males have a higher risk for both typical AMD and PCV in Asian populations.[40, 41] Other epidemiological features are predominance in relatively young men. Many hospital-based studies also found a predominance of young patients in PCV compared to typical AMD.

The most consistent shared risk factor between PCV and typical nAMD is cigarette smoking. In a hospital-based case–control study of Chinese patients, cigarette smoking was a risk factor for both PCV (odds ratio [OR] 4.4; 95% CI 2.5–7.7; $P < 0.001$) and typical nAMD (OR 4.9; 95% CI 2.7–8.8; $P < 0.001$).[42] Other hospital-based studies also support these findings.[40, 43, 44] In a population-based study, the Hisayama Study found that smoking was a significant risk factor for PCV. Possible mechanisms include increased oxidative stress, decreased choroidal blood flow, decreased macular pigment density, and the promotion of angiogenesis.[45–49]

Until recently, there was a long debate as to whether serum high-density lipoprotein cholesterol (HDL-c) is different between AMD patients and controls. However, the EYE-RISK and European Eye Epidemiology consortia clearly demonstrated that HDL-c is associated with an increased risk of AMD and that triglycerides are negatively associated.[50] Additionally, recent studies using Mendelian randomization support that increased HDL-c is a causal risk factor for AMD.[51] Lipid metabolism pathway is implicated in both PCV and typical nAMD.

Distinct differences in systemic risk factor associations between PCV and typical nAMD have been reported in a few studies. In particular, the association of diabetes mellitus (DM), with or without diabetic retinopathy (DR), appears to differ between PCV and typical nAMD. In a hospital-based, cross-sectional study of 227 cases of PCV and typical nAMD, the prevalence of DM was reportedly greater in typical nAMD than in PCV (24.7% vs. 13.0%; $P = 0.027$), whereas a previous history of CSC was more frequently detected in PCV than in typical nAMD, while no significant differences existed between the two subtypes with regard to other systemic risk factors, including body mass index (BMI), hypertension, stroke, ischemic heart disease, hyperlipidemia, smoking, and alcohol consumption.[52] A different group also found a higher prevalence of DM (OR 2.29; 95% CI 1.50–3.52; $P < 0.001$) and end-stage renal disease (OR 12.3; 95% CI 1.45–104; $P = 0.021$) in patients with typical nAMD than in PCV.[53] Furthermore, another study compared characteristics of exudative AMD in 26 eyes with DR and also found a lower prevalence of PCV than typical nAMD (15.4% vs. 80.8%).[54]

Associations with other systemic factors such as hypertension, stroke, and coronary artery disease are less consistent. A comparative study including 314 subjects with typical nAMD or PCV found that older age (OR per year 0.914; 95% CI 0.880–0.949; $P = < 0.0001$), higher BMI (OR 0.891; 95% CI 0.812–0.979; $P = 0.0159$), and higher education level were more strongly associated with PCV than with typical nAMD.[43] It is also reported that there was a significant negative association between diastolic blood pressure and typical nAMD (OR 0.7; 95% CI 0.5–0.9; $P = 0.017$, adjusted for age, gender, smoking, diabetes, and hypercholesterolemia), but diastolic blood pressure was not associated

with PCV.[42] In addition, higher BMI and raised serum levels of C-reactive protein were known to increase the risk for both typical nAMD and PCV.

Systemic inflammation is also associated with PCV as well as typical nAMD.[55] In several hospital-based studies, serum concentration of high-sensitive C-reactive protein (hs-CRP), a surrogate marker of systemic inflammation, was found to be upregulated in patients with PCV compared to controls.[40] Similarly, in a population study, the Beijing Eye Study investigated potential associations between serum hs-CRP concentration and the presence and degree of eye diseases.[55] In multivariate analysis, higher serum concentration of hs-CRP was significantly (regression coefficient r: 0.21) associated with a higher level of DR ($P = 0.007$; standardized regression coefficient beta: 0.06; non-standardized regression coefficient beta: 1.35; 95% CI: 0.37–2.22) and PCV ($P = 0.002$; beta: 0.06; B: 6.22; 95% CI: 2.24–10.2) after adjusting for higher serum concentration of HDL ($P < 0.001$), higher BMI ($P = 0.01$), lower level of education ($P = 0.04$), and lower cognitive function score ($P = 0.01$), suggesting that higher serum concentration of hs-CRP is significantly associated with a higher level of DR and higher frequency of PCV.

Serum levels of VEGF have not been investigated fully, but VEGF-related mechanisms might be less important in the pathogenesis of PCV than typical nAMD. There are several studies showing lower aqueous levels of VEGF in PCV than in typical nAMD, supporting the theory that PCV pathogenesis may be less VEGF-driven than typical nAMD.[16]

Regarding ocular risk factors, characteristic features of AMD, such as drusen and pigment abnormalities, are less frequently observed in eyes with PCV compared with eyes with typical nAMD; some studies suggest that pigmentary abnormalities alone may be an important risk factor for PCV in Asians. A longitudinal study suggested that pigmentary abnormalities without large drusen were associated with PCV (age- and sex-adjusted OR 15.9; 95% CI 1.8–140.5).[36] Another study reported that PCV patients not only had RPE atrophy, but also abnormal vascular network and polypoidal formation before the clinical manifestation of exudative changes, suggesting BNN and polypoidal formation gradually grow before exudative changes.[11] Some other studies support the presence of BNN at baseline as a risk factor for developing PCV or MNV. For example, a study evaluated the risk factors of nAMD, including PCV or any type of MNV, in fellow eyes of unilateral PCV and found BNN in the fellow eye was the only significant risk factor for the development of exudative changes in a multivariate analysis (OR 24.66, P = 0.045).[38] Interestingly, a significantly higher risk for MNV was observed if RPE and outer retinal abnormalities were accompanied by pachyvessels (hazard ratio [HR] 9.3; 95% CI 1.1–75.9; P = 0.037).[37] A study focusing on ICGA features found that all the eyes that developed MNV or PCV during their follow-up period had exhibited well-demarcated geographic hyperfluorescent lesion on late phase on ICGA at baseline, although they did not find a statistically significant difference in the development of PCV between the eyes with BNN at baseline and those without (P = 0.08).[35] Refraction is also another important risk factor for both PCV and typical AMD; hyperopic shift was observed in both PCV and typical nAMD compared with controls.

Epidemiological evidence may support pachychoroid being an important risk factor for developing PCV. In population-based studies, the Beijing Eye Study showed that thicker subfoveal and central choroidal thickness was observed in PCV eyes compared with controls.[19] In line with this, soft drusen are more infrequent. Pachydrusen,[56] or peculiar large drusenoid deposits, which are reportedly associated with pachychoroid, may be found in PCV patients. However, there are no diagnostic criteria for pachychoroid. As such, the experts in this field agree that there is a need to develop multimodal imaging diagnostic criteria for pachychoroid.

13.5 GENETICS OF PCV

While PCV and typical nAMD may share the majority of genetic components, each locus has different association signals between PCV and typical nAMD.[57] A meta-analysis of the genetic associations of PCV clarified that in total 31 polymorphisms in ten genes/loci involved in the complement cascade (CFH, C2, CFB, RDBP, and SKIV2L), the inflammatory pathway (TNFRSF10A-LOC389641 and BEST-C4orf14-POLR2B-IGFBP7), extracellular matrix/basement membrane regulation pathway (ARMS2-HTRA1) and lipid metabolism pathway (CETP) were associated with PCV.[58] On the other hand, 25 polymorphisms in 13 genes previously associated with PCV (ARMS2, HTRA1, C2, CFB, ELN, LIPC, LPL, ABCA1, VEGF-A, TLR3, LOXL1, SERPING1, and PEDF) were not significantly associated with PCV. The same study identified 39 single-nucleotide polymorphisms (SNPs) in 16 genes that were compared between PCV and typical nAMD. Of these, only SNPs in the ARMS2-HTRA1 locus showed significantly weaker association with PCV than with typical nAMD. A more recent multi-center case–control study included a total of 1,062 PCV patients,

1,157 typical nAMD patients and 5,275 controls in Singapore, Hong Kong, Korea, and Japan from the Genetics of AMD in Asians Consortium. It showed that a eight loci were associated with PCV (ARMS2-HTRA1), CFH, C2-CFB-SKIV2L, CETP, VEGFA, ADAMTS9-AS2, and TGFBR1 from SNP-based test, and COL4A3 from gene-based tests.[57] ARMS2-HTRA1 was weakly associated with PCV compared with typical nAMD, in line with the previous study, and KMT3E-SRPK2 was found to be associated with typical nAMD but not with PCV. Additionally, variants at CFH, CETP, and VEGFA exhibited different association signals in East Asians, in contrast to those in European individuals, presumably because of heterogeneity in allele frequencies. Several other studies have found CETP genetic variants to be associated with a high risk of PCV, corroborating the possible involvement of the HDL pathway in the pathogenesis of PCV.[41, 59–62] The CFH I62V polymorphism is associated with choroidal thickness in patients with PCV.[63] This association between a complement system gene and choroidal thickness may implicate a role of inflammation in the thickening of choroid in eyes with PCV. Whole-exome sequencing identified a rare c986A>G variant in the FGD6 gene associated with PCV but not typical nAMD.[64]

Genetic studies also have tried to identify prognostic factors. So far, most studies have employed a small-scale candidate gene approach. Such studies demonstrated that SNPs in the ARMS2 locus, among other SNPs, may be an important risk factor for severe phenotype. For example, the ARMS2 locus was associated with larger lesion size, higher likelihood of vitreous hemorrhage, and worse visual outcome 1 year after treatment with PDT or combination therapy in PCV.[65] It also confers a higher risk for second-eye involvement.[66] A prospective multicenter genome-wide association study (GWAS) including 461 treatment-naive exudative AMD patients failed to identify genetic loci associated with treatment outcomes but confirmed that ARMS2/HTRA1 polymorphism might be able to predict the frequency of injection after initial ranibizumab treatment.[67] Another GWAS study including 919 exudative AMD patients also failed to identify genetic loci associated with treatment outcomes, but found that four variants showed a suggestive level of associations with visual loss, among which three were VEGF-related pathway (KCNMA1, SOCS2, and OTX2).[68]

Cross-sectional case–control studies have clarified an association but not a causality. Recently, however, emerging genetic data have contributed to our understanding of causal risk factors for PCV and typical nAMD. To reveal a causal relationship, genetic variants that influence modifiable risk factors can be used as their proxies in Mendelian randomization. In short, in Mendelian randomization, naturally occurring random allocation of parental alleles at meiosis, which results in genetic variants independently distributed from potential confounders, is used as instrumental variables. Such genetic variants are immune to the influences of environmental factors and reverse causation. For example, it clarifies whether genetic variants that influence plasma lipid levels affect the risk of PCV, assuming that the genetic variants are independent of PCV, and clarifies whether long-term lipid levels lead to an increased risk of PCV. Studies conducted by two independent groups suggest that plasma HDL-c is causally associated with an increased risk for AMD.[51, 69] In particular, Fan et al.[69] found that a high level of plasma HDL-c is a causal risk factor for advanced AMD in European and Asian populations and a similar trend for the association of PCV with HDL-c level. Another study reported that higher serum CRP levels lead to an increased risk factor for AMD.[70] Additionally, refractive error seems to have minimal influence on AMD risk.[71]

13.6 RANDOMIZED CONTROLLED TRIALS AND REAL-WORLD DATA

13.6.1 Randomized Controlled Studies of PCV

Treatment of PCV mainly consists of focal laser photocoagulation, anti-VEGF monotherapy, PDT, and combination therapy of anti-VEGF and PDT. Treatment with anti-VEGF agents alone results in improved vision; however, when PDT was used either alone or in combination, there was a higher rate of polyp regression compared with anti-VEGF monotherapy. There are two pivotal large randomized controlled trials (RCTs) that aimed to determine the optimal treatments for PCV.

The EVEREST II study[72] aimed to compare the efficacy of PDT combined with ranibizumab (Lucentis; Genentech, San Francisco, CA), with larger sample size (including 322 patients with symptomatic macular PCV) and longer follow-up period (24 months) compared to the EVEREST study. As a primary outcome, the study demonstrated that visual acuity gain in combination therapy was 8.3 letters at month 12 compared with 5.1 of the monotherapy group ($P = 0.01$). Furthermore, complete polyp regression was significantly higher in the combination therapy arm compared with the monotherapy arm (69.3% vs. 34.7%, respectively, $P < 0.001$). In addition, the number of ranibizumab injections was smaller in the combination therapy group (4 vs. 7). Therefore, in addition

to better visual outcomes, combination therapy may lead to lower recurrence rate, which could be attributable to more frequent polyp regression. PLANET study[73] was a double-masked clinical RCT to compare the efficacy and safety of intravitreal aflibercept (Eylea; Regeneron, Tarrytown, NY) injection (IAI) monotherapy vs. IAI plus rescue PDT in PCV patients. In total, 310 symptomatic PCV patients were recruited. In both treatment arms, patients with PCV received monotherapy with 3-monthly IAI. At week 12, the patients were randomized into two arms and the patients in the first arm were followed by IAI injection every 4 weeks with active PDT if rescue therapy was needed (termed "rescue" PDT), while patients in the second arm treated with 3-monthly injections of aflibercept, which was followed by IAI plus sham rescue PDT. When the rescue criteria were no longer met during the study, injection intervals were gradually extended to 8 weeks. If rescue therapy was not needed at week 12, IAI injection extended to every 8 weeks. After 52 weeks, visual acuity gains were similar in both groups (10.8 vs. 10.7 letters). At week 52, complete polyp closure was observed in 38.9% and 44.8%, in monotherapy with IVI and combination therapy groups, respectively. In the 2-year results of the PLANET study, the same results were reported over 96 weeks. Fewer than 15% of patients in either group required PDT treatment.

These two large, prospective multicenter clinical trials gave important information regarding the treatment of PCV; however, optimal treatments remain unknown – in particular, there is no consensus regarding the optimal timing to perform PDT.

13.6.2 Disease Registries and Real-World Data of PCV

Since the RCTs so far have given inconclusive results regarding optimal treatments for PCV, we need further studies that address the optimal treatment strategy with a strong level of evidence. In this regard, real-world data (RWD) are becoming a valuable addition regarding treatment pathways and clinical outcomes of patients with retinal diseases in recent years. RWD provide information about the effectiveness of a treatment in a real-life setting in a wider patient population than in an RCT, and therefore adds to the evidence for the disease treatments. RWD also provide information such as long-term outcome, safety, and treatment patterns which are not designed to be assessed in clinical trials. For real-world research, registries, observational studies, and patient databases are used. Now that an increasing number of registry systems are available for retinal diseases, RWD are increasingly being recognized to constitute important evidence for treatment. There are several multinational registry studies that reported the real-world treatment outcomes of PCV and AMD in Asians which are worth mentioning.

The Fight Retinal Blindness! cohort,[74] comprising databases from Australia, New Zealand, Singapore, and Switzerland, compared the 12-month real-world visual and disease activity outcomes of eyes with PCV treated with a combination of PDT and anti-VEGF injections (combination group) versus eyes treated with anti-VEGF monotherapy alone with rescue PDT being used as required (monotherapy group). Fight Retinal Blindness! analyzed clinical information from a multisite, international registry of nAMD, and the primary outcome measure was the change in visual acuity in logMAR letters over 12 months between the two groups with intention-to-treat approach. The results demonstrated that 41 and 152 eyes received combination therapy and anti-VEGF monotherapy, respectively. Bevacizumab represented 66.1% of injections administered. The adjusted mean change in visual acuity between the combination group and monotherapy group was +16.9 letters (95% CI, 10.6–23.3 letters) and +8.2 letters (95% CI, 5.2–11.3 letters), respectively ($P = 0.02$). The proportion of inactive lesions and mean time to inactivity was 85.3% and 80.7 days (95% CI, 62.8–98.5 days), respectively, in the combination group compared with 76.8% and 150.4 days (95% CI, 132.8–168.0 days), respectively, in the monotherapy group ($P = 0.01$). The mean number of injections of anti-VEGF agent between the combination and monotherapy groups was 4.3 injections (95% CI, 3.6–5.2 injections) and 6.4 injections (95% CI, 5.9–6.9 injections), respectively ($P = 0.01$). The authors demonstrated that the real-world outcomes for treatment of PCV showed larger gains in vision, higher proportion of inactive lesions, quicker time to inactivity, and fewer injections administered in the combination group compared with the monotherapy group, consistent with current evidence reporting the advantages of combination therapy for PCV.

The LUMINOUS study,[75] a 5-year prospective study (conducted from March 2011 to April 2016), was designed to evaluate the long-term effectiveness, safety, and treatment patterns associated with ranibizumab injection in real-world practice for all approved indications. The LUMINOUS study reported the real-world effectiveness and safety of ranibizumab injection in treatment-naive patients with and without PCV. Outcome measures were visual acuity and central retinal thickness changes from baseline, and the rate of ocular adverse events in nAMD patients with or without PCV after 12 months of ranibizumab treatment during the LUMINOUS study. At baseline, 572 and 5,644 patients were diagnosed with and without PCV, respectively. The mean visual acuity gain from baseline in the PCV and non-PCV groups was +5.0 and +3.0 letters, respectively; these gains were achieved with a mean of 4.4 and 5.1 ranibizumab injections. Eighty percent of PCV patients and 72.2% of non-PCV patients who had baseline visual acuity ≥73 letters maintained this level of vision at month 12; 20.6% and 17.9% of patients with baseline visual acuity <73 letters achieved visual acuity ≥73 letters in these groups. Greater reductions in central retinal thickness from baseline were also observed for the PCV group versus the non-PCV group. The rate of serious ocular adverse events was 0.7% (PCV group) and 0.9% (non-PCV group), confirming the effectiveness and safety of ranibizumab in treatment-naive patients with PCV.

In addition, there are small-scale registry studies that took a look at the treatment outcomes of PCV in Asian countries.

In a 12-month single-center, retrospective, comparative, non-randomized cohort study conducted in Singapore, patients with typical nAMD or PCV who initiated intravitreal anti-VEGF therapy during 2015 were included (a total of 364 patients: 165 AMD and 199 PCV).[76] Baseline vision was 41 and 43 letters for typical nAMD and PCV patients, respectively. Patients with typical nAMD and PCV received 5.5 and 5.3 injections (5.0 monotherapy vs. 5.6 combination therapy; mean, 1.2 PDT sessions), respectively. Patients with typical nAMD gained 4.7 letters after 12 months ($P = 0.002$), whereas PCV patients gained 6.6 letters ($P = 0.001$) and 10.8 letters ($P < 0.001$) for monotherapy and combination therapy, respectively. Only patients with presenting visual acuity of fewer than 35 letters achieved significant visual improvement (10.4 letters for typical nAMD, 17.1 letters for PCV with monotherapy, and 35.5 letters for PCV with combination therapy). Predictors of visual acuity gain included number of intravitreal injections and baseline visual acuity of 20 letters or fewer (adjusted OR, 3.8 and 10.6 for typical nAMD and PCV, respectively). The study concluded that, for PCV eyes, anti-VEGF monotherapy and combination therapy with PDT yielded comparable outcomes as those of controlled clinical trials.

A study conducted in Japan reported the 4-year outcome of aflibercept for nAMD and PCV, recruiting 98 AMD patients.[77] During the 4 years, 25 patients dropped out. The survivors received a mean of 7.0 injections during the first year and 8.0 injections in the following 3 years. The logMAR at baseline, year 1, and year 4 was 0.28, 0.14 ($P = 0.033$), and 0.22 ($P = 0.697$), respectively. The gain of vision was not different among AMD subtypes. Among the investigated factors, the presence of external limiting membrane, the absence of vitreoretinal adhesion, and thicker choroid at baseline were associated with better logMAR values at year 4 (coefficient beta = –0.388, 0.201, and –0.001; $P = 7.34 \times 10^{-6}$; 0.01, and 0.028, respectively).

While the aforementioned results reflect real-world outcome, further comprehensive clinical information will be required in future real-world studies to provide scientifically robust evidence for treatment, safety, as well as human and economic outcomes.

13.7 NEW TECHNOLOGIES IN EPIDEMIOLOGICAL RESEARCH OF PCV

New technologies in the imaging tools have revolutionized our understanding of PCV. As mentioned previously, polypoidal vascular lesions are typically observed as red-orange nodules with fundus examinations, but a red-orange nodule is not always clear in many cases. Therefore, ICGA is the most sensitive examination for detecting polypoidal lesions and is the gold-standard investigation tool to diagnose PCV. Clinically, diagnosis of PCV is made when ICGA detects a characteristic polypoidal dilation which shows either a coil-like or aneurysmal shape. However, ICGA is an invasive examination, and therefore has not been incorporated into epidemiological researches. With the advent of newer imaging modalities such as OCT and OCTA, diagnosis of PCV can be made without ICGA.

OCT is a very useful tool in diagnosing PCV. Although it is not included in the diagnostic criteria, polypoidal lesions are observed distinctly with steep elevation of RPE, which is described as thumb-like, peaked, or notched PED. It is generally agreed that polypoidal lesions are attached to the back side of the RPE, and can be visualized as hyperreflective materials just below the elevated RPE. BNN is located between RPE and Bruch's membrane, and can be observed as shallow irregular PED. Furthermore, double-layer PED consist of a hyperreflective ring around a low internal reflective area. Several studies have confirmed the utility of OCT in the diagnosis of PCV when ICGA is not available. Several epidemiological studies, such as the Beijing Eye Study,[19] Jiangning Eye Study,[78] Kailuan Study, and Ural Eye and Medical Study,[79] used OCT to diagnose AMD and other studies have deployed OCT for population studies.[80]

OCTA is a new technology that enables non-invasive visualization of retinal choroidal vascular structure and has been rapidly spreading in recent years. OCTA is advantageous for detecting

BNN that crawls between RPE and Bruch's membrane compared to ICGA partly because OCTA has no fluorescence leakage.[81] Although it is difficult to detect all polypoidal lesions by OCTA alone, it is possible to increase the diagnosis accuracy in combination with *en face* imaging of OCT.[82–84] Some population studies, such as that conducted in Hong Kong[85] and the Singapore Chinese Eye Study,[80] are incorporating OCTA for retinal examinations.

As newer imaging techniques become available, the definition of PCV is evolving. Incorporation of such non-invasive imaging tools in epidemiological studies will further our understanding of its prevalence in the general population, as well as the underlying pathology. In this regard, it is worth mentioning that the combination of three OCT-based major criteria (sub-retinal pigment epithelium [RPE] ring-like lesion, en face OCT complex RPE elevation, and sharp-peaked PED) achieved an area under the receiver operating characteristic curve of 0.90 for the diagnosis of PCV.[86]

REFERENCES

1. Yannuzzi LA. *Idiopathic Polypoidal Choroidal Vasculopathy*. Presented at the February 1982 Macula Society Meeting, Miami, Florida.

2. Yannuzzi LA, Sorenson J, Spaide RF, Lipson B. Idiopathic polypoidal choroidal vasculopathy (IPCV). *Retina* 1990;10:1–8.

3. Pang CE, Freund KB. Pachychoroid neovasculopathy. *Retina* 2015;35:1–9.

4. Stern RM, Zakov ZN, Zegarra H, Gutman FA. Multiple recurrent serosanguineous retinal pigment epithelial detachments in black women. *Am J Ophthalmol* 1985;100:560–569.

5. Yanagi Y, Ting DSW, Ng WY, et al. Choroidal vascular hyperpermeability as a predictor of treatment response for polypoidal choroidal vasculopathy. *Retina* 2018;38:1509–1517.

6. Balaratnasingam C, Lee WK, Koizumi H, Dansingani K, Inoue M, Freund KB. Polypoidal choroidal vasculopathy: a distinct disease or manifestation of many? *Retina* 2016;36:1–8.

7. Okubo A, Sameshima M, Uemura A, Kanda S, Ohba N. Clinicopathological correlation of polypoidal choroidal vasculopathy revealed by ultrastructural study. *Br J Ophthalmol* 2002;86:1093–1098.

8. Kawamura A, Yuzawa M, Mori R, Haruyama M, Tanaka K. Indocyanine green angiographic and optical coherence tomographic findings support classification of polypoidal choroidal vasculopathy into two types. *Acta Ophthalmol* 2013;91:e474–e481.

9. Warrow DJ, Hoang QV, Freund KB. Pachychoroid pigment epitheliopathy. *Retina* 2013;33:1659–1672.

10. Gallego-Pinazo R, Dolz-Marco R, Gomez-Ulla F, Mrejen S, Freund KB. Pachychoroid diseases of the macula. *Med Hypothesis Discov Innov Ophthalmol* 2014;3:111–115.

11. Ueta T, Iriyama A, Francis J, et al. Development of typical age-related macular degeneration and

polypoidal choroidal vasculopathy in fellow eyes of Japanese patients with exudative age-related macular degeneration. *Am J Ophthalmol* 2008;146:96–101.

12. Miyake M, Ooto S, Yamashiro K, et al. Pachychoroid neovasculopathy and age-related macular degeneration. *Sci Rep* 2015;5:16204.

13. Jung BJ, Kim JY, Lee JH, Baek J, Lee K, Lee WK. Intravitreal aflibercept and ranibizumab for pachychoroid neovasculopathy. *Sci Rep* 2019;9:2055.

14. Lee WK, Baek J, Dansingani KK, Lee JH, Freund KB. Choroidal morphology in eyes with polypoidal choroidal vasculopathy and normal or subnormal subfoveal choroidal thickness. *Retina* 2016;36 Suppl 1:S73–S82.

15. Lee MY, Lee WK, Baek J, Kwon OW, Lee JH. Photodynamic therapy versus combination therapy in polypoidal choroidal vasculopathy: changes of aqueous vascular endothelial growth factor. *Am J Ophthalmol* 2013;156:343–348.

16. Tong JP, Chan WM, Liu DT, et al. Aqueous humor levels of vascular endothelial growth factor and pigment epithelium-derived factor in polypoidal choroidal vasculopathy and choroidal neovascularization. *Am J Ophthalmol* 2006;141:456–462.

17. Zhou H, Zhao X, Yuan M, et al. Comparison of cytokine levels in the aqueous humor of polypoidal choroidal vasculopathy and neovascular age-related macular degeneration patients. *BMC Ophthalmol* 2020;20:15.

18. Hyungtaek Rim T, Ryo K, Tham YC, et al. Prevalence and pattern of geographic atrophy in Asia: the Asian Eye Epidemiology Consortium. *Ophthalmology* 2020;127(10):1371–1381.

19. Li Y, You QS, Wei WB, et al. Polypoidal choroidal vasculopathy in adult chinese: the Beijing Eye Study. *Ophthalmology* 2014;121:2290–2291.

20. Fujiwa K, Yasuda M, Hata J, et al. Prevalence and risk factors for polypoidal choroidal vasculopathy in a general Japanese population: the Hisayama Study. *Semin Ophthalmol* 2018;33:813–819.

21. Liu Y, Wen F, Huang S, et al. Subtype lesions of neovascular age-related macular degeneration in Chinese patients. *Graefes Arch Clin Exp Ophthalmol* 2007;245:1441–1445.

22. Wen F, Chen C, Wu D, Li H. Polypoidal choroidal vasculopathy in elderly Chinese patients. *Graefes Arch Clin Exp Ophthalmol* 2004;242:625–629.

23. Byeon SH, Lee SC, Oh HS, Kim SS, Koh HJ, Kwon OW. Incidence and clinical patterns of polypoidal choroidal vasculopathy in Korean patients. *Jpn J Ophthalmol* 2008;52:57–62.

24. Chang YC, Wu WC. Polypoidal choroidal vasculopathy in Taiwanese patients. *Ophthalmic Surg Lasers Imaging* 2009;40:576–581.

25. Cheung CM, Lai TY, Chen SJ, et al. Understanding indocyanine green angiography in polypoidal choroidal vasculopathy: the group experience with digital fundus photography and confocal scanning laser ophthalmoscopy. *Retina* 2014;34:2397–2406.

26. Maruko I, Iida T, Saito M, Nagayama D, Saito K. Clinical characteristics of exudative age-related macular degeneration in Japanese patients. *Am J Ophthalmol* 2007;144:15–22.

27. Sho K, Takahashi K, Yamada H, et al. Polypoidal choroidal vasculopathy: incidence, demographic features, and clinical characteristics. *Arch Ophthalmol* 2003;121:1392–1396.

28. Mori K, Horie-Inoue K, Gehlbach PL, et al. Phenotype and genotype characteristics of age-related macular degeneration in a Japanese population. *Ophthalmology* 2010;117:928–938.

29. Coscas G, Yamashiro K, Coscas F, et al. Comparison of exudative age-related macular degeneration subtypes in Japanese and French patients: multicenter diagnosis with multimodal imaging. *Am J Ophthalmol* 2014;158:309–318 e302.

30. Lafaut BA, Leys AM, Snyers B, Rasquin F, De Laey JJ. Polypoidal choroidal vasculopathy in Caucasians. *Graefes Arch Clin Exp Ophthalmol* 2000;238:752–759.

31. Ladas ID, Rouvas AA, Moschos MM, Synodinos EE, Karagiannis DA, Koutsandrea CN. Polypoidal choroidal vasculopathy and exudative age-related macular degeneration in Greek population. *Eye (Lond)* 2004;18:455–459.

32. Scassellati-Sforzolini B, Mariotti C, Bryan R, Yannuzzi LA, Giuliani M, Giovannini A. Polypoidal choroidal vasculopathy in Italy. *Retina* 2001;21:121–125.

33. Ciardella AP, Donsoff IM, Huang SJ, Costa DL, Yannuzzi LA. Polypoidal choroidal vasculopathy. *Surv Ophthalmol* 2004;49:25–37.

34. Lorentzen TD, Subhi Y, Sorensen TL. Prevalence of polypoidal choroidal vasculopathy in white patients with exudative age-related macular degeneration: systematic review and meta-analysis. *Retina* 2018;38:2363–2371.

35. Kim YT, Kang SW, Chung SE, Kong MG, Kim JH. Development of polypoidal choroidal vasculopathy in unaffected fellow eyes. *Br J Ophthalmol* 2012;96:1217–1221.

36. Sasaki M, Kawasaki R, Uchida A, et al. Early signs of exudative age-related macular degeneration in Asians. *Optom Vis Sci* 2014;91:849–853.

37. Baek J, Cheung CMG, Jeon S, Lee JH, Lee WK. Polypoidal choroidal vasculopathy: outer retinal and choroidal changes and neovascularization development in the fellow eye. *Invest Ophthalmol Vis Sci* 2019;60:590–598.

38. Kim K, Kim JM, Kim DG, Yu SY, Kim ES. Five-year follow-up of unaffected fellow eyes in patients with polypoidal choroidal vasculopathy. *Ophthalmologica* 2020;243:172–177.

39. Honda S, Matsumiya W, Negi A. Polypoidal choroidal vasculopathy: clinical features and genetic predisposition. *Ophthalmologica* 2014;231:59–74.

40. Kikuchi M, Nakamura M, Ishikawa K, et al. Elevated C-reactive protein levels in patients with polypoidal choroidal vasculopathy and patients with neovascular age-related macular degeneration. *Ophthalmology* 2007;114:1722–1727.

41. Meng Q, Huang L, Sun Y, et al. Effect of High-density lipoprotein metabolic pathway gene variations and risk factors on neovascular age-related macular degeneration and polypoidal choroidal vasculopathy in China. *PLoS One* 2015;10:e0143924.

42. Cackett P, Yeo I, Cheung CM, et al. Relationship of smoking and cardiovascular risk factors with polypoidal choroidal vasculopathy and age-related macular degeneration in Chinese persons. *Ophthalmology* 2011;118:846–852.

43. Woo SJ, Ahn J, Morrison MA, et al. Analysis of genetic and environmental risk factors and their interactions

in Korean patients with age-related macular degeneration. *PLoS One* 2015;10:e0132771.

44. Laude A, Cackett PD, Vithana EN, et al. Polypoidal choroidal vasculopathy and neovascular age-related macular degeneration: same or different disease? *Prog Retin Eye Res* 2010;29:19–29.

45. Beatty S, Koh H, Phil M, Henson D, Boulton M. The role of oxidative stress in the pathogenesis of age-related macular degeneration. *Surv Ophthalmol* 2000;45:115–134.

46. Solberg Y, Rosner M, Belkin M. The association between cigarette smoking and ocular diseases. *Surv Ophthalmol* 1998;42:535–547.

47. Hammond BR, Jr., Wooten BR, Snodderly DM. Cigarette smoking and retinal carotenoids: implications for age-related macular degeneration. *Vision Res* 1996;36:3003–3009.

48. Hammond BR, Jr., Caruso-Avery M. Macular pigment optical density in a Southwestern sample. *Invest Ophthalmol Vis Sci* 2000;41:1492–1497.

49. Suner IJ, Espinosa-Heidmann DG, Marin-Castano ME, Hernandez EP, Pereira-Simon S, Cousins SW. Nicotine increases size and severity of experimental choroidal neovascularization. *Invest Ophthalmol Vis Sci* 2004;45:311–317.

50. Colijn JM, den Hollander AI, Demirkan A, et al. Increased high-density lipoprotein levels associated with age-related macular degeneration: evidence from the EYE-RISK and European Eye Epidemiology Consortia. *Ophthalmology* 2019;126:393–406.

51. Burgess S, Davey Smith G. Mendelian randomization implicates high-density lipoprotein cholesterol-associated mechanisms in etiology of age-related macular degeneration. *Ophthalmology* 2017;124:1165–1174.

52. Ueta T, Obata R, Inoue Y, et al. Background comparison of typical age-related macular degeneration and polypoidal choroidal vasculopathy in Japanese patients. *Ophthalmology* 2009;116:2400–2406.

53. Sakurada Y, Yoneyama S, Imasawa M, Iijima H. Systemic risk factors associated with polypoidal choroidal vasculopathy and neovascular age-related macular degeneration. *Retina* 2013;33:841–845.

54. Yoshikawa T, Ogata N, Wada M, Otsuji T, Takahashi K. Characteristics of age-related macular degeneration in patients with diabetic retinopathy. *Jpn J Ophthalmol* 2011;55:235–240.

55. Jonas JB, Wei WB, Xu L, Wang YX. Systemic inflammation and eye diseases. The Beijing Eye Study. *PLoS One* 2018; 13:e0204263.

56. Lee J, Byeon SH. Prevalence and clinical characteristics of pachydrusen in polypoidal choroidal vasculopathy: multimodal image study. *Retina* 2019;39:670–678.

57. Fan Q, Cheung CMG, Chen LJ, et al. Shared genetic variants for polypoidal choroidal vasculopathy and typical neovascular age-related macular degeneration in East Asians. *J Hum Genet* 2017;62:1049–1055.

58. Ma L, Li Z, Liu K, et al. Association of genetic variants with polypoidal choroidal vasculopathy: a systematic review and updated meta-analysis. *Ophthalmology* 2015;122:1854–1865.

59. Momozawa Y, Akiyama M, Kamatani Y, et al. Low-frequency coding variants in CETP and CFB are associated with susceptibility of exudative age-related macular degeneration in the Japanese population. *Hum Mol Genet* 2016;25:5027–5034.

60. Nakata I, Yamashiro K, Kawaguchi T, et al. Association between the cholesteryl ester transfer protein gene and polypoidal choroidal vasculopathy. *Invest Ophthalmol Vis Sci* 2013;54:6068–6073.

61. Liu K, Chen LJ, Lai TY, et al. Genes in the high-density lipoprotein metabolic pathway in age-related macular degeneration and polypoidal choroidal vasculopathy. *Ophthalmology* 2014;121:911–916.

62. Zhang X, Li M, Wen F, et al. Different impact of high-density lipoprotein-related genetic variants on polypoidal choroidal vasculopathy and neovascular age-related macular degeneration in a Chinese Han population. *Exp Eye Res* 2013;108:16–22.

63. Jirarattanasopa P, Ooto S, Nakata I, et al. Choroidal thickness, vascular hyperpermeability, and complement factor H in age-related macular degeneration and polypoidal choroidal vasculopathy. *Invest Ophthalmol Vis Sci* 2012;53:3663–3672.

64. Huang L, Zhang H, Cheng CY, et al. A missense variant in FGD6 confers increased risk of polypoidal choroidal vasculopathy. *Nat Genet* 2016;48:640–647.

65. Chen H, Liu K, Chen LJ, Hou P, Chen W, Pang CP. Genetic associations in polypoidal choroidal vasculopathy: a systematic review and meta-analysis. *Mol Vis* 2012;18:816–829.

66. Tateno Y, Sakurada Y, Yoneyama S, et al. Risk factors for second eye involvement in eyes with unilateral polypoidal choroidal vasculopathy. *Ophthalmic Genet* 2016;37:177–182.

67. Yamashiro K, Mori K, Honda S, et al. A prospective multicenter study on genome wide associations to ranibizumab treatment outcome for age-related macular degeneration. *Sci Rep* 2017;7:9196.

68. Akiyama M, Takahashi A, Momozawa Y, et al. Genome-wide association study suggests four variants influencing outcomes with ranibizumab therapy in exudative age-related macular degeneration. *J Hum Genet* 2018;63:1083–1091.

69. Fan Q, Maranville JC, Fritsche L, et al. HDL-cholesterol levels and risk of age-related macular degeneration: a multiethnic genetic study using Mendelian randomization. *Int J Epidemiol* 2017;46:1891–1902.

70. Han X, Ong JS, An J, Hewitt AW, Gharahkhani P, MacGregor S. Using Mendelian randomization to evaluate the causal relationship between serum C-reactive protein levels and age-related macular degeneration. *Eur J Epidemiol* 2020;35:139–146.

71. Wood A, Guggenheim JA. Refractive error has minimal influence on the risk of age-related macular degeneration: a mendelian randomization study. *Am J Ophthalmol* 2019;206:87–93.

72. Koh A, Lai TYY, Takahashi K, et al. Efficacy and safety of ranibizumab with or without verteporfin photodynamic therapy for polypoidal choroidal vasculopathy: a randomized clinical trial. *JAMA Ophthalmol* 2017;135:1206–1213.

73. Wong TY, Ogura Y, Lee WK, et al. Efficacy and safety of intravitreal aflibercept for polypoidal choroidal vasculopathy: two-year results of the aflibercept in polypoidal choroidal vasculopathy study. *Am J Ophthalmol* 2019;204:80–89.

74. Chong Teo KY, Squirrell DM, Nguyen V, et al. A multicountry comparison of real-world management

and outcomes of polypoidal choroidal vasculopathy: Fight Retinal Blindness! cohort. *Ophthalmol Retina* 2019;3:220–229.

75. Koh A, Lai TYY, Wei WB, et al. Real-world effectiveness and safety of ranibizumab treatment in patients with and without polypoidal choroidal vasculopathy: twelve-month results from the LUMINOUS study. *Retina* 2020;40:1529[N]1539.

76. Fenner BJ, Ting DSW, Tan ACS, et al. Real-world treatment outcomes of age-related macular degeneration and polypoidal choroidal vasculopathy in Asians. *Ophthalmol Retina* 2020;4:403–414.

77. Nishikawa K, Oishi A, Hata M, et al. Four-year outcome of aflibercept for neovascular age-related macular degeneration and polypoidal choroidal vasculopathy. *Sci Rep* 2019;9:3620.

78. Ye H, Zhang Q, Liu X, et al. Prevalence of age-related macular degeneration in an elderly urban Chinese population in China: the Jiangning Eye Study. *Invest Ophthalmol Vis Sci* 2014;55:6374–6380.

79. Bikbov MM, Zainullin RM, Gilmanshin TR, et al. Prevalence and associated factors of age-related macular degeneration in a Russian population: the Ural Eye and Medical study. *Am J Ophthalmol* 2020;210:146–157.

80. Majithia S, Tham YC, Chee ML, et al. Singapore Chinese Eye Study: key findings from baseline examination and the rationale, methodology of the 6-year follow-up series. *Br J Ophthalmol* 2020;104:610–615.

81. Inoue M, Balaratnasingam C, Freund KB. Optical coherence tomography angiography of polypoidal choroidal vasculopathy and polypoidal choroidal neovascularization. *Retina* 2015;35:2265–2274.

82. Tomiyasu T, Nozaki M, Yoshida M, Ogura Y. Characteristics of polypoidal choroidal vasculopathy evaluated by optical coherence tomography angiography. *Invest Ophthalmol Vis Sci* 2016;57: 324–330.

83. Cheung CMG, Yanagi Y, Akiba M, et al. Improved detection and diagnosis of polypoidal choroidal vasculopathy using a combination of optical coherence tomography and optical coherence tomography angiography. *Retina* 2018; 39(9):1655–1663.

84. Chan SY, Wang Q, Wang YX, Shi XH, Jonas JB, Wei WB. Polypoidal choroidal vasculopathy upon optical coherence tomographic angiography. *Retina* 2018;38:1187–1194.

85. You QS, Chan JCH, Ng ALK, et al. Macular vessel density measured with optical coherence tomography angiography and its associations in a large population-based study. *Invest Ophthalmol Vis Sci* 2019;60:4830–4837.

86. Cheung CMG, Lai TYY, Teo K, et al. Polypoidal choroidal vasculopathy: consensus nomenclature and non-indocyanine green angiograph diagnostic criteria from the Asia-Pacific Ocular Imaging Society PCV Workgroup. *Ophthalmology* 2021;128:443–452.

14 Diabetic Retinopathy

Charumathi Sabanayagam and Tien Yin Wong

14.1 INTRODUCTION

Diabetes is a major public health problem associated with micro- and macrovascular complications, poor quality of life, and premature mortality. Diabetes is estimated to affect 415 million people worldwide in 2015 and is projected to increase to 642 million by 2040.[1] With the aging of the population and growing prevalence of diabetes, the number of those affected by diabetic retinopathy (DR), an important microvascular complication of diabetes, is also expected to increase substantially. DR is a leading cause of preventable blindness in working-age adults worldwide. In 2015, an estimated one in three adults with diabetes globally had some form of DR and nearly one in ten had sight-threatening levels of DR, including proliferative DR and diabetic macular edema (DME).[2] Of all the people worldwide with moderate or severe visual impairment, estimated to be 217 million in 2015, DR ranked fifth, affecting 2.6 million adults.[3] Early detection and timely intervention have been shown to prevent blindness due to DR by about 98%. This review summarizes the epidemiology, impact, and prevention strategies of DR and DME.

14.2 CLASSIFICATION OF DR

The classical retinal microvascular signs of DR include presence of microaneurysms, hemorrhages, hard exudates, cotton-wool spots, intraretinal microvascular abnormalities, venous beading, and new vessels.[4] These signs are broadly classified into two phases: non proliferative DR (NPDR) and proliferative DR (PDR). Several classification systems for DR severity exist based on grading from retinal photographs for use in research and clinical practice (Table 14.1). These include the Early Treatment of Diabetic Retinopathy Study (ETDRS) scale,[5] the International Clinical Diabetic Retinopathy and DME Severity Scale,[6] and the UK National Guidelines on Screening for Diabetic Retinopathy.[7] The ETDRS system classifies DR severity into 13 levels ranging from none (level 10) to minimal NPDR (level 20), mild NPDR (level 35), moderate NPDR (level 43–47), severe NPDR (level 53), and PDR (level >60). DME is classified into presence or absence. Clinically significant macular edema (CSME) is considered present when the macular edema involved or was within 500 μm of the foveal center, or if focal photocoagulation scars were present in the macular area. The ETDRS system is considered the gold standard but due to complexity, it is mostly used in research settings.[8] The International Clinical DR Severity Scale simplifies the classification of DR into five stages for clinical use: no DR, mild NPDR, moderate NPDR, severe NPDR, and PDR. DME is classified into presence or absence. DME severity is classified into mild, moderate, and severe based on the distance of retinal thickening/hard exudates from the fovea. The UK system proposed for use in population screening classifies DR into none (R0), R1 (background), R2 (preproliferative), and R3 (proliferative). DME is classified into focal, diffuse, ischemic, or mixed.

14.3 EPIDEMIOLOGY AND IMPACT OF DR

14.3.1 Blindness Due to DR

Vision loss in DR occurs due to PDR or DME. In 2012, Yau et al. estimated that ~93 million people with diabetes had some DR, of which ~28 million people had vision-threatening stages of DR.[2] Despite improvement in screening and intervention, the prevalence of DR and blindness due to DR/DME is expected to increase, as a result of aging of the population and increased life expectancy of people with diabetes due to advances in medical treatment. In 2015, 2.6 million people were estimated to have moderate to severe visual loss due to DR and this number is projected to increase to 3.2 million within 5 years in 2020.[3] While the global prevalence of blindness due to age-related eye diseases such as cataract, uncorrected refractive error, and glaucoma decreased from 1990 to 2015, blindness due to DR has been shown to increase from 0.8% in 1990 to 1.2% in 2015. While the incidence of PDR has been shown to decline from 19.5% to 2.6% in 20 years (1975–1985 to 1986–2008) in developed countries due to improved awareness and management of DR risk factors, early identification, and initiation of timely intervention for DR,[9] more than two-thirds reduction in the prevalence of vision impairment and blindness was observed in Europe after the introduction of free screening services.[10] The Vision Loss Expert Group of the Global Burden of Disease Study estimated the prevalence of blindness due to DR in adults aged 50 years and above was highest in African regions, including West sub-Saharan, North Africa, and East sub-Saharan Africa (0.14–0.19%) compared to 0.1% or less in other regions.[11] Likewise the prevalence of moderate to severe

DOI: 10.1201/9781315146737-16

Table 14.1 Classification systems for diabetic retinopathy severity

ETDRS classification of DR severity (modified Airlie House)	International Classification of Clinical DR Severity Scale	UK National Guidelines on Screening for DR
10: No retinopathy	No DR	R0: None
14–15: Questionable DR		
20: Minimal NPDR	Mild NPDR	R1: Background
35: Mild NPDR		
43: Moderate NPDR	Moderate NPDR	R2: Preproliferative
47: Moderately severe NPDR		
53: Severe NPDR	Severe NPDR	
61: Mild PDR	PDR	R3: Proliferative
65: Moderate PDR		
71: Severe PDR		
81, 85: Advanced PDR		

Abbreviations: ETDRS, Early Treatment Diabetic Retinopathy Study; NPDR, non-proliferative diabetic retinopathy; PDR, proliferative diabetic retinopathy.

visual loss due to DR was found to be highest in North Africa/Middle East (1%), south Asia, and sub-Saharan Africa, with 0.5% each.[11]

14.3.2 Prevalence of DR and DME

Although diabetes prevalence is increasing worldwide, the brunt of the burden is borne by low- and middle-income countries, in particular, China and India, which together contribute 43% of diabetes cases globally. In 2012, Yau et al. estimated the global prevalence of DR in 2010 by pooling data from 35 studies across 16 countries, of which 13 were from developed countries and three from developing countries.[2] Global prevalence of any DR and VTDR were 35% and 10%. Prevalence of PDR was 7% and of DME was 6.8%. The study reported the prevalence of any DR and VTDR to be lower in Asians, at 19.9% and 5.3%. Since the study by Yau et al. in 2012, several studies have published meta-analyses of DR prevalence worldwide, in specific regions or populations, as shown in Table 14.2. A more recent review of the global prevalence of DR in studies published after 2015 utilizing retinal photographs by Thomas et al.[12] for the *IDF Atlas* reported lower prevalence of DR (27%), PDR (1.4%), and DME (4.6%) compared to Yau et al., with estimates suggesting overall improvement in DR control and management. When stratified by IDF regions, prevalence of any DR was found to be lowest in Europe at 20.6%, while Africa (33.8%), Middle East and North Africa (MENA: 33.8%) and the Western Pacific Region (36.2%) had the highest prevalence. PDR prevalence was highest in Africa

at 4.0% and lowest in the Western Pacific at 0.6%. In an updated meta-analysis including 50 studies across 25 countries, we found the VTDR prevalence worldwide to be 7.3%.[13] Similar to the IDF study, VTDR prevalence was highest in Africa (14.4%) and the MENA region (11.2%). But prevalence was found to be lowest in South East Asia at 3%. Ruta et al. in a systematic review including 72 studies from developing and developed countries concluded that the prevalence of DR in most of the developing countries (15 of the 23 studies) was higher than the global average of 35% reported by Yau et al.[14] The higher prevalence in developing countries could be explained by differential access to healthcare, delay in diagnosis of diabetes and DR, lack of awareness of diabetes and DR, poor facilities, and so on. In support of this finding, another study pooling data from 41 studies including Asian adults with type 2 diabetes reported the prevalence of DR to be higher than Yau et al. had estimated (28%), although VTDR prevalence was similar, at 6%.[15] In countrywide meta-analyses, any-DR prevalence was found to be lowest in China (18.5%)[16] and Ethiopia (19.5%),[17] whereas Europe had an intermediate prevalence of 25.7%.[18] Both any-DR and PDR prevalence were highest in Iran (37.8% and 13.2%).[19] Similar to any-DR, PDR prevalence was lowest in China at 1%.[16]

With improvement in screening and management strategies of DR, prevalence of PDR has been shown to decline in countries with good public health systems. On the other hand, following the rising prevalence of type 2 diabetes, blindness due to DME is on the rise. In

Table 14.2 Review of prevalence of diabetic retinopathy and diabetic macular edema in systematic reviews and meta-analyses

Author and publication year	Type of study	Number of primary studies and location	Sample size, study population	Findings
Yau et al. 2012[2]	Individual-level meta-analysis	35 studies from 21 countries worldwide	22,896 people with diabetes	Any DR 34.6% PDR 7.0%; VTDR 10.2% DME 6.8%
Liu et al. 2012[73]	Meta-analysis of published studies from China	18 primary studies from mainland China	11,996 Chinese with diabetes	Any DR 23% PDR 2.8%
Kaidonis et al. 2014[20]	Review of Australian studies	11 primary studies (six indigenous and five non-indigenous)	12,666 Australians with diabetes; 2,865 of them were indigenous	Indigenous vs. non-indigenous Any DR 23.6% vs. 32.3% PDR 3.2% vs. 4.7% VTDR 10.4% vs. 11.2% DME 7.6% vs. 9.4%
Maroufizadeh et al. 2017[74]	Meta-analysis of published studies from Iran	31 primary studies from Iran	23,729 participants with type 1 and type 2 diabetes	Any DR 41.9% PDR 13.2%
Song et al. 2018[16]	Meta-analysis of published studies from 1990 to 2017 in China	31 primary studies from China	Participants with diabetes. Total sample size not given	Any DR 18.5% PDR 1%
Thomas et al. 2019[12]	Individual-level meta-analysis of studies from 2015 to 2018	32 studies from 21 countries worldwide	543,448 people with diabetes that had retinal photography	Any DR 27% PDR 1.4% DME- 4.6%
Yang et al. 2019[15]	Meta-analysis of published studies	41 primary studies involving Asians	48,995 participants with type 2 diabetes	Any DR 28% PDR 6%
Li et al. 2019[75]	Meta-analysis of published studies from Europe	35 primary studies from Europe	205,743 participants with diabetes	Any DR 25.7% DME 3.7%
Fite et al. 2019[17]	Meta-analysis of published studies from Ethiopia	16 primary studies from Ethiopia	4,801 (calculated) participants with diabetes	Any DR 19.5%
Mohammadi et al. 2019[19]	Meta-analysis of published studies from Iran	34 primary studies from Iran	17,079 participants with type 2 diabetes	Any DR 37.8%
Teo et al. 2019[13]	Meta-analysis of published studies on VTDR	50 primary studies from 26 countries	41,712 adults with diabetes	VTDR 7.3%

Abbreviations: VTDR, vision-threatening diabetic retinopathy; PDR, proliferative diabetic retinopathy.

the meta-analysis by Yau et al. global prevalence of DME in type 2 diabetes was estimated to be 5.6%. In the *IDF Atlas Review*, DME prevalence was reported to be 4.3% worldwide.[2] Africa (41.0%) and Western Pacific (19.1%) had the highest prevalence of DME in type 2 diabetes.[12] In the Australian review, DME prevalence in indigenous Australians was reported to be higher than in non-indigenous populations (7.6% vs. 4.9%) in studies published after 1990.[20] As shown in Table 14.2, prevalence of DME was found to be lowest in Europe at 3.7%.

14.3.3 Incidence and Progression of DR

In a recent systematic review of prospective population-based studies,[21] we found that the annual incidence of DR ranged from 2.2% to 3.5% in Asian studies from India,[22] China,[23] and Singapore and a study from sub-Saharan Africa (3.4%).[24] Annual incidence was higher in the US Los Angeles Latino Eye study (LALES) at 10.4%[5] and the Barbados Incidence Study of Eye Diseases at 9%.[25] We found that most of the recent studies published after year 2000 came from developing countries, including India and China, while prospective data from developed countries were limited. This surge in DR studies in India and China could be driven by the excessive prevalence of diabetes in these countries. Although most of the initial studies (before 2000) that provided improved understanding of the incidence, progression, and risk factors of DR came from the US,[26-28] no recent study estimating incidence in whites and blacks from the US is available. In a recent meta-analysis including four prospective studies from Europe, pooled annual incidence of any DR, vision-threatening DR (VTDR), and DME was 4.6%, 0.5%, and 0.4%.[18] In a study comparing incidence of DR in migrant Indians living in Singapore to that in Indians living in urban India, we found DR incidence (21.9% vs. 9.3%) as well as progression (33.5% vs. 12.6%) to be higher in migrant Indians living in Singapore.[29] This increase could possibly be explained by a slightly longer period of follow-up in Singapore Indians (6 years vs. 4 years in the Indian study), earlier identification of more DR patients through systematic screening programs, and acculturation to western lifestyle in Singapore. In a worldwide review of prospective studies, we found the annual progression of DR to range from 3.4% to 5.3% in Asian and African studies (4.1%). Similar to higher incidence, annual DR progression was also high (12.3%) in the LALES Study in the US, including in Hispanic Americans.[21]

14.3.4 Awareness of DR

Awareness of DR remains low in developing as well as developed countries. More than half of the population with DR were found to be unaware of their condition in China, Egypt, Singapore, and the US.[30] In 2017, it was estimated that of the 451 million adults aged ≥18 years with diabetes worldwide, 224 million people were unaware of their condition.[31] Awareness of DR among physicians was also found to be suboptimal in developing countries.[32] Adherence to evidence-based guidelines for screening and managing patients with DR was not widely available in several developing countries.[33] Diabetic patients who received guidelines on recommended care had lower visual loss compared to those who did not receive recommended care.[32]

14.3.5 Risk Factors of DR

Younger age, minority ethnicity, type 1 diabetes, and longer duration of diabetes are established non-modifiable risk factors for DR. Younger age is a risk factor, presumably because of the selective mortality of older adults with DR. Alternatively younger adults were shown not to comply with screening guidelines and present with referable DR at first screen[34] and also may not adhere to a diabetes regime, resulting in increased prevalence and poor control of DR. While most of the studies did not find significant differences by sex in the prevalence[2] or incidence of DR,[21] the recent analysis of the Global Vision Database by the Vision Loss Expert Group found blindness and visual impairment due to DR to be significantly higher in women than in men (odds ratio of 2.5 in women).[3]

DR has been shown to disproportionately affect minority ethnic groups and migrant populations in several studies. African Americans compared to non-Hispanic whites (39% vs. 31%) in the US,[35] South Asians compared to whites in the UK (45% vs. 37%)[36] and Indians compared to Malays and Chinese in Singapore (30.7% vs. 25.5% and 26.2%)[37] had significantly higher prevalence of DR. In Australia, a review comparing the prevalence of DR in indigenous Australians to non-indigenous Australians in 11 studies reported that indigenous Australians, who made up only 3% of the total population, accounted for 23% of all those with VTDR.[20] Apart from higher prevalence of metabolic risk factors, differences in access to care and health-seeking behavior between ethnic groups, ethnicity-specific factors such as differences in adiposity measurements, access to care, differential susceptibility to insulin resistance, epigenetics, and genetic susceptibility have been proposed to contribute to ethnic differences in DR prevalence.[38] However, incidence of DR was reported to be similar between whites and blacks in the San Luis Study in the US[28] and Indians and Malays in Singapore.[21]

Type 1 diabetes is a known risk factor for DR. Adults with type 1 diabetes have been shown to have three times higher prevalence of DR than those with type 2 diabetes (77.3% vs. 25.2%) in a global meta-analysis study.[2] In the Wisconsin Epidemiological Study of DR (WESDR), after 25 years of follow-up, almost all those with type 1 diabetes had some form of DR while a third of them had VTDR.[39] Menarche[40] and pregnancy[41] have been shown to increase risk of DR in people with type 1 diabetes. Incidence and progression of DR increase with increasing duration of diabetes.[42, 43] The meta-analysis by Yau et al. showed DR prevalence to be 3.6 times higher in those with diabetes for more than 20 years vs. those with diabetes of less than 10 years.[2]

Among the modifiable risk factors, poor glycemic control and hypertension are well-known risk factors of DR. Associations of smoking,[44] hyperlipidemia,[45] and obesity with DR are not consistent.[46–49] In the WESDR higher levels of HbA1c were associated with long-term incidence of PDR, progression of DR,[39] and incidence of DME[50] in those with type 1 diabetes. Poor glycemic control indicated by higher HbA1c[21] and use of insulin therapy[25, 42] has been shown to be associated with onset and progression of DR in several studies. Apart from hyperglycemia, glycemic variability has been shown to increase the risk of DR in patients with type 1 diabetes. A meta-analysis including seven studies found HbA1c variability to increase the risk of DR by more than twice in type 1 diabetes.[51]

Hypertension has been shown to be associated with long-term incidence of PDR[39] and DME[26] and higher systolic or diastolic blood pressure (BP) with 4-year incidence and progression of DR in the WESDR type 1 cohort.[52] Higher systolic BP or diastolic BP was associated with incident DR in type 2 diabetes in the Beixinjing community study in China[53] and antihypertensive medication use reduced the risk of DR in type 2 diabetes by 50% in the Barbados Eye Study.[25] However, hypertension was not associated with 4-year incidence or progression of DR in type 2 diabetes in the WESDR cohort.[52] Our recent review of contemporary studies on incident DR in type 2 diabetes also failed to identify hypertension as a risk factor for DR in three out of four prospective studies with follow-up ranging from 4 to 6 years.[21]

Association between dyslipidemia and DR or DME is not consistent across studies. A meta-analysis of observational studies evaluating the associations between blood lipid levels and DR found mean levels of total cholesterol, low-density lipoprotein cholesterol, and triglycerides to be separately and significantly associated with DR in case–control studies.[45] Obesity has been shown to be positively associated with DR in most studies including Western populations,[46, 49] while higher body mass index and obesity showed a protective association in most of the Asian studies.[47, 48, 54]

14.3.6 Impact of DR on Quality of Life

DR is asymptomatic in the early stages of the disease. In those with mild or NPDR, visual acuity and visual functioning are usually not affected. With progression to vision-threatening stages of DR, vision-related daily activities such as reading, routine household work, driving, and mobility are affected, leading to poor vision-related quality of life, risk of falls, psychosocial stress, and depression.[55] Strategies preventing the onset of DR or progression to vision-threatening stages will be rewarding in maintaining a satisfactory vision-related functioning.

14.4 PREVENTION OF DR

Depending upon the stage of the diseases process, public health-based prevention strategies are classified into primary, secondary, and tertiary (Figure 14.1). Primary and secondary prevention strategies have greater impact at population level while tertiary prevention refers to only a small proportion of patients with severe stages of the disease. As per the recent estimates, 65% of those with diabetes do not have DR while

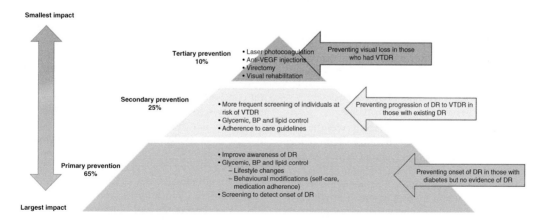

Figure 14.1 Public health approach to diabetic retinopathy (DR) prevention. BP, blood pressure; DR, diabetic retinopathy; VEGF, vascular endothelial growth factor; VTDR, vision threatening DR.

35% have some DR, of which 10% have VTDR.[2] Primary prevention strategies such as health education and risk factor control are aimed at preventing the onset of DR in those with diabetes but who do not have DR (65%). Secondary prevention targets those with early stages of DR and aims to prevent or slow progression to vision-threatening stages of DR (25%). The strategies include screening at frequent intervals for DR progress, control of systemic risk factors, improving adherence to guideline recommended care, and so on. Tertiary prevention strategies are aimed at targeting those with VTDR (10%) and include ophthalmologist care such as laser treatment or vitrectomy or use of anti-vascular endothelial growth factor (anti-VEGF) injections for PDR and DME. In current settings, tertiary prevention has been the main focus of DR management among the ophthalmologist community. However, primary and secondary prevention strategies, which can be managed by primary care physicians and endocrinologists, are cost-effective and impactful in reducing the burden of DR at population level.

14.4.1 Improve Awareness

Patient education is a key factor that influences adherence to physician recommendations. Educational materials, including knowledge about diabetes, eye complication, self-care management, and regular screening for DR, should be made available in all community and primary care centers. Vision loss from DR can be prevented by broad public health strategies but they have to suit. The International Council of Ophthalmology (ICO) recently updated its guidelines for managing DR with a specific focus on screening, referral, and follow-up schedules and timely treatment for DR according to different resource settings. The guidelines provide the minimum requirements for a screening vision and retinal examination, follow-up care, appropriate use of intravitreal anti-VEGF inhibitors, suggestions for monitoring outcomes, and indicators of success at a population level.[4]

14.4.2 Lifestyle Changes and Behavioral Modifications

Lifestyle interventions, including weight loss and increased physical activity, have been shown to reduce hyperglycemia and the need for medications in diabetic patients.[56] Physical activity was found to have a protective effect on DR (risk reduction by 6%) in patients with diabetes and the effect was more pronounced in those with VTDR (risk reduction by 11%) in a meta-analysis.[57] Improving self-care behaviors, including adherence to recommended diet,

exercise, antidiabetic and antihypertensive medication, self-monitoring of blood glucose, and regular retinal screening, improve diabetes care and management.[32]

14.4.3 Control of Systemic Risk Factors: Evidence from Meta-Analyses of Randomized Controlled Trials and Cohort Studies

Control of hyperglycemia, BP, and lipids is key for preventing the onset as well as progression of DR. Intensive glycemic control targeting an HbA1c of 6.5% has shown beneficial effects in reducing the risk of DR. A meta-analysis of seven trials, including 10,793 participants with type 2 diabetes, showed that intensive glycemic control reduced the risk of retinopathy by 20%. However, the risk of hypoglycemia increased by 30%.[58] Another meta-analysis of six trials showed that intensive glycemic control reduced the progression of retinopathy by 20%, but risk of hypoglycemia increased by 139%.[59] Although optimal glycemic goal is <6.5%, balancing benefits and risk, guidelines recommend a glycemic goal of <7% HbA1c in most diabetic patients and relaxing glycemic goals to <8% in elderly patients who are at higher risk of hypoglycemia.[60] Similar to glycemic control, BP control has also been shown to have beneficial effects on risk of DR. A meta-analysis of eight randomized controlled trials (RCTs) showed intensive BP control reduced the incidence of DR by 17% compared to conventional BP targets[61] and the finding was subsequently confirmed by trial sequential analysis. However, benefit of intensive BP control in reducing progression of DR, incidence of PDR and DME was not evident in the meta-analysis as well as the trial sequential analysis. In a meta-analysis including 13 RCTs enrolling 37,736 participants with type 2 diabetes or impaired fasting glucose, a more aggressive goal of <130/80 mmHg reduced mortality by 10% but failed to show any benefit on the risk of renal, retinal, and cardiovascular events besides increasing serious adverse events.[62] Most guidelines thus recommend a BP goal of <140/90 mmHg in diabetic patients.

Although associations of lipid with DR are not consistent across studies, statin therapy has been shown to have a beneficial effect on DR and cardiovascular disease in diabetic patients. Thus treatment of dyslipidemia is recommended in diabetic patients.[60] A meta-analysis of six cohort studies evaluated the evidence for the role of statins in reducing the risk of DR and the need for interventions, including retinal laser treatment, anti-VEGF injections, and vitrectomy in 558,177 patients with diabetes.[63] Five studies included type 2 diabetes and one study included both type 1 and type 2 patients. The study reported that statin use was associated with a 32% risk reduction for incidence of DR (hazard ratio [HR] and 95% confidence interval [CI] of 0.68 [0.55–0.84]). Risk reduction was consistently observed across subtypes of DR: 31% for PDR, 20% for NPDR, 44% for DME, and 28% risk reduction for need for interventions.[63] In a pooled analysis of two RCTs, fenofibrate reduced the risk of DME by 45%.[64]

In addition to isolated glycemic or BP control, studies have also evaluated the effect of multi-factorial interventions. A meta-analysis of 22 RCTs targeting interventions of modifiable risk factors of DR, including blood glucose, BP, lipid, dietary, physical activity, and smoking, showed beneficial effects of interventions in reducing the risk of DR by 40% and worsening of DR by 38%. Multifactorial interventions had better effect on DR onset while BP control only had an effect on reducing worsening of DR. Also interventions with follow-up durations >5 years had better effect on DR onset while interventions with >2 years of follow-up had better effect on reducing the risk of worsening of DR.[65]

14.5 DR SCREENING FOR DETECTING ONSET AND MONITORING PROGRESSION OF DR

DR remains asymptomatic in the early stages and onset may not be perceived by patients till late stage. In patients with DR, early detection, regular follow-up, and prompt treatment of VTDR prevent up to 98% of visual loss due to DR.[66] The American Diabetes Association and the American Academy of Ophthalmology recommend that people with type 2 diabetes should have an initial dilated eye examination at the time of their diabetes diagnosis and subsequent examinations should be yearly or more frequently if retinopathy is progressing.[60] Despite recommendations, ~60% only adhere to screening recommendations even in high-income countries.[67] Factors influencing screening adherence include the patient's knowledge about diabetes, younger age, availability of insurance, and access to ophthalmologists and care facilities.[30]

Telemedicine-based DR screening with remote reading by professional graders is being adopted by several countries, including the UK, US, Europe, China, India, and Singapore.[32, 68] In a meta-analysis including 1,960 participants from 20 studies, the pooled sensitivity for detecting any DR was 95% while specificity was 86%. Sensitivity for detecting mild NPDR was 74% even with mydriasis. For detecting absence of DR and mild NPDR, accuracy was higher when images were acquired through mydriasis than through non-mydriasis and using a wide-angle

camera (100–200°) than a narrow-angle one (45° or 35°).[69] DR screening using a telemedicine platform has been shown to improve screening rates in all resource settings and reduce vision loss due to DR.[70] However, repeated manual grading by graders is strenuous and not sustainable in the long run, even in high-resource settings.

Artificial intelligence-based deep learning systems for detecting referable DR/DME have been gaining traction recently with great potential to reduce cost of screening, manpower for grading, and variability in grading.[71] In a meta-analysis of 24 studies including 235,235 subjects with diabetes, the accuracy of neural network-based deep learning systems in detecting clinically significant DR was excellent, with pooled sensitivity and specificity of 92% and 91%.[72] Deep learning-based DR screening is a promising tool for scaling up DR screening to rural and remote areas but challenges, including infrastructure, dealing with poor image quality, and ethical concerns in implementation, need to be sorted out.

14.6 CONCLUSION

Despite improvement in screening and treatment strategies, prevalence of DR and blindness due to DR is increasing globally, in particular in low- and middle-income countries which bore the highest burden of diabetes. Prevention efforts should be more focused towards primary and secondary prevention strategies, including improving awareness of DR, promoting self-care, achieving recommended glycemic control, and BP goal and adherence to screening recommendations, which have more impact at the population level. More studies evaluating the effect of behavioral modifications, cost-effectiveness of artificial intelligence-based screening programs, and qualitative research studies identifying the extent of the emotional and social impact of DR are warranted to assist policy planners, healthcare workers, and researchers in developing suitable interventions to improve outcomes associated with DR.

REFERENCES

1. Ogurtsova K, da Rocha Fernandes JD, Huang Y, et al. IDF diabetes atlas: Global estimates for the prevalence of diabetes for 2015 and 2040. *Diabetes Res Clin Pract* 2017;128:40–50. doi: 10.1016/j.diabres.2017.03.024

2. Yau JW, Rogers SL, Kawasaki R, et al. Global prevalence and major risk factors of diabetic retinopathy. *Diabetes Care* 2012;35(3):556–64. doi: 10.2337/dc11-1909

3. Flaxman SR, Bourne RRA, Resnikoff S, et al. Global causes of blindness and distance vision impairment 1990–2020: a systematic review and meta-analysis.

Lancet Global Health 2017;5(12):e1221–e34. doi: 10.1016/S2214-109X(17)30393-5

4. Wong TY, Sun J, Kawasaki R, et al. Guidelines on diabetic eye care: the International Council of Ophthalmology recommendations for screening, follow-up, referral, and treatment based on resource settings. *Ophthalmology* 2018;125(10):1608–22. doi: 10.1016/j.ophtha.2018.04.007

5. Varma R, Choudhury F, Klein R, et al. Four-year incidence and progression of diabetic retinopathy and macular edema: the Los Angeles Latino Eye Study. *Am J Ophthalmol* 2010;149(5):752–61 e1–3. doi: 10.1016/j.ajo.2009.11.014

6. Wilkinson CP, Ferris FL, 3rd, Klein RE, et al. Proposed international clinical diabetic retinopathy and diabetic macular edema disease severity scales. *Ophthalmology* 2003;110(9):1677–82. doi: 10.1016/S0161-6420(03)00475-5

7. Taylor D. Diabetic eye screening revised grading definitions. To provide guidance on revised grading definitions for the NHS diabetic eye screening programme. 2012. Available at: Diabetic-Screening-Service-Revised-Grading-Definitions-November-2012.pdf (swbh.nhs.uk).

8. Wu L, Fernandez-Loaiza P, Sauma J, et al. Classification of diabetic retinopathy and diabetic macular edema. *World J Diabetes* 2013;4(6):290–4. doi: 10.4239/wjd.v4.i6.290

9. Wong TY, Mwamburi M, Klein R, et al. Rates of progression in diabetic retinopathy during different time periods: a systematic review and meta-analysis. *Diabetes Care* 2009;32(12):2307–13. doi: 10.2337/dc09-0615

10. Arun CS, Ngugi N, Lovelock L, et al. Effectiveness of screening in preventing blindness due to diabetic retinopathy. *Diabet Med* 2003;20(3):186–90. doi: 899 [pii]

11. Leasher JL, Bourne RR, Flaxman SR, et al. Global estimates on the number of people blind or visually impaired by diabetic retinopathy: a meta-analysis from 1990 to 2010. *Diabetes Care* 2016;39(9):1643–9. doi: 10.2337/dc15-2171

12. Thomas RL, Halim S, Gurudas S, et al. IDF diabetes atlas: a review of studies utilising retinal photography on the global prevalence of diabetes related retinopathy between 2015 and 2018. *Diabetes Res Clin Pract* 2019; 157:107840. doi: 10.1016/j.diabres.2019.107840

13. Teo ZL, Tham YC, Yu M, et al. Do we have enough ophthalmologists to manage vision-threatening diabetic retinopathy? A global perspective. *Eye (Lond England)* 2020;34(7):1255–61. doi: 10.1038/s41433-020-0776-5

14. Ruta LM, Magliano DJ, Lemesurier R, et al. Prevalence of diabetic retinopathy in type 2 diabetes in developing and developed countries. *Diabet Med* 2013;30(4):387–98. doi: 10.1111/dme.12119

15. Yang QH, Zhang Y, Zhang XM, et al. Prevalence of diabetic retinopathy, proliferative diabetic retinopathy and non-proliferative diabetic retinopathy in Asian T2DM patients: a systematic review and meta-analysis. *Int J Ophthalmol* 2019;12(2):302–11. doi: 10.18240/ijo.2019.02.19

16. Song P, Yu J, Chan KY, et al. Prevalence, risk factors and burden of diabetic retinopathy in China: a systematic review and meta-analysis. *J Glob Health* 2018;8(1):010803. doi: 10.7189/jogh.08.010803

17. Fite RO, Lake EA, Hanfore LK. Diabetic retinopathy in Ethiopia: a systematic review and meta-analysis. *Diabetes Metab Syndr* 2019;13(3):1885–91. doi: 10.1016/j.dsx.2019.04.016

18. Li JQ, Welchowski T, Schmid M, et al. Prevalence, incidence and future projection of diabetic eye disease in Europe: a systematic review and meta-analysis. *Eur J Epidemiol* 2020;35(1):11–23. doi: 10.1007/s10654-019-00560-z

19. Mohammadi M, Raiegani AAV, Jalali R, et al. The prevalence of retinopathy among type 2 diabetic patients in Iran: a systematic review and meta-analysis. *Rev Endocr Metab Disord* 2019;20(1):79–88. doi: 10.1007/s11154-019-09490-3

20. Kaidonis G, Mills RA, Landers J, et al. Review of the prevalence of diabetic retinopathy in Indigenous Australians. *Clin Exp Ophthalmol* 2014;42(9):875–82. doi: 10.1111/ceo.12338

21. Sabanayagam C, Banu R, Chee ML, et al. Incidence and progression of diabetic retinopathy: a systematic review. *Lancet Diabetes Endocrinol* 2019;7(2):140–9. doi: 10.1016/S2213-8587(18)30128-1

22. Raman R, Ganesan S, Pal SS, et al. Incidence and progression of diabetic retinopathy in urban India: Sankara Nethralaya-Diabetic Retinopathy Epidemiology and Molecular Genetics Study (SN-DREAMS II), report 1. *Ophthalmic Epidemiol* 2017:1–9. doi: 10.1080/09286586.2017.1290257

23. Xu J, Xu L, Wang YX, et al. Ten-year cumulative incidence of diabetic retinopathy. The Beijing Eye Study 2001/2011. *PLoS One* 2014;9(10):e111320. doi: 10.1371/journal.pone.0111320

24. Bastawrous A, Mathenge W, Wing K, et al. The incidence of diabetes mellitus and diabetic retinopathy in a population-based cohort study of people age 50 years and over in Nakuru, Kenya. *BMC Endocr Disord* 2017;17(1):19. doi: 10.1186/s12902-017-0170-x

25. Leske MC, Wu SY, Hennis A, et al. Nine-year incidence of diabetic retinopathy in the Barbados Eye Studies. *Arch Ophthalmol* 2006;124(2):250–5. doi: 124/2/250 [pii];10.1001/archopht.124.2.250 [doi]

26. Klein R, Klein BE, Moss SE, et al. The Wisconsin Epidemiologic Study of Diabetic Retinopathy. XV. The long-term incidence of macular edema. *Ophthalmology* 1995:7–16.

27. Klein R, Klein BE, Moss SE, et al. The Wisconsin Epidemiologic Study of Diabetic Retinopathy: XVII. The 14-year incidence and progression of diabetic retinopathy and associated risk factors in type 1 diabetes. *Ophthalmology* 1998:1801–15.

28. Tudor SM, Hamman RF, Baron A, et al. Incidence and progression of diabetic retinopathy in Hispanics and non-Hispanic whites with type 2 diabetes. San Luis Valley Diabetes Study, Colorado. *Diabetes Care* 1998:53–61.

29. Kumari N, Bhargava M, Nguyen DQ, et al. Six-year incidence and progression of diabetic retinopathy in Indian adults: the Singapore Indian Eye study. *Br J Ophthalmol* 2019;103(12):1732–9. doi: 10.1136/bjophthalmol-2018-313282

30. Huang OS, Tay WT, Ong PG, et al. Prevalence and determinants of undiagnosed diabetic retinopathy and vision-threatening retinopathy in a multiethnic Asian cohort: the Singapore Epidemiology of Eye Diseases (SEED) study. *Br J Ophthalmol* 2015;99(12):1614–21. doi: 10.1136/bjophthalmol-2014-306492

31. Cho NH, Shaw JE, Karuranga S, et al. IDF diabetes atlas: global estimates of diabetes prevalence for 2017 and projections for 2045. *Diabetes Res Clin Pract* 2018;138:271–81. doi: 10.1016/j.diabres.2018.02.023

32. Wong TY, Sabanayagam C. The war on diabetic retinopathy: where are we now? *Asia-Pac J Ophthalmol (Philadelphia, Pa)* 2019;8(6):448–56. doi: 10.1097/apo.0000000000000267

33. Wang LZ, Cheung CY, Tapp RJ, et al. Availability and variability in guidelines on diabetic retinopathy screening in Asian countries. *Br J Ophthalmol* 2017;101(10):1352–60. doi: 10.1136/bjophthalmol-2016-310002

34. Scanlon PH, Stratton IM, Leese GP, et al. Screening attendance, age group and diabetic retinopathy level at first screen. *Diabet Med* 2016;33(7):904–11. doi: 10.1111/dme.12957

35. Zhang X, Saaddine JB, Chou CF, et al. Prevalence of diabetic retinopathy in the United States, 2005–2008. *JAMA* 2010;304(6):649–56. doi: 10.1001/jama.2010.1111

36. Raymond NT, Varadhan L, Reynold DR, et al. Higher prevalence of retinopathy in diabetic patients of South Asian ethnicity compared with white Europeans in the community: a cross-sectional study. *Diabetes Care* 2009;32(3):410–15. doi: 10.2337/dc08-1422

37. Tan GS, Gan A, Sabanayagam C, et al. Ethnic differences in the prevalence and risk factors of diabetic retinopathy: the Singapore Epidemiology of Eye Diseases study. *Ophthalmology* 2018;125(4):529–36. doi: 10.1016/j.ophtha.2017.10.026

38. Sivaprasad S, Gupta B, Crosby-Nwaobi R, et al. Prevalence of diabetic retinopathy in various ethnic groups: a worldwide perspective. *Surv Ophthalmol* 2012;57(4):347–70. doi: 10.1016/j.survophthal.2012.01.004

39. Klein R, Knudtson MD, Lee KE, et al. The Wisconsin Epidemiologic Study of Diabetic Retinopathy: XXII the twenty-five-year progression of retinopathy in persons with type 1 diabetes. *Ophthalmology* 2008:1859–68.

40. Klein BE, Moss SE, Klein R. Is menarche associated with diabetic retinopathy? *Diabetes Care* 1990;13(10):1034–8. doi: 10.2337/diacare.13.10.1034

41. Klein BE, Moss SE, Klein R. Effect of pregnancy on progression of diabetic retinopathy. *Diabetes Care* 1990;13(1):34–40. doi: 10.2337/diacare.13.1.34

42. Dutra MM, Mesquita E, Gardete-Correia L, et al. First incidence and progression study for diabetic retinopathy in portugal, the RETINODIAB study: evaluation of the screening program for Lisbon region. *Ophthalmology* 2015;122(12):2473–81. doi: S0161-6420(15)00781-2 [pii];10.1016/j.ophtha.2015.08.004 [doi]

43. Cikamatana L, Mitchell P, Rochtchina E, et al. Five-year incidence and progression of diabetic retinopathy in a defined older population: the Blue Mountains Eye Study. *Eye (Lond)* 2007;21(4):465–71. doi: 6702771 [pii];10.1038/sj.eye.6702771 [doi]

44. Cai X, Chen Y, Yang W, et al. The association of smoking and risk of diabetic retinopathy in patients with type 1 and type 2 diabetes: a meta-analysis. *Endocrine* 2018;62(2):299–306. doi: 10.1007/s12020-018-1697-y

45. Das R, Kerr R, Chakravarthy U, et al. Dyslipidemia and diabetic macular edema: a systematic review and meta-analysis. *Ophthalmology* 2015;122(9):1820–7. doi: 10.1016/j.ophtha.2015.05.011

46. Dirani M, Xie J, Fenwick E, et al. Are obesity and anthropometry risk factors for diabetic retinopathy? The diabetes management project. *Invest Ophthalmol Vis Sci* 2011;52(7):4416–21. doi: 10.1167/iovs.11-7208

47. Raman R, Rani PK, Gnanamoorthy P, et al. Association of obesity with diabetic retinopathy: Sankara Nethralaya Diabetic Retinopathy Epidemiology and Molecular Genetics Study (SN-DREAMS report no. 8). *Acta Diabetol* 2010;47(3):209–15. doi: 10.1007/s00592-009-0113-8

48. Rooney D, Lye WK, Tan G, et al. Body mass index and retinopathy in Asian populations with diabetes mellitus. *Acta Diabetol* 2015;52(1):73–80. doi: 10.1007/s00592-014-0602-2

49. van Leiden HA, Dekker JM, Moll AC, et al. Blood pressure, lipids, and obesity are associated with retinopathy: the Hoorn study. *Diabetes Care* 2002;25(8):1320–5.

50. Klein R, Knudtson MD, Lee KE, et al. The Wisconsin Epidemiologic Study of Diabetic Retinopathy XXIII: the twenty-five-year incidence of macular edema in persons with type 1 diabetes. *Ophthalmology* 2009:497–503.

51. Gorst C, Kwok CS, Aslam S, et al. Long-term glycemic variability and risk of adverse outcomes: a systematic review and meta-analysis. *Diabetes Care* 2015;38(12):2354–69. doi: 10.2337/dc15-1188

52. Klein R, Klein BE, Moss SE, et al. Is blood pressure a predictor of the incidence or progression of diabetic retinopathy? *Arch Intern Med* 1989;149(11):2427–32.

53. Jin P, Peng J, Zou H, et al. The 5-year onset and regression of diabetic retinopathy in Chinese type 2 diabetes patients. *PLoS One* 2014;9(11):e113359. doi: 10.1371/journal.pone.0113359

54. Lu J, Hou X, Zhang L, et al. Association between body mass index and diabetic retinopathy in Chinese patients with type 2 diabetes. *Acta Diabetol* 2015;52(4):701–8. doi: 10.1007/s00592-014-0711-y

55. Fenwick E, Rees G, Pesudovs K, et al. Social and emotional impact of diabetic retinopathy: a review. *Clin Exp Ophthalmol* 2012;40(1):27–38. doi: 10.1111/j.1442-9071.2011.02599.x

56. Look ARG, Wing RR, Bolin P, et al. Cardiovascular effects of intensive lifestyle intervention in type 2 diabetes. *N Engl J Med* 2013;369(2):145–54. doi: 10.1056/NEJMoa1212914

57. Ren C, Liu W, Li J, et al. Physical activity and risk of diabetic retinopathy: a systematic review and meta-analysis. *Acta Diabetol* 2019;56(8):823–37. doi: 10.1007/s00592-019-01319-4

58. Hemmingsen B, Lund SS, Gluud C, et al. Intensive glycaemic control for patients with type 2 diabetes: systematic review with meta-analysis and trial sequential analysis of randomised clinical trials. *BMJ* 2011;343:d6898. doi: 10.1136/bmj.d6898

59. Buehler AM, Cavalcanti AB, Berwanger O, et al. Effect of tight blood glucose control versus conventional control in patients with type 2 diabetes mellitus: a systematic review with meta-analysis of randomized controlled trials. *Cardiovasc Ther* 2013;31(3):147–60. doi: 10.1111/j.1755-5922.2011.00308.x

60. American Diabetes Association. Improving care and promoting health in populations: standards of medical care in diabetes-2020. *Diabetes Care* 2020;43(Suppl 1):S7–S13. doi: 10.2337/dc20-S001

61. Zhou JB, Song ZH, Bai L, et al. Could intensive blood pressure control really reduce diabetic retinopathy outcomes? Evidence from meta-analysis and trial sequential analysis from randomized controlled trials. *Diabetes Ther* 2018;9(5):2015–27. doi: 10.1007/s13300-018-0497-y

62. Bangalore S, Kumar S, Lobach I, et al. Blood pressure targets in subjects with type 2 diabetes mellitus/impaired fasting glucose: observations from traditional and bayesian random-effects meta-analyses of randomized trials. *Circulation* 2011;123(24):2799–810. doi: 10.1161/CIRCULATIONAHA.110.016337

63. Pranata R, Vania R, Victor AA. Statin reduces the incidence of diabetic retinopathy and its need for intervention: a systematic review and meta-analysis. *Eur J Ophthalmol* 2020;1120672120922444. doi: 10.1177/1120672120922444

64. Mozetic V, Pacheco RL, Latorraca COC, et al. Statins and/or fibrates for diabetic retinopathy: a systematic review and meta-analysis. *Diabetol Metab Syndr* 2019;11:92. doi: 10.1186/s13098-019-0488-9

65. Yusufu M, Zhang X, Sun X, et al. How to perform better intervention to prevent and control diabetic retinopathy among patients with type 2 diabetes: a meta-analysis of randomized controlled trials. *Diabetes Res Clin Pract* 2019;156:107834. doi: 10.1016/j.diabres.2019.107834

66. Ferris FL, 3rd. How effective are treatments for diabetic retinopathy? *JAMA* 1993;269(10):1290–1.

67. AAO/PPP Retina/Vitreous Committee. *Diabetic Retinopathy Preferred Practice Pattern 2019*. Available from: www.aao.org/preferred-practice-pattern/diabetic-retinopathy-ppp.

68. Wong TY, Sabanayagam C. Strategies to tackle the global burden of diabetic retinopathy: from epidemiology to artificial intelligence. *Ophthalmologica* 2020;243(1):9–20. doi: 10.1159/000502387

69. Shi L, Wu H, Dong J, et al. Telemedicine for detecting diabetic retinopathy: a systematic review and meta-analysis. *Br J Ophthalmol* 2015;99(6):823–31. doi: 10.1136/bjophthalmol-2014-305631

70. Tozer K, Woodward MA, Newman-Casey PA. Telemedicine and diabetic retinopathy: review of published screening programs. *J Endocrinol Diabetes* 2015;2(4) doi: 10.15226/2374-6890/2/4/00131

71. Nielsen KB, Lautrup ML, Andersen JKH, et al. Deep learning-based algorithms in screening of diabetic retinopathy: a systematic review of diagnostic performance. *Ophthalmol Retina* 2019;3(4):294–304. doi: 10.1016/j.oret.2018.10.014

72. Wang S, Zhang Y, Lei S, et al. Performance of deep neural network-based artificial intelligence method in diabetic retinopathy screening: a systematic review and meta-analysis of diagnostic test accuracy. *Eur J Endocrinol* 2020;183(1):41–9. doi: 10.1530/EJE-19-0968

73. Liu L, Wu X, Liu L, et al. Prevalence of diabetic retinopathy in mainland China: a meta-analysis. *PLoS One* 2012;7(9):e45264. doi:10.1371/journal.pone.0045264

74. Maroufizadeh S, Almasi-Hashiani A, Hosseini M, et al. Prevalence of diabetic retinopathy in Iran: a systematic review and meta-analysis. *Int J Ophthalmol* 2017;10(5):782–789. doi:10.18240/ijo.2017.05.21

75. Li JQ, Welchowski T, Schmid M, et al. Prevalence, incidence and future projection of diabetic eye disease in Europe: a systematic review and meta-analysis. *Eur J Epidemiol* 2020;35(1):11–23. doi:10.1007/s10654-019-00560-z

15 Non-DR Retinal Vascular Diseases

Sobha Sivaprasad, Luke Nicholson, and Shruti Chandra

15.1 INTRODUCTION

In addition to diabetic retinopathy, there are several other retinal vascular diseases. Herein we describe the epidemiology of various retinal vascular diseases, including retinal vein occlusion (RVO), hypertensive retinopathy, retinal arterial occlusion, and ocular ischemic syndrome. Many of these diseases have shared modifiable risk factors, but there are specific risk factors for these conditions too. With the increasing prevalence of hypertension, hyperlipidemia, and diabetes around the world, no countries are spared from these disorders. The anatomy and pathology of the retinal vasculature provide significant insight into the general health of an individual. Although these retinal vascular conditions are not directly linked to mortality, the abnormalities in the retinal vasculature are usually the first signs that can be used to predict the vascular health of an individual. Therefore, with advances in machine learning, it is an opportunity to utilize the health of retinal vasculature as a screening tool for cardiovascular and cerebrovascular morbidities.

15.2 RETINAL VEIN OCCLUSION

15.2.1 Epidemiology of Retinal Vein Occlusion

RVO affected approximately 16 million people worldwide in 2008 and in 2015, it was estimated that 28 million people were living with the condition (1, 2). In the United Kingdom, RVO was recorded as the primary cause of blindness in 2% of certifications for sight impairment in 2013 (3). The prevalence of any form of RVO is approximately 5.20 per 1,000 adults (1). Branch RVO (BRVO) is five times more common, with 4.4 per 1,000 affected, while central RVO (CRVO) affects 0.8 per 1,000 (1). Hemiretinal vein occlusion (HRVO) is uncommon, comprising only 5% of all RVO cases (1).

The 5-year incidence of any form of RVO is 0.86%, increasing to 1.63% over a 10-year period (2, 4). The 15-year cumulative incidence of BRVO is 1.8% and 0.5% for CRVO (5). In BRVO, more than 50% of cases involved the superior temporal quadrant and only 38.5% affected the inferior temporal quadrant (5). Nasal involvement was uncommon, affecting only 9.2% of cases (5).

In the work done by Hayreh et al., observing 1,229 eyes, the cumulative probability for patients with RVO developing a second episode of RVO in the same eye was 0.9% in 2 years and 2.5% in 4 years (6). As for developing any subtype of RVO in the fellow eye, this was reported to be 7.7% in 2 years and 11.9% in 4 years (6). For patients with CRVO, in the Central Vein Occlusion Study, 9% of patients with CRVO had some form of vascular occlusion in the fellow eye and only 1.4% of fellow eyes developed incident CRVO in 3 years (7). For patients with CRVO, the risk of any form of RVO in the second eye is approximately 0.9% per year (7).

There are no gender or laterality differences in the prevalence of RVO (1, 2, 5, 8). The prevalence of RVO increases with age (2, 5, 6). However, RVO is not a disease exclusive to the elderly. The prevalence of BRVO is 0.2% in ages 43–54 years and rises to 1.3% in those above 75 years (8). This is mirrored in CRVO with a prevalence of 0.1% for ages 43–54 years; however, it only rises to 0.4% in patients above 75 years of age (8). In a separate large Australian population-based study, the increasing prevalence with age is also evident at 0.7% in patients under 60 years, rising to 4.6% of patients above 80 years (4, 9). It is worth noting the variation in the age distribution between CRVO and BRVO. Although CRVO, HRVO, and BRVO affect the elderly predominantly, with more than half older than 65 years, 13–16% of patients with CRVO were younger than 45 years old while this was the case for 10% of patients with HRVO and only 5% in BRVO (6, 10). There is no racial predilection for CRVO, but there exists a higher prevalence of BRVO in Asians and Hispanics compared to whites (1). Prevalence of BRVO in Asians and Hispanics was 4.98/1,000 and 5.98/1,000 respectively while it was only 2.82/1,000 in whites (1). In the Singapore Malay Eye Study, the general prevalence among three different Asian ethnicities was 7.2/1,000 with no differences between the three major ethnic groups: Chinese, Indian, and Malay (11).

15.2.2 Pathogenesis and Risk Factors of Retinal Vein Occlusion

RVO is caused by a thrombosis of the retinal veins and understandably is associated with systemic cardiovascular diseases (12). People with systemic hypertension or a history of myocardial infarction or stroke are more than twice as likely to develop an RVO (2). Advancing age is also a risk factor: every decade increase is associated with an odds ratio of 1.6–1.7 (2, 5). Interestingly, the association between diabetes and RVO is only unique to CRVO (5, 10). Several large population-based studies, including the

Blue Mountains Eye Study and Beaver Dam Eye Study, have concluded that diabetes was not a significant risk factor for RVO in general (2, 5, 9, 13). However, when studied specifically for subtype of RVO, diabetes was a risk factor for HRVO and CRVO while not for BRVO (5, 10). The opposite was noted in patients with raised systolic blood pressure in the first 5 years of observation; it had a significant association with BRVO although not CRVO (5, 8). Hypertension was found to have an odds ratio of 3.2 for BRVO, 2.9 for HRVO, and 2.1 for CRVO (10). Almost half of patients with BRVO may be attributed to systemic hypertension. As for ocular risk factors, patients with glaucoma – specifically open-angle glaucoma – are 3–4 times more likely to develop an RVO (5, 9, 13, 14).

There are similarities between risk factors for venous thromboembolism (VTE) and RVO, such as age, cancer, thrombophilia, oral contraceptive use, and immobilization; however, the literature is varied. Advancing age is a common risk factor for VTE and RVO (15). In a Danish study that studied the absolute cancer risk within 6 months of an RVO it was found that it was similar to the general population and patients with RVO are not at increased risk (16). As for thrombophilia and its association with RVO, the reports are varied. Among common thrombophilic risk factors, only hyperhomocysteinemia and anticardiolipin antibodies were associated with RVO, factor V Leiden only confers a weak correlation, and deficiencies in protein C and S antithrombin were not related to RVO (17, 18). As for antiphospholipid antibodies, anticardiolipin antibodies and not lupus anticoagulant were correlated with RVO in both BRVO and CRVO (19). Raised total homocysteine levels have been observed and found to be associated with RVO (18–21). Interestingly, only a raised total homocysteine was found to be related and homozygosity for methylenetetrahydrofolate reductase (MTHFR) C677T genotype, which is essential in the metabolism of homocysteine, was not found to be related to RVO (21).

The use of oral contraceptives has been associated with VTE and stroke (22). However, in a large cohort study of 63,000 women accumulating over 850,000 person-years, studying the relationship between oral contraceptive use and eye disease found an association between recent oral contraceptive use and retinal vascular lesions, however, not specific to RVO (23). Although evidence of immobilization and RVO is lacking, the relationship between dehydration and RVO is not absent. Dehydration as a risk factor was not reported in large-scale studies; instead, there exist only case series and reports of patients with RVO following an episode of severe exercise and/or dehydration. These cases do share similarities in that all were diagnosed with CRVO and were young (24–28).

There does not appear to be an increased mortality risk in patients with RVO in general; however, reports are conflicting. There is a trend that younger patients may be at an increased risk (29, 30). In the Beijing Eye Study, mortality was identified to be related to diabetic retinopathy but not RVO (31). In another cohort study from the United States, patients with CRVO were not at an increased mortality risk compared to the general population (32). This was also the case for BRVO; in the Beaver Dam Eye Study, patients with BRVO were not found to have an increased 8-year mortality rate (8). In a large population-based study from Taiwan (n = 22,919), it was concluded that RVO does not increase the mortality risk (33). Contradictory to this, Bertelsen et al. reported that mortality was increased in patients with CRVO (34). In an earlier report from the Beijing Eye Study, RVO was associated with an increased mortality in patients under 70 (30). This appears to be the case in another pooled population-based study from the Beaver Dam Eye Study; the Blue Mountains Eye Study reported that RVO was not associated with increased mortality for participants of all ages but for patients aged 70 or less, there was an association with higher cardiovascular mortality (29).

RVO and cardiovascular disease share the same risk factors and it is reasonable to postulate that RVO may be a harbinger for future cardiovascular events. However, the literature is inconclusive in this but tends to favor an association. In the same Taiwanese study, it was revealed that patients with RVO had a higher risk of developing a stroke (33). Wu et al. concluded following a meta-analysis of 15 cohort studies that patients with RVO had an increased risk of stroke and myocardial infarction (35). Zhong et al. performed a meta-analyies of nine cohort studies and identified that RVO patients are at increased risk of future stroke and myocardial infarction (36). In another study from the United Kingdom, there was no significant association between RVO and ischemic heart disease or stroke (37).

15.3 HYPERTENSIVE RETINOPATHY

Hypertensive retinopathy is defined as retinal arteriosclerotic changes secondary to systemic arterial hypertension, first described by Marcus Gunn in the 19th century in a group of patients with hypertension and renal disease (38). It is characterized by a spectrum of retinal vascular signs, including generalized or focal arteriolar narrowing, arterio-venous nicking, increased arteriolar wall opacity, retinal hemorrhages, microaneurysms, cotton-wool spots, hard exudates, and optic disc swelling (39). Even though the name implies retinal involvement alone, based on the chronicity and severity of the disease significant changes occur in both the choroid and the optic nerve. In 2018, the American College of Cardiology/American Heart Association (ACC/AHA) defined various stages of hypertension: elevated blood pressure (120–129 / <80 mmHg), stage 1 hypertension (130–139/80–89 mmHg), and stage 2 hypertension (≥140 / ≥90 mmHg) (40). In response to elevated blood pressure the retinal circulation undergoes various pathophysiological changes. Hypertensive retinopathy incorporates two disease processes – acute elevation of blood pressure triggers vasospasm to auto-regulate perfusion, resulting in acute hypertensive retinopathy, whereas chronically elevated systemic blood pressure sequentially causes vasoconstrictive, sclerotic, and exudative histologic changes in ocular vessels (41).

15.3.1 Epidemiology, Pathogenesis, and Risk Factors

Systemic arterial hypertension is a major global chronic non-communicable disease causing diverse complications (cardiovascular, stroke, kidney disease, and retinopathy) and affecting about one-fourth of the world population. This number is expected to rise to 29% by 2025 (42). In developing nations, hypertension is a significant public health problem and a leading cause of death and disability. At present the absolute prevalence of hypertension is estimated at ~37.7% in the economically developed nations versus 22.9% in developing countries (43). However, the absolute number of individuals affected in the developing nations is significantly higher due to the larger population living in these countries. Based on modeled projections, Kearney et al. estimated that by 2025 there would be about 1.17 billion individuals with hypertension living in the developing countries, comprising as high as three-fourths of the global burden of hypertension (43). Substantial variability is seen in the prevalence across countries as well: hypertension is present in ~35% of the Latin American population, 20–30% of the Chinese and Indian population, and ~14% in sub-Saharan African countries (42). Apart from racial and ethnic differences globally, increasing urbanization, changes in lifestyle, nutritional status, lack of awareness regarding the complications and insufficient treatment are contributing causes for this heterogeneity in the prevalence.

Medical literature subdivides hypertension into various groups; however essential hypertension and malignant hypertension are primarily relevant to the discussion of hypertensive retinopathy. A recording of systolic blood pressure of 140 mmHg and diastolic pressure of 90 mmHg on at least two occasions leads to a diagnosis of essential hypertension (44). Almost 25% of all the adult population and as high as 60% of adults over the age of 60 years are affected with hypertension in the United States alone (45). Hypertension is more prevalent among blacks than whites (46). Studies show that African Americans are more likely to develop hypertensive-related complications, higher mortality rates, and poorer access to anti-hypertensive treatment (47–50). Men are affected more than women; however among adults older than 50 years hypertension is more prevalent among females (46, 51). Lifestyle affects the prevalence of hypertension with agrarian societies and in individuals who are physically active (46).

As hypertension essentially is an asymptomatic disease, most patients remain undiagnosed or inadequately treated through the course of the disease. A survey done in the United States in 2011–2012 found that 82.8% of adults were aware of their hypertension, 75.7% were currently taking medication to lower their blood pressure, and 51.9% had their blood pressure controlled to less than 140/90 mmHg (52). Young adults aged 18–39 had lower awareness, treatment, and control of their hypertension compared with older adults. Hypertension carries a significant risk of cardiovascular mortality in untreated or inadequately treated hypertension. Risk of end-organ damage is twice as high in patients with "borderline" hypertension when compared to those with "optimal" blood pressure (53).

Seven large epidemiologic population studies involving a total of 26,477 participants from the community, both with and without hypertension, studied various signs of hypertensive retinopathy from retinal photographs (39, 54–60). The authors found that signs of hypertensive retinopathy can be reliably identified with standardized examination of these photographs. Good reproducibility was noted for signs like retinal hemorrhages and microaneurysms (κ = 0.80–0.99) and fair reproducibility for arteriovenous nicking and focal arteriolar narrowing (κ = 0.40–0.79) (59, 61). Using digitized photographs, the assessment of vessel diameter narrowing had high reproducibility in four of the seven population studies (59, 61). Signs of hypertensive retinopathy are common in people 40 years of age or older, even in those without a history of hypertension (44). These population studies estimated prevalence rates from 2% to 15% for various signs of retinopathy, in contrast to the report from the Framingham Eye Study that found a prevalence of less than 1% among participants who underwent an ophthalmoscopic examination with dilation (54, 55, 62). The incidence of hypertensive retinopathy is variable and is often confounded by the presence of retinal vascular diseases associated with comorbidities. The Beaver Dam Eye Study evaluated hypertensive retinopathy patients without confounding effect of coexistent vascular disease. The overall incidence of hypertensive retinopathy was about 15%, 8% showed retinopathy, 13% showed arteriolar narrowing, and 2% showed arteriovenous nicking (39).

Black people of African descent are known to have high prevalence of hypertensive retinopathy. This is likely secondary to increased prevalence of hypertension itself among blacks. Wong et al. examined racial differences in the prevalence of and risk factors for hypertensive retinopathy in a population-based sample of 1,860 African Americans and 7,874 white persons, aged 49–73 years, without diabetes (63). The retinal photographs of either eye of the subjects were evaluated for signs of hypertensive retinopathy. The prevalence of retinopathy was twice as high in African Americans than in whites (7.7% versus 4.1%, age- and gender-adjusted odds ratio [OR] 2.03, 95% confidence intervals [CI] 1.65, 2.49). After controlling for 6-year mean arterial blood pressure, use of antihypertensive medications and left ventricular hypertrophy by electrocardiogram (ECG) criteria, the excess prevalence of retinopathy in African Americans was reduced by 40% (adjusted OR 1.61, 95% CI 1.26, 2.06) (63). Variations in the prevalence of specific signs of hypertensive retinopathy according to age and sex have not been consistently demonstrated.

Apart from chronic hypertensive retinopathy changes, sudden elevation of arterial pressure can lead to a rare clinical syndrome called malignant hypertension. It presents with rapid and severe elevation of blood pressure with the systolic component above 200 mmHg or the diastolic reading greater than 140 mmHg. Apart from absolute blood pressure recordings, systemic features that define malignant hypertension include ocular, cardiac, renal, and cerebral injury. If left untreated, persistently elevated malignant hypertension can lead to a rapidly fatal course due to end-organ failure, e.g., myocardial infarction, stroke, renal or cardiac failure (46). Malignant hypertension is seen in nearly 1% of hypertensive patients and is rarely the presenting symptom for hypertension. Well-controlled hypertensive patients seldom manifest with malignant hypertension, and survival rates with effective antihypertensive treatment are nearly 50% for more than 5 years (64). The average age at diagnosis for malignant hypertension is 40 years and most patients have pre-existing primary or secondary hypertension at presentation.

15.4 RETINAL ARTERIAL OCCLUSION

The retina has a dual circulation with the branches of ophthalmic artery supplying the inner retina. Retinal arterial obstruction is a retinal vascular disorder caused secondary to a thrombotic or embolic occlusion of the arteries supplying the retina. It can be central, branch, cilioretinal, or ophthalmic artery obstruction depending on the anatomical location of occlusion. Retinal arterial obstructions cause visual loss that tends to be severe and permanent. In a central retinal artery occlusion (CRAO) the obstruction generally lies posterior to the lamina cribrosa, is usually not visible on ophthalmoscopy, and a third of the central artery occlusions tend to be embolic in nature. In comparison, branch retinal artery occlusions (BRAOs) are mostly embolic, with the obstruction seen in the branches of the central retinal artery after it emerges from the optic nerve head. The embolus is invariably visible on ophthalmoscopy. More proximal occlusions in the ophthalmic artery and even in the internal carotid artery may also lead to visual symptoms; however the symptoms are more chronic in nature. An essential feature to be kept in mind when dealing with retinal arterial obstruction is their frequent association with systemic abnormalities and the need for detailed systemic evaluation.

15.4.1 Types of Retinal Arterial Occlusion

15.4.1.1 Central Retinal Artery Occlusion

A CRAO is an ophthalmic emergency as it causes sudden, massive visual loss due to abrupt disruption of the blood supply to the entire inner retina. This entity was first described by Von Graefe back in 1859 secondary to embolism, and then in 1864 Schweigger described its features on ophthalmoscopy (65). Hayreh and Zimmerman in their study of 260 eyes with CRAO have described four distinct clinical entities under the broad umbrella of CRAO (66). These include:

1. *Non-arteritic CRAO*: This was the classical and most common presentation, with 67% of eyes falling into this group. It is caused by permanent occlusion of the central retinal artery due to an impacted embolus at the narrowest part in the course of the artery, which is at the point of its entry into the optic nerve sheath (and not at the lamina cribrosa, as often erroneously described). The mean age (range) of these patients was 68 (26–90) years with clinical features of permanent CRAO including

retinal infarction, cherry red spot, retinal arterial changes, absence of or reduced circulation on angiography, and no evidence of giant cell arteritis on systemic evaluation. The emboli causing non-arteritic CRAO originate proximally from the larger vessels in the neck like the carotid artery or even the heart. Inflammatory disorders affecting the vessel wall, chronic autoimmune diseases, and hypercoagulable disorders are rare causes of CRAO.

2. *Non-arteritic CRAO with cilioretinal artery sparing*: This entity was noted in 14% of eyes and clinical features were same as non-arteritic CRAO except for sparing of the cilioretinal artery. The mean age (range) was similar to non-arteritic CRAO at 67 (39–87) years. The preservation of cilioretinal artery circulation, however, has significant impact on the visual outcomes and prognosis in these eyes.

3. *Transient non-arteritic CRAO*: As the name suggests, the occlusion in this subtype of CRAO is transient, varying from several minutes to many hours. The duration of occlusion depends on the etiology and therefore determines the visual acuity, clinical presentation, and prognosis. It was recorded in 16% of eyes with the mean age at presentation being 63 (20–89) years. A fluctuation in intraocular pressure, either an acute marked drop in perfusion pressure or a steep rise in intraocular pressure, or a migrating embolus are frequent causes of transient non-arteritic CRAO.

4. *Arteritic CRAO*: This is a frequently seen subtype of CRAO affecting only 4% of the cohort. Giant cell arteritis affecting the common trunk of the posterior ciliary artery or ophthalmic artery is a common cause of arteritic CRAO. As the pathology affects the circulation proximally, the ischemia is not just limited to the retina but also involves the optic nerve head. These eyes frequently have associated arteritic anterior ischemic neuropathy. The clinical signs on fundoscopy are similar to classical non-arteritic CRAO with a significant absence of disc edema due to coexistent optic neuropathy. It is imperative to perform fluorescein angiography in these cases as it confirms the involvement of posterior ciliary artery circulation; otherwise it is possible to miss the diagnosis of arteritic CRAO. The importance lies in the fact that, if not treated with high-dose steroid therapy for giant cell arteritis, eventually the patient could suffer from bilateral blindness due to

CRAO in both eyes. The mean age (range) of patients affected with arteritic CRAO was slightly older than the other subtypes, i.e., 74 (62–87) years.

15.4.1.2 Branch Retinal Artery Occlusion

BRAO is a common vascular occlusive disorder. As the name suggests, it causes inner retinal ischemia secondary to occlusion of a branch of the central retinal artery. The cause of occlusion in almost two-thirds of cases is an embolus which is invariably visible on fundoscopy. However, it might not be the case every time. The various types of emboli and their incidence are mentioned further ahead in the chapter. The usual site for impaction of an embolus is either at the bifurcation of an arteriole or at the point of anatomical narrowing. Based on the natural history of the disease, BRAOs can be either of these two clinical entities: (1) permanent BRAO or (2) transient BRAO (67). Visual acuity of 20/40 or better is seen in almost 74% of patients with permanent BRAO and 94% of patients with transient BRAO, and these numbers improve to 89% and 100% respectively on follow-up (68).

15.4.1.3 Cilioretinal Artery Occlusion

Cilioretinal artery occlusion (CLRAO) is often included under the umbrella of BRAOs. However, this is anatomically incorrect as the cilioretinal artery is a branch of the posterior ciliary artery, unlike branch retinal arteries that are branches of the central retinal artery (68). The natural history studies have defined the course of this particular form of retinal arterial occlusion and classified CLRAOs as a distinct entity. Etiologically CLRAO can be of three types: (1) non-arteritic CLRAO alone; (2) arteritic CLRAO associated with giant cell arteritis; and (3) non-arteritic CLRAO associated with CRVO or hemi-central vein occlusion (hemi-CRVO) (69–73).

15.4.2 Epidemiology of Retinal Arterial Occlusion

CRAO is quite rare in the population. The incidence is estimated to be about 1–2 per 100,000 per year according to various studies. A study done in the United States gave an overall incidence of 1.9 per 100,000 per year after adjusting for age and sex. The same study reported the incidence to be higher among males at 1.67 per 100,000 per year when compared to females, who had an incidence of 1.02 per 100,000 per year (74). Another study looking at the incidence of CRAO in a Taiwanese population reported the rate to be 1.64 per 100,000 per year. Males are affected twice as commonly as females (75).

As already mentioned, the age group of patients with CRAO varies considerably depending on the etiology; however the most common age group of patients is 60 years or older. As described by Hayreh et al., the non-arteritic subtypes occur at a mean age of 63 years (range 20–90 years). However, the arteritic subtype, due to its association with giant cell arteritis, has been documented to occur in an older population, mean age 74 years (range 62–87 years). Between the two eyes, some studies have shown higher incidence in the right eye whereas some have shown a higher incidence in the left, and some studies show both eyes to be equally affected (66, 74, 76). However, considering the multiple papers published regarding CRAO there has been no evidence to support increased incidence on either side. Bilateral involvement is seen in about 1–2% of cases. There is no evidence in the literature to suggest that race or any other demographic feature predisposes to CRAO development (65).

15.4.3 Pathogenesis of Retinal Arterial Occlusion

The most common cause of retinal artery occlusions is embolism. The emboli travel from the original source to the retinal vessels and are impacted at the sites of anatomical narrowing or bifurcation. The central retinal artery has a lumen diameter of roughly 2 mm, and the most common points of embolus impaction are two points of narrowing – the point where it enters the optic nerve and the point where it enters the globe as it crosses the lamina cribrosa (77). As both these points lie behind the globe, the embolus is not visible on fundoscopy in CRAO eyes. The most common sources for retinal artery embolism have been described to be cardiac and carotid artery (78). Retinal emboli are usually of three types – calcific, cholesterol (Hollenhorst plaques), or platelet-fibrin debris (Fisher plaques) – and can be detected in 60–70% of patients with retinal artery occlusion (79, 80). Their prevalence in population studies has been estimated at 1.3–1.4%, with 10-year incidence being almost 2.9% (81, 82). Asymptomatic retinal emboli are prevalent in the population aged 40 years and older and are often transient; in one study 90% of retinal emboli detected in baseline photographs were not present 5 years later (81).

The major sources of emboli are plaques in the carotid artery and Hayreh et al. documented the presence of plaques in 71% of eyes with CRAO and 60% of eyes with BRAO on carotid Doppler/angiography. In the heart the sources of emboli are valvular lesions, congenital cardiac abnormalities, or tumor in the left atrium or myxoma (83). It is important to know that carotid artery disease can lead to retinal artery occlusion by other mechanisms as well. Hemodynamic changes reducing ocular perfusion could result from a severely stenosed carotid artery (≥70%) or nocturnal arterial hypotension coexisting with a markedly stenosed carotid artery (66). These changes effectively reduce the blood supply to the globe, leading to either a transient retinal arterial occlusion or chronic ischemia.

An important discussion however is that even though extracranial internal carotid artery stenosis is the most commonly identified cause of retinal and ocular ischemia, it is not the most common cause of retinal artery occlusion. Various studies have demonstrated that significant carotid artery stenosis has been identified using Doppler/angiography in only 14–18.7% of branch and central retinal artery occlusions (78, 84). The explanation for this is multifactorial (78). Firstly, the carotid Doppler study only studies the part of the vessel exposed in the neck; however it is possible that severe stenosis could lie proximal or distal to the same. Secondly, the "microemboli" are the cause of obstruction in the vast majority of retinal artery occlusion cases. The atherosclerotic plaques are the most common source for these microemboli, which may be present in vessels with or without any significant stenosis. Another possible pathomechanism for central artery occlusion is arterial spasm induced by the serotonin released from platelet aggregation in atherosclerotic plaques (85).

15.4.4 Risk Factors for Retinal Arterial Occlusion

Aside from carotid artery disease as the etiology responsible for central retinal artery occlusion, there are a plethora of systemic risk factors that predispose an eye to arterial occlusion.

Elevated cholesterol levels are responsible for atherosclerotic plaque build-up in the blood vessels. These plaques eventually throw microemboli responsible for retinal arterial occlusion. It is essential to note that high body mass index and triglycerides have a less important role in the atherogenic pathogenesis of retinal artery occlusion, while the low-density lipoproteins is the fraction that has a more potent role in the etiology.

15.4.4.1 Comorbidities Like Diabetes Mellitus and Systemic Hypertension

Several pathogenic mechanisms are common to diabetes and retinal artery occlusion at both macrovascular and microvascular levels (86). They include arterial stiffening, atherosclerotic change, arteriolar narrowing, and microvascular nicking (87, 88). It is understandable therefore that patients with diabetes mellitus are at a higher risk of retinal arterial occlusion than the non-diabetic population. Chang et al. have reported the incidence of retinal arterial occlusion in patients with diabetes to be 2.30 times (95% CI 1.89–2.80) higher than those without diabetes. After adjustment for confounders the incidence was found to be 2.11 times (95% CI 1.71–2.59) higher (89). Retinal artery occlusion also occurs commonly in patients with systemic hypertension (90, 91). A systematic, longitudinal, prospective study from 1973 to 2000 on 439 patients (499 eyes) with CRAO found a significantly higher prevalence of systemic hypertension in patients with hypertension (52%; 95% CI 45%, 58%) than in age- and period-matched healthy controls (30.1%) (78).

Retinal artery occlusion has also been reported with cardiovascular risk factors and with both subclinical and clinical stroke (90, 92–94). Nearly half the patients with retinal artery occlusion in one study were reported to have echocardiographic abnormalities, and 10% needed systemic treatment (95). The disorder has been associated with an increased risk of cardiovascular disease and mortality (94). In a prospective study of 99 patients with retinal artery occlusions followed up for a mean duration of 4.2 years, the absolute risk of death was estimated at 8% per year; coronary events caused 60% of the deaths (96). Mortality rates might also vary due to the presence of retinal emboli; a study of 86 patients with retinal artery occlusions showed that mortality rates for those without visible retinal emboli were similar to age–sex controls, whereas patients with visible emboli had substantially higher mortality than controls (97). In young adults with retinal arterial occlusion, cardiac valvular disease was the most commonly recognized etiology (in 19% of cases) (98).

The risk of stroke following a central retinal artery occlusion is also higher if the embolic source was known as opposed to being undetermined (80). A Taiwanese study found that approximately 20% of patients with retinal artery occlusion suffered a cerebrovascular accident within 3 years of the incident ocular event (75). Another Korean study also proved higher risk of stroke in patients with retinal arterial occlusion as almost 8% of the subjects had an ischemic stroke within 1 year prior to or after their incident ocular event (99).

Hematological disorders like thrombophilia (protein C pathway deficiency, lupus anticoagulant), antiphospholipid antibodies, and homocystenemia are systemic risk factors for retinal arterial occlusion (100–104). Thrombophilia associated with exogenous estrogens, oral contraceptives, clomiphene citrate, estrogen progestin oral contraceptives, and selective estrogen receptor modulators (SERMS) may lead to central retinal artery occlusion (105–107). Other prothrombotic conditions like factor V Leiden, prothrombin 20210A, and homozygosity for MTHFR C677T are not found to be associated with retinal artery occlusion (103, 108). Case reports of central retinal artery occlusion in patients with sickle cell hemoglobinopathy, leukemia, systemic non-Hodgkin's lymphoma, and orbital lymphoma have also been reported (109–112).

Central retinal artery occlusion is known to occur perioperatively following ophthalmic, orbital, or head and neck surgical procedures. Reports of central retinal artery occlusion associated with peribulbar or retrobulbar injection and intraocular gas injection are present in the literature. One of the most frequently practiced procedures in medical retina is intravitreal injections of anti-vascular growth factor injections for various macular diseases. Gao et al. observed a cohort of 16,686 patients who received a cumulative number of 125,108 injections over a 2-year period (113). Twelve patients in total (8 with CRAO, 4 with BRAO) developed retinal artery occlusion within 90 days of injection. They reported an incidence of one retinal artery occlusion per 1,389 patients, i.e., 0.072%.

Anecdotal reports of central branch or cilioretinal artery occlusion associated with Fabry's disease, incontinentia pigmenti, cocaine usage, migraine, Marfan's syndrome, nephrotic syndrome, and snake bite have been made (114–119). There are numerous case reports of Susac syndrome (retinocochleocerebral syndrome), which is a triad of encephalopathy, cochlear hearing loss, and BRAO (120).

Vasculitis, especially giant cell arteritis, is an important cause of central artery occlusion and CLRAO, especially in the elderly (71). Other inflammatory and infective causes for retinal artery occlusion include systemic lupus erythematosus, polyarteritis nodosa, Takayasu arteritis, Churg–Strauss syndrome, ocular Behçet's disease, autoimmune deficiency syndrome, dengue fever, and West Nile virus (78).

15.5 OCULAR ISCHEMIC SYNDROME

Ocular ischemic syndrome is a condition characterized by ocular signs secondary to severe and chronic arterial hypoperfusion. Severe carotid artery disease (stenosis or occlusion) is usually the most common cause for ocular hypoperfusion in these eyes. One of the first descriptions of this disease came in the year 1963 when Hedges described it in a 48-year-old woman with complete obstruction of her left internal carotid artery (121). The ophthalmoscopy findings were described as peripheral hemorrhages with dilated retinal veins and Hedges attributed these findings to retinal hypoxia. In the same year Kearns and Hollenhorst described a case with similar signs in the presence of advanced carotid artery stenosis and named it venous stasis retinopathy (122). They reported about 5% of their patients with unilateral stenosis occlusion of the carotid artery had features of venous stasis retinopathy.

As some authors used the same term to describe non-ischemic CRVO, which is a clinical entity with entirely different pathogenesis, the use of this nomenclature was discontinued to describe signs of ocular ischemia (123). Over subsequent years various other terms were employed to best illustrate the signs of ocular ischemia secondary to carotid artery stenosis. Additional names introduced include hypoperfusion retinopathy, hypotensive retinopathy, ischemic ocular inflammation, and ischemic oculopathy (124, 125). Eventually the term ocular ischemic syndrome was coined to describe all anterior- and posterior-segment signs associated with ocular hypoperfusion secondary to carotid occlusive disease (126). Due to a varied combination of signs and subtle presentation, ocular ischemic syndrome is unfortunately often missed or misdiagnosed (127).

15.5.1 Epidemiology of Ocular Ischemic Syndrome, Pathogenesis, and Risk Factors

The precise incidence of ocular ischemic syndrome in the population is undetermined. Sturrock and Mueller estimated an incidence of 7.5 cases per million population annually based on their work on patients with chronic ocular ischemia (128). However, due to frequent misdiagnosis of the entity, this incidence rate could be falsely low. Ocular ischemic syndrome occurs most commonly in the elderly at a mean age of 65 years (129, 130). It generally does not occur in individuals younger than 50 years of age (126, 131). Males are affected twice as frequently as females, which mirrors the higher incidence of atherosclerotic disease among males. There is no evidence of racial predilection for disease. Bilateral involvement may occur in up to 22% of cases (126, 132, 133).

15.5.2 Pathogenesis and Risk Factors of Ocular Ischemic Syndrome

Long-standing decrease in arterial inflow is the basic pathogenetic mechanism of ocular ischemic syndrome. The period and extent of impairment in blood flow to develop the syndrome are still unknown. It is important to understand that clinical features of ocular ischemia do not develop in all eyes with carotid occlusive disease and are dependent on the efficiency of the collateral circulation between the external and internal carotid arteries or between the two internal carotid arteries (130). In fact it has been reported that those patients with well-established collateral circulation may not manifest signs of ocular ischemia even in the presence of complete internal carotid artery occlusion. In contrast, poor collateral circulation with even 50% carotid artery stenosis can result in ocular ischemic syndrome (127). Contemporaneous occurrence of neurologic signs and cerebral infarctions in patients with ocular ischemic syndrome is also a result of insufficient collateral circulation (134). It is relevant to mention that patterns of occlusion can vary in the terms of degree of stenosis (50% to complete occlusion), vessels involved (common carotid artery, internal carotid artery) or laterality (unilateral or bilateral carotid arterial system involvement) (135–137).

The evidence of effect of collateralization in eyes with ocular ischemic syndrome was demonstrated in the work of Ho et al. (138). They used color Doppler imaging to understand the blood flow velocity and vascular resistance in ocular circulation. Twelve out of 16 eyes showed reversal of vascular flow in the ophthalmic artery, indicating collateral formation through external carotid artery systems due to obstructions in the internal carotid artery (138). All the eyes with ocular ischemic syndrome in the study had reduced peak systolic flow velocity in the central retinal artery. In rare cases, Doppler imaging studies have shown isolated ophthalmic artery stenosis leading to ocular ischemic syndrome in the absence of carotid artery stenosis. Almost 29% of patients with symptomatic carotid artery occlusion manifest retinal vascular changes but are asymptomatic; however annually about 1.5% of these patients progress to manifest symptomatic ocular ischemic syndrome (139). Ocular ischemic syndrome has been noted in 18% of patients secondary to surgical anastomotic treatments for carotid occlusive disease (131).

Key features frequently seen in patients with ocular ischemic syndrome include blot retinal hemorrhages, dilated beaded retinal veins, ocular neovascularization, and decreased ocular perfusion pressure in the setting of severe ipsilateral or bilateral carotid artery obstruction (130). Ischemic changes to the optic nerve, choroid, retinal pigment epithelium, and outer segments of photoreceptors have also been demonstrated in eyes with ocular ischemic syndrome (140). Posterior ciliary artery hypoperfusion is the rationale for involvement of these structures. Experimental studies by McFazdean et al. have corroborated these findings, suggesting posterior ciliary artery hypoperfusion leads to visual loss in eyes with ocular ischemic syndrome (141). In eyes with reversal of blood flow in ophthalmic artery and reduced flow in retrobulbar vessels, the ophthalmic artery behaves as a steal artery and shunts blood flow away from the globe to the low-resistance extracranial circuit, causing further worsening of ocular tissue ischemia (142–144).

REFERENCES

1. Rogers S, McIntosh RL, Cheung N, Lim L, Wang JJ, Mitchell P, et al. The prevalence of retinal vein occlusion: pooled data from population studies from the United States, Europe, Asia, and Australia. *Ophthalmology.* 2010;117(2):313–19.e1.

2. Song P, Xu Y, Zha M, Zhang Y, Rudan I. Global epidemiology of retinal vein occlusion: a systematic review and meta-analysis of prevalence, incidence, and risk factors. *J Glob Health.* 2019;9(1):010427.

3. Quartilho A, Simkiss P, Zekite A, Xing W, Wormald R, Bunce C. Leading causes of certifiable visual loss in England and Wales during the year ending 31 March 2013. *Eye (Lond).* 2016;30(4):602–7.

4. Cugati S, Wang JJ, Rochtchina E, Mitchell P. Ten-year incidence of retinal vein occlusion in an older population: the Blue Mountains Eye Study. *Arch Ophthalmol.* 2006;124(5):726–32.

5. Klein R, Moss SE, Meuer SM, Klein BE. The 15-year cumulative incidence of retinal vein occlusion: the Beaver Dam Eye Study. *Arch Ophthalmol.* 2008;126(4):513–18.

6. Hayreh SS, Zimmerman MB, Podhajsky P. Incidence of various types of retinal vein occlusion and their recurrence and demographic characteristics. *Am J Ophthalmol.* 1994;117(4):429–41.

7. The Central Vein Occlusion Study Group. Natural history and clinical management of central retinal vein occlusion. *Arch Ophthalmol.* 1997;115(4):486–91.

8. Klein R, Klein BE, Moss SE, Meuer SM. The epidemiology of retinal vein occlusion: the Beaver Dam Eye Study. *Trans Am Ophthalmol Soc.* 2000;98:133–41; discussion 41–3.

9. Mitchell P, Smith W, Chang A. Prevalence and associations of retinal vein occlusion in Australia. The Blue Mountains Eye Study. *Arch Ophthalmol.* 1996;114(10):1243–7.

10. Sperduto RD, Hiller R, Chew E, Seigel D, Blair N, Burton TC, et al. Risk factors for hemiretinal vein occlusion: comparison with risk factors for central and branch retinal vein occlusion: the eye disease case-control study. *Ophthalmology.* 1998;105(5):765–71.

11. Koh V, Cheung CY, Li X, Tian D, Wang JJ, Mitchell P, et al. Retinal vein occlusion in a multi-ethnic Asian population: the Singapore Epidemiology of Eye Disease study. *Ophthalmic Epidemiol.* 2016;23(1):6–13.

12. Green WR, Chan CC, Hutchins GM, Terry JM. Central retinal vein occlusion: a prospective histopathologic study of 29 eyes in 28 cases. *Retina.* 2005;25(5 Suppl):27–55.

13. Rath EZ, Frank RN, Shin DH, Kim C. Risk factors for retinal vein occlusions. A case-control study. *Ophthalmology.* 1992;99(4):509–14.

14. The Eye Disease Case-control Study Group. Risk factors for branch retinal vein occlusion. *Am J Ophthalmol.* 1993;116(3):286–96.

15. Wong P, Baglin T. Epidemiology, risk factors and sequelae of venous thromboembolism. *Phlebology.* 2012;27 Suppl 2:2–11.

16. Hansen AT, Veres K, Prandoni P, Adelborg K, Sørensen HT. Retinal vein thrombosis and risk of occult cancer: a nationwide cohort study. *Cancer Med.* 2018;7(11):5789–95.

17. Janssen MC, den Heijer M, Cruysberg JR, Wollersheim H, Bredie SJ. Retinal vein occlusion: a form of venous thrombosis or a complication of atherosclerosis? A meta-analysis of thrombophilic factors. *Thromb Haemost.* 2005;93(6):1021–6.

18. Bucciarelli P, Passamonti SM, Gianniello F, Artoni A, Martinelli I. Thrombophilic and cardiovascular risk factors for retinal vein occlusion. *Eur J Intern Med.* 2017;44:44–8.

19. Zhu W, Wu Y, Xu M, Wang JY, Meng YF, Gu Z, et al. Antiphospholipid antibody and risk of retinal vein occlusion: a systematic review and meta-analysis. *PLoS One.* 2014;10(4):e0122814.

20. Cahill MT, Stinnett SS, Fekrat S. Meta-analysis of plasma homocysteine, serum folate, serum vitamin B(12), and thermolabile MTHFR genotype as risk factors for retinal vascular occlusive disease. *Am J Ophthalmol.* 2003;136(6):1136–50.

21. McGimpsey SJ, Woodside JV, Cardwell C, Cahill M, Chakravarthy U. Homocysteine, methylenetetrahydrofolate reductase C677T polymorphism, and risk of retinal vein occlusion: a meta-analysis. *Ophthalmology.* 2009;116(9):1778–87.e1.

22. Bassuk SS, Manson JE. Oral contraceptives and menopausal hormone therapy: relative and attributable risks of cardiovascular disease, cancer, and other health outcomes. *Ann Epidemiol.* 2015;25(3):193–200.

23. Vessey MP, Hannaford P, Mant J, Painter R, Frith P, Chappel D. Oral contraception and eye disease: findings in two large cohort studies. *Br J Ophthalmol.* 1998;82(5):538–42.

24. Rouhani B, Mandava N, Olson JL. Central retinal vein occlusion after intense exercise in healthy patients. *Retin Cases Brief Rep.* 2010;4(2):105–8.

25. Moisseiev E, Sagiv O, Lazar M. Intense exercise causing central retinal vein occlusion in a young patient: case report and review of the literature. *Case Rep Ophthalmol.* 2014;5(1):116–20.

26. Weiss KD, Kuriyan AE, Flynn HW, Jr. Central retinal vein occlusion after prolonged vomiting and repeated Valsalva maneuvers associated with gastroenteritis and dehydration. *Ophthalmic Surg Lasers Imaging Retina.* 2014;45 Online:e23–5.

27. Jacobs DJ, Ahmad F, Pathengay A, Flynn HW, Jr. Central retinal vein occlusion after intense exercise: response to intravitreal bevacizumab. *Ophthalmic Surg Lasers Imaging.* 2011;42:e59–62.

28. Francis PJ, Stanford MR, Graham EM. Dehydration is a risk factor for central retinal vein occlusion in young patients. *Acta Ophthalmol Scand.* 2003;81(4):415–16.

29. Cugati S, Wang JJ, Knudtson MD, Rochtchina E, Klein R, Klein BE, et al. Retinal vein occlusion and vascular mortality: pooled data analysis of 2 population-based cohorts. *Ophthalmology.* 2007;114(3):520–4.

30. Xu L, Liu WW, Wang YX, Yang H, Jonas JB. Retinal vein occlusions and mortality: the Beijing Eye Study. *Am J Ophthalmol*. 2007;144(6):972–3.

31. Wang YX, Zhang JS, You QS, Xu L, Jonas JB. Ocular diseases and 10-year mortality: the Beijing Eye Study 2001/2011. *Acta Ophthalmol*. 2014;92(6):e424–8.

32. Elman MJ, Bhatt AK, Quinlan PM, Enger C. The risk for systemic vascular diseases and mortality in patients with central retinal vein occlusion. *Ophthalmology*. 1990;97(11):1543–8.

33. Chen YY, Yen YF, Lin JX, Feng SC, Wei LC, Lai YJ, et al. Risk of ischemic stroke, hemorrhagic stroke, and all-cause mortality in retinal vein occlusion: a nationwide population-based cohort study. *J Ophthalmol*. 2018;2018:8629429.

34. Bertelsen M, Linneberg A, Christoffersen N, Vorum H, Gade E, Larsen M. Mortality in patients with central retinal vein occlusion. *Ophthalmology*. 2014;121(3):637–42.

35. Wu CY, Riangwiwat T, Limpruttidham N, Rattanawong P, Rosen RB, Deobhakta A. Association of retinal vein occlusion with cardiovascular events and mortality: a systematic review and meta-analysis. *Retina*. 2019;39(9):1635–45.

36. Zhong C, You S, Zhong X, Chen GC, Xu T, Zhang Y. Retinal vein occlusion and risk of cerebrovascular disease and myocardial infarction: a meta-analysis of cohort studies. *Atherosclerosis*. 2016;247:170–6.

37. Tsaloumas MD, Kirwan J, Vinall H, O'Leary MB, Prior P, Kritzinger EE, et al. Nine year follow-up study of morbidity and mortality in retinal vein occlusion. *Eye (Lond)*. 2000;14(Pt 6):821–7.

38. Gunn M. Ophthalmoscopic evidence of general arterial disease. *Trans Ophthalmol Soc UK*. 1898;18:356–81.

39. Klein R, Klein BE, Moss SE. The relation of systemic hypertension to changes in the retinal vasculature: the Beaver Dam Eye Study. *Trans Am Ophthalmol Soc*. 1997;95:329–48; discussion 48–50.

40. Whelton PK, Carey RM, Aronow WS, Casey DE, Collins KJ, Himmelfarb CD, et al. 2017 ACC/AHA/AAPA/ABC/ACPM/AGS/APhA/ASH/ASPC/NMA/PCNA guideline for the prevention, detection, evaluation, and management of high blood pressure in adults: a report of the American College of Cardiology/American Heart Association task force on clinical practice guidelines. *Hypertension*. 2018;71(6):e13–e115.

41. Harjasouliha A, Raiji V, Garcia Gonzalez JM. Review of hypertensive retinopathy. *Dis Mon*. 2017;63(3):63–9.

42. Mittal BV, Singh AK. Hypertension in the developing world: challenges and opportunities. *Am J Kidney Dis*. 2010;55(3):590–8.

43. Kearney PM, Whelton M, Reynolds K, Muntner P, Whelton PK, He J. Global burden of hypertension: analysis of worldwide data. *Lancet*. 2005;365(9455):217–23.

44. Wong TY, Mitchell P. Hypertensive retinopathy. *N Engl J Med*. 2004;351(22):2310–17.

45. Strait JB, Lakatta EG. Aging-associated cardiovascular changes and their relationship to heart failure. *Heart Fail Clin*. 2012;8(1):143–64.

46. Oparil S, Acelajado MC, Bakris GL, Berlowitz DR, Cífková R, Dominiczak AF, et al. Hypertension. *Nat Rev Dis Primers*. 2018;4:18014.

47. Gillum RF. Pathophysiology of hypertension in blacks and whites. A review of the basis of racial blood pressure differences. *Hypertension*. 1979;1(5):468–75.

48. Alexander M, Grumbach K, Selby J, Brown AF, Washington E. Hospitalization for congestive heart failure. Explaining racial differences. *JAMA*. 1995;274(13):1037–42.

49. Perneger TV, Klag MJ, Feldman HI, Whelton PK. Projections of hypertension-related renal disease in middle-aged residents of the United States. *JAMA*. 1993;269(10):1272–7.

50. Otten MW, Jr., Teutsch SM, Williamson DF, Marks JS. The effect of known risk factors on the excess mortality of black adults in the United States. *JAMA*. 1990;263(6):845–50.

51. The sixth report of the Joint National Committee on prevention, detection, evaluation, and treatment of high blood pressure. *Arch Intern Med*. 1997;157(21):2413–46.

52. Nwankwo T, Yoon SS, Burt V, Gu Q. Hypertension among adults in the United States: National Health and Nutrition Examination Survey, 2011–2012. *NCHS Data Brief*. 2013(133):1–8.

53. National High Blood Pressure Education Program Working Group report on primary prevention of hypertension. *Arch Intern Med*. 1993;153(2):186–208.

54. Klein R, Klein BE, Moss SE, Wang Q. Hypertension and retinopathy, arteriolar narrowing, and arteriovenous nicking in a population. *Arch Ophthalmol*. 1994;112(1):92–8.

55. Sharp PS, Chaturvedi N, Wormald R, McKeigue PM, Marmot MG, Young SM. Hypertensive retinopathy in Afro-Caribbeans and Europeans. Prevalence and risk factor relationships. *Hypertension*. 1995;25(6):1322–5.

56. Stolk RP, Vingerling JR, de Jong PT, Dielemans I, Hofman A, Lamberts SW, et al. Retinopathy, glucose, and insulin in an elderly population. The Rotterdam Study. *Diabetes*. 1995;44(1):11–15.

57. Yu T, Mitchell P, Berry G, Li W, Wang JJ. Retinopathy in older persons without diabetes and its relationship to hypertension. *Arch Ophthalmol*. 1998;116(1):83–9.

58. Klein R, Sharrett AR, Klein BE, Chambless LE, Cooper LS, Hubbard LD, et al. Are retinal arteriolar abnormalities related to atherosclerosis? The Atherosclerosis Risk in Communities Study. *Arterioscler Thromb Vasc Biol*. 2000;20(6):1644–50.

59. Wong TY, Klein R, Sharrett AR, Manolio TA, Hubbard LD, Marino EK, et al. The prevalence and risk factors of retinal microvascular abnormalities in older persons: the Cardiovascular Health Study. *Ophthalmology*. 2003;110(4):658–66.

60. van Leiden HA, Dekker JM, Moll AC, Nijpels G, Heine RJ, Bouter LM, et al. Risk factors for incident retinopathy in a diabetic and nondiabetic population: the Hoorn study. *Arch Ophthalmol*. 2003;121(2):245–51.

61. Wang JJ, Mitchell P, Leung H, Rochtchina E, Wong TY, Klein R. Hypertensive retinal vessel wall signs in a general older population: the Blue Mountains Eye Study. *Hypertension*. 2003;42(4):534–41.

62. Leibowitz HM, Krueger DE, Maunder LR, Milton RC, Kini MM, Kahn HA, et al. The Framingham Eye Study monograph: an ophthalmological and epidemiological study of cataract, glaucoma, diabetic retinopathy, macular degeneration, and visual acuity in a general population of 2631 adults, 1973–1975. *Surv Ophthalmol*. 1980;24(Suppl):335–610.

63. Wong TY, Klein R, Duncan BB, Nieto FJ, Klein BE, Couper DJ, et al. Racial differences in the prevalence of hypertensive retinopathy. *Hypertension*. 2003;41(5):1086–91.

64. Laragh J. Laragh's lessons in pathophysiology and clinical pearls for treating hypertension. *Am J Hypertens*. 2001;14(9 Pt 1):837–54.

65. Hayreh SS. Central retinal artery occlusion. *Indian J Ophthalmol*. 2018;66(12):1684–94.

66. Hayreh SS, Zimmerman MB. Central retinal artery occlusion: visual outcome. *Am J Ophthalmol*. 2005;140(3):376–91.

67. Hayreh SS. Ocular vascular occlusive disorders: natural history of visual outcome. *Prog Retin Eye Res*. 2014;41:1–25.

68. Hayreh SS, Podhajsky PA, Zimmerman MB. Branch retinal artery occlusion: natural history of visual outcome. *Ophthalmology*. 2009;116(6):1188–94.e1–4.

69. Hayreh SS. Anterior ischaemic optic neuropathy. II. Fundus on ophthalmoscopy and fluorescein angiography. *Br J Ophthalmol*. 1974;58(12):964–80.

70. Hayreh SS. Anterior ischaemic optic neuropathy. Differentiation of arteritic from non-arteritic type and its management. *Eye (Lond)*. 1990;4 (Pt 1):25–41.

71. Hayreh SS, Podhajsky PA, Zimmerman B. Ocular manifestations of giant cell arteritis. *Am J Ophthalmol*. 1998;125(4):509–20.

72. Hayreh SS, Zimmerman B. Management of giant cell arteritis. Our 27-year clinical study: new light on old controversies. *Ophthalmologica*. 2003;217(4):239–59.

73. Hayreh SS, Fraterrigo L, Jonas J. Central retinal vein occlusion associated with cilioretinal artery occlusion. *Retina*. 2008;28(4):581–94.

74. Leavitt JA, Larson TA, Hodge DO, Gullerud RE. The incidence of central retinal artery occlusion in Olmsted County, Minnesota. *Am J Ophthalmol*. 2011;152(5):820–3.e2.

75. Chang YS, Jan RL, Weng SF, Wang JJ, Chio CC, Wei FT, et al. Retinal artery occlusion and the 3-year risk of stroke in Taiwan: a nationwide population-based study. *Am J Ophthalmol*. 2012;154(4):645–52.e1.

76. Brown GC, Magargal LE. Central retinal artery obstruction and visual acuity. *Ophthalmology*. 1982;89(1):14–19.

77. Lavin P, Patrylo M, Hollar M, Espaillat KB, Kirshner H, Schrag M. Stroke risk and risk factors in patients with central retinal artery occlusion. *Am J Ophthalmol*. 2018;196:96–100.

78. Hayreh SS, Podhajsky PA, Zimmerman MB. Retinal artery occlusion: associated systemic and ophthalmic abnormalities. *Ophthalmology*. 2009;116(10):1928–36.

79. Cho KH, Ahn SJ, Cho JH, Jung C, Han MK, Park SJ, et al. The characteristics of retinal emboli and its association with vascular reperfusion in retinal artery occlusion. *Invest Ophthalmol Vis Sci*. 2016;57(11):4589–98.

80. Egan RA, Lutsep HL. Prevalence of retinal emboli and acute retinal artery occlusion in acute ischemic stroke. *J Stroke Cerebrovasc Dis*. 2020;29(2):104446.

81. Klein R, Klein BE, Jensen SC, Moss SE, Meuer SM. Retinal emboli and stroke: the Beaver Dam Eye Study. *Arch Ophthalmol*. 1999;117(8):1063–8.

82. Mitchell P, Wang JJ, Li W, Leeder SR, Smith W. Prevalence of asymptomatic retinal emboli in an Australian urban community. *Stroke*. 1997;28(1):63–6.

83. Schmidt D, Hetzel A, Geibel-Zehender A. Retinal arterial occlusion due to embolism of suspected cardiac tumors – report on two patients and review of the topic. *Eur J Med Res*. 2005;10(7):296–304.

84. Sharma S, Pater JL, Lam M, Cruess AF. Can different types of retinal emboli be reliably differentiated from one another? An inter- and intraobserver agreement study. *Can J Ophthalmol*. 1998;33(3):144–8.

85. Hayreh SS, Piegors DJ, Heistad DD. Serotonin-induced constriction of ocular arteries in atherosclerotic monkeys. Implications for ischemic disorders of the retina and optic nerve head. *Arch Ophthalmol*. 1997;115(2):220–8.

86. Klein R, Klein BE, Moss SE, Wong TY. Retinal vessel caliber and microvascular and macrovascular disease in type 2 diabetes: XXI: the Wisconsin Epidemiologic Study of Diabetic Retinopathy. *Ophthalmology*. 2007;114(10):1884–92.

87. Stehouwer CD, Henry RM, Ferreira I. Arterial stiffness in diabetes and the metabolic syndrome: a pathway to cardiovascular disease. *Diabetologia*. 2008;51(4):527–39.

88. Song YJ, Cho KI, Kim SM, Jang HD, Park JM, Kim SS, et al. The predictive value of retinal vascular findings for carotid artery atherosclerosis: are further recommendations with regard to carotid atherosclerosis screening needed? *Heart Vessels*. 2013;28(3):369–76.

89. Chang YS, Ho CH, Chu CC, Wang JJ, Tseng SH, Jan RL. Risk of retinal artery occlusion in patients with diabetes mellitus: a retrospective large-scale cohort study. *PLoS One*. 2018;13(8):e0201627.

90. Recchia FM, Brown GC. Systemic disorders associated with retinal vascular occlusion. *Curr Opin Ophthalmol*. 2000;11(6):462–7.

91. Hayreh SS. Prevalent misconceptions about acute retinal vascular occlusive disorders. *Prog Retin Eye Res*. 2005;24(4):493–519.

92. Wong TY, Mitchell P. The eye in hypertension. *Lancet*. 2007;369(9559):425–35.

93. Wijman CA, Gomes JA, Winter MR, Koleini B, Matjucha IC, Pochay VE, et al. Symptomatic and asymptomatic retinal embolism have different mechanisms. *Stroke*. 2004;35(5):e100–2.

94. Patz A. Current concepts in ophthalmology. Retinal vascular diseases. *N Engl J Med*. 1978;298(26):1451–4.

95. Sharma S, Naqvi A, Sharma SM, Cruess AF, Brown GC. Transthoracic echocardiographic findings in patients with acute retinal arterial obstruction. A retrospective review. Retinal Emboli of Cardiac Origin Group. *Arch Ophthalmol*. 1996;114(10):1189–92.

96. Hankey GJ, Slattery JM, Warlow CP. Prognosis and prognostic factors of retinal infarction: a prospective cohort study. *BMJ*. 1991;302(6775):499–504.

97. Savino PJ, Glaser JS, Cassady J. Retinal stroke. Is the patient at risk? *Arch Ophthalmol*. 1977;95(7):1185–9.

98. Greven CM, Slusher MM, Weaver RG. Retinal arterial occlusions in young adults. *Am J Ophthalmol*. 1995;120(6):776–83.

99. Park SJ, Choi NK, Yang BR, Park KH, Lee J, Jung SY, et al. Risk and risk periods for stroke and acute myocardial infarction in patients with central retinal artery occlusion. *Ophthalmology*. 2015;122(11):2336–43.e2.

100. Glueck CJ, Hutchins RK, Jurantee J, Khan Z, Wang P. Thrombophilia and retinal vascular occlusion. *Clin Ophthalmol*. 2012;6:1377–84.

101. Greiner K, Hafner G, Dick B, Peetz D, Prellwitz W, Pfeiffer N. Retinal vascular occlusion and deficiencies in the protein C pathway. *Am J Ophthalmol*. 1999;128(1):69–74.

102. Palmowski-Wolfe AM, Denninger E, Geisel J, Pindur G, Ruprecht KW. Antiphospholipid antibodies in ocular arterial and venous occlusive disease. *Ophthalmologica*. 2007;221(1):41–6.

103. Weger M, Stanger O, Deutschmann H, Leitner FJ, Renner W, Schmut O, et al. The role of hyperhomocysteinemia and methylenetetrahydrofolate reductase (MTHFR) C677T mutation in patients with retinal artery occlusion. *Am J Ophthalmol*. 2002;134(1):57–61.

104. Chua B, Kifley A, Wong TY, Mitchell P. Homocysteine and retinal emboli: the Blue Mountains Eye Study. *Am J Ophthalmol*. 2006;142(2):322–4.

105. Vastag O, Tornóczky J. [Arterial occlusion in the ocular fundus induced by oral contraceptives.] *Orv Hetil*. 1984;125(51):3121–5.

106. Paufique L, Lequin M. [Thrombosis of the retinal artery and oral contraceptives.] *Bull Soc Ophtalmol Fr*. 1968;68(4):512–15.

107. Blade J, Darleguy P, Chanteau Y. [Early thrombosis of the central retinal artery and oral contraceptives.] *Bull Soc Ophtalmol Fr*. 1971;71(1):48–9.

108. Weger M, Renner W, Pinter O, Stanger O, Temmel W, Fellner P, et al. Role of factor V Leiden and prothrombin 20210A in patients with retinal artery occlusion. *Eye (Lond)*. 2003;17(6):731–4.

109. Fine LC, Petrovic V, Irvine AR, Bhisitkul RB. Spontaneous central retinal artery occlusion in hemoglobin sickle cell disease. *Am J Ophthalmol*. 2000;129(5):680–1.

110. Salazar Méndez R, Fonollá Gil M. Unilateral optic disk edema with central retinal artery and vein occlusions as the presenting signs of relapse in acute lymphoblastic leukemia. *Arch Soc Esp Oftalmol*. 2014;89(11):454–8.

111. Gass JD, Trattler HL. Retinal artery obstruction and atheromas associated with non-Hodgkin's large cell lymphoma (reticulum cell sarcoma). *Arch Ophthalmol*. 1991;109(8):1134–9.

112. Rubin PA, Rumelt S. Central retinal artery occlusion due to rapidly expanding orbital lymphoma. *Eye (Lond)*. 1998;12 (Pt 1):159–61.

113. Gao X, Borkar D, Obeid A, Hsu J, Ho AC, Garg SJ. Incidence of retinal artery occlusion following intravitreal antivascular endothelial growth factor injections. *Acta Ophthalmol*. 2019;97(6):e938–e9.

114. Ersoz MG, Ture G. Cilioretinal artery occlusion and anterior ischemic optic neuropathy as the initial presentation in a child female carrier of Fabry disease. *Int Ophthalmol*. 2018;38(2):771–3.

115. Sharma P, Ramirez-Florez S. Consumption of cannabis and cocaine: correct mix for arterial occlusions. *BMJ Case Rep*. 2009;2009.

116. Gutteridge IF, McDonald RA, Plenderleith JG. Branch retinal artery occlusion during a migraine attack. *Clin Exp Optom*. 2007;90(5):371–5.

117. Butt Z, Dhillon B, McLean H. Central retinal artery occlusion in a patient with Marfan's syndrome. *Acta Ophthalmol (Copenh)*. 1992;70(2):281–4.

118. Sinha S, Rau ATK, Kumar RV, Jayadev C, Vinekar A. Bilateral combined central retinal artery and vein occlusion in a 3-year-old child with nephrotic syndrome. *Indian J Ophthalmol*. 2018;66(10):1498–501.

119. Hayreh SS. Transient central retinal artery occlusion following viperine snake bite. *Arch Ophthalmol*. 2008;126(6):870–1; author reply 871.

120. Dörr J, Krautwald S, Wildemann B, Jarius S, Ringelstein M, Duning T, et al. Characteristics of Susac syndrome: a review of all reported cases. *Nat Rev Neurol*. 2013;9(6):307–16.

121. Hedges TR, Jr. Ophthalmoscopic findings in internal carotid artery occlusion. *Am J Ophthalmol*. 1963;55:1007–12.

122. Kearns TP, Hollenhorst RW. Venous-stasis retinopathy of occlusive disease of the carotid artery. *Proc Staff Meet Mayo Clin*. 1963;38:304–12.

123. Hayreh SS. So-called "central retinal vein occlusion". I. Pathogenesis, terminology, clinical features. *Ophthalmologica*. 1976;172(1):1–13.

124. Knox DL. Ischemic ocular inflammation. *Am J Ophthalmol*. 1965;60(6):995–1002.

125. Young LH, Appen RE. Ischemic oculopathy. A manifestation of carotid artery disease. *Arch Neurol*. 1981;38(6):358–6.

126. Brown GC, Magargal LE. The ocular ischemic syndrome. Clinical, fluorescein angiographic and carotid angiographic features. *Int Ophthalmol*. 1988;11(4):239–51.

127. Mizener JB, Podhajsky P, Hayreh SS. Ocular ischemic syndrome. *Ophthalmology*. 1997;104(5):859–64.

128. Sturrock GD, Mueller HR. Chronic ocular ischaemia. *Br J Ophthalmol*. 1984;68(10):716–23.

129. Terelak-Borys B, Skonieczna K, Grabska-Liberek I. Ocular ischemic syndrome – a systematic review. *Med Sci Monit*. 2012;18(8):Ra138–44.

130. Mendrinos E, Machinis TG, Pournaras CJ. Ocular ischemic syndrome. *Surv Ophthalmol*. 2010;55(1):2–34.

131. Kearns TP, Siekert RG, Sundt TM. The ocular aspects of carotid artery bypass surgery. *Trans Am Ophthalmol Soc*. 1978;76:247–65.

132. Brown GC, Brown MM, Magargal LE. The ocular ischemic syndrome and neovascularization. *Trans Pa Acad Ophthalmol Otolaryngol*. 1986;38(1):302–6.

133. De Graeve C, Van de Sompel W, Claes C. Ocular ischemic syndrome: two case reports of bilateral involvement. *Bull Soc Belge Ophtalmol*. 1999;273:69–74.

134. Costa VP, Kuzniec S, Molnar LJ, Cerri GG, Puech-Leão P, Carvalho CA. Clinical findings and hemodynamic changes associated with severe occlusive carotid artery disease. *Ophthalmology*. 1997;104(12):1994–2002.

135. Carter JE. Chronic ocular ischemia and carotid vascular disease. *Stroke*. 1985;16(4):721–8.

136. Berguer R. Idiopathic ischemic syndromes of the retina and optic nerve and their carotid origin. *J Vasc Surg*. 1985;2(5):649–53.

137. Foncea Beti N, Mateo I, Díaz La Calle V, Ruiz J, Gomez Beldarrain M, Garcia-Monco JC. The ocular ischemic syndrome. *Clin Neurol Neurosurg*. 2003;106(1):60–2.

138. Ho AC, Lieb WE, Flaharty PM, Sergott RC, Brown GC, Bosley TM, et al. Color Doppler imaging of the ocular ischemic syndrome. *Ophthalmology*. 1992;99(9):1453–62.

139. Klijn CJ, Kappelle LJ, van Schooneveld MJ, Hoppenreijs VP, Algra A, Tulleken CA, et al. Venous stasis retinopathy in symptomatic carotid artery occlusion: prevalence, cause, and outcome. *Stroke*. 2002;33(3):695–701.

140. Sivalingam A, Brown GC, Magargal LE, Menduke H. The ocular ischemic syndrome. II. Mortality and systemic morbidity. *Int Ophthalmol*. 1989;13(3):187–91.

141. McFadzean RM, Graham DI, Lee WR, Mendelow AD. Ocular blood flow in unilateral carotid stenosis and hypotension. *Invest Ophthalmol Vis Sci*. 1989;30(3):487–90.

142. Boto de los Bueis A, Fernández-Prieto A, Ruiz-Martín MM, Gorospe L, Amorena Santesteban G, Fonseca Sandomingo A. [Bilateral carotid occlusion in young woman. Clinical and hemodynamic ocular results.] *Arch Soc Esp Oftalmol*. 2003;78(4):227–30.

143. Costa VP, Kuzniec S, Molnar LJ, Cerri GG, Puech-Leão P, Carvalho CA. Collateral blood supply through the ophthalmic artery: a steal phenomenon analyzed by color Doppler imaging. *Ophthalmology*. 1998;105(4):689–93.

144. Galle G, Lang GK, Ruprecht KW, Lang GE. [Importance of the orbital collateral circulation for the origin of ischemic ophthalmopathy in stenotic diseases of the internal carotid artery.] *Fortschr Neurol Psychiatr*. 1983;51(8):261–9.

16 Uveitis

De-Kuang Hwang and Yih-Shiou Hwang

16.1 INTRODUCTION

Uveitis is an intraocular inflammatory disorder primarily involving the iris, ciliary body, and choroid. Compared with other common ocular diseases such as cataract, glaucoma, or macular degeneration, uveitis may occur at any age.[1] However, it is noteworthy that this disorder is often sight-threatening. Uveitis is estimated to be responsible for 5–20% of cases of legal blindness in developed countries.[2–5] Because uveitis is more common in middle-aged or younger adults, it is one of the leading causes of visual impairment among the working-age population, with substantial socioeconomic impact globally.[6–9]

16.1.1 Visual Impairment Due to Uveitis

More than one-third of uveitis patients experience significant visual impairment in the affected eyes.[10–12] Irreversible visual decline in uveitis may be caused directly by ocular media opacity, tissue ischemia or infarction, atrophy of retinal tissue, and death or dysfunction of the neurosensory retinal cells. Visual impairment could also be a consequence of various ocular complications associated with inflammation. Different visual outcomes are observed in uveitis patients, depending on the primary inflammatory site, etiology, course, and clinical severity of the disease.

16.1.2 Clinical Diagnosis of Uveitis

Uveitis is typically diagnosed on the basis of history-taking, system review, and intraocular signs observed through various ophthalmic examination techniques, including slit-lamp examination, indirect ophthalmoscopy, and numerous ophthalmological imaging studies. Uveitis can be classified into four anatomical types: *anterior*, when the primary inflammatory site is located in the anterior chamber; *intermediate*, when the inflammatory site is located in the vitreous body and ciliary body; *posterior*, when the uveitis is restricted to the retina and choroid; and *panuveitis*, when the inflammation is not restricted to any of the uveal tissues. According to most epidemiological studies, anterior uveitis is the most common type of uveitis across the world, whereas the proportions of intermediate uveitis, posterior uveitis, and panuveitis vary by country. One reason for this is that the incidence of uveitis due to certain etiologies differs greatly according to country and geographic location.

16.1.3 Etiologies of Uveitis

More than 60 diseases are associated with or directly cause the inflammation of uveal tissue.[13] These etiologies can be categorized into three groups: infectious, noninfectious, and idiopathic. *Infectious uveitis* refers to intraocular inflammation caused mainly by pathogens, which can be identified intraocularly. Pathogens, including viruses, bacteria, parasites, and mycobacteria, may directly infect intraocular tissues or trigger host immune responses, leading to various degrees of uveal inflammation. *Noninfectious uveitis* results from the immune-mediated inflammation associated with systemic or intraocular rheumatological diseases. Systemic rheumatological disorders such as seronegative spondyloarthropathy, Behçet's disease, sarcoidosis, Vogt–Koyanagi–Harada (VKH) disease, juvenile idiopathic arthritis, and multiple sclerosis have been reported to be strongly associated with uveitis. In several situations, the autoimmune or autoinflammatory response can occur with specific presentations that are all restricted to the eyes, such as multifocal choroiditis, birdshot chorioretinopathy, serpiginous choroiditis, and sympathetic ophthalmia (Table 16.1). Exogenous stimulation such as trauma to the eyeball, intraocular surgical procedures, and medications may also induce uveitis. Uveitis cases in which the exact etiologies cannot be identified on the basis of recent knowledge are categorized under "idiopathic uveitis" or "uveitis with unidentified etiology." Idiopathic uveitis is more commonly noninfectious, but could occasionally be infectious with unidentifiable pathogens.

16.1.4 Clinical Presentation of Uveitis

The clinical presentation of uveitis varies. The onset of symptoms may be sudden or insidious. The duration of inflammation may be limited or persistent. The disease course may be acute if the onset is sudden and the duration limited. It may be recurrent if the inflammatory episodes repeat a few months after inactivity. The inflammation may also be chronic and persistent. Studies have suggested that uveitis with a chronic or recurrent course is more likely associated with ocular complications, including disorders of the cornea, lens, retina, and optic nerve.[12, 14–16] Glaucoma is one of the most common complications, with irreversible damage. In particular, the literature has shown that 3.6–29.8% of uveitis patients

DOI: 10.1201/9781315146737-18

Table 16.1 Common etiologies of noninfectious uveitis

Anatomical classification	With systemic diseases	Without systemic diseases
Anterior uveitis	Human leukocyte antigen type B27-related uveitis Juvenile idiopathic arthritis-associated uveitis Behçet's disease Sarcoidosis Diabetic uveitis Tubulointerstitial nephritis and uveitis syndrome	Fuchs heterochromic iridocyclitis Posner–Schlossman syndrome Uveitis–glaucoma–hyphema syndrome
Intermediate uveitis	Sarcoidosis Tubulointerstitial nephritis and uveitis syndrome Multiple sclerosis-related uveitis	Pars planitis
Posterior uveitis	Vogt–Koyanagi–Harada disease Sarcoidosis	Birdshot chorioretinopathy Punctate inner choroidopathy Multiple choroiditis White-dot syndromes[a] Serpiginous choroiditis
Panuveitis	Behçet's disease Sarcoidosis Vogt–Koyanagi–Harada disease	Sympathetic ophthalmia

Note: [a] White-dot syndromes include various diseases such as multiple evanescent white-dot syndrome, acute posterior multifocal placoid pigment epitheliopathy, and acute zonal occult outer retinopathy.

might experience ocular hypertension or glaucoma.[17–20] The elevation of intraocular pressure in eyes with uveitis can occur through numerous different mechanisms.[21, 22] Cataract is another common complication. Up to 38% of uveitis patients will experience cataract.[15, 17] Surgery is typically more complicated if the cataract in the affected eye is comorbid with corneal opacity, shallow anterior chamber, or secluded pupil.[23] Retinal complications such as retinal detachment, macular edema, and neovascularization are most commonly assocated with severe visual loss in uveitis patients.[14, 24]

16.2 EPIDEMIOLOGY OF UVEITIS

Uveitis entities are rare, episodic, and sometimes self-limiting. These factors make it difficult to estimate the incidence and prevalence of uveitis. Limited studies have estimated the epidemiology of uveitis in specific countries, and three main methodologies have been used. First, patients from one or more relevant hospitals in an area may be enrolled and reviewed, and the incidence of uveitis can be estimated according to the total population of the area. Second, a cross-sectional population-based survey may be conducted and the prevalence of uveitis evaluated by the detection of any evidence of intraocular inflammation. Lastly, patients with uveitis may be identified from a large registration database, with or without chart review. Generally, studies based on the first method have

reported relatively low incidence rates of uveitis, whereas community surveys have reported high prevalence rates. The crude incidence and prevalence of uveitis entities are shown in Table 16.2.

16.2.1 Patterns and Distributions of Uveitis Etiologies

Studies have shown that, in general, infectious uveitis is more common in developing countries, whereas noninfectious uveitis is more common in developed countries. However, with certain pathogens, differences in environment, genetic distribution, and catering cultures may also lead to differences in uveitis incidence. For example, ocular toxoplasmosis is reported to constitute 10% of patients with uveitis in China, but less than 0.1% in the United States.[25] Similarly, incidences of Behçet's disease and VKH disease are much higher in the Asian population than in Caucasians.[26, 27] Because gender and age distributions of all disease entities differ greatly, the epidemiologic findings of uveitis vary worldwide.

The distribution of uveitis etiologies varies across the world (Table 16.3). Numerous factors such as genetic distribution, area of endemicity of a pathogen, and catering cultures are associated with certain uveitis entities. Differences in the incidence of various diseases may influence screening protocols and treatment strategies in different countries. For example, hospitals in Asian countries rarely test for the human

Table 16.2 Incidence and prevalence of uveitis in population-based studies

Country	Published year	Sample size	Incidence (1/100,000)	Prevalence (1/100,000)	Anatomical classification (%) Ant.[a]	Int.[b]	Pos.[c]	Pan.[d]	Gender (F: M[e])	Methodology
Africa										
South Africa[27]	1974	652,259	27	–	89.3	–	10.7	–	1: 1.11	Single-center series
America										
USA	1962	29,885	17	204	69.2	–	17.3	13.5	1: 0.98	Single-center series
USA	2004	731,898	52	115	70.1	2.9	2.1	5.0	1: 0.80	Registry database
USA	2008	152,267	26	83	79.0	4.8	9.5	1.0	1: 14.0	Registry database
USA	2013	217,061	25	58	72.3	6.3	21.4	–	1: 1.08	Registry database
USA[f]	2016	3,994,054	–	121	80.9	0.9	8.6	9.6	1: 0.76	Registry database
USA	2018	5,106	–	529	–	–	–	–	1: 0.59	Community survey
Asia										
Japan	1996	1,800,000	–	40	–	–	–	–	–	Questionnaires
India	2000	2,522	–	730	17.8	34.2	43.8	4.1	1: 0.91	Community survey
India	2011	5,150	–	317	21.7	0	47.8	30.4	1: 2.76	Community survey
China	2002	10,500	–	152	40	–	10	50	1: 1.00	Community survey
Taiwan	2012	956,147	111	194	77.7	0.4	6.7	15.2	1: 1.23	Registry database
South Korea	2018	1,094,440	106	173	85.7	14.3			1: 1.18	Registry database
Europe										
Switzerland	1995	600,000	17	-	61.6	10.8	20.5	7.1	1: 1.35	Single-center series
Finland	1995	459,515	23	75	94.2	1.4	3.5	0.9	1: 0.87	Single-center series
Finland	1997	613,426	20	-	87.5	–	8.3	4.2	1: 1.00	Multi-center series
Italy	2001	788.363	11	–	58.0	2.9	26.1	13.0	1: 1.09	Single-center series
Sweden	2019	352,603	108	700	93.0	1.0	5.0	1.0	1: 1.00	Registry database
Oceania										
Australia	2012	1,884	–	80	26.7	0	73.3	0	n/a[g]	Community survey
Australia	2019	3,408,068	22	36	81.1	5.0%	11.0	2.9	1: 1.04	Single-center series

Note: [a] ant., anterior uveitis; [b] int., intermediate uveitis; [c] pos., posterior uveitis; [d] pan., panuveitis; [e] F, female; M, male; [f] epidemiology of noninfectious uveitis in adults was estimated; [g] data not available.

Table 16.3 Large case series of uveitis in different countries

Country	Year	Cases n	Etiology Inf.	Non.	Und.	Specific disease entity (%) B27	Beh.	VKH	Sar.	Bird.
Africa										
Egypt[51]	2010–2017	1,315	27.8%	41.8%	30.4%	6.2	7.4	4.3	11.1	0.0
Ethiopia[52]	2013–2014	98	15.3%	7.1%	77.6%	0.0	1.0	0.0	0.0	0.0
South Africa[53]	2014–2016	198	47.0%	18.2%	34.8%	10.6	0.5	0.0	4.0	0.0
America										
Brazil[55]	2012–2013	1,053	46.3%	37.1%	16.6%	6.4	3.5	7.5	2.3	0.0
Chile[56]	2002–2012	611	28.7%	24.7%	41.2%	4.3	2.1	17.2	1.0	0.5
United States[54]	1984–2014	491	15.7%	48.0%	36.3%	7.7	N/A[a]	N/A[a]	6.7	1.4
Asia										
Bangladesh	2009–2015	652	54.4%	–	46.6%	10.1	0.7	8.4	7.3	0.0
China	1996–2003	1,752	3.1%	52.1%	44.8%	3.3	16.5	15.9	0.2	0.0
India	1996–2001	8,759	30.5%	24.9%	44.6%	4.1	0.6	1.4	4.0	0.0
Iran	2005–2011	475	23.1%	38.9%	38.0%	2.9	12.4	5.3	1.3	0.2
Iraq	2007–2011	318	28.9%	37.1%	34.0%	0.9	8.2	12.3	0.3	0.6
Japan	1994–2003	1,240	8.3%	41.9%	49.8%	4.0	6.7	9.7	14.9	0.0
Myanmar	2013–2014	139	54.7%	10.8%	34.5%	3.6	0.0	1.4	0.0	0.0
Nepal	2014	1,113	24.2%	19.4%	56.4%	6.6	0.4	1.8	1.7	0.0
Philippines	2010–2015	595	25.5%	74.5%[a]	0.0%	0.0	1.3	9.2	0.0	0.0
Saudi Arabia	2001–2010	888	20.3%	52.6%	27.1%	1.1	14.9	22.0	0.6	0.0
Singapore	1997–2010	2,200	29.9%	35.2%	34.9%	8.0	1.2	3.0	1.3	0.0
South Korea	2013	602	17.1%	24.8%	58.1%	8.8	7.1	2.3	2.7	0.0
Sri Lanka	2010–2014	750	16.6%	18.7%	64.7%	3.3	1.2	1.3	6.0	0.0
Taiwan	2001–2014	450	16.3%	57.3%	26.4%	24.9	3.8	10.4	2.7	0.0
Thailand	2014–2015	758	42.5%	41.0%	16.5%	12.4	5.7	13.5	1.2	0.0
Vietnam	2011–2015	212	27.1%	36.3%	36.3%	1.9	6.6	14.2	3.3	0.0
Qatar	2007–2011	310	39.3%	30.4%	30.3%	5.5	7.4	6.8	2.2	0.0
Europe										
France[79]	1991–1996	927	30.6%	36.4%	33.0%	5.0	6.1	2.0	6.4	4.4
Germany[84]	2012–2013	474	17.1%	42.0%	40.9%	10.1	1.9	0.6	11.4	0.6
Ireland[85]	2016–2017	255	18.8%	42.8%	38.4%	2.0	3.5	0.4	12.5	4.3
Italy[50]	2013–2015	990	30.4%	46.4%	23.2%	7.7	4.8	4.1	4.3	0.8
Netherlands[80]	1993	750	N/A	N/A	38.6%	13.1	1.7	0.4	6.4	1.5
Poland[81]	2005–2015	279	26.9%	49.4%	23.7%	9.3	N/A	N/A	6.1	N/A[a]
Spain[82]	2009–2012	1,022	29.2%	45.3%	25.5%	14.0	5.4	1.9	3.5	3.5
Switzerland[39]	1990–1993	435	N/A	N/A	28.3%	15.4	1.1	0.7	6.7	0.9
Turkey[83]	2008–2011	4,863	15.6%	76.1%	8.3%	9.7	24.9	1.5	2.1	N/A[a]
Oceania										
Australia[87]	2009–2015	1,165	21.4%	45.2%	33.4%	22.7	2.1	1.8	6.7	0.4
New Zealand	2008–2014	1,148	25.9%	74.1%[a]	–	28.7	1.6	1.0	5.0	1.0

Note: Inf., infectious; Non., noninfectious; Und., idiopathic; B27, human leukocyte antigen B27-related uveitis (including ankylosing spondylitis); Beh., Behçet's disease; VKH, Vogt–Koyanagi–Harada disease; Sar., sarcoidosis; Bird., birdshot chorioretinopathy; N/A, cases might be presented, but the case numbers were few and not shown.

leukocyte antigen type A29; similarly, serum antibodies to human T-cell lymphoma virus are seldom assayed in Western countries.

Changing patterns and shifting etiologies of uveitis have been observed in several countries. For example, compared with previous case series before 2010, patients in Singapore exhibited a higher percentage of infectious etiologies. Other case series have also demonstrated that the incidence of specific uveitis entities, such as infectious endophthalmitis, sarcoidosis, Behçet's disease, and VKH disease, have changed with time.[28–31]

16.2.2 Incidence and Prevalence of Uveitis in Africa

To date, only one epidemiologic study has estimated the incidence of uveitis in South Africa. Freedman conducted a prospective study to determine the incidence of uveitis at a Johannesburg hospital and reported an incidence of 27 cases per 100,000 person-years in 1974.[32] Most of the uveitis cases involved the anterior chamber (89.3% versus 10.7% in the posterior segment). Regarding uveitis etiology, case series from Africa have reported that infectious etiologies were more commonly diagnosed in South Africa than in Egypt and Ethiopia.[33–35] Human leukocyte antigen (HLA)-B27–related anterior uveitis, sarcoidosis, and Behçet's disease were common causes of noninfectious uveitis in these African countries.

16.2.3 Incidence and Prevalence of Uveitis in North America

The epidemiology of uveitis in the United States has been estimated by various methods. In 1962, Dr. Darrell and colleagues retrospectively enrolled all uveitis patients in a Minnesota community and reported an estimated incidence of 17 cases per 100,000 person-years and a prevalence of 204 per 100,000.[36] Following this study, several epidemiological studies were conducted using medical databases. The databases of Kaiser–Permanente health maintenance system, Veterans Integrated Service Networks, and OptumHealth Reporting and Insights were used in investigating the epidemiology of uveitis in North California, Hawaii, Pacific Northwest region, and a broad range of US regions.[37–40]

Gritz and Acharya and colleagues identified uveitis patients from subsets of the Kaiser–Permanente database and reviewed their medical records. They reported an incidence of 52 and 25 cases per 100,000 person-years in California and Hawaii, respectively, and an estimated prevalence of 115 and 58 per 100,000 population, respectively.[37, 39] Suhler and colleagues reviewed cases from the Veterans Integrated Service

Networks database to estimate the epidemiology of uveitis. Their study revealed an incidence of 26 cases per 100,000 person-years and a prevalence of 83 per 100,000 population in the Pacific Northwest region.[38] Thorne et al. used the OptumHealth Reporting and Insights database without medical chart review; they reported a prevalence of 121 and 29 cases per 100,000 population in adults and children, respectively.[40]

González and colleagues used the National Health and Nutrition Examination Survey to evaluate the prevalence of uveitis in the United States. From the 5,106 randomly selected representative population, 27 patients had a history of uveitis, amounting to a prevalence of 529 per 100,000 population in this survey.[41] No gender predominance in the incidence or prevalence of uveitis was reported in the US studies except in the study by Suhler et al., in which male patients were dominant.[38] These studies revealed that anterior uveitis represented 70–80% of all uveitis cases, whereas intermediate uveitis represented only 1–6%.

Only 16% of all uveitis cases in the United States are caused by infection, whereas the rest are due to mainly noninfectious etiologies. Ankylosing spondylitis and HLA-B27–related uveitis remain the most common cause of anterior uveitis in the United States. Sarcoidosis and juvenile idiopathic arthritis-related uveitis are also common causes. Birdshot chorioretinopathy represents 1–2% of all uveitis cases in the United States.[42]

On the basis of ethnic and genetic factors, more uveitis patients were diagnosed as having Behçet's disease and VKH disease in South America.[43, 44]

16.2.4 Incidence and Prevalence of Uveitis in Asia

Although numerous studies have both demonstrated and discussed the pattern change of uveitis entities in Japan, only one study, conducted in 1996, has estimated the prevalence of uveitis.[45] Nakao and Ohba collected questionnaires from all ophthalmologic clinics in Kagoshima Prefecture and estimated that the prevalence of endogenous uveitis was 40 per 100,000 population in southwest Japan.

Two population-based surveys were conducted in southern India: the Andhra Pradesh Eye Disease Study and the Aravind Comprehensive Eye Survey.[46, 47] The prevalence of uveitis in these areas was estimated at 317–730 per 100,000 population. A population-based survey in southern China also reported a prevalence of 152 per 100,000.[48] Together, these surveys reported a relatively low proportion of anterior uveitis cases (18–40%) and higher proportions of posterior uveitis and panuveitis.

Two teams in Taiwan and South Korea have investigated the epidemiology of uveitis using their respective national health insurance databases. After identifying patients with uveitis who sought medical help, they estimated that the incidence of uveitis was 111 cases and 106 cases per 100,000 person-years in Taiwan and South Korea, respectively.[49, 50] They also estimated the prevalence as 194 and 173 per 100,000 population in Taiwan and South Korea, respectively. One limitation of both studies was that the medical records of the identified patients could not be adequately reviewed to confirm the diagnoses. Both studies reported a higher incidence of anterior uveitis (78% in Taiwan and 86% in South Korea). No gender predominance in the incidence or prevalence of uveitis was reported in the Asian studies.

Noninfectious etiologies are the most common cause of uveitis in most Asian countries. However, uveitis case series from Myanmar and Nepal showed that only 11% and 19%, respectively, were noninfectious.[51, 52] Infections are the most common cause of uveitis in Myanmar, yet the etiologies of most uveitis cases in Myanmar, Bangladesh, South Korea, and Sri Lanka cannot be diagnosed.[53-55] Most uveitis cases in the Philippines are noninfectious, and infectious uveitis represents only 25% of cases.[56] In Vietnam, approximately one-third of uveitis patients are infectious, and one-third of patients are idiopathic.[57]

Studies in Japan have reported that 35–63% of uveitis cases were noninfectious, and 31–50% were idiopathic.[26, 30, 58-62] Case series from Taiwan, China, and Thailand reported similar patterns, with noninfectious uveitis representing 41–55% of cases in China, 38–44% in Thailand, and 47–83% in Taiwan.[25, 27, 63-70]

Birdshot chorioretinopathy was reported in case series in all Asian countries, except two cases in a series from Iraq and one case from Iran.[71, 72]

16.2.5 Incidence and Prevalence of Uveitis in Europe

Most European epidemiologic studies of uveitis were conducted using hospital-based case series. Tran et al. reviewed all uveitis patients at the Hôpital Jules Gonin, Lausanne, Switzerland, and reported an annual uveitis incidence of 17 cases per 100,000 person-years. Anterior uveitis represented 60% of uveitis cases, followed by posterior uveitis (20%).[73] Miettinen and Paivonsalo-Hietanen and colleagues reviewed cases in the University Eye Clinic in Turku and three major referral hospitals in northern Finland.[74, 75] Their studies reported a uveitis incidence of

20–23 cases per 100,000 person-years. Anterior uveitis was the most common form (88–94%).

Mercanti et al. reviewed 655 new uveitis cases in a referral center in Italy and estimated that the average incidence of uveitis in northeastern Italy was 11 cases per 100,000 person-years from 1986 to 1993.[76] Anterior uveitis represented 58% of the cases, and posterior uveitis represented 26%. More recently, Bro and Tallstedt analyzed a computerized health-care information system in Sweden without medical chart review. Their results revealed that the incidence and 5-year prevalence of uveitis in southern Sweden were 108 cases per 100,000 person-years and 700 per 100,000 population, respectively.[77] Anterior uveitis was the most common form in this case series (93%).

Patterns of uveitis in Europe vary. Infectious etiologies are less common than noninfectious ones, which represented 35–70% of all cases. Birdshot chorioretinopathy is a common cause of uveitis in many European countries.[31, 73, 78-81] Patients with Behçet's disease can often be found in the Middle-East region, with a high prevalence in Turkey.[82] Regarding the other areas in Europe, sarcoidosis remains one of the most common causes of uveitis in several countries, including Germany and Ireland.[83, 84]

16.2.6 Incidence and Prevalence of Uveitis in Oceania

Only two studies have been conducted in Australia. The population-based Central Australian Ocular Health Study was a cross-sectional study conducted in Central Australia. Using this survey, Chang and colleagues reported estimated anterior uveitis and posterior uveitis prevalence rates of 210 and 590 per 100,000 persons, respectively.[85] Later, Hart and colleagues reviewed all uveitis cases that were treated in a referral center in urban Melbourne and estimated the incidence as 21 cases per 100,000 person-years and a 1-year prevalence of 36 per 100,000 persons. Anterior uveitis was the most common form of uveitis (81%), followed by posterior uveitis (11%), in their series.[86]

In Australia, 42–45% of uveitis cases are noninfectious, and 33–46% are idiopathic.[87, 88] Case series in New Zealand showed that infectious uveitis represents only a quarter of all cases.[89]

16.3 CONDITIONS IN SPECIFIC DISEASE ENTITIES

16.3.1 Behçet's Disease

Behçet's disease is a systemic inflammatory disorder mainly characterized by oral and genital ulcers, skin lesions, and uveitis. Ocular features of

Behçet's disease may include anterior uveitis, vitreous haze, occlusive retinal vasculitis, macular edema, and retinochoroiditis. The exact pathogenic mechanism of this disease remains unclear, although genetic and immunologic factors have been identified to be strongly associated with it. Behçet's disease typically affects younger adults and threatens vision, leading to a final visual acuity worse than 20/200 in 20% of patients.[18, 90] Most reports indicate that this disease affects predominantly males, although in some countries, female patients are more common.

Although Behçet's disease occurs worldwide, it is most prevalent in the ancient Silk Road area, which links Asia, the Middle East, and the Mediterranean. The highest prevalence has been reported in China and Japan: 104–110 and 12–22 per 10,000 population, respectively.[91, 92] The incidence of Behçet's disease has been estimated at 0.2 cases per 10,000 person-years in Taiwan and 0.4 cases per 10,000 person-years in South Korea according to their respective population-based databases.[93, 94]

Behçet's disease is a major cause of non-infectious uveitis in several Asian countries. Approximately 5–28% of uveitis cases in Asia could be associated with Behçet's disease.[25, 27, 54, 57, 60, 61, 63, 64, 67, 70, 95] Nevertheless, a decreasing trend in the prevalence and severity of uveitis in Behçet's disease has been noticed in Japan, Korea, China, and Taiwan. Although the exact reason for this trend is unclear, changes in unknown environmental factors may be a possible explanation.

16.3.2 Sarcoidosis

Sarcoidosis can affect any organ system. Sarcoidosis-related uveitis typically presents with intraocular granulomatous inflammation. Anterior-chamber cells, mutton-fat keratic precipitates, iris nodules, tent-shaped peripheral anterior synechiae, vitreous haze, snowballs (or snowbanks), retinal vasculitis, retinitis, and chorioretinal granulomas are the most common presentations.

Studies have revealed that 30–70% of patients with systemic sarcoidosis may develop uveitis.[96, 97] Sarcoidosis represents 3–10% of uveitis cases in Western countries and 2–15% in Asian countries. Current literature has suggested that patients with sarcoidosis more frequently developed uveitis in Japan (50–94%) than in any other country.[98, 99]

16.3.3 Vogt–Koyanagi–Harada Disease

In VKH disease, uveitis could be comorbid with various neurologic symptoms (e.g., headache, orbital pain, fever, nausea, meningism, vertigo, and tinnitus) and skin change (e.g., alopecia,

poliosis, and vitiligo). Ocular presentations of VKH disease include bilateral exudative retinal detachment, granulomatous inflammation in the anterior chamber, and sunset glow fundus.

VKH disease is prevalent in Asian, Middle Eastern, Hispanic, and Native American populations, but not in blacks of sub-Saharan African descent. VKH disease has been reported as being the most common noninfectious uveitis in Vietnam and the second most common uveitis entity in China, constituting 16% and 14% of all uveitis cases in both countries, respectively.[25, 57] There is no consensus on gender predilection in VKH disease.

16.4 CONCLUSION

Uveitis is a sight-threatening ocular disease, and its epidemiology varies according to the incidence of each specific etiology of the intraocular inflammation. Information on uveitis is relatively scarce, compared with that of other ocular diseases. More epidemiological studies employing modern methods, including registration databases, are needed in the future.

REFERENCES

1. Jabs DA, Nussenblatt RB, Rosenbaum JT, Standardization of Uveitis Nomenclature Working Group. Standardization of uveitis nomenclature for reporting clinical data. Results of the First International Workshop. *Am J Ophthalmol* 2005;140(3):509–16.

2. Couto C MJ. *Epidemiological Study of Patients with Uveitis in Buenos Aires*. Argentina: Kugler, 1993.

3. Tabe Tambi F. Causes of blindness in the western province of Cameroon. *Rev Int Trach Pathol Ocul Trop Subtrop Sante Publique* 1993;70:185–97.

4. Kaimbo wa Kaimbo D, Missotten L. Eye diseases and the causes of blindness in the southwestern Equator (equatorial forest) in Zaire, data from an eye camp in three rural centers. *Bull Soc Belge Ophtalmol* 1997;265:59–65.

5. Al-Salem M, Arafat AF, Ismail L, Jaradat M. Causes of blindness in Irbid, Jordan. *Ann Saudi Med* 1996;16(4):420–3.

6. Krumpaszky HG, Klauss V. [Cause of blindness in Bavaria. Evaluation of a representative sample from blindness compensation records of Upper Bavaria.] *Klin Monbl Augenheilkd* 1992;200(2):142–6.

7. Iwase A, Araie M, Tomidokoro A, et al. Prevalence and causes of low vision and blindness in a Japanese adult population: the Tajimi Study. *Ophthalmology* 2006;113(8):1354–62.

8. de Smet MD, Taylor SR, Bodaghi B, et al. Understanding uveitis: the impact of research on visual outcomes. *Prog Retin Eye Res* 2011;30(6):452–70.

9. Gardiner AM, Armstrong RA, Dunne MC, Murray PI. Correlation between visual function and visual ability in patients with uveitis. *Br J Ophthalmol* 2002;86(9):993–6.

10. Durrani OM, Meads CA, Murray PI. Uveitis: a potentially blinding disease. *Ophthalmologica* 2004;218(4):223–36.

11. Suttorp-Schulten MS, Rothova A. The possible impact of uveitis in blindness: a literature survey. *Br J Ophthalmol* 1996;80(9):844–8.

12. Fanlo P, Heras H, Espinosa G, Adan A. Complications and visual acuity of patients with uveitis: epidemiological study in a reference unit in northern Spain. *Arch Soc Esp Oftalmol* 2019;94(9):419–25.

13. Nussenblatt RB, Whitcup SM. *Uveitis E-Book: Fundamentals and Clinical Practice.* Amsterdam: Elsevier Health Sciences, 2010.

14. Massa H, Pipis SY, Adewoyin T, et al. Macular edema associated with non-infectious uveitis: pathophysiology, etiology, prevalence, impact and management challenges. *Clin Ophthalmol* 2019;13:1761–77.

15. AlBloushi AF, Alfawaz AM, Al-Dahmash SA, et al. Incidence, risk factors and surgical outcomes of cataract among patients with uveitis in a university referral hospital in Riyadh, Saudi Arabia. *Ocul Immunol Inflamm* 2019;27(7):1105–13.

16. Hwang DK, Chou YJ, Pu CY, Chou P. Risk factors for developing glaucoma among patients with uveitis: a nationwide study in Taiwan. *J Glaucoma* 2015;24(3):219–24.

17. Prieto-del-Cura M, Gonzalez-Guijarro J. [Complications of uveitis: prevalence and risk factors in a series of 398 cases.] *Arch Soc Esp Oftalmol* 2009;84(10):523–8.

18. Pathanapitoon K, Kunavisarut P, Saravuttikul FA, Rothova A. Ocular manifestations and visual outcomes of Behcet's uveitis in a Thai population. *Ocul Immunol Inflamm* 2017;1–5.

19. Heinz C, Koch JM, Zurek-Imhoff B, Heiligenhaus A. Prevalence of uveitic secondary glaucoma and success of nonsurgical treatment in adults and children in a tertiary referral center. *Ocul Immunol Inflamm* 2009;17(4):243–8.

20. Paikal D, Yu F, Holland GN, Coleman AL. Coding of glaucoma for patients with uveitis in the Medicare database. *J Glaucoma* 2006;15(1):13–16.

21. Moorthy RS, Mermoud A, Baerveldt G, et al. Glaucoma associated with uveitis. *Surv Ophthalmol* 1997;41(5):361–94.

22. Kuchtey RW, Lowder CY, Smith SD. Glaucoma in patients with ocular inflammatory disease. *Ophthalmol Clin North Am* 2005;18(3):421–30, vii.

23. Moshirfar M, Somani AN, Motlagh MN, Ronquillo YC. Management of cataract in the setting of uveitis: a review of the current literature. *Curr Opin Ophthalmol* 2020;31(1):3–9.

24. Lardenoye CW, van Kooij B, Rothova A. Impact of macular edema on visual acuity in uveitis. *Ophthalmology* 2006;113(8):1446–9.

25. Yang P, Zhang Z, Zhou H, et al. Clinical patterns and characteristics of uveitis in a tertiary center for uveitis in China. *Curr Eye Res* 2005;30(11):943–8.

26. Kotake S, Furudate N, Sasamoto Y, et al. Characteristics of endogenous uveitis in Hokkaido, Japan. *Graefes Arch Clin Exp Ophthalmol* 1996;234(10):599–603.

27. Silpa-Archa S, Noonpradej S, Amphornphruet A. Pattern of uveitis in a referral ophthalmology center in the central district of Thailand. *Ocul Immunol Inflamm* 2015;23(4):320–8.

28. Biswas J, Kharel Sitaula R, Multani P. Changing uveitis patterns in South India – comparison between two decades. *Indian J Ophthalmol* 2018;66(4):524–7.

29. Yang PZ. [Concern on the changes of clinical pattern and etiological factors in uveitis in China.] *Zhonghua Yan Ke Za Zhi* 2008;44(10):865–6.

30. Wakabayashi T, Morimura Y, Miyamoto Y, Okada AA. Changing patterns of intraocular inflammatory disease in Japan. *Ocul Immunol Inflamm* 2003;11(4):277–86.

31. Luca C, Raffaella A, Sylvia M, et al. Changes in patterns of uveitis at a tertiary referral center in Northern Italy: analysis of 990 consecutive cases. *Int Ophthalmol* 2018;38(1):133–42.

32. Freedman J. Incidence of uveitis in Bantu-speaking negroes of South Africa. *Br J Ophthalmol* 1974;58(6):595–9.

33. Abd El Latif E, Ammar H. Uveitis referral pattern in upper and lower Egypt. *Ocul Immunol Inflamm* 2019;27(6):875–82.

34. Tolesa K, Abateneh A, Kempen JH, Gelaw Y. Patterns of uveitis among patients attending Jimma University Department of Ophthalmology, Jimma, Ethiopia. *Ocul Immunol Inflamm* 2019;1–7.

35. Rautenbach W, Steffen J, Smit D, et al. Patterns of uveitis at two university-based referral centres in Cape Town, South Africa. *Ocul Immunol Inflamm* 2019;27(6):868–74.

36. Darrell RW, Wagener HP, Kurland LT. Epidemiology of uveitis. Incidence and prevalence in a small urban community. *Arch Ophthalmol* 1962;68:502–14.

37. Gritz DC, Wong IG. Incidence and prevalence of uveitis in Northern California; the Northern California Epidemiology of Uveitis Study. *Ophthalmology* 2004;111(3):491–500; discussion.

38. Suhler EB, Lloyd MJ, Choi D, et al. Incidence and prevalence of uveitis in Veterans Affairs Medical Centers of the Pacific Northwest. *Am J Ophthalmol* 2008;146(6):890–6 e8.

39. Acharya NR, Tham VM, Esterberg E, et al. Incidence and prevalence of uveitis: results from the Pacific Ocular Inflammation Study. *JAMA Ophthalmol* 2013;131(11):1405–12.

40. Thorne JE, Suhler E, Skup M, et al. Prevalence of non-infectious uveitis in the United States: a claims-based analysis. *JAMA Ophthalmol* 2016;134(11):1237–45.

41. González MM, Solano MM, Porco TC, et al. Epidemiology of uveitis in a US population-based study. *J Ophthalmic Inflamm Infect* 2018;8(1):6.

42. Bajwa A, Osmanzada D, Osmanzada S, et al. Epidemiology of uveitis in the mid-Atlantic United States. *Clin Ophthalmol* 2015;9:889–901.

43. Gonzalez Fernandez D, Nascimento H, Nascimento C, et al. Uveitis in Sao Paulo, Brazil: 1053 new patients in 15 months. *Ocul Immunol Inflamm* 2017;25(3):382–7.

44. Liberman P, Gauro F, Berger O, Urzua CA. Causes of uveitis in a tertiary center in Chile: a cross-sectional retrospective review. *Ocul Immunol Inflamm* 2015;23(4):339–45.

45. Nakao K, Ohba N. [Prevalence of endogenous uveitis in Kagoshima Prefecture, Southwest Japan.] *Nippon Ganka Gakkai Zasshi* 1996;100(2):150–5.

46. Rathinam SR, Krishnadas R, Ramakrishnan R, et al. Population-based prevalence of uveitis in Southern India. *Br J Ophthalmol* 2011;95(4):463–7.

47. Dandona L, Dandona R, John RK, et al. Population based assessment of uveitis in an urban population in southern India. *Br J Ophthalmol* 2000;84(7):706–9.

48. Hu SXC, Yang P, Huang X. An epidemiological survey of uveitis in Southern China. *Chin J Ophthalmol* 2002;2:1–3.

49. Hwang DK, Chou YJ, Pu CY, Chou P. Epidemiology of uveitis among the Chinese population in Taiwan: a population-based study. *Ophthalmology* 2012;119(11):2371–6.

50. Rim TH, Kim SS, Ham DI, et al. Incidence and prevalence of uveitis in South Korea: a nationwide cohort study. *Br J Ophthalmol* 2018;102(1):79–83.

51. Manandhar A. Patterns of uveitis and scleritis in Nepal: a tertiary referral center study. *Ocul Immunol Inflamm* 2017;25(suppl):S54–S62.

52. Win MZA, Win T, Myint S, et al. Epidemiology of uveitis in a tertiary eye center in Myanmar. *Ocul Immunol Inflamm* 2017;25(suppl):S69–S74.

53. Rahman Z, Ahsan Z, Rahman NA, Dutta Majumder P. Pattern of uveitis in a referral hospital in Bangladesh. *Ocul Immunol Inflamm* 2017;1–4.

54. Lee JY, Kim DY, Woo SJ, et al. Clinical patterns of uveitis in tertiary ophthalmology centers in Seoul, South Korea. *Ocul Immunol Inflamm* 2017;25(suppl):S24–S30.

55. Siak J, Jansen A, Waduthantri S, et al. The pattern of uveitis among Chinese, Malays, and Indians in Singapore. *Ocul Immunol Inflamm* 2017;25(suppl):S81–S93.

56. Abano JM, Galvante PR, Siopongco P, et al. Review of epidemiology of uveitis in Asia: pattern of uveitis in a tertiary hospital in the Philippines. *Ocul Immunol Inflamm* 2017;25(suppl):S75–S80.

57. Nguyen M, Siak J, Chee SP, Diem VQH. The spectrum of uveitis in Southern Vietnam. *Ocul Immunol Inflamm* 2017;25(suppl):S100–S6.

58. Hikita S, Sonoda KH, Hijioka K, et al. [Incidence of uveitis in the northern Kyushu region of Japan – comparison between the periods of 1996–2001 and 2003–2008.] *Nippon Ganka Gakkai Zasshi* 2012;116(9):847–55.

59. Ohguro N, Sonoda KH, Takeuchi M, et al. The 2009 prospective multi-center epidemiologic survey of uveitis in Japan. *Jpn J Ophthalmol* 2012;56(5):432–5.

60. Takahashi R, Yoshida A, Inoda S, et al. Uveitis incidence in Jichi Medical University Hospital, Japan, during 2011–2015. *Clin Ophthalmol* 2017;11:1151–6.

61. Nakahara H, Kaburaki T, Tanaka R, et al. Frequency of uveitis in the central Tokyo Area (2010–2012). *Ocul Immunol Inflamm* 2017;25(suppl):S8–S14.

62. Kitamei H, Kitaichi N, Namba K, et al. Clinical features of intraocular inflammation in Hokkaido, Japan. *Acta Ophthalmol* 2009;87(4):424–8.

63. Gao F, Zhao C, Cheng G, et al. Clinical patterns of uveitis in a tertiary center in north China. *Ocul Immunol Inflamm* 2017;25(suppl):S1–S7.

64. Zheng Y, Zhang LX, Meng QL, et al. Clinical patterns and characteristics of uveitis in a secondary hospital in southern China. *Int J Ophthalmol* 2015;8(2):337–41.

65. Pathanapitoon K, Kunavisarut P, Ausayakhun S, et al. Uveitis in a tertiary ophthalmology centre in Thailand. *Br J Ophthalmol* 2008;92(4):474–8.

66. Sittivarakul W, Bhurayanontachai P, Ratanasukon M. Pattern of uveitis in a university-based referral center in southern Thailand. *Ocul Immunol Inflamm* 2013;21(1):53–60.

67. Sukavatcharin S, Kijdaoroong O, Lekhanont K, Arj-Ong Vallipakorn S. Pattern of uveitis in a tertiary ophthalmology center in Thailand. *Ocul Immunol Inflamm* 2017;25(suppl):S94–9.

68. Chung YM, Yeh TS, Liu JH. Endogenous uveitis in Chinese—an analysis of 240 cases in a uveitis clinic. *Jpn J Ophthalmol* 1988;32(1):64–9.

69. Chou LC, Sheu SJ, Hong MC, et al. Endogenous uveitis: experiences in Kaohsiung Veterans General Hospital. *J Chin Med Assoc* 2003;66(1):46–50.

70. Chen SC, Chuang CT, Chu MY, Sheu SJ. Patterns and etiologies of uveitis at a tertiary referral center in Taiwan. *Ocul Immunol Inflamm* 2017;25(suppl):S31–8.

71. Al-Shakarchi FI. Pattern of uveitis at a referral center in Iraq. *Middle East Afr J Ophthalmol* 2014;21(4):291–5.

72. Rahimi M, Mirmansouri G. Patterns of uveitis at a tertiary referral center in southern iran. *J Ophthalmic Vis Res* 2014;9(1):54–9.

73. Tran VT, Auer C, Guex-Crosier Y, et al. Epidemiological characteristics of uveitis in Switzerland. *Int Ophthalmol* 1994;18(5):293–8.

74. Miettinen R. Incidence of uveitis in Northern Finland. *Acta Ophthalmol (Copenh)* 1977;55(2):252–60.

75. Paivonsalo-Hietanen T, Tuominen J, Vaahtoranta-Lehtonen H, Saari KM. Incidence and prevalence of different uveitis entities in Finland. *Acta Ophthalmol Scand* 1997;75(1):76–81.

76. Mercanti A, Parolini B, Bonora A, et al. Epidemiology of endogenous uveitis in north-eastern Italy. Analysis of 655 new cases. *Acta Ophthalmol Scand* 2001;79(1):64–8.

77. Bro T, Tallstedt L. Epidemiology of uveitis in a region of southern Sweden. *Acta Ophthalmol* 2020;98(1):32–5.

78. Bodaghi B, Cassoux N, Wechsler B, et al. Chronic severe uveitis: etiology and visual outcome in 927 patients from a single center. *Medicine (Baltimore)* 2001;80(4):263–70.

79. Smit RL, Baarsma GS, de Vries J. Classification of 750 consecutive uveitis patients in the Rotterdam Eye Hospital. *Int Ophthalmol* 1993;17(2):71–6.

80. Brydak-Godowska J, Moskal K, Borkowski PK, et al. A retrospective observational study of uveitis in a single center in Poland with a review of findings in Europe. *Med Sci Monit* 2018;24:8734–49.

81. Llorenc V, Mesquida M, Sainz de la Maza M, et al. Epidemiology of uveitis in a Western urban multiethnic population. The challenge of globalization. *Acta Ophthalmol* 2015;93(6):561–7.

82. Yalcindag FN, Ozdal PC, Ozyazgan Y, et al. Demographic and clinical characteristics of uveitis in Turkey: the first national registry report. *Ocul Immunol Inflamm* 2018;26(1):17–26.

83. Grajewski RS, Caramoy A, Frank KF, et al. Spectrum of uveitis in a German tertiary center: review of 474 consecutive patients. *Ocul Immunol Inflamm* 2015;23(4):346–52.

84. Gray CF, Quill S, Compton M, et al. Epidemiology of adult uveitis in a Northern Ireland tertiary referral centre. *Ulster Med J* 2019;88(3):170–3.

85. Chang JH, Raju R, Henderson TR, McCluskey PJ. Incidence and pattern of acute anterior uveitis in Central Australia. *Br J Ophthalmol* 2010;94(2):154–6.

86. Hart CT, Zhu EY, Crock C, et al. Epidemiology of uveitis in urban Australia. *Clin Exp Ophthalmol* 2019;47(6):733–40.

87. Wakefield D, Dunlop I, McCluskey PJ, Penny R. Uveitis: aetiology and disease associations in an Australian population. *Aust N Z J Ophthalmol* 1986;14(3):181–7.

88. Zagora SL, Symes R, Yeung A, et al. Etiology and clinical features of ocular inflammatory diseases in a tertiary referral centre in Sydney, Australia. *Ocul Immunol Inflamm* 2017;25(suppl):S107–14.

89. Wong A, McKelvie J, Slight C, Sims J. Land of the long white cloud: the spectrum of uveitis at a tertiary referral center in New Zealand. *Ocul Immunol Inflamm* 2017;25(suppl):S115–21.

90. Chung YM, Lin YC, Tsai CC, Huang DF. Behcet's disease with uveitis in Taiwan. *J Chin Med Assoc* 2008;71(10):509–16.

91. Yazici H, Seyahi E, Hatemi G, Yazici Y. Behcet syndrome: a contemporary view. *Nat Rev Rheumatol* 2018;14(2):107–19.

92. Cho SB, Cho S, Bang D. New insights in the clinical understanding of Behcet's disease. *Yonsei Med J* 2012;53(1):35–42.

93. Lin YH, Tai TY, Pu CY, et al. Epidemiology of Behcet's disease in Taiwan: a population-based study. *Ophthalmic Epidemiol* 2018;25(4):323–9.

94. Lee YB, Lee SY, Choi JY, et al. Incidence, prevalence, and mortality of Adamantiades-Behcet's disease in Korea: a nationwide, population-based study (2006–2015). *J Eur Acad Dermatol Venereol* 2018;32(6):999–1003.

95. Al-Baker ZM, Bodaghi B, Khan SA. Clinical patterns and causes of uveitis in a referral eye clinic in Qatar. *Ocul Immunol Inflamm* 2018;26(2):249–58.

96. Choi SY, Lee JH, Won JY, et al. Ocular manifestations of biopsy-proven pulmonary sarcoidosis in Korea. *J Ophthalmol* 2018;2018:9308414.

97. Ohara K. [Clinical manifestations of ocular sarcoidosis in Japanese patients.] *Nihon Rinsho* 1994;52(6):1577–81.

98. Matsuo T, Fujiwara N, Nakata Y. First presenting signs or symptoms of sarcoidosis in a Japanese population. *Jpn J Ophthalmol* 2005;49(2):149–52.

99. Birnbaum AD, French DD, Mirsaeidi M, Wehrli S. Sarcoidosis in the national veteran population: association of ocular inflammation and mortality. *Ophthalmology* 2015;122(5):934–8.

17 Ocular Tumors

*Vishal Raval, Alexander Melendez, Hansell Soto, Alléxya Affonso, Rubens Belfort Neto,
and Arun D. Singh*

17.1 INTRODUCTION

Ocular tumors are rare. Yet, because of the survival implications, study of these tumors is vital. Various ocular tissues can undergo malignant transformation, accounting for a large variety of primary malignant tumors, in contrast with metastatic tumors (distant primary) or be affected by contiguous spread (secondary tumors). For inclusion in this chapter, we have limited the review to incidence and etiologic risk factors of three primary tumors that occur in the pediatric population (retinoblastoma) and adult population (uveal melanoma) and an ocular surface tumor (conjunctival squamous cell carcinoma [CSCC]). Using these three examples we review data derived from national cancer registries (Surveillance, Epidemiology and End Result [SEER], United States) and International Agency for Research on Cancer (World Health Organization). Etiologic factors such as host factors, genetic predisposition, sunlight exposure, and role of occupational hazards are also reviewed.

17.2 RETINOBLASTOMA

Retinoblastoma is the most common intraocular tumor in children, accounting for approximately 11% of cancers occurring in the first year of life, with 95% diagnosed before 5 years of age. Retinoblastoma is a genetic disease; inactivation of both alleles of the retinoblastoma susceptibility gene (*RB1*) predisposes an individual to the disease.[1] It is a prototype of hereditary cancers and the paradigm for the "two-hit hypothesis" proposed by Alfred Knudson in 1971.[2] The *RB1* gene located on the long arm of chromosome 13 (13q14) is a negative regulator element in the cell cycle process and was the first tumor suppressor gene to be identified.[3] In developed countries, the goal of treatment has shifted from globe salvage to vision preservation, whereas in underdeveloped countries, which account for more than 90% of retinoblastoma children, the intraocular tumor often goes undiagnosed and presents with advanced disease threatening the globe.[4, 5] The key to globe salvation and vision preservation in retinoblastoma depends on early diagnosis and appropriate treatment.[6] In this chapter, the incidence of retinoblastoma and various etiological factors implicated in the pathogenesis of retinoblastoma are discussed.

17.2.1 Genetic Types

The disease can be categorized as heritable and sporadic. The heritable type can be further classified as familial or new-onset germ line retinoblastoma.

17.2.1.1 Heritable Familial Retinoblastoma

This genetic form occurs in 10% of children. These children are born with a change in one copy of the *RB1* gene in every cell in the body ("first hit"). The mutation in the other copy of the *RB1* gene, the "second hit," occurs in a retinal cell some time after conception. The inherited gene mutation is highly penetrant and nearly all – about 90% – of such children develop retinoblastoma. Most children with the genetic form develop bilateral retinoblastoma. Some children with the familial form develop pinealoblastoma (trilateral retinoblastoma).[7] The other clinical variant, retinoma, is an uncommon benign form of retinoblastoma.

17.2.1.2 Heritable New-Onset Germ Line Retinoblastoma

Most children (90%) with the hereditary form do not have a parent with retinoblastoma. Although these children (30%) did not inherit the gene from an affected parent, they will be able to pass the mutation on to their children due to new-onset germ line mutation. Having the genetic form of the disease also increases a child's risk of developing other cancers later in life.

17.2.1.3 Nonheritable Sporadic Retinoblastoma

This form of retinoblastoma is the most common (60%), resulting from somatic mutations (i.e., mutations that occur in nonreproductive cells) in the *RB1* gene. Patients with nonheritable retinoblastoma have unilateral, unifocal disease and tend to be diagnosed at a later age compared with heritable cases.

17.2.2 Incidence

17.2.2.1 Incidence in the United States

In the United States the reported incidence of retinoblastoma in children aged 0–4 years is 12.4 cases per million.[8, 9] Worldwide incidence of retinoblastoma is constant at one case per 15,000–20,000 live births, which corresponds to about 9,000 new cases every year.[10] With a well-established genetic origin, no significant

DOI: 10.1201/9781315146737-19

changes in overall US retinoblastoma rates from the mid-1970s through 2004 have been reported.[5] A steady improvement in survival (US) over the same 30-year interval was reported.[5, 9] Tamboli et al. examined the effects of trends of treatment modality on survival with an increase in chemotherapy utilization and a decrease in radiation therapy from 1975 to 2010.[11] The specific longitudinal associations and disease patterns were evaluated in a recent report based upon the SEER program tumor registry:[12] 1,452 cases of retinoblastoma were analyzed. The mean patient age at diagnosis was 1.44 years. The tumor was unilateral in 71.0% or bilateral in 29.0%. Patients with bilateral tumors were diagnosed at an earlier age (0.46 years) than patients with unilateral disease (1.77 years; $P < 0.0001$). Smaller tumors, bilateral retinoblastoma, and the lowest-grade lesions were associated with younger age at diagnosis. While there was a decrease in the proportion of high-grade tumors over the study interval, the authors did not observe a decrease in the mean age at diagnosis. T4-stage tumors were associated with decreased survival in comparison to lower-stage lesions. Bilateral retinoblastoma was associated with decreased overall survival and an increased incidence of second, non-ocular malignancies, most notably pineoblastoma and osteosarcoma, compared with unilateral retinoblastoma.

17.2.2.2 Incidence Globally

A 10-year population-based cancer registry data analysis has shown the overall incidence of cancer in the pediatric age group (0–14 years) reported as age-standardized rate (world standard rate, WSR) of 4.5 per million person-years with the highest number reported from Southeast Asia countries (WSR 6.0) (Figure 17.1).[10, 13] About 43% (3,452 of 8,099 children) of the global burden of retinoblastoma lives in the Asia-Pacific region, with India alone contributing to 1,500–2,000 cases per year.[14] Other countries with a large proportion of global RB cases include China (1,103), Indonesia (277), Pakistan (260), Bangladesh (184), and the Phillipines (142) (Figure 17.2).[14]

The recent data from Cancer Incidence in 5 Continents (CI5) from 1988 to 2012 (CI5 volumes VII–XI) evaluated trends in cancer incidence in children under 5 years of age, overall and by type, which included retinoblastoma.[15] Overall, in children under 5 years of age, retinoblastoma incidence has decreased in northern Europe and southern Asia, but no changes in incidence were observed when analyzed as per subregion or human development index (HDI) category (Table 17.1).

17.2.2.3 Age and Sex-Specific Incidence

In a study by Broaddus et al., there was no significant trend in age-adjusted incidence of

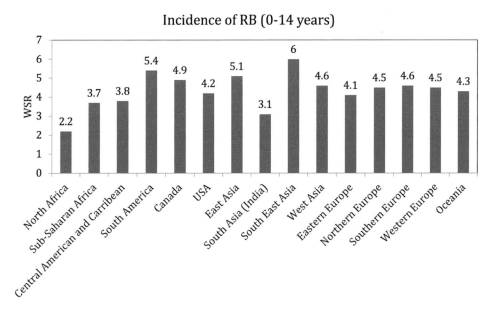

Figure 17.1 Global incidence of retinoblastoma (RB) reported as age-standardized rate (world standard rate, WSR) in the pediatric age group (0–14 years). (Data derived from: Steliarova-Foucher E, Colombet M, Ries LAG, et al. International incidence of childhood cancer, 2001–10: A population-based registry study. *The Lancet Oncology* 2017;18(6):719–731.)

Retinoblastoma : Global Distribution

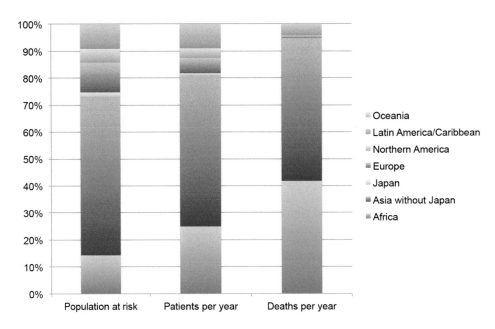

Figure 17.2 Global distribution of retinoblastoma. (Data derived from: Kivela T. The epidemiological challenge of the most frequent eye cancer: Retinoblastoma, an issue of birth and death. *British Journal of Ophthalmology* 2009;93(9):1129–1131.)

Table 17.1 Estimated average annual percent change (AAPC) and incidence (per million) of retinoblastoma by human development index (HDI) category and year of diagnosis.

HDI level	1988–1992	1993–1997	1998–2002	2003–2007	2008–2012	AAPC (95% CI)
Low to medium	9.1	10.6	7.6	8.7	6.6	−1.92 (−3.68, −0.14)
Low/medium to high	6.8	6.8	12.1	8.8	8.8	0.85 (−2.03, 3.82)
Medium to very high	6.7	2.6	7.5	10.8	9.5	3.31 (−1.38, 8.23)

CI, confidence interval.

Note: [a] There were five countries with low HDI, seven countries with medium HDI, 21 countries with high HDI, and 53 countries with very high HDI.

retinoblastoma for all races/genders, nor was there any significant variation of incidence between races or between genders (US).[5] The proportion of bilateral cases (26.7%) versus unilateral cases (71.9%) remained stable over the 30-year period.[5] Patient's age at diagnosis varied with tumor characteristics. Patients with bilateral tumors were diagnosed earlier (0.46 years) than those with unilateral disease (1.77 years). Age at diagnosis also differed by tumor histological grade, with grade 1 tumors diagnosed at a younger age (0.94 years) than grade 3 tumors (2.24 years) or grade 4 tumors (2.14 years).[12] However, the recent population-based cancer registry collected from 153 registries from 62 countries, departments, and territories for the entire decade of 2001–10 found that the incidence of retinoblastoma was higher in boys than girls (incidence sex ratio of 1.0 in age group 0–4 years).[13] Similarly the SEER data from 2000 to 2009 also showed the incidence rate was 13.2 among boys and 11.2 among girls, giving a significantly elevated male:female ratio of 1.18 (95% confidence interval [CI], 1.02–1.36).[8]

17.2.3 Environmental and Host Risk Factors

There is no clear pattern, but there is a suggestion that environmental factors may play a role, though genetic susceptibility to a particular environmental risk factor and behavioral risk factors may explain some of the observed differences.

17.2.3.1 Heritable Retinoblastoma

Heritable retinoblastoma results from a new germ line mutation that is of paternal origin in over 90% of patients.[16] The mutation occurs before the child's conception. Based on these two facts, it seems logical that the search for genetic and nongenetic risk factors for heritable retinoblastoma should focus on the father's genes and his exposures before the child's conception.[17]

A number of studies[18, 19] have examined paternal age with a wide range of results, with the most methodologically sound studies observing paternal age difference of only about 1 year between those with retinoblastoma and the general population. Therefore, the results are yet not convincing until much more research has been done. Exposure to germ line mutagens increases the frequency of germ line mutations in animals.[17] In individuals exposed to radiation or chemotherapeutic drugs and families of cancer survivors and atomic bomb survivors there have been reports of a new germ line mutation which could put them at a higher risk of developing cancer as compared to the general population.[20-22] However there is no strong evidence in relation to etiology or higher incidence of retinoblastoma among such populations.

17.2.3.2 Sporadic Retinoblastoma

Nonheritable retinoblastoma occurs as a result of somatic mutation. The child does not have a germ line RB1 mutation and, as the mutations are somatic, they must occur after the child's conception, either during gestation or in early postnatal life. Therefore, the search for risk factors should focus on exposures of the mother that would affect the child in utero and the child after birth.

A mother's use of insect or garden sprays during pregnancy, diagnostic X-ray with direct fetal exposure, and father's employment as a welder, machinist, or related metal worker are associated with increased risk of sporadic retinoblastoma.[20, 21, 23-25] In a case–control study in central Mexico, lower intake of vegetables and fruits during pregnancy was associated with increased risk of retinoblastoma in the child.[26] A study in the Netherlands estimated that children born after in vitro fertilization had a five- to seven-fold increased risk of retinoblastoma.[27] Some viral proteins bind to and inactivate the retinoblastoma protein that is coded by RB1, and thus, it is hypothesized that viruses may contribute to the development of retinoblastoma. One such viral protein is the human papillomavirus (HPV) protein, E7. In support of the viral hypothesis, DNA sequences from oncogenic HPV subtypes were detected in approximately one-third of retinoblastoma tumor samples studied in central Mexico.[28]

17.2.4 Conclusions

Although these associations may turn out not to be real, our understanding of retinoblastoma genetics and etiology is still evolving. Based on molecular understanding of the disease, we can identify the critical time period (before vs. after conception) and the family member in which the critical event occurred (father, mother, or child) for heritable and sporadic retinoblastoma. Epidemiological studies should be designed that recognize distinctions between the genetic forms of retinoblastoma and investigate events that surround the critical time period in the individuals at risk. Such studies will improve our knowledge of possible risk factors and could lead to prevention of retinoblastoma.

17.3 UVEAL MELANOMA

Ocular melanomas are non-cutaneous melanomas that account for 5% of all melanoma cases.[29] Within this group, uveal melanoma (iris, ciliary body, and choroid) accounts for most ocular melanomas cases (82.5%) compared to adnexal melanomas, which are rare.[30, 31] While being the most common malignant eye tumor in adults, uveal melanoma also has a higher predisposition in involving the choroid of the eye.[32]

17.3.1 Incidence

Within the past five decades in the United States, the overall number of annual cases reported for uveal melanoma has remained stable, with an estimated 5.2 per million per year (Figure 17.3).[30, 33] Various studies across Europe report lower incidences within southern territories (Spain and Italy) with cases averaging a minimum of 2 per million per year, while countries further to the north (England, Ireland, Norway, Denmark) report a higher incidence of the disease with a maximum of 8 per million per year.[34-36] Areas of higher exposure to ultraviolet (UV) light, such as Australia, have a similar incidence when compared with Northern European countries, with an estimated 9 per million per year, respectively.[37] Currently, the lowest incidence rates for uveal melanoma have been reported

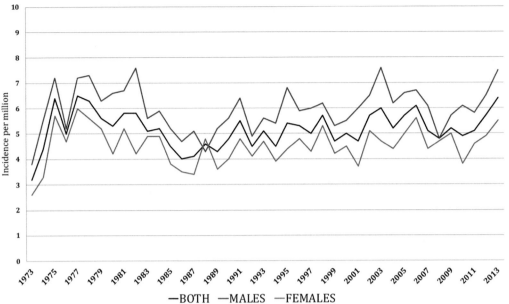

Figure 17.3 Age-adjusted incidence of uveal melanoma, 1973–2013. Number of persons per million population (*y*-axis) adjusted to the US 2000 population (uveal melanoma C69.2–C69.4 only). (Adapted from: Aronow ME, Topham AK, Singh AD. Uveal melanoma: 5-Year update on incidence, treatment, and survival (SEER 1973–2013). *Ocular Oncology and Pathology* 2018;4(3):145–151.)

in Asia, Africa, and Pacific countries with incidence rates as low as 0.6 per million per year (Figure 17.4).[38, 39]

17.3.1.1 Age and Sex-Specific Incidence

There is an age difference in the incidence of uveal melanoma within the population. The older population is more commonly affected than younger individuals.[30, 33, 40] The mean age at diagnosis is 62 years, and the peak incidence age is at 70 years (Figure 17.5).[30, 33] This age-specific incidence rate has also been described in previous studies around the world, such as in Canada, England, and Europe.[34–36, 41] However, in Asian countries uveal melanoma incidence is reported to be prevalent in younger individuals averaging 42.9 years in age.[42] In addition, iris melanoma tends to be reported more commonly in younger patients.[43, 44] Furthermore, the incidence of uveal melanoma in males is greater compared to females.[30, 33, 35, 36, 41]

17.3.2 Host Factors

17.3.2.1 Skin Color and Race

An important risk factor is skin color and race. Caucasian (whites) are predominantly affected (98% of all cases).[30, 45] In contrast, uveal melanoma is far less prevalent in Hispanics, Asians, and African American populations with 1%, <1%,

and <1%, respectively.[44] Expressed differently, the relative risk in comparison to blacks: 19.2 for non-Hispanic whites, 5.4 for Hispanics, and 1.2 for Asian and Pacific Islanders.[46] It is thought that the difference in incidence of uveal melanoma is due to the variable amount of melanin within the distinct populations.[47, 48]

17.3.2.2 Iris Color

It has been reported that iris color is a risk factor for the development of uveal melanoma.[45, 47] The most affected eye colors are light-color irises while brown-colored eyes are the least affected.[45, 49] Recent studies have determined the potential link of higher risk to the difference of melanin molecules in the iris. Eumelanin and pheomelanin both are present in the iris; the distinction lies with the ratio of these types of melanin. Lighter-colored eyes contain a higher degree of pheomelanin and lower amounts of eumelanin, while in darker eyes the distribution is opposite.[50] Pheomelanin is more phototoxic than eumelanin, causing an increased propensity of developing radical oxygen species and decreased antioxidant potential when exposed to light, both of which can cause damage to DNA.[51, 52] Additionally, recent studies have identified three single-nucleotide polymorphisms in pigment genes *HERC2*, *OCA4*, and *IRF4*, which are known risk factors linked to

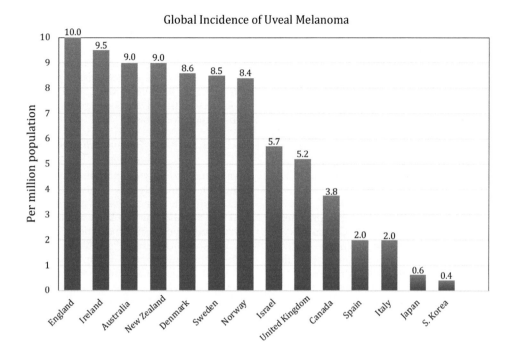

Figure 17.4 Global incidence of uveal melanoma.

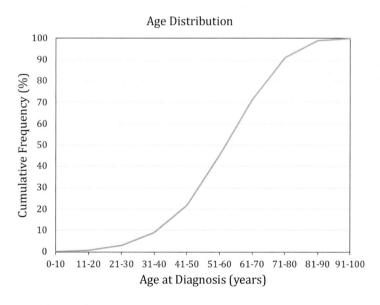

Figure 17.5 Cumulative frequency of uveal melanoma by age. (Data from: Surveillance, Epidemiology, and End Results (SEER) Program Research Data (1975–2016), National Cancer Institute, DCCPS, Surveillance Research Program, Surveillance Systems Branch (www.seer.cancer. gov), released April 2019, based on the November 2018 submission.)

cutaneous melanoma; however, further studies are needed to confirm these observations reading uveal melanoma.[53]

17.3.2.3 Cutaneous Nevi

The incidence of uveal melanoma has also been linked with cutaneous and uveal nevi. It has been reported that cutaneous nevi and freckles are risk factors.[45] Most notably, atypical nevi have a higher risk for uveal melanoma, which has been related to a higher susceptibility of developing cutaneous melanoma and possible uveal melanoma due to relation with familial atypical mole and melanoma (FAM-M) syndrome.[54, 55]

17.3.2.4 Uveal Nevi

Choroidal nevi are common, with a prevalence of 4.7% in the United States. Caucasians are more affected than blacks.[56] Similar to uveal melanoma, choroidal nevi are more prevalent in adults than in children.[56] Furthermore, the annual risk for malignant transformation of choroidal nevi was determined to be 1 in 8,845.[57] The youngest age group were shown to have a lower rate of 1 in 269,565, while the oldest age group showed a higher rate of 1 in 3,664 in malignant transformation.[57]

17.3.2.5 Oculodermal Melanocytosis

Oculodermal melanocytosis (ODM) is a well-recognized risk factor for the development of uveal melanoma.[58–60] It is characterized by congenital hyperpigmentation of the skin, episclera, meninges, and uvea, while being more prevalent in African American, Hispanic, and Asian populations.[43] It affects roughly 0.04% of the Caucasian population. Within patients with ODM, around 1.4% have developed uveal melanoma; it is 35 times more common in patients with the disease.[60] Lifetime risk for developing uveal melanoma in ODM has been estimated to be 1 in 400 in the Caucasian population.[60] Furthermore, the risk of metastasis is reported to be 60% higher in patients with uveal melanoma associated with ODM compared to patients without melanocytosis.[58]

17.3.2.6 BAP1 Tumor Predisposition Syndrome

Germ line *BAP1* gene mutations have been identified in roughly 5% of uveal melanoma cases, with the gene located in chromosome 3p21.1.[61, 62] This gene has been related to *BAP1* tumor predisposition syndrome (*BAP1* TPS), an autosomal-dominant condition associated with the development of multiple cancers such as uveal melanoma, cutaneous melanoma, mesothelioma, lung adenocarcinoma, and renal cell carcinoma.[63] The syndrome has also been implicated with the occurrence of phenotypic variants of uveal melanoma, such as familial uveal melanoma and bilateral primary uveal melanoma (Table 17.2).[64, 65] In a recent study, the point prevalence of uveal melanoma in patients with germ line *BAP1* pathogenic variants was estimated at 2.8% (95% CI, 0.88–4.81%) in the US population.[66]

17.3.3 Environmental Factors

17.3.3.1 Ultraviolet Light

UV light has been associated as a risk factor for development of cutaneous melanoma.[67] On the

Table 17.2 BAP1 tumor predisposition syndrome: Phenotypes of uveal melanoma

Feature		Subtype
Tumor characteristics	Multiple	Multi-focal primary uveal melanoma
	Bilateral	Bilateral primary uveal melanoma
Clinical features	Occurrence at an earlier age	Uveal melanoma in young individual
	Familial occurrence	Familial uveal melanoma
	Metastasis	High risk of metastasis
Systemic associations	Skin lesions	*BAP1*-inactivated melanocytic tumors (BIMT) [a]
	Systemic tumors	Renal cell carcinoma, mesothelioma, skin melanoma, other cancers
Family history	Other cancers	Uveal melanoma, renal cell carcinoma, mesothelioma, skin melanoma, and other cancers

Note: [a] Other nomenclatures: nevoid melanomas and highly atypical nevoid melanoma-like melanocytic proliferations (NEMMP), melanocytic *BAP1*-mutated atypical intradermal tumor (MBAIT), and atypical Spitz tumor (AST).

Source: Modified from: Singh N, Singh R, Bowen RC, Abdel-Rahman MH, Singh AD. Uveal Melanoma in BAP1 Tumor Predisposition Syndrome: Estimation of Risk. *Am J Ophthalmol* 2020;224:172–177.

contrary, the role of UV light in the formation of uveal melanoma has been inconclusive and unclear. Multiple studies finding a link between UV light and uveal melanoma have shown no correlation.[45, 68, 69] However, recent studies have determined that UV light exposure may be a possible risk factor.[70] Mutations that were previously implicated only in cutaneous melanoma and attributed to UV light exposure (*BRAF, NRAS, CDKN2A, PTEN, TP53, TERT, ARID2,* and *KMT2C*) have now been identified in a minority of cases of uveal melanoma.[71]

17.3.3.2 Occupational Exposure

In relation to occupational UV light exposure, no conclusive evidence has been determined for its influence on developing uveal melanoma.[45] Previous reports have suggested that artificial UV light is a potential risk factor in arc welders.[45, 72] Moreover, the use of sunlamps and cooking has also been reported as risk factors for uveal melanoma. On the contrary, pesticides and mobile phone usage have not yielded any significant association.[73–76] Further research is needed to study the relationship of UV light exposure in the development of uveal melanoma.

17.3.4 Conclusion

Uveal melanoma comprises the majority (82.5%) of ocular melanomas. Throughout decades, the incidence within the United States has remained stable with an estimated incidence of 5.2 per million per year. Higher incidence of uveal melanoma has been reported in Northern European countries in contrast to Asia and Africa. Various host risk factors, such as light skin color, light-colored irises, ODM, atypical cutaneous nevi, and *BAP1* germ line mutation (*BAP1* TPS) are important contributors. *BAP1* TPS can underlie

familial uveal melanoma, bilateral primary uveal melanoma, and pediatric uveal melanoma. Exposure to UV light as a potential risk factor remains to be established. Recent studies have identified mutations attributed to UV light exposure in a minority of uveal melanoma cases. Finally, occupational risk factors such as arc welders, sunlamp exposure, and cooking have been reported in a few studies.

17.4 CONJUNCTIVAL SQUAMOUS CELL CARCINOMA

CSCC, a subset of ocular surface squamous neoplasia (OSSN), is a malignant neoplasia arising from the conjunctival epithelium and can be found in all races and both sexes. It is more common in males. The mean age-standardized rate (ASR) worldwide is 0.18 and 0.08 cases/year/100,000 among males and females, respectively.[77] The incidence of CSCC is highest in Africa, followed by Central and South America (Table 17.3).[78]

Over time, the incidence rate has shown a tendency to increase among different regions. In Zimbabwe, the ASR of CSCC rose more than 10-fold, from 0.17 to 1.8 per 100,000 between 1990 and 1999.[77] In Canada, the average annual increase in incidence of 4.5% was reported between 1992 and 2010.[79] Overall, CSCC is becoming more frequent, especially in countries near to the equator.[77, 79–81]

17.4.1 Etiology and Risk Factors

Several possible factors have been studied and attempted to correlate with the development of CSCC.[82] However, exposure to UV radiation, HPV, human immunodeficiency virus (HIV) infection and other types of immunosuppression are the most important ones.[81–84]

Table 17.3 Age-standardized incidence rates of squamous cell carcinoma in the eye (ICD-O-3 C.69) by continent for the period 2008–2012

| Region | Age-standardized incidence rate (cases/year/100,000 population) | | |
	Males mean (95% CI)	Females mean (95% CI)	*P*-value
Africa	1.37 (–0.46–3.20)	1.94 (–0.53–4.41)	0.622
Central and South America	0.23 (0.16–0.29)	0.17 (0.07–0.27)	0.316
Oceania	0.41 (0.20–0.63)	0.13 (0.04–0.22)	0.017
North America	0.08 (0.07–0.09)	0.01 (0.01–0.02)	<0.001
Asia	0.07 (0.05–0.10)	0.04 (0.02–0.05)	0.032
Europe	0.06 (0.05–0.08)	0.01 (0.00–0.02)	<0.001
Worldwide estimate	0.37 (–0.16–0.9)	0.38 (–0.42–1.19)	0.972

CI, confidence interval.

Source: Derived from Bray F, Colombet M, Mery L, Piñeros M, Znaor A, Zanetti R, Ferlay J, editors (2021). *Cancer Incidence in Five Continents*, Vol. XI. IARC Scientific Publication.

17.4.1.1 Sunlight Exposure

The rarity of OSSN in Europe and North America and its higher incidence in sub-Saharan African countries and in Australia,[85] where people are more exposed to sunlight, suggests an important role for solar UV light in the development of OSSN. This is supported by studies that have observed a relationship between exposure to solar UV light and the development of OSSN.[81, 84, 85] Newton et al.[86] noted that the occurrence of ocular squamous cell carcinoma was affected depending on the latitude. The incidence was found to reduce by 49% for every 10° increase in latitude from 1.2 cases/year/100,000 in Uganda (latitude 0.3°) to <0.02/year/100,000 in the UK (latitude >50°).[77, 86]

It is well known that UV-B radiation causes direct DNA damage by crosslinking adjacent bases to form cyclobutane pyrimidine dimers (CPDs) and 6-4 photoproducts (6-4 PPs). This produces a mutation in the p53 tumor supressor gene, allowing cells with damaged DNA past the G1-S cell cycle checkpoint. In recent years, several studies have demonstrated that UV light signature – telomerase reverse transcriptase (TERT) promoter mutations – are common in OSSN lesions, supporting UV induction as the major source of mutagenesis in these lesions.[87, 88]

17.4.1.2 Human Papillomavirus

Although HPV has been demonstrated to be present in samples of OSSN, the relationship between the two is still controversial.[77, 83] DNA of HPV was found in fresh tissue of OSSN, using amplification with polymerase chain reaction (PCR) and sequencing of the DNA, in ocular surface swabs of patients with OSSN, and in studies of formalin-fixed paraffin-embedded tissue, using immunostaining. However, HPV was also detected in uninvolved eyes with apparently healthy conjunctiva and in cases of persistence of infection many years after successful eradication of OSSN lesions. In one study, where evidence for HPV was analyzed by immunohistochemistry and multiplex PCRPCR, no HPV was detected in OSSN lesions.[89] A study where a sensitive in situ hybridization technique that uses an enzyme-catalyzed deposition of reporter molecules was carried out to determine presence of DNA specific for HPV-6/ 11, HPV-16, and HPV-18 within histologically examined biopsy specimens detected DNA from HPV-16 and HPV-18 in a substantial percentage of conjunctival premalignant and malignant lesions, but failed to identify these findings as risk factors for developing OSSN.[83] Another study showed no statistically significant association between anti-HPV antibody status and the risk of conjunctival neoplasia.[90] These facts

lead to the assumption that HPV alone may be incapable of causing OSSN,[82, 91] and that other factors in conjunction with HPV are involved in the causation of OSSN, such as concomitant nonidentified HIV infection.[82]

17.4.1.3 Acquired Immunodeficiency Syndrome

The incidence of OSSN has increased significantly since the eruption of the AIDS epidemic, especially in sub-Saharan African countries.[92] In studies from Rwanda, Uganda, Congo, Kinshasa, and Zimbabwe, HIV infection was strongly associated with an apparent increase in the incidence of OSSN. In a study from Kenya 74% of patients with OSSN were HIV-positive.[93] Uganda reported a sixfold increase of CSCC shortly after the outbreak of HIV/AIDS, from 0.6 cases/year/100,000 between 1970 and 1988 to 3.5/year/100,000 by 1992.[77] In these countries the OSSN occurs at a younger age than was previously reported and the disease tends to be aggressive. The association with HIV suggests that immunosuppression plays a role in OSSN; however, a linear association between the CD4 lymphocyte count and OSSN has not been confirmed.[77]

Although HIV infection seems to be an obvious risk factor by itself, its interaction with UV light and HPV may accelerate the development of OSSN. A study conducted in Uganda found an increased tendency of infection with HPV-8 as the conjunctival lesions worsened, but only among HIV-positive patients.[94]

17.4.1.4 Post-Transplantation and Immunosuppression

Solid organ transplantation and consequent immunosuppression are important risk factors for the development of squamous cell carcinoma, basal cell carcinoma, melanoma, and lymphoma.[95-97] The incidence of squamous cell carcinoma varies with the type, intensity, and duration of the immunosuppressive treatment.[98] OSSN have also been observed in the setting of immunosuppression.[99] Such tumors tend to be bilateral, multifocal, aggressive, and nonresponsive to topical interferon therapy.[100, 101]

17.4.1.5 Chronic Inflammation

It is well known that inflammation enables many essential hallmarks of cancer. While tumor-intrinsic inflammation promotes tumor growth, survival, and invasion, tumor-extrinsic inflammation can contribute to carcinogenesis.[102] Interleukins (ILs) can influence tumor cell functions and affect tumor initiation and progression. Eghtedari et al.[103] found expressed interleukin-6 (IL-6) in conjunctival samples with

OSSN, suggesting chronic inflammation and therefore promotion of dysplastic cell growth. There have been few reports of OSSN associated with atopic keratoconjunctivitis and other chronic inflammatory conditions, including a case in an anophthalmic socket several years after enucleation,[104–106] supporting the idea of chronic inflammation being a risk factor.

17.4.1.6 Xeroderma Pigmentosum and Other DNA Repair Disorders

Xeroderma pigmentosum (XP) is a rare autosomal-recessive condition characterized by hypersensitivity to sunlight, resulting in early photoaging and photocarcinogenesis. The prevalence in Europe and the United States is estimated at 1/1,000,000.[107] Patients with XP are a clinically heterogeneous group with wide variability in clinical features between and within XP complementation groups. The clinical manifestations, severity of disease, and age of onset are in part dependent on the cumulative UVR exposure, the complementation group, and the precise nature of the pathogenic mutation(s).[108]

According to the genotype, XP can be divided into classical XP or XP variant. Classical XP refers to cases with a mutation in seven different genes (XP-A, XP-B, XP-C, XP-D, XP-E, XP-F, and XP-G), leading to a defective nucleotide excision repair (NER) pathway. The XP variant is associated with a mutation in the XP-V gene presenting a normal NER pathway but a defective replication system of UV light-damaged and XP-V. Mutations on groups A, B, D, F, and G are characterized by late disease onset, severe sunburn reactions on minimal sun exposure, and a higher frequency of neurological abnormalities. Mutations in groups C, E, and V, on the other hand, are characterized by an earlier disease onset, normal sunburn reactions to sun exposure, and lower frequency of neurological abnormalities.[109]

Ocular disease in XP is almost exclusively limited to the anterior, UV-exposed structures of the eye: the eyelids, conjunctiva, and cornea.[110,111] Those manifestations occur in 40–100% of patients.[110,111] Compared to the general population, patients with XP up to 20 years of age have a 1,000-fold increase in cancer of the sun-exposed ocular tissues.[108,109] Squamous cell carcinoma and basal cell carcinoma are reported as the most common tumors on the ocular surface and eyelids, respectively.[110,111] The prevalence rates of ocular surface cancer in this population vary considerably in the literature. Prevalence of OSSN up to 72% is described. In addition to early onset, the rate of recurrence, despite adequate treatment with surgery with complete excision respecting the

margin associated with adjuvant cryotherapy, was 64.3%.[112] Recurrences are observed up to 8 years after the initial excision.[112] The increased risk of recurrence of OSSN and the frequent need for monitoring requires an ophthalmologist specialized in ocular oncology.

XP is an inherited disease with no available cure, and the primary prevention of disease development remains genetic counseling, whereas progression is attenuated by protection against UV exposure. The patient prognosis depends on how early a definite diagnosis of XP is established to initiate strict protection from sunlight, control of neurologic symptoms, early skin cancer detection, and prompt treatment and provision to prevent the progress of tumors. Specifically, for the eyes, ocular protection from sunlight is essential to prevent ocular surface tumors.

REFERENCES

1. Murphree AL, Benedict WF. Retinoblastoma: clues to human oncogenesis. *Science (New York).* 1984;223(4640):1028–1033.

2. Knudson AG, Jr. Mutation and cancer: statistical study of retinoblastoma. *Proc Natl Acad Sci U S A.* 1971;68(4):820–823.

3. Hong FD, Huang HJ, To H, et al. Structure of the human retinoblastoma gene. *Proc Natl Acad Sci U S A.* 1989;86(14):5502–5506.

4. Rodriguez-Galindo C, Wilson MW, Chantada G, et al. Retinoblastoma: one world, one vision. *Pediatrics.* 2008;122(3):e763–770.

5. Broaddus E, Topham A, Singh AD. Incidence of retinoblastoma in the USA: 1975–2004. *Br J Ophthalmol.* 2009;93(1):21–23.

6. Abramson DH, Beaverson K, Sangani P, et al. Screening for retinoblastoma: presenting signs as prognosticators of patient and ocular survival. *Pediatrics.* 2003;112(6 Pt 1):1248–1255.

7. Zimmerman LE, Burns RP, Wankum G, Tully R, Esterly JA. Trilateral retinoblastoma: ectopic intracranial retinoblastoma associated with bilateral retinoblastoma. *J Pediatr Ophthalmol Strabismus.* 1982;19(6):320–325.

8. Wong JR, Tucker MA, Kleinerman RA, Devesa SS. Retinoblastoma incidence patterns in the US Surveillance, Epidemiology, and End Results program. *JAMA Ophthalmol.* 2014;132(4):478–483.

9. Fernandes AG, Pollock BD, Rabito FA. Retinoblastoma in the United States: a 40-year incidence and survival analysis. *J Pediatr Ophthalmol Strabismus.* 2018;55(3):182–188.

10. Kivela T. The epidemiological challenge of the most frequent eye cancer: retinoblastoma, an issue of birth and death. *Br J Ophthalmol.* 2009;93(9):1129–1131.

11. Tamboli D, Topham A, Singh N, Singh AD. Retinoblastoma: a SEER dataset evaluation for treatment patterns, survival, and second malignant neoplasms. *Am J Ophthalmol.* 2015;160(5):953–958.

12. Andreoli MT, Chau FY, Shapiro MJ, Leiderman YI. Epidemiological trends in 1452 cases of

retinoblastoma from the Surveillance, Epidemiology, and End Results (SEER) registry. *Can J Ophthalmol J Can Ophtalmol.* 2017;52(6):592–598.

13. Steliarova-Foucher E, Colombet M, Ries LAG, et al. International incidence of childhood cancer, 2001–10: a population-based registry study. *Lancet Oncol.* 2017;18(6):719–731.

14. Usmanov RH, Kivelä T. Predicted trends in the incidence of retinoblastoma in the Asia-Pacific region. *Asia-Pac J Ophthalmol (Philadelphia, Pa).* 2014;3(3):151–157.

15. Hubbard AK, Spector LG, Fortuna G, Marcotte EL, Poynter JN. Trends in international incidence of pediatric cancers in children under 5 years of age: 1988–2012. *JNCI Cancer Spectrum.* 2019;3(1):pkz007.

16. Dryja TP, Mukai S, Petersen R, Rapaport JM, Walton D, Yandell DW. Parental origin of mutations of the retinoblastoma gene. *Nature.* 1989;339(6225):556–558.

17. Allen JW, Ehling UH, Moore MM, Lewis SE. Germ line specific factors in chemical mutagenesis. *Mutation Res.* 1995;330(1–2):219–231.

18. Moll AC, Imhof SM, Kuik DJ, et al. High parental age is associated with sporadic hereditary retinoblastoma: the Dutch retinoblastoma register 1862–1994. *Hum Genet.* 1996;98(1):109–112.

19. Matsunaga E, Minoda K, Sasaki MS. Parental age and seasonal variation in the births of children with sporadic retinoblastoma: a mutation-epidemiologic study. *Hum Genet.* 1990;84(2):155–158.

20. Bunin GR, Petrakova A, Meadows AT, et al. Occupations of parents of children with retinoblastoma: a report from the Children's Cancer Study Group. *Cancer Res.* 1990;50(22):7129–7133.

21. Abdolahi A, van Wijngaarden E, McClean MD, et al. A case-control study of paternal occupational exposures and the risk of childhood sporadic bilateral retinoblastoma. *Occup Environm Med.* 2013;70(6):372–379.

22. Senturia YD, Peckham CS, Peckham MJ. Children fathered by men treated for testicular cancer. *Lancet (Lond, England).* 1985;2(8458):766–769.

23. Bunin GR, Tseng M, Li Y, Meadows AT, Ganguly A. Parental diet and risk of retinoblastoma resulting from new germline RB1 mutation. *Environm Mol Mutagenesis.* 2012;53(6):451–461.

24. Omidakhsh N, Ganguly A, Bunin GR, von Ehrenstein OS, Ritz B, Heck JE. Residential pesticide exposures in pregnancy and the risk of sporadic retinoblastoma: a report from the Children's Oncology Group. *Am J Ophthalmol.* 2017;176:166–173.

25. Omidakhsh N, Bunin GR, Ganguly A, et al. Parental occupational exposures and the risk of childhood sporadic retinoblastoma: a report from the Children's Oncology Group. *Occup Environm Med.* 2018;75(3):205–211.

26. Orjuela MA, Titievsky L, Liu X, et al. Fruit and vegetable intake during pregnancy and risk for development of sporadic retinoblastoma. *Cancer Epidemiol Biomarkers Prevent.* 2005;14(6):1433–1440.

27. Moll AC, Imhof SM, Cruysberg JR, Schouten-van Meeteren AY, Boers M, van Leeuwen FE. Incidence of retinoblastoma in children born after in-vitro fertilisation. *Lancet (Lond, England).* 2003;361(9354):309–310.

28. Orjuela M, Castaneda VP, Ridaura C, et al. Presence of human papilloma virus in tumor tissue from children with retinoblastoma: an alternative

mechanism for tumor development. *Clin Cancer Res.* 2000;6(10):4010–4016.

29. Chang AE, Karnell LH, Menck HR. The National Cancer Data Base report on cutaneous and noncutaneous melanoma: a summary of 84,836 cases from the past decade. The American College of Surgeons Commission on Cancer and the American Cancer Society. *Cancer.* 1998;83(8):1664–1678.

30. Aronow ME, Topham AK, Singh AD. Uveal melanoma: 5-year update on incidence, treatment, and survival (SEER 1973–2013). *Ocul Oncol Pathol.* 2018;4(3):145–151.

31. McLaughlin CC, Wu X-C, Jemal A, Martin HJ, Roche LM, Chen VW. Incidence of noncutaneous melanomas in the U.S. *Cancer.* 2005;103(5):1000–1007.

32. Shields CL, Kaliki S, Shah SU, Luo W, Furuta M, Shields JA. Iris melanoma: features and prognosis in 317 children and adults. *J AAPOS.* 2012;16(1):10–16.

33. Singh AD, Turell ME, Topham AK. Uveal melanoma: trends in incidence, treatment, and survival. *Ophthalmology.* 2011;118(9):1881–1885.

34. Virgili G, Gatta G, Ciccolallo L, et al. Incidence of uveal melanoma in Europe. *Ophthalmology.* 2007;114(12):2309–2315.

35. Baily C, O'Neill V, Dunne M, et al. Uveal melanoma in Ireland. *Ocul Oncol Pathol.* 2019;5(3):195–204.

36. Keenan TD, Yeates D, Goldacre MJ. Uveal melanoma in England: trends over time and geographical variation. *Br J Ophthalmol.* 2012;96(11):1415–1419.

37. Vajdic CM, Kricker A, Giblin M, et al. Incidence of ocular melanoma in Australia from 1990 to 1998. *Int J Cancer.* 2003;105(1):117–122.

38. Park SJ, Oh C-M, Kim BW, Woo SJ, Cho H, Park KH. Nationwide incidence of ocular melanoma in South Korea by using the National Cancer Registry Database (1999–2011). *Investig Opthalmol Vis Sci.* 2015;56(8):4719.

39. Tomizuka T, Namikawa K, Higashi T. Characteristics of melanoma in Japan: a nationwide registry analysis 2011–2013. *Melanoma Res.* 2017;27(5):492–497.

40. Nittmann M, Margo CE. Age conditional probability of ocular and ocular adnexal malignancies. *Ocul Oncol Pathol.* 2021;7(1):70–73.

41. Ghazawi FM, Darwich R, Le M, et al. Uveal melanoma incidence trends in Canada: a national comprehensive population-based study. *Br J Ophthalmol.* 2019;103(12):1872–1876.

42. Wong W, Sundar G, Chee C, Zhao P, Rajagopalan R, Gopal L. Clinical spectrum, treatment and outcomes of uveal melanoma in a tertiary centre. *Singapore Med J.* 2019;60(9):474–478.

43. Yonekawa Y, Kim IK. Epidemiology and management of uveal melanoma. *Hematol Oncol Clin North Am.* 2012;26(6):1169–1184.

44. Shields CL, Kaliki S, Cohen MN, Shields PW, Furuta M, Shields JA. Prognosis of uveal melanoma based on race in 8100 patients: the 2015 Doyne lecture. *Eye (Lond).* 2015;29(8):1027–1035.

45. Nayman T, Bostan C, Logan P, Burnier MN, Jr. Uveal melanoma risk factors: a systematic review of meta-analyses. *Curr Eye Res.* 2017;42(8):1085–1093.

46. Hu DN, Yu GP, McCormick SA, Schneider S, Finger PT. Population-based incidence of uveal melanoma

in various races and ethnic groups. *Am J Ophthalmol.* 2005;140(4):612–617.

47. Weis E. The association between host susceptibility factors and uveal melanoma. *Arch Ophthalmol.* 2006;124(1):54.

48. Kaliki S, Shields CL. Uveal melanoma: relatively rare but deadly cancer. *Eye (Lond).* 2017;31(2):241–257.

49. Houtzagers LE, Wierenga APA, Ruys AAM, Luyten GPM, Jager MJ. Iris colour and the risk of developing uveal melanoma. *Int J Mol Sci.* 2020;21(19).

50. Wakamatsu K, Hu DN, McCormick SA, Ito S. Characterization of melanin in human iridal and choroidal melanocytes from eyes with various colored irides. *Pigment Cell Melanoma Res.* 2008;21(1):97–105.

51. Tanaka H, Yamashita Y, Umezawa K, Hirobe T, Ito S, Wakamatsu K. The pro-oxidant activity of pheomelanin is significantly enhanced by UVA irradiation: benzothiazole moieties are more reactive than benzothiazine moieties. *Int J Mol Sci.* 2018;19(10).

52. Meredith P, Sarna T. The physical and chemical properties of eumelanin. *Pigment Cell Res.* 2006;19(6):572–594.

53. Ferguson R, Vogelsang M, Ucisik-Akkaya E, et al. Genetic markers of pigmentation are novel risk loci for uveal melanoma. *Sci Rep.* 2016;6(1):31191.

54. Singh AD, Damato B, Howard P, Harbour JW. Uveal melanoma: genetic aspects. *Ophthalmol Clin North Am.* 2005;18(1):85–97, viii.

55. Singh AD, Shields CL, Shields JA, Eagle RC, De Potter P. Uveal melanoma and familial atypical mole and melanoma (FAM-M) syndrome. *Ophthalmic Genet.* 1995;16(2):53–61.

56. Qiu M, Shields CL. Choroidal nevus in the United States adult population: racial disparities and associated factors in the National Health and Nutrition Examination Survey. *Ophthalmology.* 2015;122(10):2071–2083.

57. Singh AD, Kalyani P, Topham A. Estimating the risk of malignant transformation of a choroidal nevus. *Ophthalmology.* 2005;112(10): 1784–1789.

58. Shields CL, Kaliki S, Livesey M, et al. Association of ocular and oculodermal melanocytosis with the rate of uveal melanoma metastasis: analysis of 7872 consecutive eyes. *JAMA Ophthalmol.* 2013;131(8):993–1003.

59. Gonder JR, Ezell PC, Shields JA, Augsburger JJ. Ocular melanocytosis. A study to determine the prevalence rate of ocular melanocytosis. *Ophthalmology.* 1982;89(8):950–952.

60. Singh AD, De Potter P, Fijal BA, Shields CL, Shields JA, Elston RC. Lifetime prevalence of uveal melanoma in white patients with oculo(dermal) melanocytosis. *Ophthalmology.* 1998;105(1):195–198.

61. Singh M, Durairaj P, Yeung J. Uveal melanoma: a review of the literature. *Oncol Ther.* 2018;6(1):87–104.

62. Gupta MP, Lane AM, DeAngelis MM, et al. Clinical characteristics of uveal melanoma in patients with germline BAP1 mutations. *JAMA Ophthalmol.* 2015;133(8):881–887.

63. Pilarski R, Carlo M, Cebulla C, Abdel-Rahman M. BAP1 tumor predisposition syndrome. In: Adam MP, Ardinger HH, Pagon RA, et al., eds. *GeneReviews.* Seattle, WA: University of Washington, 1993.

64. Rai K, Pilarski R, Boru G, et al. Germline BAP1 alterations in familial uveal melanoma. *Genes Chromosomes Cancer.* 2017;56(2):168–174.

65. Yu MD, Masoomian B, Shields JA, Shields CL. BAP1 germline mutation associated with bilateral primary uveal melanoma. *Ocul Oncol Pathol.* 2020;6(1):10–14.

66. Singh N, Singh R, Bowen RC, Abdel-Rahman MH, Singh AD. Uveal melanoma in BAP1 tumor predisposition syndrome: estimation of risk. *Am J Ophthalmol.* 2020;224:172–177.

67. van den Bosch T, Kilic E, Paridaens D, de Klein A. Genetics of uveal melanoma and cutaneous melanoma: two of a kind? *Dermatol Res Pract.* 2010;2010:360136.

68. Shah CP, Weis E, Lajous M, Shields JA, Shields CL. Intermittent and chronic ultraviolet light exposure and uveal melanoma: a meta-analysis. *Ophthalmology.* 2005;112(9):1599–1607.

69. Singh AD, Rennie IG, Seregard S, Giblin M, McKenzie J. Sunlight exposure and pathogenesis of uveal melanoma. *Surv Ophthalmol.* 2004;49(4):419–428.

70. Johansson PA, Brooks K, Newell F, et al. Whole genome landscapes of uveal melanoma show an ultraviolet radiation signature in iris tumours. *Nature Commun.* 2020;11(1):2408.

71. Goh AY, Ramlogan-Steel CA, Jenkins KS, Steel JC, Layton CJ. Presence and prevalence of UV related genetic mutations in uveal melanoma: similarities with cutaneous melanoma. *Neoplasma.* 2020;67(5):958–971.

72. Guénel P, Laforest L, Cyr D, et al. Occupational risk factors, ultraviolet radiation, and ocular melanoma: a case-control study in France. *Cancer Causes Control.* 2001;12(5):451–459.

73. Ge YR, Tian N, Lu Y, Wu Y, Hu QR, Huang ZP. Occupational cooking and risk of uveal melanoma: a meta-analysis. *Asian Pac J Cancer Prev.* 2012;13(10):4927–4930.

74. Stang A, Schmidt-Pokrzywniak A, Lash TL, et al. Mobile phone use and risk of uveal melanoma: results of the risk factors for uveal melanoma case-control study. *J Natl Cancer Inst.* 2009;101(2):120–123.

75. Behrens T, Lynge E, Cree I, et al. Pesticide exposure in farming and forestry and the risk of uveal melanoma. *Cancer Causes Control.* 2012;23(1):141–151.

76. Tucker MA, Shields JA, Hartge P, Augsburger J, Hoover RN, Fraumeni JF, Jr. Sunlight exposure as risk factor for intraocular malignant melanoma. *N Engl J Med.* 1985;313(13):789–792.

77. Gichuhi S, Sagoo MS, Weiss HA, Burton MJ. Epidemiology of ocular surface squamous neoplasia in Africa. *Trop Med Int Health.* 2013;18(12):1424–1443.

78. Bray F, Colombet M, Mery L, et al. *Cancer Incidence in Five Continents.* Vol XI. Lyon: IARC Scientific Publication No. 166; 2021.

79. Darwich R, Ghazawi FM, Le M, et al. Epidemiology of invasive ocular surface squamous neoplasia in Canada during 1992–2010. *Br J Ophthalmol.* 2020;104(10):1368–1372.

80. Hämmerl L, Ferlay J, Borok M, Carrilho C, Parkin DM. The burden of squamous cell carcinoma of the conjunctiva in Africa. *Cancer Epidemiol.* 2019;61:150–153.

81. Merz LE, Afriyie O, Jiagge E, et al. Clinical characteristics, HIV status, and molecular biomarkers in squamous cell carcinoma of the conjunctiva in Ghana. *Health Sci Rep.* 2019;2(2):e108.

82. Newton R, Ziegler J, Ateenyi-Agaba C, et al. The epidemiology of conjunctival squamous cell carcinoma in Uganda. *Br J Cancer.* 2002;87(3):301–308.

83. Moubayed P, Mwakyoma H, Schneider DT. High frequency of human papillomavirus 6/11, 16, and 18 infections in precancerous lesions and squamous cell carcinoma of the conjunctiva in subtropical Tanzania. *Am J Clin Pathol.* 2004;122(6):938–943.

84. Sun EC, Fears TR, Goedert JJ. Epidemiology of squamous cell conjunctival cancer. *Cancer Epidemiol Biomarkers Prevent.* 1997;6(2):73–77.

85. Lee GA, Hirst LW. Ocular surface squamous neoplasia. *Surv Ophthalmol.* 1995;39(6):429–450.

86. Newton R, Ferlay J, Reeves G, Beral V, Parkin DM. Effect of ambient solar ultraviolet radiation on incidence of squamous-cell carcinoma of the eye. *Lancet (Lond, England).* 1996;347(9013):1450–1451.

87. Lin SY, Liao SL, Hong JB, et al. TERT promoter mutations in periocular carcinomas: implications of ultraviolet light in pathogenesis. *Br J Ophthalmol.* 2016;100(2):274–277.

88. Scholz SL, Thomasen H, Reis H, et al. Frequent TERT promoter mutations in ocular surface squamous neoplasia. *Invest Ophthalmol Vis Sci.* 2015;56(10):5854–5861.

89. Guthoff R, Marx A, Stroebel P. No evidence for a pathogenic role of human papillomavirus infection in ocular surface squamous neoplasia in Germany. *Curr Eye Res.* 2009;34(8):666–671.

90. Waddell K, Magyezi J, Bousarghin L, et al. Antibodies against human papillomavirus type 16 (HPV-16) and conjunctival squamous cell neoplasia in Uganda. *Br J Cancer.* 2003;88(12):2002–2003.

91. Hanbazazh M, Gyure KA. Ocular human papillomavirus infections. *Arch Pathol Lab Med.* 2018;142(6):706–710.

92. Goedert JJ, Coté TR. Conjunctival malignant disease with AIDS in USA. *Lancet (Lond, England).* 1995;346(8969):257–258.

93. Gichuhi S, Macharia E, Kabiru J, et al. Clinical presentation of ocular surface squamous neoplasia in Kenya. *JAMA Ophthalmol.* 2015;133(11):1305–1313.

94. Ateenyi-Agaba C. Conjunctival squamous-cell carcinoma associated with HIV infection in Kampala, Uganda. *Lancet (Lond, England).* 1995;345(8951):695–696.

95. Perry JD, Polito SC, Chundury RV, et al. Periocular skin cancer in solid organ transplant recipients. *Ophthalmology.* 2016;123(1):203–208.

96. Dahlke E, Murray CA, Kitchen J, Chan AW. Systematic review of melanoma incidence and prognosis in solid organ transplant recipients. *Transplant Res.* 2014;3:10.

97. Clarke CA, Morton LM, Lynch C, et al. Risk of lymphoma subtypes after solid organ transplantation in the United States. *Br J Cancer.* 2013;109(1):280–288.

98. Kim C, Cheng J, Colegio OR. Cutaneous squamous cell carcinomas in solid organ transplant recipients:

emerging strategies for surveillance, staging, and treatment. *Semin Oncol.* 2016;43(3):390–394.

99. Shields CL, Ramasubramanian A, Mellen PL, Shields JA. Conjunctival squamous cell carcinoma arising in immunosuppressed patients (organ transplant, human immunodeficiency virus infection). *Ophthalmology.* 2011;118(11):2133–2137. e2131.

100. Ashkenazy N, Karp CL, Wang G, Acosta CM, Galor A. Immunosuppression as a possible risk factor for interferon nonresponse in ocular surface squamous neoplasia. *Cornea.* 2017;36(4):506–510.

101. Shome D, Honavar SG, Manderwad GP, Vemuganti GK. Ocular surface squamous neoplasia in a renal transplant recipient on immunosuppressive therapy. *Eye (Lond).* 2006;20(12):1413–1414.

102. Green MD, Zou W. Inflammation. In: DeVita J, Vincent T., Lawrence TS, Rosenberg SA, eds. *Cancer Principles and Practice of Oncology.* 11th ed. United States: Wolters Kluwer; 2019:276–286.

103. Eghtedari M, Beigi V, Maalhagh M, Ashraf H. Expression of interleukin-6 in ocular surface squamous neoplasia. *Clin Ophthalmol.* 2019;13:1675–1680.

104. Akpek EK, Polcharoen W, Chan R, Foster CS. Ocular surface neoplasia masquerading as chronic blepharoconjunctivitis. *Cornea.* 1999;18(3):282–288.

105. Shah A, Espana EM, Singh AD. Ocular surface squamous neoplasia associated with atopic keratoconjunctivitis. *Ocul Oncol Pathol.* 2017;3(1):22–27.

106. Espana EM, Levine M, Schoenfield L, Singh AD. Ocular surface squamous neoplasia in an anophthalmic socket 60 years after enucleation. *Surv Ophthalmol.* 2011;56(6):539–543.

107. Kleijer WJ, Laugel V, Berneburg M, et al. Incidence of DNA repair deficiency disorders in western Europe: Xeroderma pigmentosum, Cockayne syndrome and trichothiodystrophy. *DNA Repair (Amst).* 2008;7(5):744–750.

108. Bradford PT, Goldstein AM, Tamura D, et al. Cancer and neurologic degeneration in xeroderma pigmentosum: long term follow-up characterises the role of DNA repair. *J Med Genet.* 2011;48(3):168–176.

109. DiGiovanna JJ, Kraemer KH. Shining a light on xeroderma pigmentosum. *J Invest Dermatol.* 2012;132(3 Pt 2):785–796.

110. Lim R, Sethi M, Morley AMS. Ophthalmic manifestations of xeroderma pigmentosum: a perspective from the United Kingdom. *Ophthalmology.* 2017;124(11):1652–1661.

111. Brooks BP, Thompson AH, Bishop RJ, et al. Ocular manifestations of xeroderma pigmentosum: long-term follow-up highlights the role of DNA repair in protection from sun damage. *Ophthalmology.* 2013;120(7):1324–1336.

112. Gupta N, Sachdev R, Tandon R. Ocular surface squamous neoplasia in xeroderma pigmentosum: clinical spectrum and outcome. *Graefes Arch Clin Exp Ophthalmol.* 2011;249(8):1217–1221.

PART III
EPIDEMIOLOGICAL METHODS FOR EVALUATION AND INTERVENTION

18 Systematic Review and Meta-Analysis

Gianni Virgili, Jennifer Evans, and Tianjing Li

18.1 INTRODUCTION

A systematic review identifies and synthesizes all relevant studies to answer a research question based on pre-specified criteria (IOM 2011; Lasserson 2019). A systematic review differs from a narrative review in that it follows a research protocol which defines standardized, rigorous, and in theory, replicable methods to minimize bias and errors. Systematic review methods can be used to answer many types of research question, such as questions about the effectiveness and safety of a preventive or therapeutic intervention (intervention reviews), etiology and/or prognosis of a disease, and accuracy of a screening or diagnostic test.

Developing and publishing a structured protocol prior to embarking on a systematic review is important as it ensures that reproducible methodology is used during the conduct of the review; the overarching final aim is to reduce the variability of systematic review results (IOM 2011). The first step is to specify the research question in terms of PICO, i.e., the population, intervention(s), comparator(s), and outcomes. This is followed by developing a comprehensive search strategy to identify all potentially relevant studies, including searching multiple electronic bibliographic databases, trial registries, conference proceedings, and other resources that may be more difficult to access. The next step is to collect data and assess the risk of bias in included studies. Ideally, data extraction should be done independently by at least two reviewers, with a clear process for adjudicating discordances. Generally, but not always, a systematic review may include a meta-analysis (i.e., a statistical combination of the results from multiple independent studies), which may improve the precision of the estimate of effect and can quantify the amount of heterogeneity among studies. Finally, the overall qualitative and quantitative data extracted and synthesized from the studies are used to form conclusions with an indication of certainty of the evidence.

18.2 STEPS IN COMPLETING A SYSTEMATIC REVIEW OF INTERVENTIONS

Like any other type of well-conducted research, systematic reviews should follow a set of rigorous steps, which should be detailed *a priori* in a protocol. It is recommended that protocols of systematic reviews are registered in a registry, such as the International Prospective Register of Systematic Reviews (PROSPERO; available at www.crd.york.ac.uk/prospero/). Cochrane review protocols are published in *The Cochrane Library* (www.cochrane.org).

Before a systematic review is initiated, an appropriate team should be formed, including context and clinical expertise, information specialists or librarians, a methodologist, and a team of reviewers that is able to ensure its timely completion. The involvement of patient or caregiver stakeholders is highly desirable to ensure the relevance of the review, especially regarding outcome measures. Systematic reviews commissioned by public health decision makers often have an external advisory group, especially in the context of guideline development.

Research questions in systematic reviews are typically framed using the PICO framework (AHRQ 2015; IOM 2011; Thomas 2019), which determines study eligibility. Additional elements that can be considered are timing (T) and setting (S). For example, the duration of intervention/comparator and, especially, the timepoints of outcome measurement are often considered. The setting in the population and/or interventions/comparators can also be specified, such as the inclusion of patients admitted to an intensive care unit or the home delivery of treatment. Studies should not be excluded, particularly in the title and abstract selection phase, because some outcomes are not analyzed or not reported; such studies should be included in the review, even if they do not contribute data to the analyses. Finally, the PICO framework can be adapted to different systematic review designs, such as in the context of a systematic review that focuses on exposures or risk factors, the interventions (I) element is replaced by exposures (E). Clearly, non-intervention systematic reviews will not generally include only randomized trials, but also cohort studies and case–control studies.

Systematic reviewers design a search strategy with the objective of identifying all relevant studies that address the research question(s). The objective to summarize *all* existing relevant studies that address the research question is the first and main distinction between systematic and narrative reviews. The search strategy should be designed with the input of an experienced information specialist. A balance will need to be struck between a comprehensive search and a feasible workload.

DOI: 10.1201/9781315146737-21

The search strategy used should be documented in full in the review to ensure transparency and reproducibility. The searches usually include both free-text words and controlled vocabulary terms that are coded in each database.

Systematic review authors generally search multiple electronic databases, usually starting with MEDLINE. The strategy is then adapted at least to EMBASE, but content-specific databases may be needed, such as PSYCHINFO.

Clinical trial registries (such as ClinicalTrials.gov) are commonly used to search for ongoing studies, but also to obtain pre-publication study results or to check for deviations from the protocol for individual studies. Furthermore, systematic review authors are encouraged to search 'gray' literature that is outside of traditional peer-reviewed journals, such as conference abstracts, websites, materials from regulatory bodies (e.g., the US Food and Drug Administration), and clinical study reports. The references of studies included in the systematic review and of other systematic reviews are routinely 'hand-searched.'

The next step is to conduct title and abstract screening, typically independently by two screeners (preferably one topic area expert and one methodological expert), with a third screener addressing discrepancies. This is often done using systematic review platforms, such as AbstrackR, DistillerSR, Rayyan, and Covidence, some of which employ advanced machine-learning algorithms that learn to predict the likelihood of relevance of the remaining abstracts. However, the number of titles in eyes and vision reviews is generally easily manageable. The full text report of titles of potential interest is reviewed and the selection process is repeated, documenting the reasons for exclusion at each step.

After the identification of studies eligible for inclusion in the review, the following step is to extract all relevant data and assess the risk of bias from each study. Data that are relevant for extraction for each study should have been pre-specified, including details of all PICO components and information supporting the risk of bias assessment.

Various tools for assessing risk of bias have been developed for different study designs by Cochrane methodologists, such as the revised Cochrane Risk of Bias tool for randomized trials (RoB 2) (Sterne et al. 2019) and the Risk of Bias in Nonrandomized Studies of Interventions (ROBINS-I) (Sterne 2016). The Newcastle–Ottawa Scale is still widely used for observational studies of exposure–outcome associations, but also for non-randomized comparative studies (available at www.ohri.ca/programs/clinical_epidemiology/oxford.asp).

RoB 2 has been developed for individually randomized parallel-group trials, cluster-randomized parallel-group trials, and individually randomized crossover trials. For each trial, the tool requires a separate assessment of each outcome (or group of similar outcomes). RoB 2 includes several signaling questions grouped in five main domains:

1. Risk of bias arising from the randomization process

2. Risk of bias due to deviations from the intended interventions

3. Risk of bias due to missing outcome data

4. Risk of bias in measurement of the outcome

5. Risk of bias in selection of the reported result

Each signaling question is part of an algorithm that guides reviewers to arrive at a judgment regarding the risk of bias, categorized as low risk of bias, some concerns, and high risk of bias, with the aim of minimizing subjectivity, while still allowing room for uncertainty in responses. Finally, the tool guides systematic reviewers in summarizing the five domain-specific judgments of risk bias into an overall risk of bias judgment for each trial (and outcome), usually based on the weakest rating for domain. Even with structured tools, such as RoB 2, part of the challenge with assessing risk of bias in included studies remains the poor quality of reporting in many studies.

Before conducting a meta-analysis of the included studies, systematic reviewers summarize the existing evidence narratively as a 'qualitative synthesis.' This is a very different concept from 'qualitative research,' since a qualitative synthesis is the descriptive approach which allows researchers to understand the variation of PICO elements across studies and the variation of the strength of the evidence in a review, as a precursor to conducting a meta-analysis. The aim of the qualitative synthesis is 'to develop and convey a deeper understanding of the diversity of questions addressed, designs, strength of evidence, methods used in the underlying literature and the combinability of the studies' (IOM 2011).

Meta-analysis is the statistical combination of the results obtained for an outcome from two or more studies in a systematic review, which may generate effect estimates with increased precision and present and estimate any heterogeneity in the findings among individual studies. Each meta-analysis uses a measure of comparative effect which is specific to the type of outcomes, e.g., risk ratio, odds ratio, mean difference, hazard ratio. The measure of effect and its uncertainty, usually as 95% confidence intervals, are presented from each study and as a meta-analytic or pooled estimate, when appropriate.

After the evidence from the included studies has been extracted, appraised and summarized, systematic reviewers grade the certainty of the evidence and draw conclusions accordingly. The certainty of the evidence is usually graded separately for the body of evidence and various systems have been proposed, such as by the GRADE Working Group (Guyatt 2011), the United States Preventive Services Task Force (USPSTF) (Krist et al. 2018), and the AHRQ Program (Berkman 2015). Each domain is assessed separately for each comparison and outcome:

- *Risk of bias*: To what extent did the relevant studies minimize the risk of bias?

- *Directness*: To what extent is the evidence presented in the relevant studies directly applicable to this particular comparison in the systematic review?

- *Consistency*: To what extent were the relevant studies consistent in their results?

- *Precision*: How narrow is the range of uncertainty associated with the results in the relevant studies?

- *Publication bias*: Is it likely that some relevant studies were not published and therefore missing from the evidence identified? Is this missingness likely to have impacted the results of the synthesis?

GRADE assumes that randomized controlled trials are high-certainty evidence and then certainty of the evidence is downgraded once a domain is identified as having a challenge, usually scaling down ratings from 'high' to 'moderate,' 'low,' or 'very low' certainty. The certainty of evidence is usually presented in summary of findings tables or 'evidence profiles' (Schünemann 2019).

The final step of a systematic review is presenting the findings of the review in a clear, accurate, and comprehensive report. This involves a description of the various methods used in the systematic review (including any changes to the methods from those detailed in the protocol), characteristics of the included studies, results of individual included studies, risk of bias in individual included studies, the qualitative synthesis, any quantitative syntheses, and the evidence profiles reflecting the certainty of the evidence. The discussion should summarize the key findings and interpret them in the context of the review question, acknowledging its strengths and limitations as well as its applicability to the review question. The findings are compared with those of any previous systematic review and the conclusions summarize the implications of the findings for current practice and further research, avoiding recommendations that may be context-specific and should be developed by guideline committees, rather than by systematic review authors.

Cochrane reviews are highly structured, but all reviews should follow the Preferred Reporting Items for Systematic Reviews and Meta-Analyses (PRISMA) as a framework for reporting (Moher 2009; Liberati 2009). Extensions of PRISMA to systematic reviews of other types, as well as for review protocols, are available from the Enhancing the Quality and Transparency Of health Research (EQUATOR) Network (www.equator-network.org/).

18.3 SYSTEMATIC REVIEWS OF OTHER TYPES OF RESEARCH QUESTIONS

Review questions are not limited to comparing interventions and also concern, for instance, questions on the accuracy of diagnostic tests, on etiology and prognosis of a disease. The following sections focus on specific systematic review designs, pointing to reading material regarding the fundamentals of newer review methodology.

Reading existing systematic reviews is useful to learn their methodology and structure. Readers can refer to the *Cochrane Library* for a complete list of all Eyes and Vision systematic reviews on www.cochranelibrary.com/cdsr/reviews/topics.

18.3.1 Reviews of Diagnostic Test Accuracy Studies

Diagnostic test accuracy (DTA) reviews are very different from intervention reviews. In a DTA study, the diagnostic performance of an index test is verified using a reference standard test, which is assumed to be optimal or, at least, to have the best possible diagnostic performance. The population included is usually a series of consecutive patients for whom a clinical question is made regarding the presence or absence of the target condition, such as a disease or disease stage. Most DTA studies do not use randomization and study participants receive both the index and the reference test.

DTA studies use two measures of effect: sensitivity, the proportion of index test positives among the diseased; and specificity, the proportion of index test negatives among the non-diseased. These two measures are inversely correlated, meaning that sensitivity decreases while specificity increases, which happens when the diagnostic threshold, e.g., fasting glucose to diagnose diabetes, varies. This is clearly seen when pairs of sensitivities and specificities obtained at different thresholds are plotted as a receiver operating characteristic (ROC) curve in a ROC plane.

Perhaps surprisingly, the first and most important step in preparing a DTA review is a discussion of the clinical diagnostic pathway and the settings in which the test results could be used (Gopalakrishna 2016). This should ideally be done by a multidisciplinary panel involving both clinicians and methodologists. Diagnostic thinking is often implicit and test results may be different across patient subgroups depending on prior testing, disease severity, and setting. The fact that estimates of sensitivity and specificity are obtained in all DTA studies does not mean that such pairs can be compared. In fact, accuracy estimates of diagnostic studies should not be combined if they are obtained from different steps of the clinical diagnostic pathway.

When mapping the clinical pathway, the *population* to whom the test should be applied must be defined. As a minimum this includes a discussion on patient characteristics, referral scheme, and prior testing. The *index test* characteristics include not only technical variations, but also the examiner's profile and training. The *reference standard* test should ideally be the same for all study participants, but this is not always feasible or ethical; if so, the quality of multiple reference standards should be discussed. The reference test must not be considered a comparator as it is assumed to be the optimal method to verify the presence or absence of the *target condition*. Finally, *timing* issues are important and include how repeated index testing is handled and the interval between index and reference tests. These elements are the equivalent of the PICO components in an intervention review and are also assessed as risk of bias domains when the quality of each study is assessed in a DTA review.

The *search strategy* for DTA studies does not include limitations for study design and is generally broad and inclusive, although this has to be tailored to keep the number of records retrieved manageable.

As for intervention reviews, the *data extraction* comprises all the features that are used to characterize the population, index and reference tests, including what is useful to assess risk of bias. Quantitative data to be extracted are 2-by-2 data generated by the cross-classification of the index test results and disease status: true positives, false negatives, false positives, and true negatives. When a cut-off for index test positivity is possible, such as for continuous measures, the threshold(s) used to define positivity is extracted since meta-analyses are best conducted at pre-defined thresholds to improve the applicability of their results.

The *QUADAS-2 tool* (Whiting 2011) was among the first risk of bias tools to be structured in domains, with several signaling questions guiding the overall assessment of each domain. Three domains concern the clinical question or PICO components: populations, index test(s), and the reference standard(s) used to verify the target condition. These domains are not only assessed for risk of bias, rated as low, high, or unclear, but also for applicability, which means whether the study is directly relevant for the review question. The fourth risk of bias domain is on flow and timing, which assesses any timing issues and the participant flow in the study from eligible individuals to number of participants in analyses.

A critical issue regarding the *risk of bias for patient selection* in DTA studies is the inclusion of a consecutive series of patients that match the review question and avoiding a case–control design when possible. As an example, a few hundred studies have investigated the performance of optic nerve head and retinal nerve fiber layer or ganglion cell layer imaging for diagnosing manifest glaucoma, verified with glaucoma specialist decision informed by clinical examination and visual field assessment. A case–control design means that glaucoma patients are selected based on a previous diagnosis and a control group of healthy patients is then included. This design overestimates the performance of a test because the cases and the controls are very different due to inclusion criteria (Rutjes 2005). The appropriate design is a single-gate design in which a cohort of consecutive patients is enrolled with the same inclusion criteria, in a well-defined setting, to make one, or more, well-defined clinical decisions. For example, the GATE study included all referrals by optometrists to glaucoma clinics and investigated whether optical coherence tomography (OCT) could be an accurate triage tool to safely avoid referrals (Azuara-Blanco 2016; Virgili 2018). Before the GATE study was published, a Cochrane review (Michelessi 2015) included over 100 case–control studies that had assessed the accuracy of OCT and other imaging devices to diagnose manifest glaucoma. The review found highly heterogeneous estimates across studies and an overestimate of pooled accuracy due to the case–control design.

Assessing the *risk of bias for the index test* requires that its results are interpreted in a masked (or blinded) fashion. Masking may not be an issue for entirely objective test results. The threshold used to define positivity should be pre-specified since results seeking thresholds that maximize accuracy can overestimate it.

The *risk of bias for the reference standard* requires that the reference standard is valid, and also that its results are interpreted in a masked fashion. This can be difficult to achieve when an invasive reference standard is conditional on the index test results. This may also affect the validity of the reference standard, for example in cancer-screening research when follow-up is used, rather than biopsy, to confirm the absence of cancer in index test-negative patients. An effort should be made by researchers to ensure that the follow-up is long enough and uses adequate tests that maximize case detection and the validity of the different reference standard tests.

Drawing from the previous example, the use of a different reference standard for index test positives versus negatives (or differential verification) can cause *risk of bias for the flow and timing domain*. Bias also arises when not all patients included in the studies contribute to analyses, and this depends on index test positivity. This domain also covers issues regarding repeated index testing, unit of analysis (e.g., multiple lesions in the same organ), and the interval between index and reference standard.

The *meta-analysis of DTA studies* is more complex since two measures of effect, sensitivity and specificity, jointly contribute to test accuracy and are inversely correlated (Macaskill 2011). This relationship is usually represented in a ROC plot, where each study provides a pair of sensitivity and specificity estimates. Statistical techniques in DTA reviews reflect this additional complexity and statistical packages are used to pool estimates of sensitivity and specificity at specific test thresholds with statistical techniques that model simultaneously sensitivity and specificity and take into account their negative correlation, or bivariate meta-analysis models (Reitsma 2005). If no diagnostic cut-off is reported, or if the diagnosis is subjectively made, such as sometimes with imaging devices, no measurement threshold is available at which data can be combined. In such cases, statistical techniques are used that model overall accuracy, threshold effects, and the fact that accuracy may vary with threshold, or hierarchical summary ROC models (Rutter 2001). Comparisons between tests or parameters, as well as across study subgroups, are made, including variables that allow subgroup analyses to be conducted in these models.

Grading the certainty of the evidence uses the same criteria of intervention reviews, although risk of bias is assessed differently. Inconsistency, or heterogeneity of sensitivity and/or specificity estimates across studies, is much more common in DTA reviews than in intervention reviews. As in intervention reviews, using absolute frequencies, particularly of false positives and false negatives, helps with the assessment of imprecision. On the contrary, publication and reporting biases are more difficult to detect since a research protocol is rarely registered for DTA studies and no standard tests for publication bias exist.

Drawing conclusions from DTA reviews is more difficult than for intervention review. In fact, a remarkable feature of DTA studies is that any benefits on patient-centered outcomes are not collected, but they are inferred from the fact that a correct diagnosis is achieved, based on previous research. Although a DTA review does not use systematic methods to assess the consequences of incorrect diagnoses, authors should briefly present the clinical consequences of a correct diagnosis of disease, or its absence, and especially of false positives (overdiagnoses) and false negatives (missed diagnoses). Even when optimal accuracy is not achieved, a test can be useful if it is at least very sensitive or very specific, depending on the decision to be made. For example, test use for population screening often privileges specificity to avoid over-referral of healthy patients to a further level of care. On the other hand, at least high sensitivity is needed when a clinical decision is made on patients with a high probability of disease, for example to decide on further testing. Point-of-care tests, that bring the test conveniently to the patient, are sometimes used to replace existing tests that are not immediately available at the bedside. When such tests are used for replacement they should generally have both high sensitivity and high specificity.

Inferences made from DTA reviews should take into account disease prevalence. For example, a recent Cochrane review investigated the accuracy of non-contact methods for diagnosing angle closure, which can be used for screening or in primary care (Jindal 2020). Forty-seven studies (26,151 participants) often reported accuracy at a given test threshold, such as lateral anterior-chamber depth (LACD) of 25% or less to define narrow angles, but also subjective measures which have no such definition. The authors reported pooled estimates using bivariate models in studies with a relatively high prevalence of narrow angles, clustering at about 15% or 30%. For LACD 25% or less, sensitivity was 83% and specificity was 88%. Although these estimates are apparently good, a substantial fraction of false positives and false negatives would be generated at moderately high prevalence. When the test measure is continuous in primary studies, for example using

OCT parameters, researchers can explore the performance at high sensitivity or high specificity, depending on whether the aim is to rule out or rule in narrow angles, respectively.

The final interpretation of any estimate depends on the alternative decision to be made. In screening settings suboptimal accuracy is acceptable when no testing is the alternative, but specificity should be high to avoid over-referral. On the other hand, if the decision is to safely avoid referrals from optometrists to glaucoma services, sensitivity should be maximized to limit false negatives, at the expense of specificity.

18.3.2 Prognostic Reviews

Making a diagnosis is the identification of an existing condition. Predicting the onset of a condition, or the prognosis of a condition, is generally more difficult. Borderline scenarios exist in which both a diagnostic and a prognostic approach are possible. For example, diagnosing glaucoma when only a suspicion exists is a challenge, since no gold standard other than follow-up is available and the proof is given by the occurrence of manifest glaucoma within a few years. This example is ideal to present research scenarios that depend on the expectations we have on test performance. If the development of manifest glaucoma in patients with ocular hypertension could be predicted with a single high-performance test, for example an imaging test such as the OCT, we might use the accuracy framework and compute sensitivity and specificity for predicting the occurrence of glaucoma within a given time. Unfortunately, no such perfect test exists for now. Because no single test is able to predict the onset of glaucoma in people with ocular hypertension, a systematic review of predictive studies could be conducted, for example, to inform a model that compares the cost of alternative strategies to manage ocular hypertension (Takwoingi 2014).

In recent years, systematic review methodologists have developed methods to conduct prognostic reviews of disease course, single prognostic factors, and predictive models (Hemingway 2013; Hingorani 2013; Riley 2013; Steyerberg 2013). These methods include reporting standards, risk of bias tools, and statistical methods (https://methods.cochrane.org/prognosis/tools).

18.3.3 Rapid, Living and Scoping Reviews

The need for evidence syntheses in response to the COVID-19 pandemic has made researchers more aware that reviews should be conducted in a short time (www.cochrane.org/coronavirus-covid-19-cochrane-resources-and-news; Tricco et al. 2020). More generally, all reviews should

be based on questions that are important for users, thus all of them would be developed quickly. Although no established definition of a *'rapid'* review is widely accepted, Hamel (2020) have revised the underlying key themes and proposed the following definition: 'A rapid review is a rigorous and transparent form of knowledge synthesis that accelerates the process of conducting a traditional systematic review through streamlining or omitting a variety of methods to produce evidence for stakeholders in a resource-efficient manner.'

Moreover, systematic reviews should be kept up to date to remain useful. Cochrane is the only publisher of systematic reviews that specifically includes a mechanism for updating its publications. Further steps have been made with the recent development of the concept of *'living'* reviews that are updated nearly continuously with the evidence progressively made available (https://training.cochrane.org/resource/introducing-living-systematic-reviews). Although most of the actions that turn a review into a rapid or living review concern the organization of the production process and the use of coordinated professional teams, some new issues arise (Elliot 2017; Laine 2020; Millard 2019; Schünemann 2020).

At the opposite end of the spectrum of evidence production, the existing literature in a field of interest may not be well known in terms of the volume, nature, and characteristics of the primary research. *'Scoping'* reviews are used for this purpose as well as to determine the value and potential scope and cost of undertaking a full systematic review and identify research gaps in the existing literature (Arksey 2006; https://joannabriggs.org/scoping-review-network). This methodology is still in an early phase since, in 2014, a scoping review of scoping reviews (Pham 2014) found highly variable methodology, although half of the reviews made formal reference to a methodological system. The PRISMA Extension for Scoping Reviews has been released with the aim of improving the reporting of scoping reviews (Tricco 2018).

18.4 A DATABASE OF SYSTEMATIC REVIEWS

The US satellite of Cochrane Eyes and Vision (CEV) has prepared, and maintains, a dataset of existing systematic reviews in eyes and vision that is available to patients, physicians, researchers, policymakers, and others to inform decision-making and to identify gaps in eyes and vision research (https://eyes.cochrane.org/resources/cevus-database-systematic-reviews-eyes-and-vision). This database currently includes nearly 5,000 systematic reviews and

Table 18.1 Criteria for assessing the reliability of systematic reviews

Criterion	Definition applied to systematic review reports
Defined eligibility criteria	Described inclusion and/or exclusion criteria for eligible studies
Conducted comprehensive literature search	Review authors: (1) described an electronic search of two or more bibliographic databases; (2) used a search strategy comprising a mixture of controlled vocabulary and keywords; (3) reported using at least one other method of searching such as searching of conference abstracts; identified ongoing trials; complemented electronic searching by hand search methods (e.g., checking reference lists); and contacted included study authors or experts
Assessed risk of bias of studies included	Used any method (e.g., scales, checklists, or domain-based evaluation) designed to assess methodologic rigor of included studies
Used appropriate methods for meta-analysis	Used quantitative methods that: (1) were appropriate for the study design analyzed (e.g., maintained the randomized nature of trials; used adjusted estimates from observational studies); (2) correctly computed the weight for studies included
Observed concordance between review findings and conclusions	Authors' reported conclusions were consistent with findings, provided a balanced consideration of benefits and harms, and did not favor a specific intervention if there was lack of evidence

a subset of intervention reviews have been classified as 'reliable' by at least two experienced raters.

Such a database provides a central repository for researchers and other invested individuals to identify evidence that goes beyond that provided by individual primary studies. The database will serve many functions, one of which would be to avoid publication of multiple reviews on the same topic that include the same set of studies or significant overlap among the reviews. Investigators who conduct eye and vision research can use this database to support the scientific premise underlying their research questions or, as we have done previously, to identify 'research gaps' that need further investigation. Sponsors and reviewers of applications for research funding can use the database to evaluate the novelty and significance of research proposals. Journal editors and peer reviewers can access the database to gauge the scientific value of the research reported in newly submitted manuscripts. Patients and other stakeholders can use the plain-language summaries available in some systematic reviews to improve their understanding of eye or vision conditions and the effectiveness and safety of available treatments.

CEV has partnered with guideline developers such as the American Academy of Ophthalmology, European Glaucoma Society, and the UK National Institute for Health and Care Excellence (NICE) to identify reliable evidence to support the guideline recommendations they have developed and disseminated (Table 18.1) (Golozar 2018; Le 2017, 2019; Lindsley et al. 2016;

Mayo-Wilson 2017; Michelessi 2020; Qureshi 2020; Saldanha 2019). We believe that a field-specific database will play a pivotal role in fostering partnerships with research sponsors and professional societies in eyes and vision and can facilitate the identification and use of systematic reviews to inform health care decision-making in ophthalmology and optometry.

18.5 CONCLUSIONS

This chapter has presented some of the several methodological tools that are used for conducting systematic reviews. We have presented an overview as a stimulus for readers to read and use systematic reviews. The *Cochrane Handbook for Systematic Reviews* is the single, freely available, book that covers most of the needs of a systematic reviewer (Higgins et al. 2020).

REFERENCES

AHRQ 2015. *Methods Guide for Effectiveness and Comparative Effectiveness Reviews*. Available from https://effectivehealthcare.ahrq.gov/products/cer-methods-guide/overview; accessed on October 27, 2019.

Arksey H, O'Malley L. Scoping studies: towards a methodological framework. *Int J Soc Res Methodol*. 2005;8:19–32.

Azuara-Blanco A, Banister K, Boachie C, McMeekin P, Gray J, Burr J, Bourne R, Garway-Heath D, Batterbury M, Hernández R, McPherson G, Ramsay C, Cook J. Automated imaging technologies for the diagnosis of glaucoma: a comparative diagnostic study for the evaluation of the diagnostic accuracy, performance as triage tests and cost-effectiveness (GATE study). *Health Technol Assess*. 2016 Jan;20(8):1–168. doi: 10.3310/hta20080.

Berkman ND, Lohr KN, Ansari MT, Balk EM, Kane R, McDonagh M, Morton SC, Viswanathan M, Bass EB, Butler M, Gartlehner G, Hartling L, McPheeters M, Morgan

LC, Reston J, Sista P, Whitlock E, Chang S. Grading the strength of a body of evidence when assessing health care interventions: an EPC update. *J Clin Epidemiol.* 2015;68(11):1312–24.

Elliott JH, Synnot A, Turner T, et al; Living Systematic Review Network. Living systematic review: 1. Introduction – the why, what, when, and how. *J Clin Epidemiol.* 2017;91:23–30.

Golozar A, Chen Y, Lindsley K, Rouse B, Musch DC, Lum F, Hawkins BS, Li T. Identification and description of reliable evidence for 2016 American Academy of Ophthalmology preferred practice pattern guidelines for cataract in the adult eye. *JAMA Ophthalmol.* 2018;136:514–23.

Gopalakrishna G, Langendam MW, Scholten RJ, Bossuyt PM, Leeflang MM. Defining the clinical pathway in Cochrane diagnostic test accuracy reviews. *BMC Med Res Methodol.* 2016;16(1):153. doi:10.1186/s12874-016-0252-x

Guyatt G, Oxman AD, Akl EA, Kunz R, Vist G, Brozek J, Norris S, Falck-Ytter Y, Glasziou P, DeBeer H, Jaeschke R, Rind D, Meerpohl J, Dahm P, Schünemann HJ. GRADE guidelines: 1. Introduction – GRADE evidence profiles and summary of findings tables. *J Clin Epidemiol.* 2011;64(4):383–94.

Hamel C, Michaud A, Thuku M, Skidmore B, Stevens A, Nussbaumer-Streit B, Garritty C. Defining rapid reviews: a systematic scoping review and thematic analysis of definitions and defining characteristics of rapid reviews. *J Clin Epidemiol.* 2020 Oct 8;129:74–85. doi: 10.1016/j.jclinepi.2020.09.041.

Hemingway H, Croft P, Perel P, Hayden JA, Abrams K, Timmis A, Briggs A, Udumyan R, Moons KG, Steyerberg EW, Roberts I, Schroter S, Altman DG, Riley RD; PROGRESS Group. Prognosis research strategy (PROGRESS) 1: a framework for researching clinical outcomes. *BMJ.* 2013 Feb 5;346:e5595. doi: 10.1136/bmj.e5595.

Higgins JPT, Thomas J, Chandler J, Cumpston M, Li T, Page MJ, Welch VA (editors). *Cochrane Handbook for Systematic Reviews of Interventions* version 6.1 (updated September 2020). Cochrane, 2020. Available from www.training.cochrane.org/handbook.

Hingorani AD, Windt DA, Riley RD, Abrams K, Moons KG, Steyerberg EW, Schroter S, Sauerbrei W, Altman DG, Hemingway H; PROGRESS Group. Prognosis research strategy (PROGRESS) 4: stratified medicine research. *BMJ.* 2013 Feb 5;346:e5793. doi: 10.1136/bmj.e5793.

IOM 2011. *Committee on Standards for Systematic Reviews of Comparative Effectiveness Research, Board on Health Care Services, Eden J, Levit L, Berg A, Morton S, eds. Finding What Works in Health Care: Standards for Systematic Reviews.* Washington, DC: National Academies Press; 2011.

Jindal A, Ctori I, Virgili G, Lucenteforte E, Lawrenson JG. Non-contact tests for identifying people at risk of primary angle closure glaucoma. *Cochrane Database Syst Rev.* 2020 May 28;5(5):CD012947. doi: 10.1002/14651858.CD012947.pub2.

Krist AH, Wolff TA, Jonas DE, Harris RP, LeFevre ML, Kemper AR, Mangione CM, Tseng CW, Grossman DC. Update on the methods of the U.S. Preventive Services Task Force: methods for understanding certainty and net benefit when making recommendations. *Am J Prev Med* 2018;54(1S1):S11–S18.

Laine C, Taichman DB, Guallar E, Mulrow CD. Keeping up with emerging evidence in (almost) real time network meta-analyses. *Ann Intern Med.* 2020;173(2):153–4.

Lasserson TJ, Thomas J, Higgins JPT. Chapter 1: Starting a review. In: Higgins JPT, Thomas J, Chandler J, Cumpston M, Li T, Page MJ, Welch VA (editors). *Cochrane Handbook for Systematic Reviews of Interventions* version 6.0 (updated July 2019). Cochrane, 2019. Available from www.training.cochrane.org/handbook.

Le JT, Hutfless S, Li T, Bressler NM, Heyward J, Bittner AK, Glassman A, Dickersin K. Setting priorities for diabetic retinopathy clinical research and identifying evidence gaps. *Ophthalmol Retina.* 2017;1(2):94–102.

Le JT, Qureshi R, Twose C, et al. Evaluation of systematic reviews of interventions for retina and vitreous conditions. *JAMA Ophthalmol.* 2019;137(12):1399–1405.

Liberati A, Altman DG, Tetzlaff J, Mulrow C, Gøtzsche PC, Ioannidis JP, Clarke M, Devereaux PJ, Kleijnen J, Moher D. The PRISMA statement for reporting systematic reviews and meta-analyses of studies that evaluate health care interventions: explanation and elaboration. *PLoS Med.* 2009;6(7):e1000100. doi: 10.1371/journal.pmed.1000100.

Lindsley K, Li T, Ssemanda E, Virgili G, Dickersin K. Interventions for age-related macular degeneration: are practice guidelines based on systematic reviews? *Ophthalmology* 2016;123(4):884–897.

Macaskill P, Gatsonis C, Deeks JJ, Harbord RM, Takwoingi Y. Chapter 10: Analysing and presenting results. In: Deeks JJ, Bossuyt PM, Gatsonis C (editors), *Cochrane Handbook for Systematic Reviews of Diagnostic Test Accuracy* Version 1.0. *The Cochrane Collaboration,* 2010. Available from: http://srdta.cochrane.org/.

Mayo-Wilson E, Ng SM, Chuck RS, Li T. The quality of systematic reviews of interventions for refractive error can be improved: a review of systematic reviews. *BMC Ophthalmol.* 2017;17(1):164.

Michelessi M, Lucenteforte E, Oddone F, et al. Optic nerve head and fibre layer imaging for diagnosing glaucoma. *Cochrane Database Syst Rev.* 2015;2015(11):CD008803. doi:10.1002/14651858.CD008803.pub2

Michelessi M, Li T, Miele A, Azuara-Blanco A, Qureshi R, Virgili G. Multiple diagnostic test accuracy systematic reviews on optical coherence tomography for diagnosing glaucoma: an overview of systematic reviews. *Br J Ophthalmol.* 2020;Jun 3:bjophthalmol-2020-316152. doi: 10.1136/bjophthalmol-2020-316152.

Millard T, Synnot A, Elliott J, Green S, McDonald S, Turner T. Feasibility and acceptability of living systematic reviews: results from a mixed-methods evaluation. *Syst Rev.* 2019;8(1):325. doi:10.1186/s13643-019-1248-5

Moher D, Liberati A, Tetzlaff J, Altman DG; PRISMA Group. Preferred reporting items for systematic reviews and meta-analyses: the PRISMA statement. *Ann Intern Med.* 2009;151(4):264–9, W64.

Pham MT, Rajić A, Greig JD, Sargeant JM, Papadopoulos A, McEwen SA. A scoping review of scoping reviews: advancing the approach and enhancing the consistency. *Res Synth Methods.* 2014;5(4):371–85. doi:10.1002/jrsm.1123

Qureshi R, Azuara-Blanco A, Michelessi M, Virgili G, Breda J, Cutolo C, Pazos M, Katsanos A, Garhofer G, Kolko M, Prokosch V, Al Rajhi A, Lum F, Much D, Gedde S, Li T. What do we really know about the effectiveness of glaucoma interventions: an overview of systematic reviews? *Ophthalmol Glaucoma* 2021;4(5):454–62.

Reitsma JB, Glas AS, Rutjes AW, Scholten RJ, Bossuyt PM, Zwinderman AH. Bivariate analysis of sensitivity and specificity produces informative summary measures in diagnostic reviews. *J Clin Epidemiol.* 2005;58(10):982–990.

Riley RD, Hayden JA, Steyerberg EW, Moons KG, Abrams K, Kyzas PA, Malats N, Briggs A, Schroter S, Altman DG, Hemingway H; PROGRESS Group. Prognosis Research Strategy (PROGRESS) 2: prognostic factor research. *PLoS Med*. 2013;10(2):e1001380. doi: 10.1371/journal. pmed.1001380.

Rutjes AW, Reitsma JB, Vandenbroucke JP, Glas AS, Bossuyt PM. Case-control and two-gate designs in diagnostic accuracy studies. *Clin Chem*. 2005;51(8):1335–41. doi:10.1373/clinchem.2005.048595

Rutter CM, Gatsonis CA. A hierarchical regression approach to meta-analysis of diagnostic test accuracy evaluations. *Stat Med*. 2001;20:2865–2884.

Saldanha IJ, Lindsley KB, Lum F, Dickersin K, Li T. Reliability of the evidence addressing treatment of corneal diseases: a summary of systematic reviews. *JAMA Ophthalmol*. 2019;137(7):775–85.

Schünemann HJ, Higgins JPT, Vist GE, Glasziou P, Akl EA, Skoetz N, Guyatt GH. Chapter 14: Completing 'Summary of findings' tables and grading the certainty of the evidence. In: Higgins JPT, Thomas J, Chandler J, Cumpston M, Li T, Page MJ, Welch VA (editors). *Cochrane Handbook for Systematic Reviews of Interventions* version 6.0 (updated July 2019). Cochrane, 2019. Available from www.training. cochrane.org/handbook.

Schünemann HJ, Santesso N, Vist GE, et al. Using GRADE in situations of emergencies and urgencies: Certainty in evidence and recommendations matters during the COVID-19 pandemic, now more than ever and no matter what . *J Clin Epidemiol*. 2020;S0895-4356(20)30425-X. doi:10.1016/ j.jclinepi.2020.05.030

Sterne JA, Hernán MA, Reeves BC, et al. ROBINS-I: a tool for assessing risk of bias in non-randomised studies of interventions. *BMJ*. 2016;355:i4919. doi:10.1136/bmj.i4919

Sterne JAC, Savović J, Page MJ, Elbers RG, Blencowe NS, Boutron I, Cates CJ, Cheng HY, Corbett MS, Eldridge SM, Emberson JR, Hernán MA, Hopewell S, Hróbjartsson A, Junqueira DR, Jüni P, Kirkham JJ, Lasserson T, Li T, McAleenan A, Reeves BC, Shepperd S, Shrier I, Stewart LA, Tilling K, White IR, Whiting PF, Higgins JPT. RoB 2: a revised tool for assessing risk of bias in randomised trials. *BMJ. 2019* Aug 28;366:l4898. doi: 10.1136/bmj.l4898.

Steyerberg EW, Moons KG, van der Windt DA, Hayden JA, Perel P, Schroter S, Riley RD, Hemingway H, Altman DG; PROGRESS Group. Prognosis Research Strategy (PROGRESS) 3: prognostic model research. *PLoS Med*. 2013;10(2):e1001381. doi: 10.1371/journal.pmed.1001381. doi:10.1002/14651858.CD012097.pub2

Takwoingi Y, Botello AP, Burr JM, et al. External validation of the OHTS-EGPS model for predicting the 5-year risk of open-angle glaucoma in ocular hypertensives. *Br J Ophthalmol*. 2014;98(3):309–314. doi:10.1136/bjophthalmol-2013-303622

Thomas J, Kneale D, McKenzie JE, Brennan SE, Bhaumik S. Chapter 2: Determining the scope of the review and the questions it will address. In: Higgins JPT, Thomas J, Chandler J, Cumpston M, Li T, Page MJ, Welch VA (editors). *Cochrane Handbook for Systematic Reviews of Interventions* version 6.1 (updated September 2020). Cochrane, 2020. Available from www.training.cochrane.org/handbook.

Tricco AC, Lillie E, Zarin W, O'Brien KK, Colquhoun H, Levac D, Moher D, Peters MD, Horsley T, Weeks L, Hempel S, et al. PRISMA extension for scoping reviews (PRISMA-ScR): checklist and explanation. *Ann Intern Med*. 2018;169(7):467–473. doi:10.7326/M18-0850.

Tricco AC, Garritty CM, Boulos L, et al. Rapid review methods more challenging during COVID-19: commentary with a focus on 8 knowledge synthesis steps.*J Clin Epidemiol*. 2020;S0895-4356(20)30616-8. doi:10.1016/ j.jclinepi.2020.06.029

Virgili G, Michelessi M, Cook J, Boachie C, Burr J, Banister K, Garway-Heath DF, Bourne RRA, Asorey Garcia A, Ramsay CR, Azuara-Blanco A. Diagnostic accuracy of optical coherence tomography for diagnosing glaucoma: secondary analyses of the GATE study. *Br J Ophthalmol*. 2018 May;102(5):604–10. doi: 10.1136/ bjophthalmol-2017-310642.

Whiting PF, Rutjes AW, Westwood ME, Mallett S, Deeks JJ, Reitsma JB, Leeflang MM, Sterne JA, Bossuyt PM; QUADAS-2 Group. QUADAS-2: a revised tool for the quality assessment of diagnostic accuracy studies. *Ann Intern Med*. 2011 Oct 18;155(8):529–36. doi: 10.7326/ 0003-4819-155-8-201110180-00009.

19 Assessment of Vision-Related Quality of Life

Eva K. Fenwick, Preeti Gupta, and Ryan E. K. Man

19.1 INTRODUCTION

Population aging is a global phenomenon, with 1.5 billion people estimated to be aged ≥60 years worldwide by 2030,[1, 2] 60% of whom will reside in Asia.[3] As a result of this rapid demographic shift, coupled with swift urbanization and an increasingly sedentary lifestyle, there has been a considerable increase in the prevalence of ocular pathologies and associated visual impairment (VI).[4, 5] Globally, it was estimated in 2015 that 36 million people were blind and 400 million lived with VI,[4] with Asia alone accounting for ~60% of these cases.[4, 5] The global prevalence rates of blinding eye diseases, including age-related macular degeneration (AMD), diabetic retinopathy (DR), and glaucoma, are 8.7%,[6, 7] 34.6%,[8] and 3.5%,[9, 10] respectively, with Asia having the world's highest rates of AMD (35%, 59 million)[6] and glaucoma (60%, 39 million)[9] cases.

The clinical management of most common ocular pathologies and related VI is well established. Laser trabeculoplasty for glaucoma management,[11, 12] intravitreal anti-vascular endothelial growth factor (anti-VEGF, e.g., ranibizumab, aflibercept, or bevacizumab) therapy for AMD,[13] laser photocoagulation or vitrectomy for DR,[14, 15] and anti-VEGF therapy for diabetic macular edema (DME)[16] are highly effective in treating these conditions, and have markedly decreased the prevalence of VI globally.

Importantly, eye diseases, vision loss, and associated treatments can profoundly impact several aspects of a patient's vision-related quality of life (VRQoL), such as daily functioning, mobility, emotional wellbeing, ocular symptoms, social participation, and work opportunities. It is therefore imperative to understand the impact of ocular pathologies from the patient's perspective, especially as healthcare is increasingly moving from a volume-based system towards a value-based model.[17] A better understanding of the impact of ocular pathologies on VRQoL at a population level can improve patient–physician interaction, enhance treatment adherence through the adoption of targeted treatment options, and optimize long-term clinical and VRQoL prognoses. Furthermore, population-based studies can provide a better understanding of the effectiveness of current ocular treatments, screening programs, and models of care, from the patient's point of view. Indeed, the early identification of persons at risk who require escalation of treatment or rehabilitation, and optimization of new interventions or models of care, can improve both clinical and patient-reported outcomes.

This chapter focuses on the assessment of VRQoL, an important patient-reported outcome in ophthalmic epidemiology studies. Section 19.2 discusses the current patient-reported outcome measures (PROMs) that are conventionally used to assess VRQoL in ophthalmic epidemiology. Section 19.3 provides a systematic review of the impact of ocular pathologies and VI on VRQoL using these PROMs. Section 19.4 discusses the psychometric properties of currently available VRQoL PROMs and provides evidence-based advice on how to select the best PROM for use in an ophthalmic epidemiology study. The chapter concludes with a discussion on the current gaps and future challenges of PROM testing in ocular epidemiology via digital and computerized adaptive testing (CAT) methods.

19.2 MEASUREMENT OF PATIENT-REPORTED OUTCOMES

19.2.1 What Are Patient-Reported Outcomes?

Patient-reported outcomes are reports associated with health conditions, that come directly from the patient, without external interpretation.[18] They include measurable outcomes such as generic health, functioning, disease-specific quality of life (QoL), self-management, coping, and self-efficacy, as they relate to the impact of a disease or health condition from the patient's perspective.[19] Patient-reported outcomes can be measured in different ways, for example, through collection of people's subjective responses via self-reported surveys (i.e., PROMs). They can also be measured by collecting performance-based, objective data (i.e., patient-centered outcome measures [PCOMs]), where people's ability to do a task is evaluated using standardized criteria (e.g., reading tests or driving simulations). PROMs or PCOMs can be measured in absolute terms or as a differential change over time.

While PCOMs are useful for evaluating patients' capability objectively and overcome some of the bias associated with self-reported assessment of ability levels,[20] they have limited capacity to measure other aspects of QoL such as symptoms, concerns, and psychosocial wellbeing. Moreover, they sometimes require specialized laboratory environments, and are therefore difficult to implement in epidemiological settings. As such, we will focus on PROMs for the remainder of this chapter as they are more commonly employed in ophthalmic epidemiology.

DOI: 10.1201/9781315146737-22

19.2.2 Why Should PROMs Be Measured?

Incorporating the patient's perspective using PROMs in ophthalmic epidemiology is important as the data can be used to guide clinical care and management, and to inform policy decisions about healthcare and treatments.[21] Indeed, as healthcare moves rapidly towards a value-based rather than volume-based system, PROMs are becoming an essential source of data for healthcare systems to measure the quality of their services.[22] They are also frequently used by health authorities and decision-makers such as the US Food and Drug Administration (FDA) and the UK National Institute for Health and Care Excellence (NICE) to evaluate how healthcare services, interventions, or treatments impact on people's QoL.[23]

19.2.3 Vision-Related Quality of Life

One of the most commonly measured PROMs in ocular epidemiology is VRQoL. VRQoL is a holistic concept that refers to multiple constructs (domains) affected by vision, such as activity limitation (e.g., day-to-day tasks, reading, and self-care), mobility (getting out and about independently), symptoms (e.g., blurry vision), emotional (e.g., feelings of burden, worry about vision getting worse), social isolation (e.g., loss of social life), and convenience (e.g., needing more time to do things).[24] However, as paper-and-pencil PROMs are often restricted in length to avoid over-burdening participants, most VRQoL questionnaires tap into only two or three domains, predominantly activity limitation, emotional wellbeing, and mobility. PROMs with items (questions) relating only to activity limitation should be referred to measuring 'vision-specific functioning (VSF)' or 'activity limitation', rather than VRQoL. It is also important to differentiate between PROMs measuring *generic* health-related QoL and those measuring VRQoL. In generic health-related QoL instruments, items are phrased generally and are not specifically related to vision. As such, generic instruments are often not sensitive to the QoL impact of vision loss or eye conditions,[25, 26] and should be used with caution in epidemiological studies with an ocular and vision focus. Table 19.1 summarizes the characteristics of these different types of PROM.[27]

19.3 SYSTEMATIC REVIEW OF THE VRQOL IMPACT OF VI AND OCULAR PATHOLOGIES AT A POPULATION-BASED LEVEL

19.3.1 Visual Impairment

With population aging, and the fact that most leading causes of VI are age-related,[45] it is expected that the burden of vision loss/blindness will worsen. Therefore, it is imperative to understand the impact of eye conditions and related vision loss from the patient's perspective. Currently, there is compelling evidence from numerous population-based studies in both Asian[46–49] and Western populations[50–54] of a dose–response relationship between the severity spectrum of VI and poorer VRQoL outcomes. For instance, the Blue Mountains Eye Study (BMES),[51] Proyecto VER,[52, 55] and the Salisbury Eye Evaluation (SEE) study[53] have consistently reported decreased VRQoL among visually impaired community-dwelling Caucasian adults compared to their normally sighted counterparts. Similarly, the Singapore Epidemiology of Eye Disease (SEED) study,[46, 47] Aravind Comprehensive Eye Survey (ACES),[48] and Andhra Pradesh Eye Disease Study (APEDS)[49] have also demonstrated that VI is independently associated with a significant decrease in VRQoL in Asian adults across the spectrum of VI severity. In the Singapore Malay Eye Study (SiMES), compared with people with normal vision, people with mild/moderate VI were 1.6 (95% confidence interval [CI], 1.2 to –2.2; $P = 0.01$) and 2.2 (95% CI, 1.6 to –3.0; $P = 0.007$) times more likely to have moderate and poor VSF, respectively. Similarly, participants with severe VI were 3.5 (95% CI, 1.1 to –12.7; $P < 0.001$) and 13.6 (95% CI, 4.0 to –45.4; $P < 0.001$) times more likely to have moderate and poor VSF, respectively. Likewise, in the Singapore Indian Eye Study (SINDI), participants with VI had a systematic reduction in VSF scores compared to those with normal vision in both eyes, ranging from –11.2% for normal vision in one eye and low vision in the other eye, to –77.2% for blindness in both eyes. These findings suggest that even people with mild VI may benefit from referrals for low-vision rehabilitation services to optimize VRQoL outcomes.

Apart from VSF, VI is associated with substantial decrements in other constructs of VRQoL, such as mobility and independence, vision-specific emotional wellbeing, and mental health. For example, in the Singapore Chinese Eye Study (SCES), there was a clinically meaningful reduction in ability to perform tasks related to mobility and independence (–20%; $\beta = -1.44$; 95% CI, –1.75 to –1.13) in patients with severe bilateral VI compared with no VI.[56] In the SEE study, people with VI were significantly more likely to report difficulty walking up and down stairs and walking 150 feet than non-visually impaired people,[57] and in a rural Indian population, mobility losses of 5.1, 10.2, and 23.4 points of 100 were found for people with VI, low vision, and blindness, respectively.[48] Similarly, in the SCES, compared with no VI, severe bilateral

Table 19.1 Characteristics and purpose of different types of patient-reported outcome measures

Type	Examples	Characteristics	Purpose
Disease-specific QoL (vision-related)	GlauQoL[28] QIRC[29]	The items are specific to a particular eye condition and relate to a range of QoL domains	Provides measurement of the impact of a particular eye condition and associated vision loss on QoL Pros: Likely to be very sensitive to the QoL impact of the particular condition because the items are directly relevant. May be preferred by patients and clinicians and perceived as 'empathetic' Cons: Only relevant to a subset of the population, so may not be suitable for ocular epidemiological studies with a broad population
VRQoL	IVI[30–32] NEI-VFQ-25/-50[33, 34]	The items are specific to vision impairment resulting from any eye condition and relate to a range of QoL domains	Provides measurement of the impact of vision impairment in general on QoL Pros: Likely to be more sensitive to the QoL impact of vision impairment than a generic health-related QoL measure. Usually developed on, and therefore suitable for, people with various eye diseases. Provides a more holistic assessment of QoL compared to vision-specific functioning PROMs Cons: May not detect QoL issues relating to specific eye conditions, such as symptoms and treatment-related effects
VSF	VF-14[35] AI[36, 37] ADVS[38]	Items focus on activity limitation relating to vision loss. No assessment of emotional reactions or other QoL domains associated with vision loss	Provides measurement of activity limitation due to vision impairment Pros: Measures a single, simple construct and scores are easy to interpret. Instruments are usually shorter than those measuring VRQoL because fewer items are needed Cons: Is not an appropriate substitute for a QoL outcome measure
Generic health-related QoL	SF-36[39, 40] SF-12[41]	Contains a range of general health items covering various aspects of QoL, including functioning, symptoms, emotional wellbeing, social relationships, concerns, convenience	Provides measurement of QoL relating to general health Pros: Can be applied to a variety of populations and allows for broad comparisons across groups. May be of greatest interest to policy planners Cons: May be unresponsive to issues or changes relating to specific health conditions or changes in vision. A specialized QoL tool may be more appropriate when a particular health condition is under study
Utility: Preference-based and multi-attribute	TTO SG EQ-5D[42] HUI[43, 44]	Reflects the health status of a patient and the associated value of that health status through his/her preferences about health states and treatment outcomes. Health status is reflected by a single continuous score that usually ranges from death (0.0) to full	Provides a utility score which can be used to generate quality-adjusted life-years (QALYs), which are needed for cost-effectiveness analyses. Should be used when economic factors are important Pros: Allows a comparison of disutility across different disease states and can be used in cost-effectiveness analysis. Useful for guiding policy decisions

(continued)

244

Table 19.1 (continued)

Type	Examples	Characteristics	Purpose
		health (1.0). Preferences can be derived directly from patient ratings of health-related hypothetical scenarios or indirectly by patients rating their health status from a multi-attribute classification system (similar to a questionnaire)	Cons: Does not provide information about which domains of QoL are affected. Generic utilities (e.g., EQ-5D) may not be responsive to vision or eye conditions. Conversely, vision-specific utilities may not be generalizable on the health-related QALY scale and therefore are of limited application in cost-effectiveness analyses, especially if comparing against other health conditions

Abbreviations: ADVS, Activities of Daily Living Scale; AI, activity inventory; EQ-5D, EuroQol; GlauQoL, Glaucoma QoL Questionnaire; HUI, Health Utilities Index; IVI, Impact of vision impairment; NEI-VFQ, National Eye Institute Vision Function Questionnaire; QALY, quality-adjusted life years; QIRC, Quality of Life Impact of Refractive Correction; QoL, quality of life; SF, Short Form series; SG, Standard Gamble; TTO, Time Trade Off; VF-14, Visual Function-14; VRQoL, Vision-Related Quality of Life; VSF, Vision-Specific Functioning.

VI was associated with a clinically meaningful reduction in emotional wellbeing (−23%; $\beta = -1.84$; 95% CI, −2.23 to −1.43).[58] Furthermore, systematic declines in mental health and social wellbeing scores as subjects' VI worsened from moderate to severe to blindness have been reported.[48, 52] For example, in the BMES, bilateral presenting VI was significantly associated with poorer scores for the social functioning, dependency, and mental health domains of the National Eye Institute Visual Function Questionnaire (NEI-VFQ) compared to none or unilateral VI, and these scores were mainly driven by non-correctable impairment.[51] These findings emphasize that broad, preventative strategies to prevent or slow progression of VI in the population are warranted. Importantly, recent studies have found that uniocular visual acuity may underestimate the impact of vision loss on VRQoL indices compared with binocular visual acuity, suggesting the use of binocular instead of uniocular measures of visual acuity in patient-reported outcome evaluation of vision loss in ocular epidemiology studies in order to better reflect the impact of vision loss on VRQoL.[59-61]

19.3.2 Age-Related Macular Degeneration

In addition to VI, many epidemiological studies have reported the detrimental impact of common age-related ocular conditions such as AMD, DR, glaucoma, and cataract on VRQoL independently of the person's level of VI.[46-49, 51, 52, 56, 58, 62-70] For example, AMD, one of the commonest cause of irreversible blindness in older adults,[45] not only affects central visual functioning that requires fine discrimination such as reading and face recognition, but also impacts on other activities of daily living, including mobility, driving, and self-care.[71] In a population-based study by Lamoureux and colleagues, people with late AMD were twice as likely (odds ratio [OR] = 2.23; 95% CI, 1.16–7.11) to have lower overall VSF than those without AMD.[72] Similarly, community-dwelling adult Latinos with early AMD had lower mean scores for several NEI-VFQ subscales, including driving, near and distance vision, and social functioning, with these decrements more pronounced in participants with bilateral and advanced AMD.[73]

19.3.3 Diabetic Retinopathy

There is also considerable evidence from population-based studies in Asians and Caucasians that DR, particularly in its vision-threatening stages, has a profound, negative impact on people's VRQoL[47, 52, 65, 70, 74-77] including enhanced social, emotional, and financial strains such as dependency, reduced social functioning, poor mental health,[52, 75, 78] and depression.[79, 80] For instance, using data from the baseline and follow-up SEED cohort studies, people with prevalent and incident vision-threatening DR (VTDR) and proliferative DR (PDR) had substantial difficulty undertaking vision-specific daily activities, independent of presenting VI.[47, 65, 70, 74] Moreover, data from our group have also indicated that the decrement in VRQoL scores becomes significant only in the presence of bilateral, rather than unilateral, DR.[81] Collectively, these results suggest that clinical DR management strategies should include early detection and treatment to prevent progression to more severe bilateral disease, in order to mitigate multifaceted VRQoL losses.

19.3.4 Glaucoma

Many population-based studies have also demonstrated the negative impact of glaucoma on VRQoL.[46-49, 52, 62, 82, 83] Individuals with advanced glaucoma in the worse eye in SiMES had significantly reduced VSF (β = –0.65, 95% CI, –1.03 to –0.28) compared to those without the disease.[62] Similarly, those with bilateral glaucoma in the SEE study reported greater difficulty on the Activities of Daily Vision Scale (OR = 3.25; 95% CI, 1.56–6.76), compared to those without glaucoma.[82] Moreover, population-based studies in Asia[48, 58] and the West[52] have outlined an independent association between glaucoma and reduced psychosocial functioning. For example, in the SCES, glaucoma was associated with substantial decrements in vision-specific emotional wellbeing (β = –1.88, 95% CI, –3.00 to –0.76) compared to those without the disease, independent of visual acuity.[58] Additionally, reduction in mobility and independence (–13%; β = –0.94, 95% CI, –1.82 to –0.06 in the SCES; and β = –6.2, 95% CI, –9.9 to –2.5 in the ACES)[48, 56] was noted in individuals with glaucoma compared to those without the disease. Overall, data from these studies suggest programs to optimize orientation and mobility and psychological interventions to improve coping and emotional functioning are needed for people with glaucoma to ensure they can remain independent and to protect their mental health.

19.3.5 Cataract and Refractive Error

Last, numerous studies from Asia[47, 48, 56, 69, 84, 85] and the West[51, 52] have demonstrated that cataract and refractive error, the two main causes of VI globally, are associated with decreased VRQoL and increased difficulty in performing vision-related tasks. In SINDI, for instance, people with bilateral cataracts experienced difficulty performing vision-specific daily activities independent of refractive error (β = –0.11; 95% CI, –0.21 to 0.00).[69] In SiMES, uncorrected myopia was independently associated with poorer overall VSF (β = –0.34; $P \leq 0.001$),[84] and in SEED, compared with corrected presbyopia, non-correction was associated with worse overall VSF and reduced ability to perform individual near and distance vision-specific tasks, even after adjusting for distance visual acuity.[85] Similarly, in SCES, cataract was independently associated with worse mobility and independence (–6%; β = –0.43; 95%CI, –0.65 to –0.22).[56] Additionally, in the ACES, cataract contributed to poor social dependency and reduced social functioning and mental health.[48] Simple interventions such as adequate refractive correction and cataract surgery are essential to improve VSF, and real-life visual ability.

Taken together, these studies provide evidence that VI and eye diseases (AMD, DR, glaucoma, cataract, and refractive error) are associated with considerable impairment in multiple domains of VRQoL, particularly their severe stages, highlighting the importance of including PROMs in addition to traditional clinical endpoints in both epidemiological studies and clinical care. Furthermore, knowledge of the impact of different eye diseases on VRQoL will help to establish the relative burden of different eye conditions and the merits of each disease-specific intervention, and may therefore help to inform resource allocation for therapies designed to arrest or treat these diseases.

19.4 WHAT ARE THE BEST VRQOL PROMS TO USE IN OCULAR EPIDEMIOLOGY?

With over 100 available VRQoL PROMs, selecting the most appropriate one for an ophthalmic epidemiology study can be daunting. Several systematic and comprehensive reviews have been undertaken to evaluate the psychometric properties of ophthalmic PROMs and to determine the best instruments for use in specific populations.[86-89] A summary of these findings is provided in Table 19.2.

However, as some reviews may be outdated or not cover all relevant considerations for PROM selection, it is important for study teams to independently and thoroughly assess current PROMs for their specific studies. There are several important factors to consider when selecting an appropriate PROM for a specific ophthalmic epidemiological study, and these are outlined in detail in the following sections.

19.4.1 Determine the Trait to Be Measured

As described in Table 19.1, there are several different types of PROMs available, including vision-specific and disease-specific QoL questionnaires and utility measures, each with benefits and drawbacks. The choice of a suitable PROM depends on the aim of the study, the trait to be assessed and the specific research question. For instance, if the intent is to generate quality-adjusted life-years (QALYs) for economic analyses, it is important to use a utility measure rather than a QoL PROM. In contrast, if the purpose is to report on VRQoL outcomes as a study aim in a particular population, then a VRQoL PROM that has been developed for use in that specific population/setting would be most appropriate.

Tip: *How you intend to use your data will directly inform your PROM selection.*

Table 19.2 Recommended ophthalmic patient-reported outcome measures

Eye condition	Recommended instrument(s)
Vision-related QoL/vision-specific functioning[90]	IVI, VCM1
Glaucoma[86, 89, 91]	GAL-9
Cataract[92]	Catquest9SF
Refractive error[93]	QoV, QIRC, NAVQ
Amblyopia and strabismus[94]	AS-20
Diabetic retinopathy (DR)	Recognized lack of robust DR-specific instruments available[95]
Age-related macular degeneration (AMD)	Recognized lack of robust AMD-specific instruments available[96, 97]

Abbreviations: AS-20, Adult Strabismus questionnaire; GAL-9, Glaucoma Activity Limitation questionnaire; IVI, Impact of Vision Impairment; NAVQ, Near Activity Visual Questionnaire; QoL, Quality of life; QoV, Quality of Vision; QIRC, Quality of Life Impact of Refractive Correction; VCM1, Core Questionnaire of Vision-Related Quality of Life.

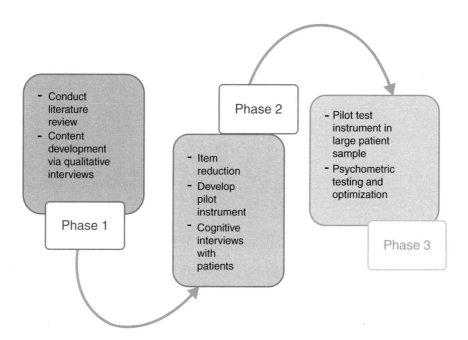

Figure 19.1 Stages of patient-reported outcome measures (PROM) development.

19.4.2 Assess the Developmental Stages of the Selected PROM

Ideally, PROMs should be developed using a mixed-methods approach, combining qualitative and quantitative phases (Figure 19.1). Evidence of well-conducted qualitative methodology (see the Consolidated Criteria for Reporting Qualitative research [COREQ] criteria guidelines for qualitative studies[98]) is important as it supports the face and content validity of the PROM. This means that the items in the PROM are more likely to be relevant because they have been developed using input from patients with the condition of interest. Cognitive interviews to test the comprehensibility of the instrument in the relevant population are also important in instrument development as they help to expose any confusing wording or phrases and provide a systematic process to improve the clarity and comprehensiveness of the tool.[99]

Tip: *Assess whether the chosen PROM has incorporated qualitative input from the patient's perspective during its development.*

19.4.3 Ascertain the Psychometric Evaluation and Validation Stages of the Selected PROM

It is important to critically review the psychometric properties of vision-specific PROMs in order to ensure that the measurement they provide is robust and reliable. Most papers reporting on PROM validation will provide at least some Classical Test Theory (CTT) metrics, such as validity (i.e., the degree to which a PROM measures what it purports to measure), and reliability (i.e., the degree to which the measurement is free from measurement error).

PROMs, developed using CTT methods are called *first-generation* instruments. *Second-generation* vision-related PROMs are those developed or subsequently validated using modern psychometric theory, particularly Rasch analysis. Rasch analysis is a form of Item Response Theory and a technique by which measurement scales to measure patient-reported outcomes can be built and/or evaluated.[100] Rasch analysis overcomes the limitations associated with simple ordinal 'summary' scoring methods used in first-generation instruments,[101] and provides a means to convert ordinal scores to estimates of interval measures. Additionally, Rasch analysis provides comprehensive psychometric evaluation not available in CTT;[102] for example, how well each item in the questionnaire assesses the latent construct being measured (e.g., activity limitation); how well the items are able to discriminate between different strata of respondents; how well the items 'target' the respondents' level of the construct; and whether the response options within the scale are working as intended (i.e., being logically selected by participants).[103]

Several VRQoL instruments, such as the Impact of Vision Impairment (IVI) and NEI-VFQ, have been developed using CTT,[30, 34] and then further validated or adapted using Rasch analysis.[31, 104–106] For example, the original domain structure of the NEI-VFQ has been shown to have several psychometric shortcomings when subjected to Rasch analysis. For instance, rather than providing an overall VRQoL score and 12 subscale scores, Marella and colleagues demonstrated that the NEI-VFQ functioned best as 'activity limitation' and 'socioemotional' scales.[105] Importantly, Rasch-scaled data have been shown to increase measurement precision compared to raw, summary scores.[107] This *improved measurement precision* increases the *sensitivity of your chosen PROM* to detect change in scores over time, which is important in longitudinal ophthalmic epidemiology studies.

Even though second-generation PROMs have already been 'validated' using Rasch analysis, it is important to conduct Rasch analysis anew on your PROM study data to *optimize* the psychometric properties of the questionnaire for your population and *convert* ordinal scores into interval-level estimates ready for use in parametric testing.

Other important measurement characteristics of PROMs to consider include responsiveness, which is the ability of a PROM to detect change over time in the construct being measured (e.g., progression of eye diseases and vision impairment); and interpretability, namely the degree to which one can assign meaning or commonly understood connotations to a PROM's quantitative scores or change in scores.[108] These are especially important measurement matrices to consider, given that epidemiological data are often used to inform disease-specific policy decisions, resource allocation, and public health and clinical management guidelines.

While few PROMs satisfy every single psychometric characteristic, it is important to evaluate the level and quality of PROM development and validation. Second-generation PROMs are preferable to first-generation ones as they have undergone more rigorous psychometric evaluation and, as such, are more likely to provide robust measurement.

Tip: *The COnsensus-based Standards for the Selection of Health Measurement INstruments (COSMIN) guidelines are a useful resource for evaluating the different types of measurement properties for PROMs.[108, 109]*

19.4.4 Cultural and Linguistic Validation of the Selected PROM

Ophthalmic epidemiology studies are often conducted in culturally and linguistically diverse populations and, as such, PROMs may need to be available in several languages other than English. Sometimes validated language versions are freely available; however, it may be necessary to have PROMs translated for use in a particular population. In such cases, it is important to professionally forward- and back-translate questionnaires to ensure that the content is linguistically, as well as grammatically, appropriate. The study team may also consider conducting some cognitive interviews in the new language version of the questionnaire in the population of interest to detect and correct any issues with comprehensibility before widespread data collection commences.

It is also important to check if items in a PROM are culturally relevant. For example, if most of the targeted population does not drive, items about driving may result in substantial missing data. Similarly, many vision-related PROMs were developed more than two decades ago and, as such, the item content may be out of date (e.g., items referring to tasks such as reading a telephone book or crocheting may not be broadly applicable any more).

Tip: *Assess whether PROM items are linguistically and culturally appropriate, and relevant to a contemporary population.*

19.4.5 Other Important Considerations in PROM Selection

Ophthalmic epidemiology studies usually comprise a battery of clinical and patient-centered tests resulting in a long testing protocol. As such, it is often necessary to select VRQoL instruments that are short and quick to administer so as to reduce burden on the interviewer and respondent. PROMs with more than 30 items may be too lengthy, unless they provide measurement of multiple constructs that are central to your study outcomes.

Mode of administration is also an important factor.[110] Generally, it is preferable for VRQoL instruments to be interviewer-administered rather than self-administered, as this reduces the risk of missing or incorrect responses and may be especially important if the participant is visually impaired and cannot read the questionnaire items clearly. Face-to-face rather than phone interviews are also usually preferable to build rapport between the interviewer and respondent and enable body language to be observed. Phone interviews may also be physically and mentally draining for participants trying to hear the questions and hold the phone handset. However, phone administration may be the most feasible and pragmatic option to conduct interviews in some instances, and indeed some PROMs have been specifically validated for use over the phone. As mode of interview may affect the PROM scores, it is important to report the interview mode in all publications arising from ophthalmic epidemiological studies.

As technology advances at a rapid rate, online administration of PROMs via video-conferencing software is also becoming a feasible option and may overcome much of the burden of face-to-face interviewing, such as travel time, and many of the problems associated with phone interviewing, such as loss of visual cues. However, barriers surrounding availability of IT infrastructure such as internet connectivity and hardware, and associated costs, must be resolved if usage of video-conferencing in ophthalmic epidemiology studies is to become widespread.

Tip: *Ensure that the chosen PROM has been validated for use in different modes of administration.*

19.5 CONCLUSIONS AND FUTURE RESEARCH

The assessment of VRQoL using ophthalmic PROMs is gaining prominence given the shift from a generalized 'one size fits all' disease management philosophy to individualized value-based care over the last decade. As such, vision-specific PROMs are increasingly being implemented in ophthalmic epidemiological studies to capture the impact of VI, associated eye diseases, and impact of treatment from the patient's perspective, as evidenced by our systematic review. Given the plethora of ophthalmic PROMs available, care has to be taken when choosing the appropriate instrument, including the outcome to be assessed, the instrument's psychometric and cultural validity, as well as its mode of administration.

The way ophthalmic epidemiological studies are conducted may be irrevocably changed following the COVID-19 pandemic and researchers must pivot to keep up with the 'new normal.' Transitioning away from traditional methods of collecting PROM data that have relied heavily on paper-and-pencil, face-to-face data interviews with participants to video-conferencing platforms incorporating online, cloud-based, digitalized entry of PROMs using laptops and tablets is likely to become the new normal. Digitalized PROMs eliminate the need for data entry and data checking, saving on resources (manpower and time), which are often in short supply in large-scale epidemiological studies. However, while overcoming some of the limitations of paper-and-pencil administration, digitalized PROMs remain lengthy and potentially poorly targeted for population-based study participants, many of whom do not have VI or eye conditions.

A nimble solution to these issues is *computerized adaptive testing*, which is a method for administering items (questions) from a calibrated item bank.[111] CAT iteratively administers from the bank to the respondent items that are selected based on their level of impairment (i.e., it choose the items that will provide the greatest amount of information).[112] Subsequent items are selected based on the examinee's previous responses and selection proceeds until a pre-defined stopping criterion (e.g., measurement precision or number of items) is reached.[113] This ensures that items are tailored to the individual's level of impairment.[111] As such, compared to PROMs with a fixed set of items, CATs require fewer items and less time to arrive at equally precise scores; and reduce test-taker burden by asking relevant questions and tailoring the test to test-taker ability level. CAT also facilitates automated data entry and scoring.

Recent advances in the area of modern psychometric methods in ophthalmology have led to the development of several vision and ophthalmic disease-specific CATs. For example, our team has developed and validated a CAT version of the IVI questionnaire (IVI-CAT) that enables measurement of VRQoL in five or ten items, on average, depending on the level of precision required, corresponding to 82.1 and 65.4% item reductions compared to the full-length IVI tool.[114] Similarly, RetCAT[TM115–118] and GlauCAT[TM119] are DR/DME- and glaucoma-specific item banks and CAT systems, respectively, that measure QoL efficiently over multiple domains, including visual symptoms, ocular comfort symptoms, activity limitation, driving, lighting, mobility, emotional wellbeing, social concerns, convenience, and economic. Similar CAT systems for other eye diseases are also under development.[120–124]

While CAT confers many advantages over paper-and-pencil PROMs, there are several technological barriers to overcome for widespread implementation into research to be successful.[125] For example, studies conducted in remote areas may lack internet access or elderly people may not be comfortable using computers or tablets. As such, a strong IT support and reliable internet infrastructure to integrate CAT within local communities are needed. Similarly, data storage is also an important issue, as is ensuring high levels of patient data security within local cloud systems. While the challenges may seem overwhelming, they are not insurmountable and digital data collection is likely to become the way of the post-pandemic future.

REFERENCES

1. Vaupel JW. Biodemography of human ageing. *Nature*. 2010;464(7288):536–542.

2. United Nations Department of Economic and Social Affairs, Population Division. *World Population Prospects: The 2017 Revision, Key Findings and Advance Tables*. ESA/P/WP/248. New York: United Nations, 2017.

3. Complete Life Tables 2008–2013 for Singapore Resident Population. 2013. www.singstat.gov.sg/docs/default-source/default-document-library/publications/publications_and_papers/births_and_deaths/lifetable08-13.pdf. Accessed 20/5/2015.

4. Bourne RRA, Flaxman SR, Braithwaite T, et al. Magnitude, temporal trends, and projections of the global prevalence of blindness and distance and near vision impairment: a systematic review and meta-analysis. *Lancet Glob Health*. 2017;5(9):e888–e897.

5. Pascolini D, Mariotti SP. Global estimates of visual impairment: 2010. *Br J Ophthalmol*. 2012;96(5):614–618.

6. Wong WL, Su X, Li X, et al. Global prevalence of age-related macular degeneration and disease burden projection for 2020 and 2040: a systematic review and meta-analysis. *Lancet Glob Health*. 2014;2(2):e106–116.

7. Jonas JB, Cheung CMG, Panda-Jonas S. Updates on the epidemiology of age-related macular degeneration. *Asia Pac J Ophthalmol (Phila)*. 2017;6(6):493–497.

8. Yau JW, Rogers SL, Kawasaki R, et al. Global prevalence and major risk factors of diabetic retinopathy. *Diabetes Care*. 2012;35(3):556–564.

9. Tham YC, Li X, Wong TY, Quigley HA, Aung T, Cheng CY. Global prevalence of glaucoma and projections of glaucoma burden through 2040: a systematic review and meta-analysis. *Ophthalmology*. 2014;121(11):2081–2090.

10. Jonas JB, Aung T, Bourne RR, Bron AM, Ritch R, Panda-Jonas S. Glaucoma. *Lancet*. 2017;390(10108):2183–2193.

11. Weinreb RN, Aung T, Medeiros FA. The pathophysiology and treatment of glaucoma: a review. *JAMA*. 2014;311(18):1901–1911.

12. Lusthaus J, Goldberg I. Current management of glaucoma. *Med J Aust*. 2019;210(4):180–187.

13. Lim LS, Mitchell P, Seddon JM, Holz FG, Wong TY. Age-related macular degeneration. *Lancet*. 2012;379(9827):1728–1738.

14. Stitt AW, Curtis TM, Chen M, et al. The progress in understanding and treatment of diabetic retinopathy. *Prog Retin Eye Res*. 2016;51:156–186.

15. Wang W, Lo ACY. Diabetic retinopathy: pathophysiology and treatments. *Int J Mol Sci*. 2018;19(6).

16. Relhan N, Flynn HW, Jr. The Early Treatment Diabetic Retinopathy Study historical review and relevance to today's management of diabetic macular edema. *Curr Opin Ophthalmol*. 2017;28(3):205–212.

17. Pesudovs K. Patient-centred measurement in ophthalmology – a paradigm shift. *BMC Ophthalmol*. 2006;6:25.

18. Food and Drug Administration. *Guidance for Industry – Patient-Reported Outcome Measures: Use in Medical Product Development to Support Labeling Claims*. Food and Drug Administration: U.S. Department of Health and Human Services; 2009.

19. Basch E. New frontiers in patient-reported outcomes: adverse event reporting, comparative effectiveness, and quality assessment. *Annu Rev Med*. 2014;65:307–317.

20. Feinstein A, Josephy B, Wells C. Scientific and clinical problems in indexes of functional disability. *Ann Intern Med*. 1986;105:416–420.

21. Basch E. Patient-reported outcomes – harnessing patients' voices to improve clinical care. *N Engl J Med*. 2017;376(2):105–108.

22. Baumhauer J, Bozic K. Value-based healthcare: patient-reported outcomes in clinical decision making. *Clin Orthop Relat Res*. 2016;474:1375–1378.

23. Snyder CF, Aaronson NK, Choucair AK, et al. Implementing patient-reported outcomes assessment in clinical practice: a review of the options and considerations. *Qual Life Res*. 2012;21(8):1305–1314.

24. WHOQOL Group. *Measuring quality of life*. Geneva: World Health Organization; 1997:1–13.

25. Fenwick EK, Xie J, Ratcliffe J, et al. The impact of diabetic retinopathy and diabetic macular edema on health-related quality of life in type 1 and type 2 diabetes. *Invest Ophthalmol Vis Sci*. 2012;53(2):677–684.

26. Kaplan RM, Tally S, Hays RD, et al. Five preference-based indexes in cataract and heart failure

patients were not equally responsive to change. *J Clin Epidemiol.* 2011;64(5):497–506.

27. Guyatt GH, Feeny DH, Patrick DL. Measuring health-related quality-of-life. *Ann Intern Med.* 1993;118(8):622–629.

28. Bechetoille A, Arnould B, Bron A, et al. Measurement of health-related quality of life with glaucoma: validation of the Glau-QoL 36-item questionnaire. *Acta Ophthalmol.* 2008;86(1):71–80.

29. Pesudovs K, Garamendi E, Elliott DB. The Quality of Life Impact of Refractive Correction (QIRC) questionnaire: development and validation. *Optom Vis Sci.* 2004;81:769–777.

30. Weih LM, Hassell JB, Keeffe J. Assessment of the impact of vision impairment. *Invest Ophthalmol Vis Sci.* 2002;43(4):927–935.

31. Lamoureux EL, Pallant JF, Pesudovs K, Hassell JB, Keeffe JE. The impact of vision impairment questionnaire: an evaluation of its measurement properties using Rasch analysis. *Invest Ophthalmol Vis Sci.* 2006;47(11):4732–4741.

32. Lamoureux E, Pallant J, Pesudovs K, Rees G, Hassell J, Keeffe J. The impact of vision impairment questionnaire: an assessment of its domain structure using confirmatory factor analysis and rasch analysis. *Invest Ophthalmol Vis Sci.* 2007;48:1001–1006.

33. Mangione CM, Berry S, Spritzer K, et al. Identifying the content area for the 51-item National Eye Institute Visual Function Questionnaire: results from focus groups with visually impaired persons. *Arch Ophthalmol.* 1998;116(2):227–233.

34. Mangione CM, Lee PP, Gutierrez PR, Spritzer K, Berry S, Hays RD. Development of the 25-item National Eye Institute Visual Function Questionnaire. *Arch Ophthalmol.* 2001;119(7):1050–1058.

35. Steinberg EP, Tielsch JM, Schein OD, et al. The VF-14: an index of functional impairment in patients with cataract. *Arch Ophthalmol.* 1994;112(5):630–638.

36. Massof RW. A systems model for low-vision rehabilitation. 1. Basic Concepts. *Optom Vis Sci.* 1995;72(10):725–736.

37. Massof RW. A systems model for low vision rehabilitation. II. Measurement of vision disabilities. *Optom Vis Sci.* 1998;75(5):349–373.

38. Mangione CM, Phillips RS, Seddon JM, et al. Development of the 'Activities of Daily Vision Scale'. A measure of visual functional status. *Med Care.* 1992;30(12):1111–1126.

39. Ware JE, Jr., Sherbourne CD. The MOS 36-item short-form health survey (SF-36). I. Conceptual framework and item selection. *Med Care.* 1992;30(6):473–483.

40. McHorney CA, Ware JE, Jr., Raczek AE. The MOS 36-Item Short-Form Health Survey (SF-36): II. Psychometric and clinical tests of validity in measuring physical and mental health constructs. *Med Care.* 1993;31(3):247–263.

41. Ware J, Jr., Kosinski M, Keller SD. A 12-Item Short-Form Health Survey: construction of scales and preliminary tests of reliability and validity. *Med Care.* 1996;34(3):220–233.

42. Williams A. EuroQol – a new facility for the measurement of health-related quality of life. *Health Policy.* 1990;16(3):199–208.

43. Furlong W, Feeny DH, Torrance G, Barr R. The Health Utilities Index (HUI) system for assessing health-related quality of life in clinical studies. *Ann Med.* 2001;33:375–384.

44. Horsman J, Furlong W, Feeny DH, Torrance G. The Health Utilities Index (HUI(R)): concepts, measurement properties and applications. *Health Qual Life Outcomes.* 2003;1:54.

45. Flaxman SR, Bourne RRA, Resnikoff S, et al. Global causes of blindness and distance vision impairment 1990–2020: a systematic review and meta-analysis. *Lancet Glob Health.* 2017;5(12):e1221–e1234.

46. Lamoureux EL, Chong EW, Thumboo J, et al. Vision impairment, ocular conditions, and vision-specific function: the Singapore Malay Eye Study. *Ophthalmology.* 2008;115(11):1973–1981.

47. Chiang PP, Zheng Y, Wong TY, Lamoureux EL. Vision impairment and major causes of vision loss impacts on vision-specific functioning independent of socioeconomic factors. *Ophthalmology.* 2013;120(2):415–422.

48. Nirmalan PK, Tielsch JM, Katz J, et al. Relationship between vision impairment and eye disease to vision-specific quality of life and function in rural India: the Aravind Comprehensive Eye Survey. *Invest Ophthalmol Vis Sci.* 2005;46(7):2308–2312.

49. Nutheti R, Keeffe JE, Shamanna BR, Nirmalan PK, Krishnaiah S, Thomas R. Relationship between visual impairment and eye diseases and visual function in Andhra Pradesh. *Ophthalmology.* 2007;114(8):1552–1557.

50. Finger RP, Fenwick E, Marella M, et al. The impact of vision impairment on vision-specific quality of life in Germany. *Invest Ophthalmol Vis Sci.* 2011;52(6):3613–3619.

51. Chia EM, Mitchell P, Ojaimi E, Rochtchina E, Wang JJ. Assessment of vision-related quality of life in an older population subsample: the Blue Mountains Eye Study. *Ophthalmic Epidemiol.* 2006;13(6):371–377.

52. Broman AT, Munoz B, Rodriguez J, et al. The impact of visual impairment and eye disease on vision-related quality of life in a Mexican–American population: proyecto VER. *Invest Ophthalmol Vis Sci.* 2002;43(11):3393–3398.

53. Rubin GS, Bandeen-Roche K, Huang GH, et al. The association of multiple visual impairments with self-reported visual disability: SEE project. *Invest Ophthalmol Vis Sci.* 2001;42(1):64–72.

54. Rahi JS, Cumberland PM, Peckham CS. Visual impairment and vision-related quality of life in working-age adults: findings in the 1958 British birth cohort. *Ophthalmology.* 2009;116(2):270–274.

55. Globe DR, Wu J, Azen SP, Varma R. The impact of visual impairment on self-reported visual functioning in Latinos: the Los Angeles Latino Eye Study. *Ophthalmology.* 2004;111(6):1141–1149.

56. Fenwick EK, Ong PG, Man RE, et al. Association of vision impairment and major eye diseases with mobility and independence in a Chinese population. *JAMA Ophthalmol.* 2016;134(10):1087–1093.

57. Swenor BK, Muñoz B, West SK. Does visual impairment affect mobility over time? The Salisbury Eye Evaluation Study. *Invest Ophthalmol Vis Sci.* 2013;54(12):7683–7690.

58. Fenwick EK, Ong PG, Man REK, et al. Vision impairment and major eye diseases reduce vision-specific emotional well-being in a Chinese population. *Br J Ophthalmol.* 2017;101(5):686–690.

59. Kidd Man RE, Liang Gan AT, Fenwick EK, et al. Using uniocular visual acuity substantially underestimates the impact of visual impairment on quality of life compared with binocular visual acuity. *Ophthalmology*. 2020;127(9):1145–1151.

60. Varma R, Wu J, Chong K, Azen SP, Hays RD. Impact of severity and bilaterality of visual impairment on health-related quality of life. *Ophthalmology*. 2006;113(10):1846–1853.

61. Vu HT, Keeffe JE, McCarty CA, Taylor HR. Impact of unilateral and bilateral vision loss on quality of life. *Br J Ophthalmol*. 2005;89(3):360–363.

62. Chan EW, Chiang PP, Wong TY, et al. Impact of glaucoma severity and laterality on vision-specific functioning: the Singapore Malay eye study. *Invest Ophthalmol Vis Sci*. 2013;54(2):1169–1175.

63. Fenwick EK, Cheung CMG, Ong PG, et al. The impact of typical neovascular age-related macular degeneration and polypoidal choroidal vasculopathy on vision-related quality of life in Asian patients. *Br J Ophthalmol*. 2017;101(5):591–596.

64. Lamoureux EL, Hassell JB, Keeffe JE. The impact of diabetic retinopathy on participation in daily living. *Arch Ophthalmol*. 2004;122(1):84–88.

65. Lamoureux EL, Tai ES, Thumboo J, et al. Impact of diabetic retinopathy on vision-specific function. *Ophthalmology*. 2010;117(4):757–765.

66. Pondorfer SG, Terheyden JH, Heinemann M, Wintergerst MWM, Holz FG, Finger RP. Association of vision-related quality of life with visual function in age-related macular degeneration. *Sci Rep*. 2019;9(1):15326.

67. Quaranta L, Riva I, Gerardi C, Oddone F, Floriani I, Konstas AG. Quality of life in glaucoma: a review of the literature. *Adv Ther*. 2016;33(6):959–981.

68. Chua J, Lim B, Fenwick EK, et al. Prevalence, risk factors, and impact of undiagnosed visually significant cataract: the Singapore Epidemiology of Eye Diseases study. *PLoS One*. 2017;12(1):e0170804.

69. Chew M, Chiang PP, Zheng Y, et al. The impact of cataract, cataract types, and cataract grades on vision-specific functioning using Rasch analysis. *Am J Ophthalmol*. 2012;154(1):29–38.e22.

70. Gupta P, Liang Gan AT, Kidd Man RE, et al. Impact of incidence and progression of diabetic retinopathy on vision-specific functioning. *Ophthalmology*. 2018;125(9):1401–1409.

71. Taylor DJ, Hobby AE, Binns AM, Crabb DP. How does age-related macular degeneration affect real-world visual ability and quality of life? A systematic review. *BMJ Open*. 2016;6(12):e011504.

72. Lamoureux EL, Mitchell P, Rees G, et al. Impact of early and late age-related macular degeneration on vision-specific functioning. *Br J Ophthalmol*. 2011;95(5):666–670.

73. Choudhury F, Varma R, Klein R, Gauderman WJ, Azen SP, McKean-Cowdin R. Age-related macular degeneration and quality of life in Latinos: the Los Angeles Latino Eye study. *JAMA Ophthalmol*. 2016;134(6):683–690.

74. Fenwick EK, Man REK, Gan ATL, et al. Beyond vision loss: the independent impact of diabetic retinopathy on vision-related quality of life in a Chinese Singaporean population. *Br J Ophthalmol*. 2019;103(9):1314–1319.

75. Mazhar K, Varma R, Choudhury F, McKean-Cowdin R, Shtir CJ, Azen SP. Severity of diabetic retinopathy and health-related quality of life: the Los Angeles Latino Eye Study. *Ophthalmology*. 2011;118(4):649–655.

76. Klein R, Moss SE, Klein BE, Gutierrez P, Mangione CM. The NEI-VFQ-25 in people with long-term type 1 diabetes mellitus: the Wisconsin Epidemiologic Study of Diabetic Retinopathy. *Arch Ophthalmol*. 2001;119(5):733–740.

77. Willis JR, Doan QV, Gleeson M, et al. Vision-related functional burden of diabetic retinopathy across severity levels in the United States. *JAMA Ophthalmol*. 2017;135(9):926–932.

78. Fenwick E, Rees G, Pesudovs K, et al. Social and emotional impact of diabetic retinopathy: a review. *Clin Exp Ophthalmol*. 2012;40(1):27–38.

79. Khoo K, Man REK, Rees G, Gupta P, Lamoureux EL, Fenwick EK. The relationship between diabetic retinopathy and psychosocial functioning: a systematic review. *Qual Life Res*. 2019;28(8):2017–2039.

80. Poongothai S, Anjana RM, Pradeepa R, et al. Association of depression with complications of type 2 diabetes—the Chennai Urban Rural Epidemiology Study (CURES-102). *J Assoc Physicians India*. 2011;59:644–648.

81. Man RE, Fenwick EK, Sabanayagam C, et al. Differential impact of unilateral and bilateral classifications of diabetic retinopathy and diabetic macular edema on vision-related quality of life. *Invest Ophthalmol Vis Sci*. 2016;57(11):4655–4660.

82. Freeman EE, Muñoz B, West SK, Jampel HD, Friedman DS. Glaucoma and quality of life: the Salisbury Eye Evaluation. *Ophthalmology*. 2008;115(2):233–238.

83. McKean-Cowdin R, Wang Y, Wu J, Azen SP, Varma R. Impact of visual field loss on health-related quality of life in glaucoma: the Los Angeles Latino Eye study. *Ophthalmology*. 2008;115(6):941–948.e941.

84. Lamoureux EL, Saw SM, Thumboo J, et al. The impact of corrected and uncorrected refractive error on visual functioning: the Singapore Malay Eye Study. *Invest Ophthalmol Vis Sci*. 2009;50(6):2614–2620.

85. Man REK, Fenwick EK, Sabanayagam C, et al. Prevalence, correlates, and impact of uncorrected presbyopia in a multiethnic Asian population. *Am J Ophthalmol*. 2016;168: 191–200.

86. Vandenbroeck S, De Geest S, Zeyen T, Stalmans I, Dobbels F. Patient-reported outcomes (PRO's) in glaucoma: a systematic review. *Eye (Lond)*. 2011;25(5):555–577.

87. Pesudovs K, Burr JM, Harley C, Elliott DB. The development, assessment, and selection of questionnaires. *Optom Vis Sci*. 2007;84(8):663–674.

88. Khadka J, Gothwal VK, McAlinden C, Lamoureux EL, Pesudovs K. The importance of rating scales in measuring patient-reported outcomes. *Health Qual Life*. 2012;10:80–93.

89. Khadka J, McAlinden C, Pesudovs K. Quality assessment of ophthalmic questionnaires: review and recommendations. *Optom Vis Sci*. 2013;90(8):720–744.

90. de Boer MR, Moll AC, de Vet HC, Terwee CB, Völker-Dieben HJ, van Rens GH. Psychometric properties of vision-related quality of life questionnaires: a systematic review. *Ophthalmic Physiol Opt*. 2004;24(4):257–273.

91. Fenwick EK, Man RE, Aung T, Ramulu P, Lamoureux EL. Beyond intraocular pressure: optimizing patient-reported outcomes in glaucoma. *Prog Retin Eye Res.* 2020;76:100801.

92. Lamoureux EL, Fenwick E, Pesudovs K, Tan D. The impact of cataract surgery on quality of life. *Curr Opin Ophthalmol.* 2011;22(1):19–27.

93. Kandel H, Khadka J, Lundström M, Goggin M, Pesudovs K. Questionnaires for measuring refractive surgery outcomes. *J Refract Surg.* 2017;33(6):416–424.

94. Kumaran SE, Khadka J, Baker R, Pesudovs K. Patient-reported outcome measures in amblyopia and strabismus: a systematic review. *Clin Exp Optom.* 2018;101(4):460–484.

95. Fenwick E, Pesudovs K, Rees G, et al. The impact of diabetic retinopathy: understanding the patient's perspective. *Br J Ophthalmol.* 2010;95(6):774–782.

96. Krezel AK, Hogg RE, Azuara-Blanco A. Patient-reported outcomes in randomised controlled trials on age-related macular degeneration. *Br J Ophthalmol.* 2015;99(11):1560–1564.

97. Finger RP, Fleckenstein M, Holz FG, Scholl HP. Quality of life in age-related macular degeneration: a review of available vision-specific psychometric tools. *Qual Life Res.* 2008;17(4):559–574.

98. Tong A, Sainsbury P, Craig J. Consolidated criteria for reporting qualitative research (COREQ): a 32-item checklist for interviews and focus groups. *Int J Qual Health Care.* 2007;19(6):349–357.

99. Collins D. Pretesting survey instruments: an overview of cognitive methods. *Qual Life Res.* 2003;12(3):229–238.

100. Boone W, Staver J, Yale M. *Rasch Analysis in the Human Sciences.* Dordrecht: Springer; 2014.

101. Lamoureux E, Pallant J, Pesudovs K, Hassell J, Keeffe J. The Impact of Vision Impairment Questionnaire: an evaluation of its measurement properties using Rasch analysis. *Invest Ophthalmol Vis Sci.* 2006;47 :4732–4741.

102. Pesudovs K. Item banking: a generational change in patient-reported outcome measurement. *Optom Vis Sci.* 2010;87(4):1–9.

103. Lamoureux E, Pesudovs K. Vision-specific quality-of-life research: a need to improve the quality. *Am J Ophthalmol.* 2011;151(2):195–197 e192.

104. Lamoureux EL, Pallant JF, Pesudovs K, Rees G, Hassell JB, Keeffe JE. The Impact of Vision Impairment Questionnaire: an assessment of its domain structure using confirmatory factor analysis and Rasch analysis. *Invest Ophthalmol Vis Sci.* 2007;48(3):1001–1006.

105. Marella M, Pesudovs K, Keeffe JE, O'Connor PM, Rees G, Lamoureux EL. The psychometric validity of the NEI VFQ-25 for use in a low-vision population. *Invest Ophthalmol Vis Sci.* 2010;51(6):2878–2884.

106. Pesudovs K, Gothwal VK, Wright T, Lamoureux EL. Remediating serious flaws in the National Eye Institute Visual Function Questionnaire. *J Cataract Refract Surg.* 2010;36(5):718–732.

107. Garamendi E, Pesudovs K, Stevens MJ, Elliott DB. The Refractive Status and Vision Profile: evaluation of psychometric properties and comparison of Rasch and summated Likert-scaling. *Vision Res.* 2006;46(8–9):1375–1383.

108. Mokkink LB, Terwee CB, Patrick DL, et al. The COSMIN checklist for assessing the methodological quality of studies on measurement properties of health status measurement instruments: an international Delphi study. *Qual Life Res.* 2010;19(4):539–549.

109. Mokkink LB, Prinsen CA, Bouter LM, Vet HC, Terwee CB. The COnsensus-based Standards for the selection of health Measurement INstruments (COSMIN) and how to select an outcome measurement instrument. *Braz J Phys Ther.* 2016;20(2):105–113.

110. Bowling A. Mode of questionnaire administration can have serious effects on data quality. *J Public Health (Oxf).* 2005; 27(3):281–291.

111. Gibbons RD, Weiss DJ, Kupfer DJ, et al. Using computerized adaptive testing to reduce the burden of mental health assessment. *Psychiatr Serv.* 2008;59(4):361–368.

112. Gershon RC. Computer adaptive testing. *J Appl Meas.* 2005;6(1):109–127.

113. Lamoureux E, Fenwick E. *Measuring quality of life quicker and better using computerized adaptive testing.* Invited talk presented at World Glaucoma Congress; 27 March 2019, 2019; Melbourne, Australia.

114. Fenwick E, Loe B, Khadka K, Man R, Rees G, Lamoureux E. Optimizing measurement of vision-related quality of life: a computerized adaptive test for the Impact of Vision Impairment questionnaire (IVI-CAT). *Qual Life Res.* 2020;29(3):765–774.

115. Fenwick E, Khadka J, Pesudovs K, Rees G, Lamoureux E. Diabetic retinopathy and macular edema quality-of-life item banks: development and initial evaluation using computerized adaptive testing. *Invest Ophthalmol Vis Sci.* 2017;58(14):6379–6387.

116. Fenwick E, Pesudovs K, Khadka J, et al. The impact of diabetic retinopathy on quality of life: qualitative findings from an item bank development project. *Qual Life Res.* 2012;21(10):1771–1782.

117. Fenwick E, Pesudovs K, Khadka J, Rees G, Wong T, Lamoureux E. Evaluation of item candidates for a diabetic retinopathy quality of life item bank. *Qual Life Res.* 2013;22(7):1851–1858.

118. Fenwick E, Barnard J, Gan A, et al. Computerised adaptive tests: an innovative, efficient and precise method to assess the patient-centred impact of diabetic retinopathy. *Transl Vis Sci Technol.* 2020;9(7):3.

119. Khadka J, McAlinden C, Craig JE, Fenwick EK, Lamoureux EL, Pesudovs K. Identifying content for the glaucoma-specific item bank to measure quality-of-life parameters. *J Glaucoma.* 2015;24(1):12–19.

120. McCloud C, Khadka J, Gilhotra JS, Pesudovs K. Divergence in the lived experience of people with macular degeneration. *Optom Vis Sci.* 2014;91(8):966–974.

121. Prem Senthil M, Khadka J, De Roach J, et al. Developing an item bank to measure the coping strategies of people with hereditary retinal diseases. *Graefes Arch Clin Exp Ophthalmol.* 2018;256(7):1291–1298.

122. Prem Senthil M, Khadka J, De Roach J, et al. Development and psychometric assessment of novel item banks for hereditary retinal diseases. *Optom Vis Sci.* 2019;96(1):27–34.

123. Prem Senthil M, Khadka J, Gilhotra JS, et al. Understanding quality of life impact in people with retinal vein occlusion: a qualitative inquiry. *Clin Exp Optom*. 2019;102(4):406–411.

124 Fenwick EK, Lee EPX, Man REK, Ho KC, Najjar RP, Milea D, Teo KYC, Tan ACS, Lee SY, Yeo IYS, Tan GSW, Mathur R, Wong TY, Cheung CMG, Lamoureux EL. Identifying the content for an item bank and computerized adaptive testing system to measure the impact of age-related macular degeneration on health-related quality of life. *Qual Life Res*. 2021; September 25. doi: 10.1007/s11136-021-02989-w.

125. Wu AW, Jensen RE, Salzberg C, Snyder CF. *Advances in the Use of Patient Reported Outcome Measures in Electronic Health Records Including Case Studies*. Atlanta, GA: In support of the PCORI National Workshop to Advance the Use of PRO measures in Electronic Health Records;2013.

20 Screening Programs

Jakob Grauslund and Malin Lundberg Rasmussen

20.1 INTRODUCTION

Screening is a well-recognized method to identify yet unrecognized disease in asymptomatic people in order to facilitate timely treatment. In the present chapter, we will present the concept of screening, including the Wilson and Jungner criteria, which paved the ground for the introduction of systematic screening programs worldwide (1). In particular, we will present evidence for ocular screening programs aimed to prevent irreversible vision loss. This includes infant and pediatric eye screening as well as screening for diabetic retinopathy (DR). Various methods will be presented, and, finally, we will look into the state of the art of future artificial intelligence (AI)-based screening options.

20.2 CONCEPTUALIZING SCREENING

Screening is a matter of finding the sick amongst the healthy in order to prevent disease or to find an early treatable state of a disease to prevent worsening. In order for a disease or condition to qualify for a screening program, requirements must be met. Wilson and Jungner set up the following requirements that need to be considered before initiating screening (1):

1. The condition should be an important health problem. The use of the term important includes diseases that affect a greater population, such as diabetes, which is presumed to affect approximately half a billion people worldwide by 2030 (2). It can, however, also include diseases that only affect a few people, but where the impact of the disease, if untreated, is very severe; examples of this include phenylketonuria (PKU) (3) and congenital/infantile cataract (4).

2. There should be an accepted treatment for patients with recognized disease and the treatment of the pre-symptomatic stage should affect the course of the disease and the prognosis positively.

3. Facilities for diagnosis and treatment should be available. Screening should not be established if adequate resources for screening and treatment are not available. Therefore, screening for some diseases might be feasible in some communities, while not in others.

4. There should be a recognizable latent or early symptomatic stage.

5. The natural history of the condition, including development from latent to declared disease, should be adequately understood in order to make sure that the screening and treatment are feasible. Knowing the natural history of a disease is crucial before implementing screening. If a disease has a latent phase, but only a small amount will progress, diagnosing the latent phase will result in unneeded concern to the population and, moreover, screening will not be cost-beneficial. Furthermore, the latent stage of the disease should optimally be long and progression slow. Screening of a highly progressive disease is likely to result in a very short screening interval in order not to miss progression and also the advantage of early treatment will probably not result in significant improvement compared to patients first treated when symptoms arise.

6. There should be a suitable test or examination. Tests for screening should have an acceptable high sensitivity and specificity in order to find the sick amongst the healthy and to avoid an excessive number of false negatives, hence missing a substantial number of patients. Likewise, too many false positives could result in increased concern for patients. It is important to make clear that a screening test is not necessarily intended to be diagnostic. The aim is to find persons in suspicion of disease and refer these persons for further investigation and/or treatment. Furthermore, it is important to realize that some patients may be falsely reassured due to false-negative screening results and some patients may be harmed by treatment not needed because of a false-positive result. It is important that the screening population and health personnel are aware and informed of these terms.

7. The test should be acceptable to the population. Side effects of the test should not overshadow the symptoms of the disease or risk causing other diseases, e.g., use of computed tomography (CT) scans in children with risk of radiation and secondary cancer (5, 6).

8. There should be an agreed policy on whom to treat as patients, including management of borderline patients.

9. The cost of case-finding (including diagnosis and treatment of patients diagnosed)

DOI: 10.1201/9781315146737-23

should be economically balanced in relation to possible expenditure on medical care as a whole. These questions/requirements have to be answered politically before implementing screening, so a case-by-case judgment is not needed by the physician.

10. Case-finding should be a continuing process and not a "once and for all" project. This means that persons tested as "normal" in one screening needs to be re-examined at periodic timeslots.

There are different types of screening settings dependent on disease and population. Mass screening is the screening of a whole population, e.g., screening of all newborns for PKU or screening of all women in a certain age-group for cervical cancer (7). In contrast, high-risk screening is the screening of individuals at risk of a disease. It has a higher likelihood of finding individuals with disease. An example is the consideration to screen high-risk patients (based on age, familiar history, ethnicity, refraction, etc.) for glaucoma (8). Finally, opportunistic screening describes the setting where patients attending a visit for one thing are screened for another. One example could be patients over 50 years visiting their general physician for any reason, where blood pressure and blood glucose are measured in order to find persons with undiagnosed hypertension and/or diabetes.

A controversial, not implemented, screening is the example of customers at the optician having intraocular pressure (IOP) measured while buying glasses/contact lenses. This screening might be feasible in finding patients without known risk factors (9, 10). However, there is the risk of a false-positive elevated IOP, which will result in unnecessary visits to the ophthalmologist and maybe unnecessary worrying for the patient and, on the other hand, false-negative normal IOP in patients at risk of glaucoma, who are falsely reassured that they are not at risk of developing glaucoma.

20.3 SCREENING PROGRAMS IN OPHTHALMOLOGY

Screening in ophthalmology is feasible for a number of reasons. Firstly, a variety of ocular diseases place a heavy burden on healthcare systems world-wide. This is in particular true for diabetes, in which DR is the most frequent complication (11, 12) and a common cause of blindness (13, 14). Secondly, detection of disease is feasible with functional and imaging examinations like visual acuity measurement and fundus photography, which are accessible in most countries. Thirdly, detection of screen

positives will have a beneficial effect given the well-established treatment options for retinopathy of prematurity (ROP), retinoblastomas, refractive errors in pre-school children, and sight-threatening DR. Finally, digital imaging in ROP and DR screening often presents the option of telemedicine screening, which is a potential way to decentralize screening units, centralize expert grading and, thus, optimize healthcare resources.

20.3.1 Pediatric Eye Screening

With the aim of preventing vision loss in children, screening programs have been implemented in multiple countries with setups varying from premature children at risk of ROP to refractive errors in pre-school and early school children.

Eye screening in children is important because patients themselves are not always able to communicate subjective complaints. This could lead to delayed diagnosis of visual impairment and, additionally, visual impairment in children may cause severe secondary educational and socioeconomic problems (15, 16).

Refractive errors, amblyopia, strabismus, ocular disease, and color vision deficits are areas of interest in ocular pediatric screening (17).

20.3.1.1 Screening for Retinopathy of Prematurity

ROP is a progressive retinal disease, which in severe untreated cases can lead to retinal detachment and blindness (18). ROP occurs in the premature infant because the retinal vasculature at the time of birth is not fully developed. In 1988, a multicenter study showed that cryotherapy of avascular retina decreased the risk of progression (19), and in 2003 guidelines were adjusted after showing even further decrease of risk if early laser photocoagulation of high-risk prethreshold retinopathy was established (20).

Hence, examining premature infants for ROP meets the criteria for high-risk screening.

According to the American Academy of Pediatrics and UK Retinopathy of Prematurity Guidelines, infants with a birth weight equal to or less than 1500 g or gestational age of 32 weeks (in the US 30 weeks) or less should be screened (18, 21). Also included in screenings are infants otherwise presumed at risk, e.g., infants with intrauterine growth inhibition.

Both societies agree that first screening should be done approximately 4 weeks after birth, but not earlier than the 31st gestational week. Once-only screening can be done if the retina is fully vascularized on the first screening. Otherwise, screening should be done weekly or biweekly until normal vascularization has occurred. In cases of progression or severe findings screening should be done twice a week. Referral to treatment is based on specific high-risk findings. Screening is done after dilation of the pupil and can be done either by direct or indirect ophthalmoscopy, digital photography, or both. The latter gives the opportunity of telemedicine or consultancy with tertiary centers. Screening should be done by an experienced ophthalmologist. To avoid discomfort for the infant, topical anesthetic agents are used and oral sucrose can be added if needed.

In developed countries, where premature children survive at an increasingly young gestational age, there is an increased risk of ROP and a higher need for screening (22).

20.3.1.2 Detection of Visual Loss and Refractive Errors in Pre-School Children

Already within the first few weeks, children should be screened to rule out congenital or infantile cataract. While incidence is very low – 2–4 per 10,000 births – it can result in severe visual impairment if left undiagnosed and untreated (4). In a matter of 30 seconds or less, general physicians or pediatricians are able to perform an examination to rule out congenital cataract within the first weeks of life.

In dimmed light, the red reflex of the retina is examined. Any obstacles shadowing the reflex will need an examination by an ophthalmologist. Patients with a family history of cataract or at increased risk of cataract (e.g., children with Down's syndrome [23]) should be referred to screening by an ophthalmologist, even if a normal red reflex has been identified at initial screening. Likewise, patients with a familial history of retinoblastoma (24) or glaucoma (25) should be screened by an ophthalmologist.

Unilateral or bilateral visual impairment in children could be due to refractive errors (myopia, hyperopia, astigmatism, or anisometropia), strabismus, or ocular disease. Myopia is the most common refractive error in younger ages, and the incidence is increasing (26).

Visual acuity is measured using the Snellen, E chart, or similar charts. It can be easily tested by minimally trained personnel. In most children, visual acuity can be examined at the age of 4 or 5 or even younger. If any suspicion of visual impairment arises, patients should be referred to an ophthalmologist, where more detailed visual acuity can be measured.

Strabismus or squint can be tested by lightning reflex test, where a light source is aimed at the nose of the child and the reflex on the cornea is assessed. The reflex should fall mirrored on the same place in both eyes. If not, non-parallel eyes should be suspected. Another test for strabismus is the cover test, in which the movement of one eye in the covering of the other eye reveals a pretest squint. This movement can sometimes be more easily seen compared to the light reflex in younger, restless children. Furthermore, stereopsis can be measured by Lang stereopsis test in older pre-school children. If it is not possible to measure visual acuity or to fully examine children, great attention must be paid to the parents' suspicions and observations and the child should be referred for expert evaluation by an ophthalmologist.

Color vision can also be tested in children, in order to guide those with color vision deficiency in terms of future job planning, as some professions are excluded if color vision deficiency is present (e.g., pilot and train driver) (27).

The screening tests mentioned above are fast and easily performed and inexpensive. On the other hand, neglecting screening can result in irreversible amblyopia. Visual impairment in a child can also affect the development of motoric and educational skills (15). Despite this a survey of pre-school children in the United States found that only 34 states had guidelines for pre-school vision, and of those, the screening was voluntary in 19 states (28). In the remaining 17 states, preschool vision screening is recommended when children enter kindergarten.

20.3.2 Screening for Diabetic Retinopathy

20.3.2.1 Rationale and Implementation

Diabetes is the global epidemic of the 21st century. It is estimated that between 2015 and 2040, the global prevalence of diabetes will increase from 415 to 642 million people (2). DR is the most common complication in diabetes, affecting one-third of patients at a given time (29). Most important, however, is the fact that one in ten patients have sight-threatening DR (proliferative diabetic retinopathy [PDR] and diabetic macular edema [DME]) (29), which may lead to irreversible visual loss, if not treated timely.

In contrast to the expectations of most people, the purpose of DR screening is not to detect DR *per se*, since treatment is not possible in the early stages. Rather, DR screening is vital in order to detect sight-threatening DR at an asymptomatic stage. This was demonstrated by landmark studies like the Diabetic Retinopathy Study (DRS) and the Early Treatment Diabetes Retinopathy Study (ETDRS). In PDR, the formation of fragile retinal new vessels, at the disc or elsewhere, may lead to vitreous hemorrhage or tractional retinal detachment with a subsequent loss of vision. To address this, the DRS demonstrated that a 29% 3-year risk of severe visual impairment in patients with high-risk PDR (30) could be reduced by 57% by prompt treatment with retinal scatter photocoagulation (31). In recent years, intravitreal vascular endothelial growth factor (VEGF) inhibitors have also been demonstrated as a viable option to preserve vision in PDR (32, 33). In DME, the ETDRS demonstrated that the risk of moderate visual impairment was reduced from 24% to 12% by macular focal/grid photocoagulation, but visual improvement was not likely (34). Since then, VEGF inhibitors have consistently been demonstrated as an efficient option to halt and reverse visual loss in DME (35).

With effective treatment options at hand, it is important to identify patients with sight-threatening PDR in order to institute timely treatment. Consequently, national screening programs have been set up in a number of countries world-wide. At the Screening for Diabetic Retinopathy in Europe meeting in 2016, all attending European countries were making progress in implementing DR screening, with national coverage of the screening programs ranging from 11% to 100% (36). In Asia, home of 60% of all patients with diabetes, national guidelines for DR screening have been published in 11 of 50 countries (37). However, less than half of the population is covered and full criteria for initiation of screening, frequency of screening, referral of screening positives, and further details for the screening process were only given for two countries.

20.3.2.2 Clinical Impact of National Screening Programs

Implementation of national programs for diabetic eye screening has proven advantageous in various countries. An important milestone for this argument was laid by Liew et al., who demonstrated that, as a consequence of the national DR-screening program in England and Wales, DR was, for the first time in five decades, no longer the leading cause of blindness in the working-age population of the UK (38). Prior to that, national screening programs had emerged in various countries, of which Iceland and Singapore were among the pioneers (39, 40).

Various studies have demonstrated cost-effectiveness of DR screening as compared to no screening (41–45). Javitt and Aiello demonstrated that screening and treatment of eye diseases in patients with diabetes had a cost of $3,190 per quality-adjusted life-year (QALY) saved, which was considered substantially lower than many routinely provided healthcare interventions (41). In extension, Javitt et al. reported that recommended eye care for all patients with type 2 diabetes in the US would lead to net savings

of $472 million and 94,304 person-years of sight (44).

20.3.2.3 Methodological Considerations for Diabetic Eye Screening

A number of methodological considerations are important prior to implementation of a DR-screening program. Among others, these include choices of screening population, fundoscopy vs. fundus photography, non-mydriatic vs. mydriatic examinations, retinal field of view, implementation of optical coherence tomography (OCT), screening intervals, usage of telemedicine, detection of concomitant ocular disease, and threshold for referral of screen positives. The present chapter will address a number of these considerations and present available evidence.

20.3.2.3.1 Screening Population

Life-long diabetic eye screening is important in all patients with diabetes, given that sight-threatening DR is feasible in all patients (46, 47). This was demonstrated in the Wisconsin Epidemiologic Study of Diabetic Retinopathy, where Klein et al. examined 996 and 1,370 patients with onset before and after 30 years of age, respectively (46, 47). While PDR in the two groups was unlikely in patients who had had diabetes below 5 years (0% and 2.0%), a longer duration of diabetes was positively associated with a higher risk of PDR (25.0% and 15.5%, respectively, in patients with a duration of 15 years or more). The studies did not identify an upper age above which progression to PDR was no longer likely. On the contrary, PDR could occur at all ages, underlining the necessity to adhere patients to the DR-screening programs.

Often in type 2 diabetes, the true onset of the disease occurs years before the diagnosis is made. Consequently, PDR might be present at the time of the diagnosis (47), and DR screening should be initiated at that point in time. On the other hand, PDR is not likely for the first 5 years in type 1 diabetes (46). In addition, progression to PDR is very unlikely in children with PDR (0% and 1.9% in patients aged 0–15 and 15–19 years, respectively) (46), and, hence, DR screening can be initiated at a later stage. Consequently, it can be recommended in type 1 diabetes to defer DR screening for the first 5 years of diabetes and no earlier than at the age of 9 years (48, 49).

20.3.2.3.2 Fundoscopy or Fundus Photography

An optimal view of the posterior pole is essential for sufficient DR screening. To achieve this, slit-lamp fundoscopy and fundus photography are the most accepted methods for DR examination. While fundoscopy has the advantages of low cost and presumably better performance in patients with vitreous opacities or poor pupillary dilation, it is difficult to master and has a limited performance in comparison with fundus photography.

In a systematic review, Hutchinson et al. recommended mydriatic retinal photography as the most effective strategy for testing with fundoscopy as a viable option for patients with ungradable retinal images (50). While non-mydriatic retinal photography did not perform better than fundoscopy, mydriatic retinal imaging consistently demonstrated higher sensitivity.

Non-Mydriatic or Mydriatic Examinations

The consideration to include mydriatic retinal imaging in a DR-screening program has different aspects. Non-mydriatic retinal imaging is a faster approach, causing less discomfort in patients. However, clinical performance is also important to consider.

In a meta-analysis Piyasena et al. reported performance in 18 studies using non-mydriatic retinal imaging (51). There was a pooled sensitivity of DR detection of 86%, increasing to 91% for two-field images. Specificity was 91–94%, and the mean proportion of ungradable images was 18.4%. In comparison, sensitivities and specificities for mydriatic retinal images were 92% and 94%, respectively, but the mean proportion of ungradables was substantially lower (6.2%). Despite the acceptable performance of non-mydriatic retinal images, the higher number of ungradable images is a clinical concern, which is important to consider when DR screening is implemented.

20.3.2.3.3 Optimal Retinal Field of View

Traditionally, the ETDRS seven-field 30° stereo images have been regarded as the gold standard for DR grading. While indirect fundoscopy only has a 34% sensitivity compared to this method (52), ETDRS imaging is time-consuming, a burden for patients, and difficult to perform for healthcare professionals. Consequently, a number of studies have evaluated if comparable performance could be achieved with fewer retinal fields.

Consensually accepted is the EURODIAB IDDM Complications Study, where Aldington et al. were able to validate the use of two-field 45° mydriatic retinal images (53). Five independent retinal experts achieved a median agreement of 77% (kappa 0.85 and 0.83 for within- and between-observer agreement). Consequently, the two-field (nasal and macular) strategy has been widely adopted in screening programs world-wide.

The introduction of ultra-wide-field (UWF) retinal imaging has provided a more contemporary solution, taking into account the availability of this method to visualize 80% of the entire retina, which is substantially more than the 30% of the retinal surface visualized by seven-field ETDRS imaging. In addition, pupil dilation is not mandatory for UWF. However, such cameras are more expensive than traditional fundus cameras, and identification of retinal lesions might be more difficult for UWF that use scanning laser ophthalmoscope instead of true colors.

To address performance, Rasmussen et al. performed a four-way comparison between non-mydriatic, mydriatic, and steered mydriatic UWF (using ETDRS as comparator) (54). All methods had a very high agreement, within one level, with ETDRS (99.0%, 98.9%, and 100.0%, respectively). Among 190 retinal images, PDR was only missed in two eyes with UWF (due to eye lashes) and three eyes with ETDRS images (neovascularization not identifiable or out of area of visualization). Along with the findings of others (55, 56), this study has, so far, led to the conclusion that UWF compares well with ETDRS standard, but does not lead to increased performance.

20.3.2.3.4 Usage of OCT in DR Screening

At the time the ETDRS study coined the term clinically significant macular edema (CSME) (34), OCT had not been invented, and classification of edema had to rely upon retinal stereo evaluation. An optimized detection of CSME in DR screening might lead to fewer false positives in the screening program and, hence, a better utilization of healthcare resources. In addition, anxiety and concerns of visual loss would be lower for patients if CSME could be ruled out at the stage of screening prior to referral for DR treatment.

Wong et al. demonstrated in 352 patients with foveal hemorrhages, hard exudates, or both, a false-positive CSME rate of 86.6% if OCT was not included in the decision (57). Mackenzie et al. confirmed this in the UK screening program, in which spectral domain OCT was able to rule on CSME in 42.1% of cases, who met the traditional screening definitions (58). While it is arguably not indicated to perform OCT in the vast majority of patients without CSME-suspected lesions in fundus photography, these studies support the inclusion of OCT in selected patients.

20.3.2.3.5 Screening Intervals

In most DR-screening programs, annual screening has initially been the standard of care for the vast majority of patients. However, evidence has emerged that individualized considerations can be used to extend screening intervals almost three times (59), while reducing the number of screening episodes by 40% (60, 61). This is in particular true for patients without DR. To exemplify, the Diabetes Control and Complications Trial and the subsequent Epidemiology of Diabetes Interventions and Complications Study demonstrated that in type 1 diabetes the screening interval needed to obtain a 5% risk of progression to PDR or CSME was 4 years, 3 years, 6 months, and 3 months for patients with no DR, mild non-proliferative DR (NPDR), moderate NPDR, and severe NPDR, respectively (62).

In extension, Thomas et al. demonstrated that, in comparison to annual screening, biennial DR screening was cost-effective for most patients (63). For patients with type 1 and 2 diabetes and HbA1c of 6.5% (47.5 mmol/mol), extending screening intervals led to savings of £94,696 and £106,075 per QALY, respectively, with decremental cost-effectiveness ratios above £20,000 per QALY considered cost-effective.

While DR-screening intervals can be safely prolonged for most patients, lower intervals are important in high-risk patients. These include patients with impaired glycemic control (64, 65), hypertension (66), pregnancy (67), bariatric surgery (68), and socioeconomic deprivation (69).

20.3.2.3.6 Usage of Telemedicine in DR Screening

Telemedicine has been proposed as a way to optimize DR screening. The notion is to capture retinal images locally and then transmit these electronically to a centralized grading center staffed by trained readers. This is a potential solution to the increasing demand of retinal experts needed for DR screening. To illustrate that retinal expertise is often centralized at larger cities and specialized hospitals, Gibson reported that 24.0% of US counties did not have any ophthalmologists or optometrists (70).

In a systematic review, Horton et al. evaluated various clinical components of telemedicine screening programs for DR (71). They identified a number of factors with the potential to influence the quality of telemedicine in DR screening, including the number and size of retinal fields imaged, mydriatic examinations, and stereoscopic imaging. Furthermore, the review supported the concept of primary care-based examinations and technical or licensed eye care providers able to perform evaluation of retinal images in centralized reading centers.

The high number of diabetes-related examinations is often a barrier for effective diabetes care. In Denmark, systemic same-day-complication screening has recently been launched for patients with diabetes in order to integrate all diabetes examinations at the same day. This is a telemedicine-based screening program embracing DR screening. Patients attend a local hospital-based diabetes clinic. Micro- and macrovascular complications are evaluated, including fundus photography-based DR screening supported by OCT, when applicable. Retinal images are transferred electronically to a centralized grading center, from which DR grading is performed by certified ophthalmic experts within an hour. At the local hospital-based diabetes clinic, evaluation of DR is integrated with evaluation of nephropathy, neuropathy, blood pressure, and glycemic control, and based upon this, individualized plans for diabetes treatment are given by the attending diabetologist.

In the Singapore Integrated Diabetic Retinopathy Program, Nguyen et al. demonstrated favorable cost-effectiveness for a telemedicine-based DR-screening program in comparison with the existing model with family physician-based assessments (72). The study estimated that telemedicine-based DR screening would lead to future cost savings of S$29.4 million over a lifetime horizon for the healthcare system in Singapore. This was confirmed in a systematic review by Avidor et al. (73), that demonstrated significant cost savings of telemedicine-based DR screening, in particular in low-income populations and rural patients with high transportation costs.

20.3.2.3.7 Referral for Ophthalmic Care of Screen Positive Patients

Reference standards are a key component in a DR-screening program. However, these are subject to considerable variations between countries given different treatment standards in the national healthcare systems.

To exemplify this, a variety of reference standards were given for different Asian countries, and in some programs these were not clearly defined (37). Most referral criteria included visual acuity measurement, level of DR (often set at moderate NPDR or worse), or inability to obtain sufficient retinal examination (74). As another example, in the Danish national DR-screening program patients are only referred at the level of PDR or CSME, given that DR treatment is not indicated at earlier stages (48).

While well-defined referral guidelines are essential in order to set up an effective screening program, national healthcare systems and standards for treatment are important to consider in order to maximize the number of true positives.

20.3.2.3.8 Detection of Glaucoma and Age-Related Macular Degeneration

It is generally stated that screening for diseases like glaucoma and AMD is not indicated except, perhaps, in selected high-risk patients. To illustrate this, the US Preventive Services Task Force did not find sufficient evidence to recommend for or against screening for glaucoma in adults (75). With respect to the World Health Organization criteria for screening programs (1), it was stated that the diagnosis of primary open-angle glaucoma is not based on the basis of a single test, the natural history of the disease is not well understood, measurements of visual fields can be difficult, and the primary treatment for glaucoma reduces IOP but has an uncertain function in visual impairment reduction. Likewise, Tamura et al. reported that a simulative screening program for AMD in Japan would be able to reduce blindness by 41% but would not be cost-effective (76).

While glaucoma and AMD do not meet the criteria for screening, early diagnosis of asymptomatic patients would still be clinically valuable in order to reduce visual impairment. Given that the optic disc and macula are available for inspection in retinal images, it would be possible to include such an evaluation in DR screening. This notion has in particular been important with recent advancements in AI-based retinal imaging. To illustrate this, Ting et al. used 125,189 and 72,610 retinal images, respectively, in a deep-learning (DL) system to detect possible glaucoma and AMD (77). Sensitivities and specificities were very high for both diseases (glaucoma: 94.4% and 87.2%; AMD: 93.2% and 88.7%), indicating that DL is a potential way to include evaluations for additional diseases in DR screening.

20.4 FUTURE ADVANCEMENTS IN OPHTHALMIC SCREENING

With recent technological developments, it has become feasible to include new scientific landmarks, which have in particular been demonstrated in DR screening. In this section, we will highlight some of the important results and put this into perspective for DR screening.

20.4.1 Screening by Machine Learning

Manual grading of DR images is a strenuous, labor-intensive, highly specialized task. With recent AI advancements, automated assessment of DR images has become possible. The early versions of this were termed automated retinal image analysis systems (ARIAS). The concept of this is computer-based identification of pathological lesions, which ultimately provide a classification of DR. In other words, the algorithm has

been trained to recognize specific patterns (e.g., retinal microaneurysms and hemorrhages) and translate these into corresponding DR categories.

In a systematic review, Nørgaard and Grauslund identified seven classification-based ARIAS in DR screening (78). In general, all studies had a high sensitivity (87.0–95.2%), which is very important, given that it is essential in DR screening not to miss patients in need of treatment. On the other hand, ARIAS were in general limited by a moderate specificity (49.6–68.8%). This implies a substantial number of false positives, which could limit the cost benefit to implementing such systems.

Tufail et al. also addressed this issue in a health technology assessment, including 102,856 retinal images from 20,258 patients tested by three ARIAS (79). The two ARIAS included in the final analysis achieved acceptable sensitivity regarding referable DR and false-positive rates and were considered cost-effective alternatives to manual grading.

20.4.2 Deep Learning

In recent years, impressive results for DR classification have been demonstrated by DL-based convolutional neural networks (CNN), which have become state of the art for automated image recognition (80). This is an efficient use of big data to improve diagnosis of DR and other retinal diseases, and recently the first DL algorithms were approved by the US Food and Drug Administration (81).

The concept of DL is experience-based learning of underlying features in data by neural networks. By back-propagation on annotated retinal images, a CNN is built based on image recognition (80). This consists of input, hidden, and output layers. The input layers specify the width of the network. The hidden layers are fully connected and use convolution (transformation of input data by applying kernel weights acting as feature sensors) and pooling to advance to the output layer (which will give the classification of the image). With the input of a high number (82) of retinal images with a given DR classification, the algorithm will run numerous iterations in order to adjust internal parameters, which will ultimately, with very high accuracy, predict the desired output of the image. This is conceptually the opposite workflow to machine learning, where retinal lesions are identified based on pre-programmed rules. In DL, there are no rules for detection, which is performed by computer experience. In a recent systematic review, Nielsen et al. demonstrated high diagnostic performance with sensitivities and specificities above 80% in previous studies of DR classification (83).

The era of DL in diabetic eye screening was entered in 2017 with a pivotal paper of Gulshan et al. utilizing 128,175 retinal images in patients with diabetes to demonstrate sensitivities and specificities of more than 90% for detecting moderate NPDR or worse (82). In comparison to ARIAS, DL algorithms are, thus, able to reduce the rate of false positives, which is one of the major challenges in DR screening. To complement these findings, Ting et al. demonstrated similarly high sensitivities and specificities in multi-ethnic populations and concluded that DL is also able to identify patients with glaucoma and AMD (77).

20.4.3 Handheld Screening Devices

While sufficient population coverage is critical for successful ophthalmic screening programs, lack of accessibility to retinal fundus cameras can often be a problem in rural areas and low-income countries. A potential way to deal with the challenge is handheld retinal cameras, which can often be used in conjunction with a smartphone.

In a prospective study, Zhang et al. concluded in 111 eyes of 56 patients that undilated retinal images were gradable in 86–94% of patients, and that sensitivity and specificity for identification of vision-threatening DR were 79% and 77%, respectively. Piyasena et al. examined 700 patients with diabetes and found a high proportion of ungradable retinal images in non-mydriatic patients (43.4%), which decreased substantially to 12.8% after pupil dilation (51). Sensitivities and specificities of referable DR were 88.7–92.5% and 94.9–96.4%, indicating that implementation could be feasible, but that the level of ungradable retinal images, in particular in eyes with non-dilated pupils, is a concern for portable screening devices.

20.5 CONCLUSIONS

Screening of sight-threatening diseases is an important task in ophthalmic care. This chapter has conceptualized the term of ocular screening and provided clinical examples of impact and challenges in this area. With a globally aging population and recent technological landmarks in hand, the ground has been laid for future ways to combat blindness in various ocular diseases.

REFERENCES

1. Wilson JMG, Jungner G. *Principles and Practice of Screening for Disease.* Geneva: World Health Organization; 1968.
2. Ogurtsova K, da Rocha Fernandes JD, Huang Y, Linnenkamp U, Guariguata L, Cho NH, et al. IDF diabetes atlas: global estimates for the prevalence of diabetes for 2015 and 2040. *Diabetes Res Clin Pract.* 2017;128:40–50.
3. van Spronsen FJ. Phenylketonuria: a 21st century perspective. *Nat Rev Endocrinol.* 2010;6(9):509–14.
4. Sheeladevi S, Lawrenson JG, Fielder AR, Suttle CM. Global prevalence of childhood cataract: a systematic review. *Eye (Lond).* 2016;30(9):1160–9.
5. Pearce MS, Salotti JA, Little MP, McHugh K, Lee C, Kim KP, et al. Radiation exposure from CT scans in childhood and subsequent risk of leukaemia and brain tumours: a retrospective cohort study. *Lancet.* 2012;380(9840):499–505.
6. Mathews JD, Forsythe AV, Brady Z, Butler MW, Goergen SK, Byrnes GB, et al. Cancer risk in 680,000 people exposed to computed tomography scans in childhood or adolescence: data linkage study of 11 million Australians. *BMJ.* 2013;346:f2360.
7. Chrysostomou AC, Stylianou DC, Constantinidou A, Kostrikis LG. Cervical cancer screening programs in Europe: the transition towards HPV vaccination and population-based HPV testing. *Viruses.* 2018;10(12).
8. Gupta D, Chen PP. Glaucoma. *Am Fam Physician.* 2016;93(8):668–74.
9. Stoutenbeek R, Jansonius NM. Glaucoma screening during regular optician visits: can the population at risk of developing glaucoma be reached? *Br J Ophthalmol.* 2006;90(10):1242–4.
10. de Vries MM, Stoutenbeek R, Müskens RP, Jansonius NM. Glaucoma screening during regular optician visits: the feasibility and specificity of screening in real life. *Acta Ophthalmol.* 2012;90(2):115–21.
11. Klein R, Knudtson MD, Lee KE, Gangnon R, Klein BE. The Wisconsin Epidemiologic Study of Diabetic Retinopathy: XXII the twenty-five-year progression of retinopathy in persons with type 1 diabetes. *Ophthalmology.* 2008;115(11):1859–68.
12. Grauslund J, Green A, Sjolie AK. Prevalence and 25 year incidence of proliferative retinopathy among Danish type 1 diabetic patients. *Diabetologia.* 2009;52(9):1829–35.
13. Klein R, Lee KE, Gangnon RE, Klein BE. The 25-year incidence of visual impairment in type 1 diabetes mellitus: the Wisconsin epidemiologic study of diabetic retinopathy. *Ophthalmology.* 2010;117(1):63–70.
14. Grauslund J, Green A, Sjolie AK. Blindness in a 25-year follow-up of a population-based cohort of Danish type 1 diabetic patients. *Ophthalmology.* 2009;116(11):2170–4.
15. Solebo AL, Teoh L, Rahi J. Epidemiology of blindness in children. *Arch Dis Child.* 2017;102(9):853–7.
16. Courtright P, Hutchinson AK, Lewallen S. Visual impairment in children in middle- and lower-income countries. *Arch Dis Child.* 2011;96(12):1129–34.
17. Rahi JS, Williams C, Bedford H, Elliman D. Screening and surveillance for ophthalmic disorders and visual deficits in children in the United Kingdom. *Br J Ophthalmol.* 2001;85(3):257–9.
18. Fierson WM. Screening examination of premature infants for retinopathy of prematurity. *Pediatrics.* 2018;142(6).
19. Cryotherapy for Retinopathy of Prematurity Cooperative Group. Multicenter trial of cryotherapy for retinopathy of prematurity. Preliminary results. *Arch Ophthalmol.* 1988;106(4):471–9.
20. Early Treatment for Retinopathy of Prematurity Group. Revised indications for the treatment of

retinopathy of prematurity: results of the early treatment for retinopathy of prematurity randomized trial. *Arch Ophthalmol.* 2003;121(12):1684–94.

21. RCPCHHealth. *Guideline for the Screening and Treatment of Retinopathy of Prematurity – Clinical Guideline.* Available from: www.rcpch.ac.uk/resources/screening-treatment-retinopathy-prematurity-clinical-guideline.

22. Harrison MS, Goldenberg RL. Global burden of prematurity. *Semin Fetal Neonatal Med.* 2016;21(2):74–9.

23. Stoll C, Dott B, Alembik Y, Roth MP. Associated congenital anomalies among cases with Down syndrome. *Eur J Med Genet.* 2015;58(12):674–80.

24. Skalet AH, Gombos DS, Gallie BL, Kim JW, Shields CL, Marr BP, et al. Screening children at risk for retinoblastoma: consensus report from the American Association of Ophthalmic Oncologists and Pathologists. *Ophthalmology.* 2018;125(3):453–8.

25. Seidman DJ, Nelson LB, Calhoun JH, Spaeth GL, Harley RD. Signs and symptoms in the presentation of primary infantile glaucoma. *Pediatrics.* 1986;77(3):399–404.

26. Holden BA, Fricke TR, Wilson DA, Jong M, Naidoo KS, Sankaridurg P, et al. Global prevalence of myopia and high myopia and temporal trends from 2000 through 2050. *Ophthalmology.* 2016;123(5):1036–42.

27. Randolph SA. Color vision deficiency. *Workplace Health Saf.* 2013;61(6):280.

28. Ciner EB, Dobson V, Schmidt PP, Allen D, Cyert L, Maguire M, et al. A survey of vision screening policy of preschool children in the United States. *Surv Ophthalmol.* 1999;43(5):445–57.

29. Yau JW, Rogers SL, Kawasaki R, Lamoureux EL, Kowalski JW, Bek T, et al. Global prevalence and major risk factors of diabetic retinopathy. *Diabetes Care.* 2012;35(3):556–64.

30. The Diabetic Retinopathy Study Research Group. Photocoagulation treatment of proliferative diabetic retinopathy: the second report of Diabetic Retinopathy Study findings. *Ophthalmology.* 1978;85(1):82–106.

31. Diabetic Retinopathy Study. Preliminary report on effects of photocoagulation therapy. The Diabetic Retinopathy Study Research Group. *Am J Ophthalmol.* 1976;81(4):383–96.

32. Sivaprasad S, Prevost AT, Vasconcelos JC, Riddell A, Murphy C, Kelly J, et al. Clinical efficacy of intravitreal aflibercept versus panretinal photocoagulation for best corrected visual acuity in patients with proliferative diabetic retinopathy at 52 weeks (CLARITY): a multicentre, single-blinded, randomised, controlled, phase 2b, non-inferiority trial. *Lancet.* 2017;389(10085):2193–203.

33. Writing Committee for the Diabetic Retinopathy Clinical Research Network, Gross JG, Glassman AR, Jampol LM, Inusah S, Aiello LP, et al. Panretinal photocoagulation vs intravitreous ranibizumab for proliferative diabetic retinopathy: a randomized clinical trial. *JAMA.* 2015;314(20):2137–46.

34. Early Treatment Diabetic Retinopathy Study Research Group. Photocoagulation for diabetic macular edema. Early Treatment Diabetic Retinopathy Study report number 1. *Arch Ophthalmol.* 1985;103(12):1796–806.

35. Wells JA, Glassman AR, Ayala AR, Jampol LM, Bressler NM, Bressler SB, et al. Aflibercept, bevacizumab, or ranibizumab for diabetic macular edema: two-year results from a comparative effectiveness randomized clinical trial. *Ophthalmology.* 2016;123(6):1351–9.

36. Screening for Diabetic Retinopathy in Europe – Progress Since 2011: Report of Meeting. www.drscreening2005.org.uk/Download%20Documents/ScreeningInEurope2016ConferenceReport_1%200.pdf

37. Wang LZ, Cheung CY, Tapp RJ, Hamzah H, Tan G, Ting D, et al. Availability and variability in guidelines on diabetic retinopathy screening in Asian countries. *Br J Ophthalmol.* 2017;101(10):1352–60.

38. Liew G, Michaelides M, Bunce C. A comparison of the causes of blindness certifications in England and Wales in working age adults (16–64 years), 1999–2000 with 2009–2010. *BMJ Open.* 2014;4(2):e004015.

39. Danielsen R, Helgason T, Jonasson F. Prognostic factors and retinopathy in type 1 diabetics in Iceland. *Acta Medica Scandinavica.* 1983;213(5):323–6.

40. Lau HC, Voo YO, Yeo KT, Ling SL, Jap A. Mass screening for diabetic retinopathy – a report on diabetic retinal screening in primary care clinics in Singapore. *Singapore Med J.* 1995;36(5):510–13.

41. Javitt JC, Aiello LP. Cost-effectiveness of detecting and treating diabetic retinopathy. *Ann Intern Med.* 1996;124(1 Pt 2):164–9.

42. Porta M, Rizzitiello A, Tomalino M, Trento M, Passera P, Minonne A, et al. Comparison of the cost-effectiveness of three approaches to screening for and treating sight-threatening diabetic retinopathy. *Diabetes Metab.* 1999;25(1):44–53.

43. James M, Turner DA, Broadbent DM, Vora J, Harding SP. Cost effectiveness analysis of screening for sight threatening diabetic eye disease. *BMJ.* 2000;320(7250):1627–31.

44. Javitt JC, Aiello LP, Chiang Y, Ferris FL, 3rd, Canner JK, Greenfield S. Preventive eye care in people with diabetes is cost-saving to the federal government. Implications for health-care reform. *Diabetes Care.* 1994;17(8):909–17.

45. Stefansson E, Bek T, Porta M, Larsen N, Kristinsson JK, Agardh E. Screening and prevention of diabetic blindness. *Acta Ophthalmol Scand.* 2000;78(4):374–85.

46. Klein R, Klein BE, Moss SE, Davis MD, DeMets DL. The Wisconsin epidemiologic study of diabetic retinopathy. II. Prevalence and risk of diabetic retinopathy when age at diagnosis is less than 30 years. *Arch Ophthalmol.* 1984;102(4):520–6.

47. Klein R, Klein BE, Moss SE, Davis MD, DeMets DL. The Wisconsin epidemiologic study of diabetic retinopathy. III. Prevalence and risk of diabetic retinopathy when age at diagnosis is 30 or more years. *Arch Ophthalmol.* 1984;102(4):527–32.

48. Grauslund J, Andersen N, Andresen J, Flesner P, Haamann P, Heegaard S, et al. Evidence-based Danish guidelines for screening of diabetic retinopathy. *Acta Ophthalmol.* 2018;96(8):763–9.

49. Lueder GT, Silverstein J, American Academy of Pediatrics Section on Ophthalmology, Section on Endocrinology. Screening for retinopathy in the pediatric patient with type 1 diabetes mellitus. *Pediatrics.* 2005;116(1):270–3.

50. Hutchinson A, McIntosh A, Peters J, O'Keeffe C, Khunti K, Baker R, et al. Effectiveness of screening and monitoring tests for diabetic retinopathy – a systematic review. *Diabet Med.* 2000;17(7):495–506.

51. Piyasena M, Murthy GVS, Yip JLY, Gilbert C, Peto T, Gordon I, et al. Systematic review and meta-analysis of diagnostic accuracy of detection of any level of diabetic retinopathy using digital retinal imaging. *Syst Rev*. 2018;7(1):182.

52. Lin DY, Blumenkranz MS, Brothers RJ, Grosvenor DM. The sensitivity and specificity of single-field nonmydriatic monochromatic digital fundus photography with remote image interpretation for diabetic retinopathy screening: a comparison with ophthalmoscopy and standardized mydriatic color photography. *Am J Ophthalmol*. 2002;134(2):204–13.

53. Aldington SJ, Kohner EM, Meuer S, Klein R, Sjolie AK. Methodology for retinal photography and assessment of diabetic retinopathy: the EURODIAB IDDM complications study. *Diabetologia*. 1995;38(4):437–44.

54. Rasmussen ML, Broe R, Frydkjaer-Olsen U, Olsen BS, Mortensen HB, Peto T, et al. Comparison between Early Treatment Diabetic Retinopathy Study 7-field retinal photos and non-mydriatic, mydriatic and mydriatic steered widefield scanning laser ophthalmoscopy for assessment of diabetic retinopathy. *J Diabetes Complications*. 2015;29(1):99–104.

55. Kernt M, Hadi I, Pinter F, Seidensticker F, Hirneiss C, Haritoglou C, et al. Assessment of diabetic retinopathy using nonmydriatic ultra-widefield scanning laser ophthalmoscopy (Optomap) compared with ETDRS 7-field stereo photography. *Diabetes Care*. 2012;35(12):2459–63.

56. Silva PS, Cavallerano JD, Sun JK, Soliman AZ, Aiello LM, Aiello LP. Peripheral lesions identified by mydriatic ultrawide field imaging: distribution and potential impact on diabetic retinopathy severity. *Ophthalmology*. 2013;120(12):2587–95.

57. Wong RL, Tsang CW, Wong DS, McGhee S, Lam CH, Lian J, et al. Are we making good use of our public resources? The false-positive rate of screening by fundus photography for diabetic macular oedema. *Hong Kong Med J*. 2017;23(4):356–64.

58. Mackenzie S, Schmermer C, Charnley A, Sim D, Vikas T, Dumskyj M, et al. SDOCT imaging to identify macular pathology in patients diagnosed with diabetic maculopathy by a digital photographic retinal screening programme. *PLoS One*. 2011;6(5):e14811.

59. Mehlsen J, Erlandsen M, Poulsen PL, Bek T. Individualized optimization of the screening interval for diabetic retinopathy: a new model. *Acta Ophthalmol*. 2012;90(2):109–14.

60. Lund SH, Aspelund T, Kirby P, Russell G, Einarsson S, Palsson O, et al. Individualised risk assessment for diabetic retinopathy and optimisation of screening intervals: a scientific approach to reducing healthcare costs. *Br J Ophthalmol*. 2016;100(5):683–7.

61. Aspelund T, Thornorisdottir O, Olafsdottir E, Gudmundsdottir A, Einarsdottir AB, Mehlsen J, et al. Individual risk assessment and information technology to optimise screening frequency for diabetic retinopathy. *Diabetologia*. 2011;54(10):2525–32.

62. The Diabetes Control and Complications Trial Research Group. Frequency of evidence-based screening for retinopathy in type 1 diabetes. *N Engl J Med*. 2017;376(16):1507–16.

63. Thomas RL, Winfield TG, Prettyjohns M, Dunstan FD, Cheung WY, Anderson PM, et al. Cost-effectiveness of biennial screening for diabetes related retinopathy in people with type 1 and type 2 diabetes compared to annual screening. *Eur J Health Econ*. 2020;21(7):993–1002.

64. The Diabetes Control and Complications Trial Research Group. The effect of intensive treatment of diabetes on the development and progression of long-term complications in insulin-dependent diabetes mellitus. *N Engl J Med*. 1993;329(14):977–86.

65. UK Prospective Diabetes Study (UKPDS) Group. Intensive blood-glucose control with sulphonylureas or insulin compared with conventional treatment and risk of complications in patients with type 2 diabetes (UKPDS 33). *Lancet*. 1998;352(9131):837–53.

66. UK Prospective Diabetes Study Group. Tight blood pressure control and risk of macrovascular and microvascular complications in type 2 diabetes: UKPDS 38. *BMJ*. 1998;317(7160):703–13.

67. The Diabetes Control and Complications Trial Research Group. Effect of pregnancy on microvascular complications in the diabetes control and complications trial. *Diabetes Care*. 2000;23(8):1084–91.

68. Kim YJ, Kim BH, Choi BM, Sun HJ, Lee SJ, Choi KS. Bariatric surgery is associated with less progression of diabetic retinopathy: A systematic review and meta-analysis. *Surg Obes Relat Dis*. 2017;13(2):352–60.

69. Kashim RM, Newton P, Ojo O. Diabetic retinopathy screening: a systematic review on patients' non-attendance. *Int J Environ Res Public Health*. 2018;15(1).

70. Gibson DM. The geographic distribution of eye care providers in the United States: implications for a national strategy to improve vision health. *Prev Med*. 2015;73:30–6.

71. Horton MB, Silva PS, Cavallerano JD, Aiello LP. Clinical components of telemedicine programs for diabetic retinopathy. *Curr Diab Rep*. 2016;16(12):129.

72. Nguyen HV, Tan GS, Tapp RJ, Mital S, Ting DS, Wong HT, et al. Cost-effectiveness of a national telemedicine diabetic retinopathy screening program in Singapore. *Ophthalmology*. 2016;123(12):2571–80.

73. Avidor D, Loewenstein A, Waisbourd M, Nutman A. Cost-effectiveness of diabetic retinopathy screening programs using telemedicine: a systematic review. *Cost Eff Resour Alloc*. 2020;18:16.

74. Arnold LW, Wang Z. The HbA1c and all-cause mortality relationship in patients with type 2 diabetes is J-shaped: a meta-analysis of observational studies. *Rev Diabet Stud*. 2014;11(2):138–52.

75. US Preventive Services Task Force. Screening for glaucoma: recommendation statement. *Ann Fam Med*. 2005;3(2):171–2.

76. Tamura H, Goto R, Akune Y, Hiratsuka Y, Hiragi S, Yamada M. The clinical effectiveness and cost-effectiveness of screening for age-related macular degeneration in Japan: a Markov modeling study. *PLoS One*. 2015;10(7):e0133628.

77. Ting DSW, Cheung CY, Lim G, Tan GSW, Quang ND, Gan A, et al. Development and validation of a deep learning system for diabetic retinopathy and related eye diseases using retinal images from multiethnic populations with diabetes. *JAMA*. 2017;318(22):2211–23.

78. Nørgaard MF, Grauslund J. Automated screening for diabetic retinopathy – a systematic review. *Ophthalmic Res*. 2018;60(1):9–17.

79. Tufail A, Rudisill C, Egan C, Kapetanakis VV, Salas-Vega S, Owen CG, et al. Automated diabetic

retinopathy image assessment software: diagnostic accuracy and cost-effectiveness compared with human graders. *Ophthalmology*. 2017;124(3):343–51.

80. LeCun Y, Bengio Y, Hinton G. Deep learning. *Nature*. 2015;521(7553):436–44.

81. Abràmoff MD, Lavin PT, Birch M, Shah N, Folk JC. Pivotal trial of an autonomous AI-based diagnostic system for detection of diabetic retinopathy in primary care offices. *NPJ Digit Med*. 2018;1(1):39.

82. Gulshan V, Peng L, Coram M, Stumpe MC, Wu D, Narayanaswamy A, et al. Development and validation of a deep learning algorithm for detection of diabetic retinopathy in retinal fundus photographs. *JAMA*. 2016;316(22):2402–10.

83. Nielsen KB, Lautrup ML, Andersen JKH, Savarimuthu TR, Grauslund J. Deep learning-based algorithms in screening of diabetic retinopathy: a systematic review of diagnostic performance. *Ophthalmol Retina*. 2019;3(4):294–304.

84. Zhang W, Nicholas P, Schuman SG, Allingham MJ, Faridi A, Suthar T et al. Screening for diabetic retinopathy using a portable, noncontact, nonmydriatic handheld retinal camera. *J Diabetes Sci Technol*. 2017;11(1):128–34.

21 Community Intervention Trials in Eye Health

*Ving Fai Chan, Prabhath Piyasena, Priya Adhisesha Reddy, Olusola Olawoye,
and Nathan Congdon*

21.1 INTRODUCTION

Making healthcare decisions on the best scientific evidence is important in any area of medical practice. While there are numerous research designs that can be used to generate evidence to determine the effectiveness of an intervention, the choice of design depends on the research hypothesis and availability of resources (1). A randomized controlled trial (RCT) design has unique benefits in evaluating the effectiveness of an intervention. Compared to case–control studies, case series, case reports, and expert opinions, RCTs have been recognized as providing the highest level of evidence for the evaluation of healthcare outcomes, after meta-analyses (1).

In recent decades, there have been a growing number of RCTs conducted at the community level, which are known as community intervention trials. Because of their strengths in generating robust evidence beyond the individual level, there is a growing trend towards conducting community intervention trials to inform policy and practice. In this chapter, we will review the methodology for conducting community intervention trials and discuss their relevance for global eye health and their implications for policy and practice.

21.2 RANDOMIZED CONTROLLED TRIALS

RCTs are considered to be the gold standard in analytical research, and are mainly designed to assess the efficacy or effectiveness of new treatments and interventions at the individual level under ideal conditions (2). Controlled trials are an especially useful research tool to examine cause and effect, by reducing bias and employing an experimental (as compared to observational) design, though they can involve high costs (3). In RCTs, the effect of an intervention is compared with a control or placebo to ascertain the impact of the intervention. Randomization, when carried out reliably on sufficiently large sample sizes, ensures similar distribution of potential confounding factors between the intervention and control groups (4). Important aspects of conducting a valid RCT are selection of a representative sample of the population, careful definition and measurement of the main study outcome, and having adequate sample size to achieve sufficient power (2).

21.3 COMMUNITY INTERVENTION TRIALS

The focus on community intervention trials has grown over the last few decades in healthcare research, shifting the paradigm from individuals to populations. Community intervention trials are also referred to in the literature as group randomized trials and field intervention trials (5, 6). This approach differs fundamentally from conventional clinical trials conducted in a healthcare facility, by focusing on what actually works and is cost-effective on the ground level and by assessing the effectiveness not just of an intervention but of a healthcare strategy (7–9) (Table 21.1). Interventions such as lifestyle modification are well studied using community trial designs (10).

One important aspect of community intervention trials is the definition of the community to be studied. Researchers have described communities using geographic and social boundaries of varying sizes or by means of socio-demographic characteristics (8). A few examples are community-based trials, work-site trials, and school-based interventions in which larger groups can be mobilized towards a desired goal at once. However, the generalizability of outcomes will depend on the degree to which the selected community is representative of the larger population, and the effects of external factors such as socio-political culture of the setting on the study design (8).

The choice of conducting a conventional RCT versus a community intervention trial involves a balancing of scientific methodological rigor and availability of resources. Many early community intervention trials were designed to assess interventions to reduce mortality due to cardiac disease, such as the North Karelia Project, conducted to identify risk factors explaining very high cardiac mortality in a particular region of Finland (10, 11). Another landmark, the largest community intervention trial ever conducted in the United States, was the Minnesota Heart Health Program (MHHP), begun in the 1980s and involving nearly 500,000 participants (10). Since then, community intervention trials have been conducted in other areas such as cancer control, an example being the Community Intervention Trial for Smoking Cessation (COMMIT) (12).

DOI: 10.1201/9781315146737-24

Table 21.1 Comparison of traditional randomized controlled trials and community intervention trials using the PICOST approach

Domain	Traditional randomized controlled trials	Community intervention trials
Participants	Participants randomized at individual level	Participants randomized in groups or communities
Intervention/objective	Assessing efficacy or effectiveness of a single or complex intervention	Assessing a public health strategy comprising an intervention or more than one intervention
Control selection	At individual level	At group or community level
Outcome	Outcomes mostly described based on clinical effectiveness leading to changes in clinical practices	Outcomes mostly described based on population attributable risk with multiple level of influences, including policy
Setting	Mostly at clinical, hospital, or other controlled environments	Mostly at community level, close to the actual living environment of the general population
Timeline	Mostly assess the intervention effect at a specified time	Mostly assess the secular trends of the overall outcome over time

21.3.1 Relevance of Community Trials to Global Eye Health

The extension from individual-based RCTs to group-based community intervention trials has been observed in eye health research over recent decades, primarily in low-income settings, where the prevalence of vision impairment and blindness is high. Availability of affordable services may be poor or low uptake may persist for other reasons. Assessing factors determining acceptance of care through community intervention trials may provide valuable information for developing preventive and curative strategies to optimize eye health outcomes.

Though it is common practice to select components of a community eye care strategy for study that have already shown required efficacy when tested separately in conventional RCTs, a community intervention trial is not simply a larger version of an RCT. Hence, there is no proscription against initially testing an intervention in a community intervention trial without first conducting a conventional RCT. Rather, community intervention trials test the overall effectiveness of an eye care strategy in achieving outcomes in the community (13). While RCTs may test biological, physiological, or pharmacological outcomes against a control, generally focusing on clinical aspects, community intervention trials also assess the effectiveness of an eye care intervention which focuses on overall eye health of a particular defined group (13). Hence, community intervention trials offer the advantage of providing the necessary information required to tailor eye health strategies according to the particular needs of various populations.

When designing a community intervention trial for eye care, various factors that are usually not considered when designing an individual-based RCT must be taken into account. The feasibility of conducting the study, sample size or number of clusters, generalizability of the findings, and acceptability of the intervention are some of the major concerns. Moreover, interventions may consist of elements not directly related to eye care, such as supply of clean water for facial hygiene in trachoma. In designing a community intervention trial, the following questions may have to be addressed at the initial stage:

- Why? Reasons for selecting a particular community

- Who? Characteristics of community and homogeneity among the participants

- Where? Site and size of the communities

- What? Intervention and outcome assessment

- When? Time line of outcome assessment and follow-up

In addition to the factors mentioned previously, one other critical aspect in designing a community trial is that eye care interventions studied must be culturally and socially relevant to the community of interest (14). Theoretically, effectiveness of an eye care intervention that resolves a pathological condition should be the same in any setting. However, it is not always the case because outcomes affecting visual status at a personal level could be related to various cultural and socio-economic factors unique to the community. Because the characteristics of communities, such as participants' attitude towards and acceptance of the intervention, differ from one setting to another, an intervention shown to be effective in one setting may not be effective in another. Therefore, community intervention trials are very useful to develop and test strategies aligned with the needs, barriers to access, and socio-demographic characteristics of specific communities of concern. To ensure successful implementation, community intervention trials are often multidisciplinary, employing mixed-methods design and involving community participation in development of the intervention.

Patterns of eye care access, utilization, and success in controlling blindness and visual impairment vary greatly from one community to another, which in some cases may be attributed to poverty in the community of concern (15). One example is factors related to gender affecting access to cataract services in low-income settings (16). In the eye health evidence base, it is shown that these types of research questions are best assessed in a community intervention trial, and may be difficult to address usefully with a conventional RCT. An example is testing the SAFE (Surgery, Antibiotics, Facial cleanliness and Environmental improvement) strategy for trachoma control at the community level (17). Another is community-based mass drug administration programs to control onchocerciasis (18). These studies have shown that health promotional strategies or even administration of a drug at the community-wide level may lead to better results in improving eye health than intervening at an individual level.

Generic stages of conducting a community intervention trial involve development of the protocol, selection of the community, baseline assessment, intervention delivery, follow-up, and surveillance or evaluation. It may be necessary to conduct a pilot study to assess the feasibility of conducting a larger community intervention trial. This may have been supported by a formative stage consisting of qualitative research. A generic format of the steps in conducting a community intervention trial is shown in Figure 21.1.

21.3.2 Challenges in Conducting Community Intervention Trials

In this subsection, we outline major methodological challenges in designing community intervention trials. These challenges are mainly related to scientific methodological issues and the local

socio-political context in the area where the study will be conducted (8).

The first factor to be considered when designing a community intervention trial is the definition of the community. Early community intervention trials commonly defined a community using geographical boundaries. More recently, socio-demographic and other factors have commonly been used to define "communities." Although the interventions are generally delivered at the individual level, the unit of randomization and allocation is "en bloc" at the level of the community (19).

The most common issue arising from randomizing communities instead of at the individual level is a reduction in statistical power due to so-called "clustering effects," resulting from similarities between persons within a given community (20). The degree of such clustering or similarity is often measured using the intraclass correlation coefficient (ICC).

A challenge for investigators is to identify methods to reduce the impact of clustering on power in community trials (20). Investigators should calculate the ICC to estimate the necessary sample size for the study early in the design phase, as otherwise an under-powered or over-powered study may result (20). As an example, if an intervention is delivered at the school level, it is the number of schools rather than the total number of children in each school (beyond a certain lower limit) which has the greatest impact on power (21). The ICC (smaller is better) and number of clusters (larger is better) are the major determinants of power in a community intervention trial.

Secondly, one has to assess variability between communities (22). Stratification and balancing can be used to assure a good balance of important covariates between communities allocated to the control vs. intervention group, though this depends on the ability to measure these covariates prior to randomization and allocation (22).

Randomization at the community cluster level and cluster variation thus lead to the third issue, complexities in estimating the required sample size and power of the community trials. Study power is inherently reduced when the unit of randomization is a community cluster or a group rather than an individual (23). Since interventions are assigned for groups or communities, investigators need to increase the number of groups or communities to improve the power of the study; increasing the absolute number of participants within a community or group will have modest effects on power (24).

Masking or blinding, a critical tool to reduce risk of bias in any trial, represents a particular

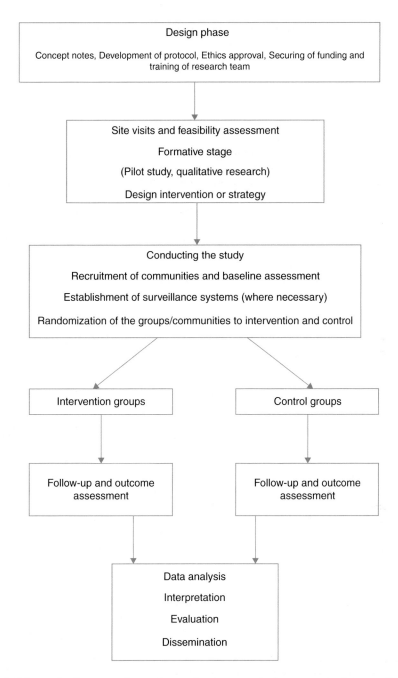

Figure 21.1 Schematic diagram of steps in conducting a typical community intervention trial.

challenge in community intervention trials. The difficulty of masking participants when they are living in their own home environment may lead to questionable validity of self-reported outcomes in a community trial (19). Frequent interactions and dynamic movements within nearby communities may cause participants from intervention and control clusters to share information, thus leading to identification of the intervention (25). A group of researchers who conducted a cluster randomized trial in India described the logistical difficulties in conducting a community intervention trial, such as assigning control clusters, blinding, implementing intervention simultaneously and minimizing leakage as *"courting real troubles"*(26). It may be practically difficult to mask community groups with the use of placebos, while service providers and participants are aware of an ongoing intervention in another nearby community, leading to cross-contamination between clusters (23). One unavoidable challenge in conducting community intervention trials is selection bias, though techniques to allow allocation concealment have been created specifically for use in community trials (27).

Researchers and statisticians have worked to resolve many challenges inherent in the design and analysis of community intervention trials. Since the outcomes of community intervention trials involve interrelated effects at the individual level, the unit of analysis should be at the community level. "Conditional" and "marginal" models are the two main approaches described in the literature (20). In conditional models, intervention effects are assessed within the same participants pre- and post-intervention while in the marginal models, intervention effects are assessed between intervention and control groups. These approaches are useful when conducting the analysis and interpreting data where there is heterogeneity among cluster observations (28).

Another challenge in community intervention trials is following up communities over the desired time period, when movements within and between communities are often dynamic, resulting in in-and-out migrations over time. Some researchers have suggested the use of repeated cross-sectional samples as opposed to longer longitudinal studies to address this challenge. However, the choice between longitudinal and repeated cross-sectional designs may depend on the objective of the study and level of attrition. From a scientific methodological perspective, longitudinal approaches are more desirable, since they confer a higher statistical power to observe a true change in the intended outcome.

When interventions are delivered at the community level, undetectable or unmeasured factors in the environment of the communities, such as social, cultural, and behavioral determinants, can influence the final outcome (29). One author described this phenomenon as "black box interventions" which may lead to replication of the identical intervention in a different population giving rise to a different outcome (19).

21.3.3 Implication of Evidence Collected from Community Intervention Trials

In this sub-section, we examine the interpretation of the results of community intervention trials. Such studies are generally conducted in community settings, workplaces, or schools where the environment is more or less similar to the actual living conditions of the participants. Therefore, results of community intervention trials are more likely to represent real-world scenarios, as compared to the outcome of RCTs conducted under tightly controlled conditions (30).

Outcomes and lessons learned from community studies in the past have led to novel approaches in conducting such trials and in improving the evaluation process (7). One of the main lessons learned from early community intervention trials such as North Karelia Project in Finland, MHHP in the US, and COMMIT is the importance of focus on policy interventions to improve health (7). These studies have shown the possibility of moving entire communities towards an intended health outcome, using multi-sectoral approaches. In addition, these studies relied on the principles and models of community organization to deliver successful research studies. Therefore, the implications of the results of a community intervention trial are far broader than those of conventional randomized controlled trials (7). Interventions should be tailored to the targeted communities to improve their effectiveness (7). Process evaluations are needed to assess the level at which intervention components are delivered, as planned at the design phase. Finally, dosing and duration of the intervention as applied at the community level are important in assessing the implications of results.

Another aspect that should be considered when applying the results of community intervention trials is the degree to which the principle of "intention to treat" has been applied during analysis. When interpreting results, it is important to note that many participants did not adhere to the intervention as called for in the study design, though they are still accounted for as part of the intervention group in strict intention-to-treat analyses.

Another concern with strict application of the results of community intervention trials is the sustainability of the intervention, and models of dissemination (7). Implementation fidelity is important in delivering interventions at the community level as intended; this is critical to effective translation of evidence into practice and must be systematically evaluated, as an estimate of the quality of implementation (31). Some authors argue that it is not the complexity of the intervention itself that is of crucial importance, but rather the complexity of systems involved (32). Early studies of cardiovascular health showed that community-based interventions are more cost-effective than individual-based interventions delivered at healthcare facilities.

To assist in understanding community intervention trials in eye care, two case studies (33, 34) conducted in sub-Saharan Africa are detailed in Table 21.2.

21.4 CONCLUSIONS

Community intervention trials have been increasingly conducted in the field of eye health to determine the effectiveness of eye care

Table 21.2 Case studies in eye health

	Case 1	Case 2
Title	Should trichiasis surgery be offered in the village? A community randomised trial of village vs. health centre-based surgery	Peek Community Eye Health-mHealth system to increase access and efficiency of eye health services in Trans Nzoia County, Kenya: study protocol for a cluster randomised controlled trial
Settings	The Gambia	Kenya
Disease focus/ topic	Trachoma	Primary eye care
Rationale	Historically, the standard care offered through the Gambian National Eye Care Programme was trichiasis surgery provided in health centers and hospitals on a weekly basis and outreach surgery in at least two rural health centers on a monthly basis. The country's strategy of providing trichiasis surgery in rural health centers by trained ophthalmic nurses at the village level aimed to improve surgical acceptance by reducing geographical distance from patients' houses to the site of surgery and removing the fixed health center levy	A large unmet need for eye health provision due to lack of access and awareness of specialist services and their overutilization for conditions that could be managed in the community or primary care. The Peek Community Screening App that enables community volunteers (CV) was used to make referral decisions about patients with eye problems, generate automated short messages service notifications to patients or guardians, and has a program dashboard for visualizing service delivery
Objectives	To estimate the effect of this strategy on surgical acceptance rates, to determine whether and by how much they could be improved by offering surgery at village level	To increase access and efficiency of eye health services using the Peek Community Eye Health-mHealth system
Design	Paired-cluster randomized trial	Single-masked, cluster-randomized controlled trial
Intervention	Patients were informed that surgery was offered free of charge by community ophthalmic nurses at the village level. Patients were given a specific time to attend for surgery within 2 weeks of the screening date. To reduce the possibility that awareness of the availability of village-based surgery might affect uptake in those allocated to health center surgery, the health center clusters were screened and treated before the village-based clusters	In each cluster, a small mobile team trained community volunteers and local community volunteers were to visit each household. The visual acuity of each eye would be measured separately using the Peek Acuity App with test algorithm prompts. Those who had reduced visual acuity on screening or reported an eye problem would be referred to a health post for triage on a specific date when the Kenyan Eye Unit (KEU) team were visiting. The system would generate several notification and reminder SMS text messages to prompt subjects to go for eye management at KEU
	Patients were informed that surgery was offered free of charge at the nearest health centers	Potential participants with eye problems at the community would be notified through community sensitization (posters and local announcements) that if they had an eye problem they should present themselves to the health facility for the triage clinic on a specified date

(continued)

Table 21.2 (continued)

	Case 1	Case 2
Sample size calculation	One of the issues identified by Bowman et al. was determining the sample size for the study because cluster had to be allocated prior to screening for trichiasis before it was known how many people would need trichiasis surgery. Hence, the study team made an estimation based on a concurrently running cohort study in another division which reported surgical attendance rates of around 10–20% for health center-based surgery with an improvement in attendance rates from 10 to 30%, which was felt to be important to the program. Prevalence surveys indicated that each cluster would contain approximately 20 surgical patients. This meant that between four and nine pairs were required, depending on inter-cluster variability, for 80% power and 95% confidence levels. Sample size = 56 villages	A typical health facility has a catchment population of 5,000 people. The number of people attending health facilities following community outreaches was estimated at an average rate of 15 per 1,000 population. Assuming an intraclass correlation coefficient of 0.001, desired power of 90%, and significance level of 5%, a sample of 36 community units (18 in each arm) would be sufficient to detect a difference of 0.5%, from 1.5% in the control arm to 2.0% in the intervention arm (a 33% relative change) in overall attendance rates. Sample size = 36 clusters
Unit of randomization	Village	Community units (catchment population of a health center)
Randomization	56 villages from two divisions were assigned to eight pairs of clusters with one cluster from each pair randomly allocated to receive village-based surgery and the other health center-based surgery (standard care)	Restricted randomization (consider the direction, cluster size, and distance from the hospital) were to be used. Community units would be allocated to receive either the Peek Community Eye Health system (intervention) or periodic health center-based outreach clinics with onward referral for further treatment (current care)
Outcomes	Surgical uptake rates during the trial period, surgical results and postoperative complication rates were assessed 1 week and 3 months after the surgery	The primary outcome is the number of people per 10,000 population attending triage at a local health facility with any confirmed eye conditions (true positives) following a community volunteer referral or by self-referral, within 4 weeks from the time of sensitization
Other unique features	An interesting feature of the study was that informed consent was sought from community leaders and subjects were offered the more effective treatment strategy if they did not accept the surgery option offered to them during the study	A data and safety monitoring committee was not considered necessary because the study presents minimal risk and the authors did not anticipate significant adverse events. An audit will be done by the trial sponsor, if it is deemed necessary No interim analysis is planned due to the relatively short duration of the study The control arm clusters will have the same screening service as the intervention arm after the end of the trial

interventions. The evidence generated from community intervention trials can be applied at a community level, making them highly relevant to test interventions implemented in low-resource settings. However, community intervention trials are resource-intensive because of the large sample size needed to ensure sufficient power. The various challenges and aspects to be considered in designing community intervention trials have been discussed above. Despite the challenges, community intervention trials remain very important in testing intervention effectiveness in a format that can have significant implications for public health practice and health policy.

REFERENCES

1. Evans D. Hierarchy of evidence: a framework for ranking evidence evaluating healthcare interventions. *J Clin Nurs*. 2002;12(1):77–84.

2. Kendall J. Designing a research project: randomised controlled trials and their principles. *Emergency Med J*. 2003;20:164–8.

3. Hariton E, Locascio J. Randomised controlled trials – the gold standard for effectiveness research. *BJOG*. 2018;125(13):1716.

4. Kabisch M, Ruckes C, Seibert-Grafe M, et al. Randomized controlled trials: part 17 of a series on evaluation of scientific publications. *Dtsch Arztebl Int*. 2011;108(39):663–8.

5. Smith P, Morrow R, Ross D. *Field Trials of Health Interventions: A Toolbox*, 3rd edn. Oxford: Oxford University Press; 2015:1–43.

6. Pais S, Murray D, Alfano C, et al. Individually randomized group treatment trials: a critical appraisal of frequently used design and analystical approaches. *Am J Public Heal*. 2008;98(8):1418.

7. Sorensen G, Emmons K, Hunt M, et al. Implications of the results of community intervention trials. *Annu Rev Public Heal*. 1998;19:379–416.

8. Atienza A, King A. Community-based health intervention trials: an overview of methodological issues. *Epidemiol Rev*. 2002;24(1):72–9.

9. Labrique A, Katz J. *Community Intervention Trials. Wiley Blackwell Encyclopedia of Health, Illness, Behaviour and Society*. John Wiley: 2014:1–23.

10. Murray D. Design and analysis of community trials: lessons from the Minnesota Heart Health Program. *Am J Epidemiol*. 1995;142(6):569–75.

11. Vartiainen E. The North Karelia Project: cardiovacular disease prevention in Finland. *Glob Cardiol Sci Pr*. 2018;2(13).

12. COMMIT Research Group. Community Intervention Trial for Smoking Cessation (COMMIT): summary of design and intervention. *J Natl Cancer Inst*. 1991;83(22):1620–8.

13. Hohmann A, Shear M. Community-based intervention research: coping with the noise of real life in study design. *Am J Psychiatry*. 2002;159:201–7.

14. Gilbert CE. The imporatnce of primary eye care. *Comm Eye Heal*. 1998;11(26):17–23.

15. Gilbert C. Poverty and blindness in Pakistan: results from the Pakistan national blindness and visual impairment survey. *BMJ*. 2008;336(7634):29–32.

16. Ramke J, Kyari F, Mwangi N, et al. Cataract service are leaving widows behind: examples from national cross-sectional surveys in Nigeria and Sri Lanka. *Int J Env Res Public Heal*. 2019;16(20):3854.

17. Ngondi J, Matthews F, Reacher M, et al. Associations between active trachoma and community intervention with Antibiotics, Facial cleanliness, and Environmental improvement (A,F,E). *PLoS Negl Trop Dis*. 2008;2(4):e229.

18. Whitworth J, Morgan D, Maude G, et al. A community trial of ivermectin for onchocerciasis in Sierra Leone: clinical and parasitological responses to the initial dose. *Trans R Soc Trop Med Hyg*. 1991;85(1):92–6.

19. Koepsell T, Wagner E, Cheadle A, et al. Selected methodological issues in evaluating community based health promotion and disease prevention programs. *Annu Rev Publ Heal*. 1992;13:31–57.

20. Murray D, Varnell S, Blistein J. Design and analysis of group-randomized trials: a review of recent methodological developments. *Am J Public Heal*. 2004;94:423–32.

21. Murray D, Short B. Intraclass correlation among measures related to alcohol use by school aged adolescents: estimates, correlates and applications in intervention studies. *J Drug Educ*. 1996;26(3):207–30.

22. Feng Z, Diehr P, Yasuri Y, et al. Explaining community-level variance in group randomized trials. *Stat Med*. 1999;18:539–56.

23. Anderson N. Community-led trials: intervention co-design in a cluster randomised controlled trial. *BMC Public Health*. 2017;17(397).

24. Whiting-O'Keefe Q, Henke C, Simborg D. Choosing the correct unit of analysis in medical care experiments. *Med Care*. 1984;22(12):1101–14.

25. Day S, Altman D. Blinding in clinical trials and other studies. *BMJ*. 2000;321(7259):504.

26. Ranson M, Sinha T, Morris S, et al. CRTs – cluster randomized trials or "courting real troubles." *Can J Public Heal*. 2006;97(1):72–5.

27. Giraudeau B, Ravaud P. Preventing bias in cluster randomised trials. *PLoS Med*. 2009;6(5):e1000065.

28. Muff S, Held L, Keller L. Marginal or conditional regression models for correlated non-normal data. *Methods Ecol Evol*. 2016;7(12):6.

29. Pearson T, Lewis C, Wall S, et al. Dissecting the "black box" of community intervention: background and rationale. *Scand J Public Heal*. 2001;29(56):5–12.

30. Blumenthal D, DiClemente R. *Community-Based Health Research – Issues and Methods*. New York: Springer, 2004:170–84.

31. Breitenstein S, Gross D, Garvey C, et al. Implementation fidelity in community-based interventions. *Res Nurs Health*. 2010;33:164–73.

32. Shiell A, Hawe P, Gold L. Complex interventions or complex systems? Implications for health economic evaluation. *BMJ*. 2008;336(1281).

33. Bowman RJC, Soma O, Alexander N, et al. Should trichiasis surgery be offered in the village? A community randomised trial of village vs. health centre-based surgery. *Trop Med Int Heal*. 2000;5(8):528–33.

34. Rono H, Bastawrous A, Macleod D, et al. Peek Community Eye Health – mHealth system to increase access and efficiency of eye health services in Trans Nzoia County, Kenya: study protocol for a cluster randomised controlled trial. *BMC Trials*. 2019;20(502):1–12.

Index

A

Administrative databases, statistical analysis 72
African Programme for Onchocerciasis Control (APOC) 115
Age-related cataracts 134–135
  classification 134
  disease-related risk factors 135
  environmental risk factors 135
  epidemiology 134
  etiology 134
  lifestyle risk factors 135
  personal and individual risk factors 135
  prevalence 134
  risk factors 134–135
  secondary cataracts 134
Age-related macular degeneration (AMD) 166–169
  aging populations and 166
  description 166
  detection during DR screening 261
  dietary risk factors 168–169
  effects on the retinal pigment epithelium (RPE) 166
  future research 169
  gender and 168
  genomic biomarkers 43–44
  impact on quality of life 245
  limitations of current population-based studies 169
  metabolomic studies 51
  microbiome research 54–55
  moderate to severe vision impairment (MSVI) 166, 167
  ocular risk factors 168
  prevalence of 166
  proteomic studies 53
  risk factors 168–169
  smoking risk factor 169
  systemic risk factors 168
  treatments 166
  underlying pathophysiological processes 43–44
  visual acuity measurement 17
  visual impairment and blindness caused by 166–168
AIDS, risk factor for OSSN 226
Altman, Doug 75, 83
Amblyopia 87, 99
Antimicrobial resistance 117
Apps *see* Smartphone apps
Artificial intelligence (AI) in ophthalmology 3, 62
  corneal disorders 113, 121
  DR and DME screening 31
  glaucoma screening 157–158
  infectious keratitis 121
  keratoconus 121

refractive surgery 121
  see also Deep learning (DL); Machine learning (ML)
Astigmatism 87, 99–100
  relationship with myopia 99–100
Atropine eye drops 99
Auckland Regional Telemedicine ROP Screening Network 34–36
Australia, Lions Outback Vision 24–25
Autoimmune uveitis 55
Automated retinal image analysis systems (ARIAS) 261

B

BAP1 tumor predisposition syndrome, risk factor for uveal melanoma 224
BCN 10 grading system for cataracts 138
Behçet's disease, uveitis in 213–214
Big Data 5
  examples of statistical methods 70–72
  future outlook and challenges 11
  future research 72
  in healthcare 62
  machine learning (ML) models 64–70
  omics data 62
  use in ophthalmology 4–11
Big Data for corneal disorders 116–120
  corneal genetic studies 118–120
  corneal transplant registries and institutions 118
  infectious keratitis studies and registries 117–118
  large-scale and EHR-based registries 116–120
Big Data sources
  disease registries 3
  electronic health records (EHRs) 3, 4
  health insurance databases 8–9
Binocular indirect ophthalmoscopy (BIO) 27
Biobanks, EHRs-linked to 6–7
Biochemical markers 41–55
Biological markers (biomarkers) 41 *see also* Epigenetic biomarkers; Genomic biomarkers
Bitot's spots 116
Blepharitis 55
Brain–computer interfaces 20
Bullous keratopathy 114

C

Cataract 87, 134–141
  age-related 134–135
  causes of lens opacity 134
  congenital cataracts 135–136
  description of 134
  impact on quality of life 246
  infantile cataracts 135, 136

U

Undetected glaucoma 151–153
  lack of access to services 152
  lack of accurate diagnosis 152
  lack of adequate resources 152–153
  lack of disease knowledge 152
  lack of effective screening tools 153
  lack of participatory effort 153
  lack of service utilization 152
  magnitude of 151–152
  reasons for 152–153
Uveal melanoma 221–225
  age and sex-specific incidence 222, 223
  BAP1 tumor predisposition syndrome, risk
    factor 224
  cutaneous nevi risk factor 224
  description 221
  environmental risk factors 224–225
  host risk factors 222–224
  incidence 221–222, 223
  iris color risk factor 222, 224
  occupational exposure to UV light 225
  oculodermal melanocytosis (ODM) risk factor
    224
  skin color and race risk factors 222
  ultraviolet light risk factor 224–225
  uveal nevi risk factor 224
Uveitis 208–214
  clinical diagnosis 208
  clinical presentation 208–209
  conditions in specific disease entities
    213–214
  description 208
  epidemiology 209–213
  etiologies 208, 209, 212–213
  in Behçet's disease 213–214
  in sarcoidosis 214
  in Vogt–Koyanagi–Harada disease 214
  incidence and prevalence 209, 210, 212–213
  Africa 212
  Asia 212–213
  Europe 213
  North America 212
  Oceania 213
  infectious uveitis 208
  noninfectious uveitis 208, 209
  patterns and distribution of etiologies 208,
    212
  types of 208, 209
  visual impairment caused by 208

V

Valuation of Lost Productivity (VOLP)
    questionnaire 130
Vertical cup-to-disc ratio (VCDR) 44, 45

Virtual reality (VR), visual acuity assessment 16,
    17, 20
Virtual Reality-Glaucoma Visual Function Test
    (VR-GVFT) 20
Vision-related quality of life (VRQoL) 15
Vision-related quality of life (VRQoL)
    assessment 242–250
  aging populations 242
  characteristics of different types of PROMs
    243, 244–245
  concept of VRQoL 243
  cultural and linguistic validation of the
    selected PROM 248–249
  determine the trait to be measured 246
  development stages of the selected PROM 247
  future research 249–250
  global prevalence of blinding eye diseases 242
  impact of age-related macular degeneration
    (AMD) 245
  impact of cataracts 246
  impact of diabetic retinopathy (DR) 245
  impact of glaucoma 246
  impact of refractive errors 246
  impact of visual impairment (VI) 242, 243, 255
  implications for treatment 242
  patient-centered outcome measures (PCOMs)
    242
  patient-reported outcome measures (PROMs)
    242–250
  psychometric evaluation and validation
    stages of the selected PROM 248
  selection of VRQoL PROMS to use in ocular
    epidemiology 246–249
  systematic review of impact of VI and ocular
    pathologies 243, 245–246
  why PROMs should be measured 243
Visual acuity (VA)
  remote measurement 14–16
  screening children for 257
Visual Fields Easy app 16, 17
Vitamin A deficiency 114, 115–116
Vogt–Koyanagi–Harada disease, uveitis in 214

W

Wearable technology, remote monitoring 14–20
WHO simplified cataract-grading system 136
Wills Eye Glaucoma app 16
Work Productivity and Activity Impairment
    (WPAI) questionnaire 130

X

Xeroderma pigmentosum, risk factor for OSSN
    227
Xerophthalmia 113, 115–116
Xerophthalmic fundus 116